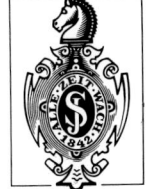

Hubert A. Sissons · Ronald O. Murray · H.B.S. Kemp

Orthopaedic Diagnosis

Clinical, Radiological and Pathological Coordinates

With 534 Figures, Many in Colour

Springer-Verlag
Berlin Heidelberg New York Tokyo 1984

Hubert A. Sissons, MD, FRCPath, FRCP, FRCS, FCAP

Director, Department of Pathology and Laboratory Medicine, Hospital for Joint Diseases Orthopaedic Institute, New York, and Professor of Pathology, Mount Sinai School of Medicine, New York; Formerly Professor of Morbid Anatomy, Institute of Orthopaedics, University of London, and Honorary Consultant in Morbid Anatomy, Royal National Orthopaedic Hospital, London and Stanmore, Middlesex

Ronald O. Murray, MBE, MD(Cantab), FRCP (Edin), FRCR, FACR(Hon), FRACR(Hon), FFRRCSI(Hon)

Honorary Consulting Radiologist, Royal National Orthopaedic Hospital and Institute of Orthopaedics, London and Stanmore, Middlesex, and Honorary Consulting Radiologist, Lord Mayor Treloar Orthopaedic Hospital, Alton, Hampshire

H.B.S. Kemp, MB, MS, FRCS, FRCS(Ed)

Consultant Orthopaedic Surgeon, Royal National Orthopaedic Hospital, London and Stanmore, Middlesex

ISBN 3-540-12795-X Springer-Verlag Berlin Heidelberg New York Tokyo
ISBN 0-387-12795-X Springer-Verlag New York Berlin Heidelberg Tokyo

Library of Congress Cataloging in Publication Data
Sissons, Hubert A. (Hubert Armand), 1920–
Orthopaedic Diagnosis.
Bibliography: p. Includes index. 1. Orthopedia—Diagnosis. I. Murray, Ronald O. II. Kemp, H.B.S. (Hubert Bond Stafford), 1925–   . III. Title. [DNLM: 1. Orthopedics—Problems. WE 18 S6230] RD734.S57 1984 617′.3
83-19631
ISBN 0-387-12795-X (U.S.)

This work is subject to copyright. All rights are reserved, whether the whole or part of the material is concerned, specifically those of translation, reprinting, re-use of illustrations, broadcasting, reproduction by photocopying machine or similar means, and storage in data banks. Under §54 of the German Copyright Law, where copies are made for other than private use, a fee is payable to 'Verwertungsgesellschaft Wort', Munich.

© Springer-Verlag Berlin Heidelberg 1984

The use of registered names, trademarks etc, in this publication does not imply, even in the absence of a specific statement, that such names are exempt from the relevant protective laws and regulations and therefore free for general use.

Filmset by Wilmaset, Birkenhead, Merseyside, England
Reproduction of illustrations by Toppan Printing Company, Singapore
Printing and binding by G. Appl, Wemding, Germany

2128/3916 543210

For
Pat, Jane and Moyra

Preface

This book was conceived with the object of presenting to doctors and medical students with a potential interest in the disciplines of orthopaedic surgery, diagnostic radiology and orthopaedic pathology, a volume which would contain basic and essential information concerning those disorders of the skeleton in which a common interest exists. Diagnosis in such conditions is dependent on close collaboration between specialists in these subjects. As medical knowledge has advanced, so the necessity for detailed specialisation has increased. As a result co-operation in a combined approach has become of great importance.

The method of presentation, in the form of Exercises, is designed to permit readers to test their own diagnostic ability. The book consists of ninety-four problems of diagnosis which might be encountered in any orthopaedic unit. The case material has been chosen to emphasise those conditions in which appreciation and integration of the clinical, radiological and pathological features are required in order to establish the diagnosis. Each Exercise consists of a number of questions and answers. The questions (**Q1**, **Q2** etc.) all refer to individual patients. They describe the initial complaint of the patient, the clinical findings and, where relevant, significant laboratory data. The appropriate radiograph is illustrated, with attention drawn to the abnormalities which are present. The histological features of the lesion are reproduced without comment. The reader is encouraged to join in this learning experience by reaching personally a diagnostic conclusion *before* turning to the answers to the problems (**A1**, **A2** etc.), which are to be found on the succeeding pages.

The answers discuss first the pre-operative diagnosis, especially when the subsequent histological findings have shown it to be incorrect. Indeed, many of the cases illustrated have been chosen for this reason. In some instances supplementary operative photographs, radiographs and pathological material from the patient concerned are illustrated. The ultimate and definitive diagnosis is established by a co-ordinated approach involving all the disciplines concerned.

In each Exercise a fuller description of the particular entity follows, headed by a short introductory paragraph referring to its incidence and its predilection for age and sex.

Important clinical features then are described, indicating the natural history of the disorder and the complications which may develop.

The radiological features are considered by reference to the skeletal sites most likely to be affected and by description of the appearances encountered most commonly. Supplementary radiographs illustrate the variety of abnormalities which may be recognised. In order to include a comprehensive selection of radiographs, a number of these have been reduced in size, illustrating only the essential features of the lesion, so that the reader can appreciate the diagnostic messages contained in their descriptive legends.

The histological features, similarly, are described in sufficient detail to allow the reader to become familiar with the characteristic appearances of the various entities discussed.

Treatment of each condition is summarised, with reference to recent advances in medical and surgical management.

References are designed to include significant developments in recent years and to lead to the literature, rather than to be comprehensive. They are to be found mainly in journals of wide circulation and are therefore available in most medical libraries. Brief mention has been made of some related or rarer entities for which space has prevented detailed description, but for each of these a leading reference has been inserted.

The book is concluded by a number of Exercises illustrating diagnostic problems of particular interest. To each of these conditions reference has been made in the preceding pages.

Finally, the authors express the hope that study of this volume will emphasise again the necessity of a co-ordinated approach by all the disciplines concerned with the diagnosis and treatment of orthopaedic disorders.

Contents

Preface VII
Acknowledgements XI
Exercises 1–57 1–397
Index 399

The omission of a conventional Table of Contents is deliberate. To identify each exercise by a diagnosis would detract from the specific purpose of presenting each exercise as an unknown case.

Acknowledgements

The authors express their thanks to their colleagues at the Royal National Orthopaedic Hospital in London and the Hospital for Joint Diseases in New York for permission to use their case material and for access to the collected material in the Departments of Radiology and Pathology of these Institutions. Many of the radiological illustrations are from the Museum of Orthopaedic Radiology in the Institute of Orthopaedics in the University of London. This Museum contains radiographs from many parts of the world and grateful acknowledgement is made to those who have contributed this material.

The authors are deeply indebted to Miss Frances Quinn, who typed the manuscript, to Mrs. Uta Boundy and Mr. John Collins, who prepared the clinical and radiographic illustrations, and to Mr. Daniel Benevento and the late Mr. Terry Davies, who were responsible for the histological illustrations. The authors also acknowledge with pleasure the unfailing co-operation of the publishers through Mr. Michael Jackson and Mr. Roger Dobbing.

Exercise 1

Q1. This 30-year-old woman presented on account of pain in the left hip for the previous 12 months.

On clinical examination the range of movement was full, but slight discomfort was elicited at the extremes of flexion and adduction. All biochemical investigations were negative.

Radiologically a large osteolytic lesion was demonstrated in the intertrochanteric region of the femur, largely surrounded by a well-defined and thick zone of sclerosis. On the lateral side of the femoral neck, however, the cortex was extremely thin and had suffered a minor infraction. Distal to this area abnormal and homogeneous density was evident in the medullary cavity. Skeletal survey revealed no other osseous abnormality.

As in the case of the other diagnostic problems presented in this volume, the histological appearance of the abnormal tissue is illustrated below, at appropriate magnifications, in Q1b and Q1c.

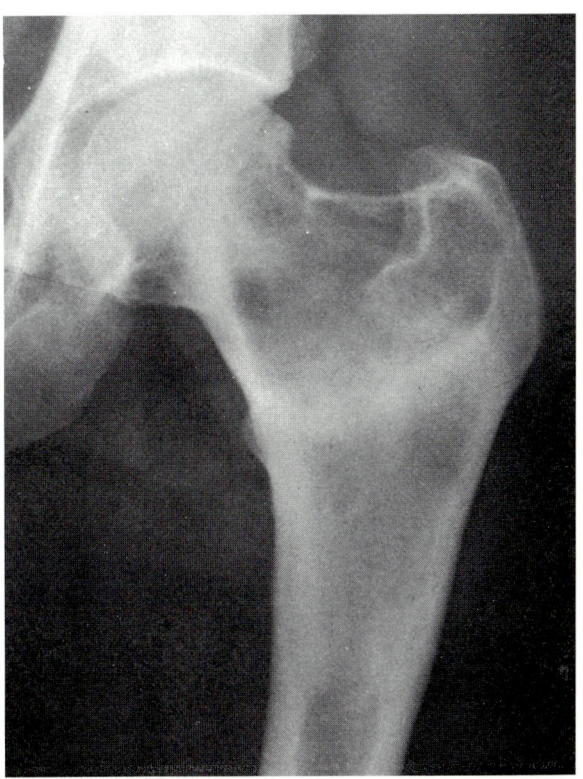

Q1a.

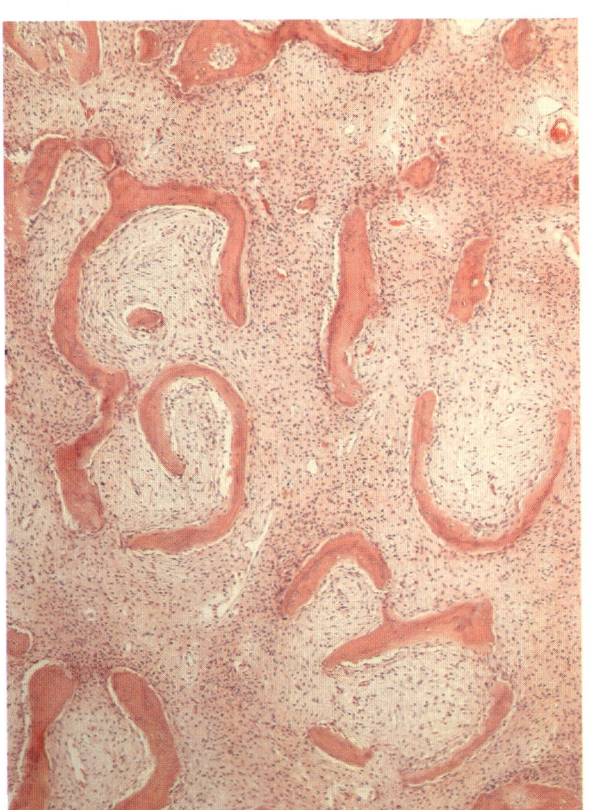

Q1b. (×44)

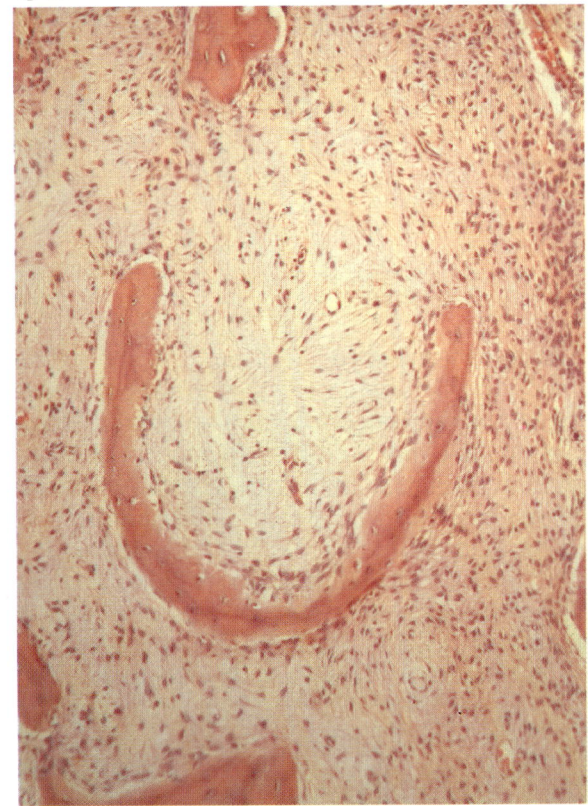

Q1c. (×100)

A1. Monostotic fibrous dysplasia

Pre-operatively this diagnosis was suggested. In view of the extensive involvement and the danger of a complete fracture occurring, replacement of the affected area by a custom built prosthesis was undertaken in preference to curettage and packing with bone chips.

The gross specimen (Figs. 1.1a and b) showed the affected portion of the femur to be replaced by a solid fibrous mass, with a large smooth-walled cyst corresponding to the radiological area of lucency. Histologically the fibrous tissue (Q1b) contains the scattered trabeculae of woven (non-lamellar) bone (Q1c), which are characteristic of fibrous dysplasia.

Five years after operation the patient was asymptomatic with normal function.

Fibrous Dysplasia

This skeletal disorder, of unknown aetiology, is characterised fundamentally by replacement of medullary bone by fibrous tissue, within which cartilaginous and osseous foci commonly develop.

Clinical Features

The condition usually becomes evident during childhood or adolescence, with an equal sex incidence, although minor manifestations are detected frequently during incidental radiological examination in the absence of symptoms or signs. The usual cause of presentation is localised pain due to a pathological infraction through a weakened bone, a frank fracture or a deformity due to alteration in shape or limb length inequality. The lesions may be solitary (monostotic) or multiple (polyostotic) and usually grow slowly; most become quiescent at the time of skeletal maturation, although continued enlargement in adult life is well recognised. Polyostotic lesions in children, usually females, may be associated with areas of cutaneous pigmentation and endocrine disturbance, especially precocious puberty (*Albright's syndrome*). Malignant change is a very rare complication, but has been reported, particularly as a sequel to previous radiation therapy.

Radiological Features

1. Site. Any bone may be affected, long bones (especially femur and tibia) being commonest, followed by pelvis, ribs, skull and facial bones.

2. Appearance. A characteristic hazy texture has been likened to 'ground glass'. Contained densities due to ossification foci may result in diffuse sclerosis. The margin often consists of a dense sclerotic rim, described as 'orange rind'. The cortex frequently is thinned and expanded with lucent areas attributed to haemorrhage or cyst formation. Premature epiphyseal fusion and deformities (particularly 'shepherd's crook' femur) often are observed in severe polyostotic forms, usually associated with former infractions or frank fractures.

3. Special Forms. The variant *leontiasis ossea* is due to involvement of facial bones and the base of the skull, resulting in densely sclerotic and asymmetrical lesions causing adult deformity. *Cherubism* is typified by expanding and osteolytic lesions in the maxilla and mandible of children. The remainder of the skeleton usually is spared.

Pathological Features

The lesions consist of fibrous tissue containing a variable amount of non-lamellar or woven bone, often arranged, as shown in Q1b and c, in curved plates which give them a distinctive pattern. Campanacci has drawn attention to a histological variant, termed *osteofibrous dysplasia*, affecting especially the tibia in young children, in which the trabeculae of woven bone are covered by layers of prominent osteoblasts. This variant is discussed in more detail in another Exercise.

The focal lesions of fibrous dysplasia are to be distinguished histologically (and indeed radiologically) from the diffuse fibrous replacement that occurs in hyperparathyroidism and which has been known clinically as 'osteitis fibrosa'. The biochemical abnormalities of hyperparathyroidism (hypercalcaemia and hypophosphataemia) are not features of fibrous dysplasia.

Treatment

Most of the lesions discovered incidentally should be left alone and not subjected to biopsy. Since they may enlarge, particularly in children, periodical re-assessment is advisable, especially if they become symptomatic or are situated in a location liable to fracture. Stress fractures which do occur tend to repair satisfactorily without surgical intervention, but prophylactic curettage and bone grafting may be indicated. For larger monostotic foci, such as that illustrated in Fig. 1.4, prosthetic replacement has proved a very valuable method of treatment. For the patient grossly deformed by widespread polyostotic lesions, external splinting and supports may be helpful. Radiotherapy is not indicated. It does not relieve pain, delays healing of fractures and may precipitate malignant change.

References

Albright F, Butler AM, Hampton AO, Smith P (1937) Syndrome characterized by osteitis fibrosa disseminata, areas of pigmentation and endocrine dysfunction, with precocious puberty in females; report of 5 cases. N Engl J Med 216: 727–746
Campanacci M, Laus M (1981) Osteofibrous dysplasia of the tibia and fibula. A new clinical entity. J Bone Jt Surg 63A: 367–375
Cornelius EA, McClendon JL (1969) Cherubism—fibrous dysplasia of the jaws. Am J Roent 106: 136–143
Gibson MJ, Middlemiss JH (1971) Fibrous dysplasia of bone. Br J Radiol 44: 1–13
Harris WH, Dudley HR, Barry RJ (1962) The natural history of fibrous dysplasia. J Bone Jt Surg 44A: 207–233
Huvos AG, Higinbotham NL, Miller TR (1972) Bone sarcomas arising in fibrous dysplasia. J Bone Jt Surg 54A: 1047–1056
Jaffe HL, Lichtenstein L (1942) Fibrous dysplasia of bone. Arch Pathol 33: 777–816

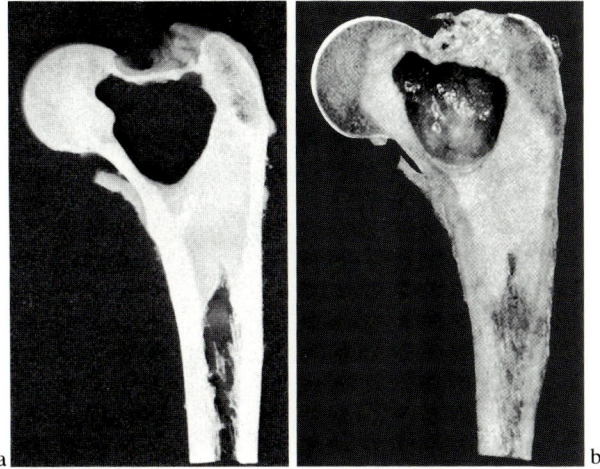

Fig. 1.1. a This radiograph of a slab of tissue from the specimen resected from the patient in Q1 illustrates the hazy appearance of the main lesion and the contained cyst, which corresponded to the radiological area of lucency, as shown also in **b** the photograph of the specimen.

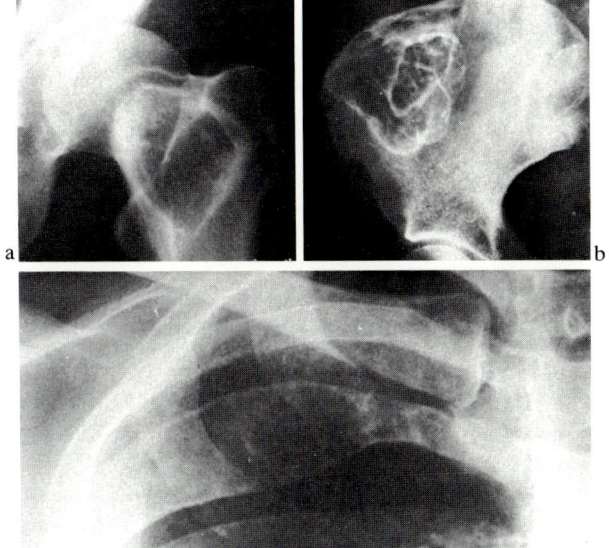

Fig. 1.2. *Monostotic fibrous dysplasia. Incidental lesions causing no symptoms.* **a** *Intertrochanteric region of femur.* The characteristic dense 'orange rind' margin was observed in a 65-year-old man with pain in the knee. Such lesions are very common and do not require biopsy. **b** *Ilium.* In this instance the loculated pattern with dense peripheral margins is characteristic. The lesion was found in a 36-year-old woman during another investigation. **c** *Rib* in a 28-year-old man. The expanding lytic lesion has thinned the cortex. Found on a routine chest film for emigration purposes, the patient was obliged to have it resected for histological confirmation.

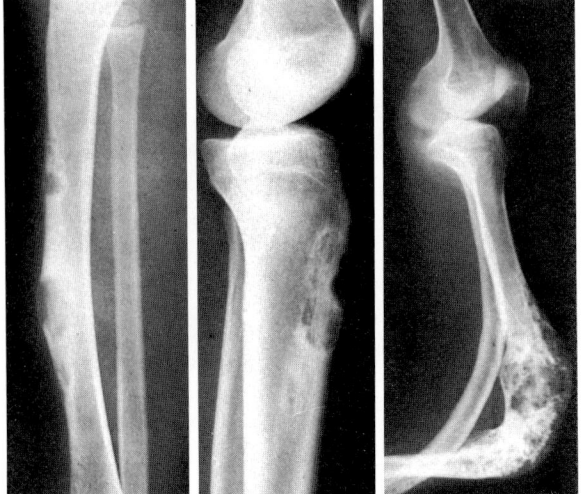

Fig. 1.3. *Fibrous dysplasia—symptomatic tibial lesions.* **a** Four-year-old girl with painful swelling. This typifies the 'osteofibrous dysplasia' variant described by Campanacci and requires continued supervision. **b** Twenty-year-old female with a painful swelling, first noticed a month before. Radiological differentiation from a chondromyxoid fibroma depended on recognition of a satellite lesion. Biopsy confirmation was obtained. **c** Nineteen-year-old male with gross anterior bowing deformity from long-standing focus of disease. Minimal involvement of the fibula is evident.

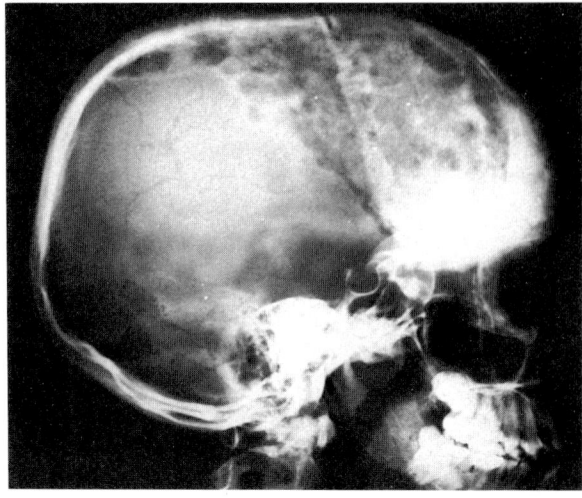

Fig. 1.5. *Monostotic fibrous dysplasia of calvarium.* For 7 years this 22-year-old female had been aware of an increasing swelling over her left eye which recently had been associated with headache. No diplopia had developed. A large area of mixed lysis and sclerosis involved the left parietal and frontal bones, with bony thickening being especially prominent in the anterior fossa. Acrylic replacement was performed with considerable correction of the deformity.

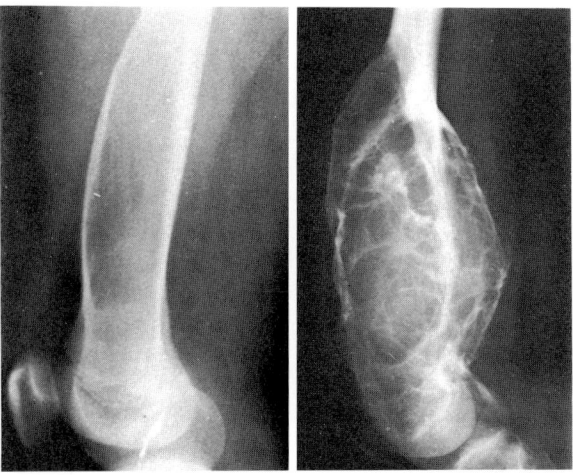

Fig. 1.4. *Aggressive monostotic fibrous dysplasia.* In 1962 this 13-year-old girl began to complain of discomfort above the right knee. The lytic, expanding lesion in the femur at first was regarded as a unicameral bone cyst. It continued to enlarge and suffered several fractures. By 1970, when review of the original biopsy material confirmed the diagnosis, great enlargement had taken place. Prosthetic replacement was very successful and the patient was well and functioning normally 11 years later.

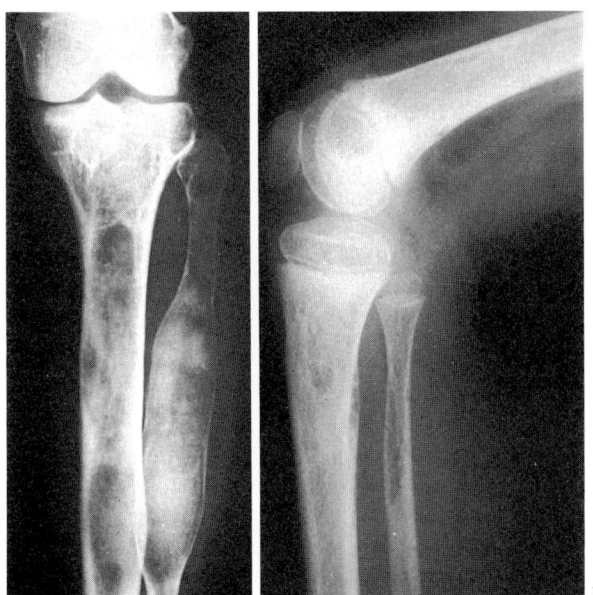

Fig. 1.6. *Polyostotic fibrous dysplasia.* **a** Typical expanding areas of fibrous replacement in the tibia and fibula of a young adult demonstrate beautifully the radiological 'ground glass' appearance. **b** In this 12-year-old boy without symptoms many little lesions with well-defined margins are characteristic of the disorder. Density of the metaphyses was physiological.

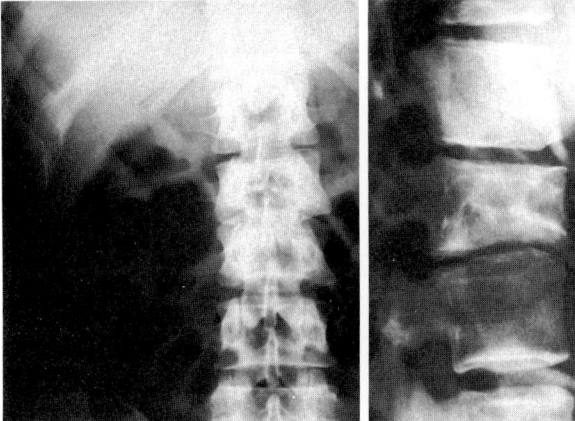

Fig. 1.7. *Polyostotic fibrous dysplasia.* This 23-year-old woman reported sporadic attacks of backache for 12 years. Clinically a mild mid-lumbar kyphos was evident. The irregular areas of lucency with marginal sclerosis within a slightly wedged body of L2 initially posed some diagnostic difficulty. Despite the narrowing of the L2/3 disc space the appearance was not consistent with simple herniation of an intervertebral disc. The clue to the diagnosis lay in the typical appearance of the right 11th rib, which was biopsied with histological confirmation. Involvement of the spine by fibrous dysplasia is unusual.

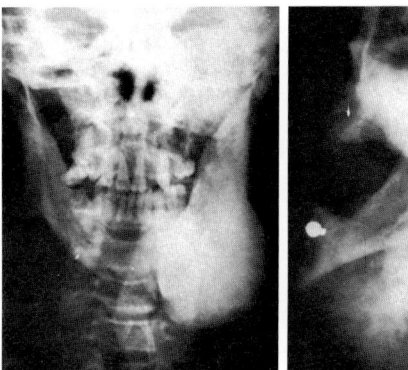

Fig. 1.9. *Leontiasis ossea.* Gross involvement of the facial bones is typical of this variant of fibrous dysplasia, causing a leonine facial deformity. These lesions grew slowly in this 41-year-old man. They are usually painless.

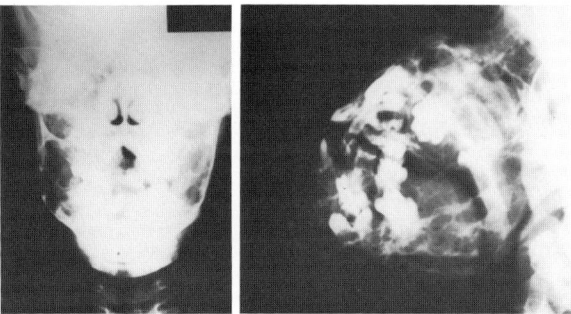

Fig. 1.8. *Cherubism.* Huge, expanding lesions of fibrous dysplasia are present in the mandible and maxilla of this young child, with displacement of the teeth. The condition may be observed in siblings and frequently is hereditary. It is aggressive in early years and then tends to become static. The deformity stretches the facial skin, pulling down the lower eyelids, so that the sclerae are exposed and the eyes appear to look upwards—hence the name.

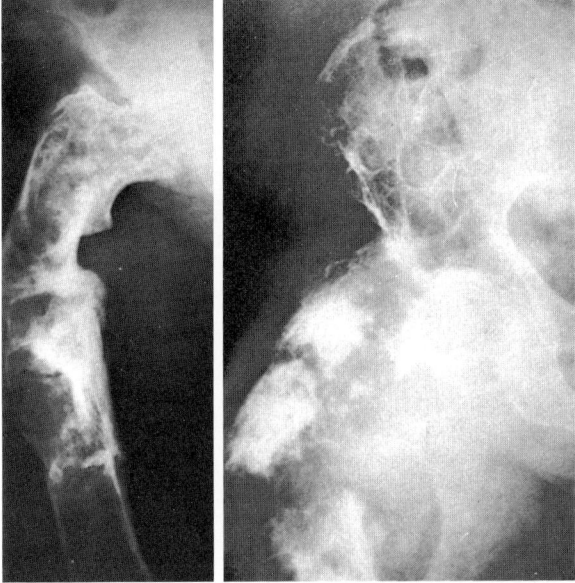

Fig. 1.10. *Sarcomatous change in polyostotic dysplasia.* This very rare complication occurred in the femur of a 74-year-old female. Many fractures had already caused a 'shepherd's crook' deformity. Observe typical involvement of the ilium. The affected femur of this patient had been treated by radiotherapy, which probably was responsible for the malignancy.

Q1. This 70-year-old man presented with a history of chronic urinary obstruction.

Clinical examination revealed no obvious abnormality. In particular no symptoms referable to the skeleton were detected.

Routine intravenous pyelography disclosed the presence of numerous rounded and oval areas of increased density in the vertebrae, pelvis and ribs. Excretion by the left kidney was delayed.

A biopsy of one of the sclerotic lesions in the pelvis was performed.

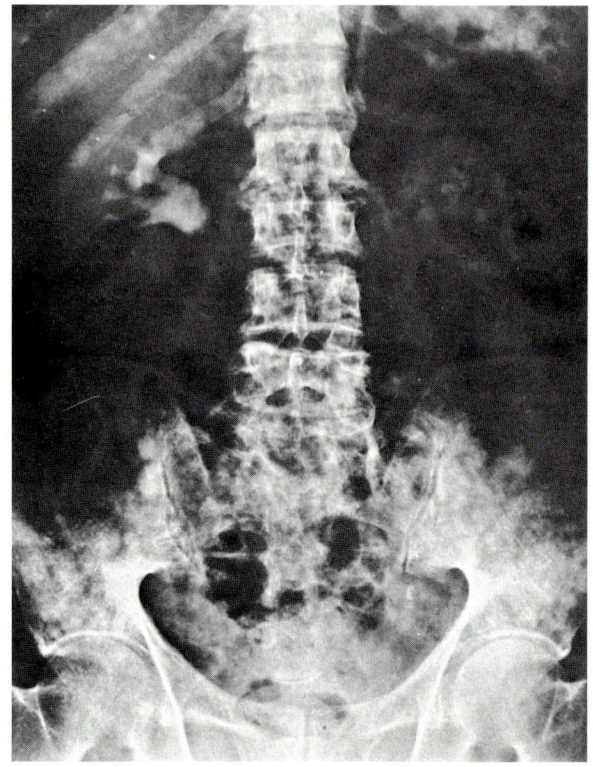

Q1a.

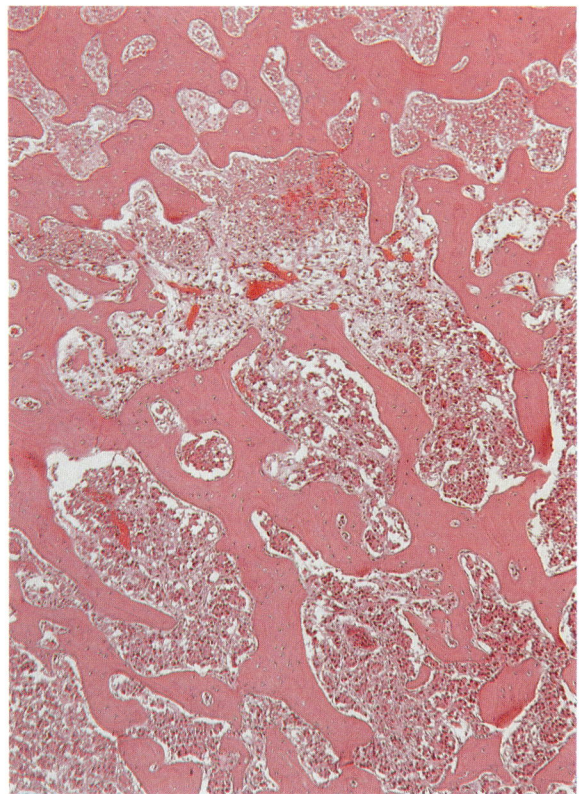

Q1b. (×50)

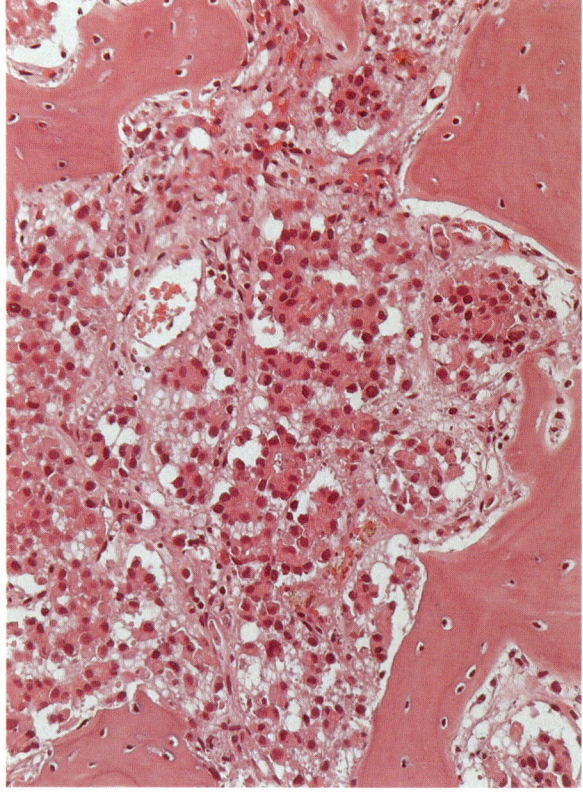

Q1c. (×155)

Exercise 2

Q2. The patient, a 60-year-old man, had complained of chronic pain in the right foot for several months.

Local tenderness was elicited on pressure over the cuboid.

Radiological examination revealed a well-defined lytic lesion in this bone.

A biopsy of this bone was performed. The patient was referred for a second opinion, a tentative diagnosis of osteoblastoma having been suggested.

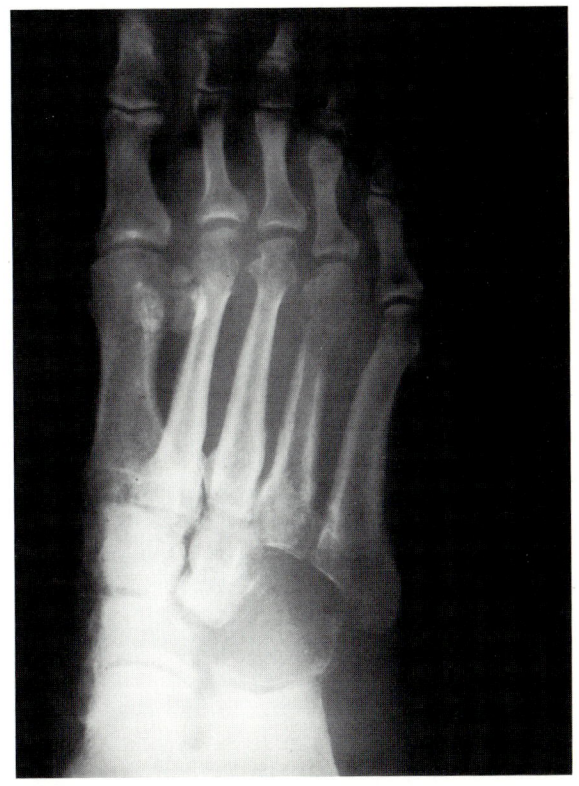

Q2a.

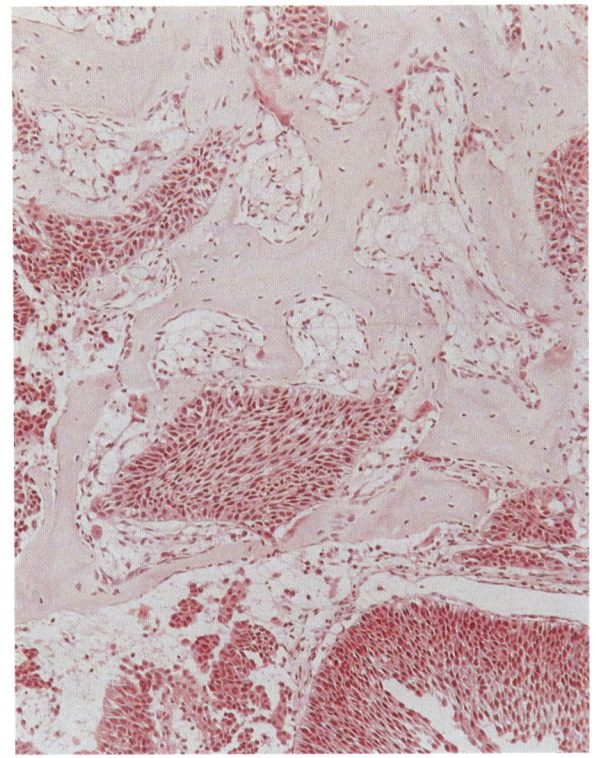

Q2b. (×98)

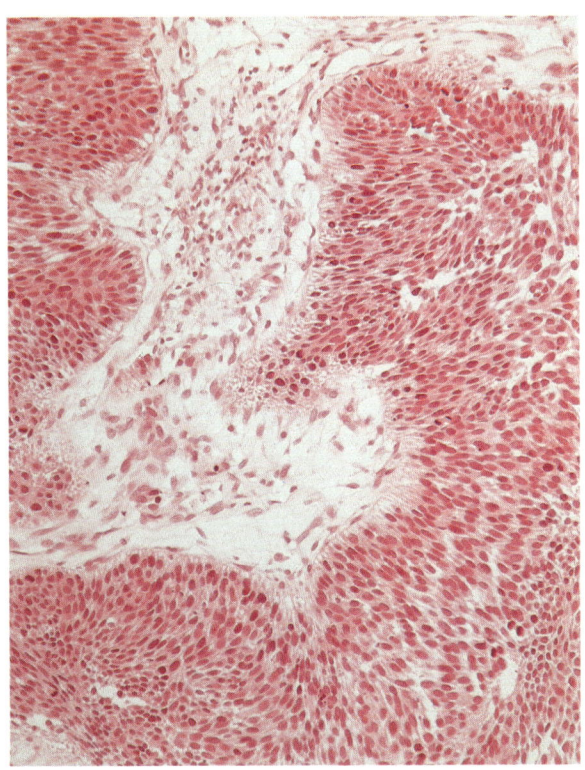

Q2c. (×148)

A1. Sclerosing metastases from carcinoma of prostate

The radiological findings are characteristic of bony metastases. The osteosclerotic appearance of the lesions, and the history of urinary obstruction, strongly suggested a diagnosis of prostatic carcinoma. This diagnosis was confirmed by a marked increase in serum acid phosphatase and the presence of a hard median lobe of the prostate on rectal examination.

Histological study of the biopsy material (Q1b and c) demonstrated a network of irregular bone trabeculae. These structures were clearly responsible for the radiological density of the affected areas of the skeleton. The spaces between the trabeculae are occupied by darkly staining tumour cells, their arrangement in small clusters indicating their epithelial nature. This appearance is completely consistent with a prostatic carcinoma, although the histological structure of this tumour is not specific. In Q1b it is evident from the absence of nuclear staining that part of the tumour tissue is necrotic, as is the bone tissue in the same area.

A2. Osteolytic metastases from carcinoma of urinary bladder

The presence of a second area of bone destruction in the neck of the 4th metatarsal had been overlooked. Review of the radiographs immediately suggested the lesions to be osteolytic metastases, despite their relatively unusual location.

More critical examination of the biopsy material showed a tumour with a recognisably epithelial pattern immediately confirming its metastatic nature (Q2b and c). The tumour cells are rounded or spindle shaped and are arranged in compact masses, the appearance of which contrasts strikingly with that of the intervening stromal connective tissue. In Q2b, a network of reactive bone, the surface of which is covered by numerous osteoblasts and osteoclasts, is present, and presumably had been responsible for the original suggestion of an osteoblastoma. The histological structure of this neoplasm, however, with masses of spindle-shaped cells arranged in some areas in a papillary fashion, is, in fact, quite characteristic. This appearance is typical of a tumour of urinary epithelium referred to as papillary (transitional cell) carcinoma. Such an origin could be suggested confidently in this patient. On the basis of these pathological findings, genito-urinary investigations established the presence of a carcinoma of the bladder.

Skeletal Metastases

The skeleton is a frequent site of metastases from many types of malignant tumour. Such secondary deposits, indeed, are the commonest type of malignant bone disease.

The primary tumours most often responsible for bone metastases are carcinomas of the breast, prostate and lung. Next in frequency are carcinomas of the colon, stomach and urinary bladder. The primary tumour responsible for bone metastases may be clinically latent, carcinomas of the kidney and thyroid having a special reputation for this type of presentation. Thyroid metastases, however, are somewhat rare in our experience. In children, neuroblastoma is the commonest source of secondary tumours in bone.

Bone metastases may be solitary or multiple. A solitary, or apparently solitary, metastasis may be confused with a primary bone tumour or a plasmacytoma, while disseminated metastases may mimic myelomatosis.

Clinical Features

The symptoms and signs of metastatic disease in the skeleton vary greatly, extending from being totally occult in the case of many solitary lesions to advanced cachexia, loss of weight, fever and all the other manifestations of disseminated malignancy. The most common symptom is localised bone pain, but attention to the presence of a metastasis is drawn often by the development of a spontaneous and painful pathological fracture. Such fractures affect especially the vertebral bodies and the major long bones of the lower limbs.

The biochemical findings are sometimes of importance in the diagnosis of bone metastases. Extensive deposits are often associated with an elevated serum alkaline phosphatase, usually ascribed to a reactive osteoblastic response to the tumour. A high serum acid phosphatase may be a clue to the presence of a prostatic carcinoma. Bone metastases may be associated with hypercalcaemia, produced either by widespread bone destruction or by the secretion of material resembling parathyroid hormone by the tumour cells. Exclusion of myelomatosis is aided by demonstrating the absence of Bence-Jone protein, and of the abnormal and excessive globulins found by electrophoresis. In children, a diagnosis of metastatic neuroblastoma may be indicated by an abnormally high urinary excretion of catecholamines, a finding of value in distinguishing this type of tumour from Ewing's sarcoma.

Radiological Features

1. Site. While any part of the skeleton may be affected, metastases usually involve areas where haemopoietic bone marrow is present, namely the spine, pelvis, ribs and calvarium. In the limbs, the proximal ends of the humerus and femur are the sites most frequently involved.

The possibility of metastasis to unusual parts of the skeleton must always be kept in mind. Metastases distal to the knee and elbow are more common than was formerly believed. Involvement of the small bones of the hands and feet is relatively unusual. Deposits in phalanges, however, frequently originate from lung, and metastases in the leg, more often than not, are derived from a primary tumour in the pelvis. Difficulty in radiological diagnosis tends to arise most often with a metastasis of very late development, or one occurring, exceptionally and with a particularly sinister prognosis, in a young adult.

It must be stressed that bone metastases may be present, particularly at an early stage, without any alteration in the radiographic appearance of the affected bone or bones. Because of this, the earliest involvement of the skeleton is more likely to be detected by radionuclide scanning (with such an agent as technetium polyphosphate) than by the time-honoured radiological skeletal survey.

2. Appearance. The great majority of bone metastases are osteolytic. When presenting as a solitary lesion, such a metastasis may appear deceptively benign, but evidence of rapid growth and extension reveals the correct diagnosis. Recognition of the aggressive characteristics of marrow infiltration, with a wide zone of transition and with destruction and expansion of the overlying cortex, is of great importance. Cortical expansion is particularly associated with solitary metastases from kidney and thyroid, which may consequently simulate closely the pattern of a plasmacytoma—a differential diagnosis always worthy of consideration.

Purely sclerotic metastases are less common than the osteolytic type. When encountered they are almost invariably multiple.

Prostatic cancer is the most common cause of sclerotic metastases. Exceptionally a large solitary metastasis of this type may simulate an osteosarcoma occurring unusually late in life. Lytic lesions from this malignant tumour occur only rarely and usually in an older age group. Sclerotic metastases may be derived also from primary malignant tumours of the alimentary tract, particularly the stomach and colon, and the bladder. In a small percentage, they may originate from the breast.

Advanced skeletal metastases not infrequently present a mixed appearance of osteolysis and osteosclerosis, the latter feature being attributable to reactive bone formation. Occasionally purely osteolytic lesions, amenable to treatment, respond by becoming sclerotic.

Pathological Features

Biopsy can be of importance in the diagnosis of bone metastases, although in some cases the presence of a primary tumour and the evidence of widespread skeletal dissemination may be so clear that histological confirmation is unnecessary. If it is intended to refer a patient with any suspected skeletal malignancy to an oncological centre, it is desirable that such referral takes place before a biopsy is performed.

Needle biopsy, as opposed to open surgical biopsy, is often used in cases of suspected bone metastases, particularly when open biopsy might interfere with subsequent treatment.

With a malignant lesion of bone, the histological recognition of the tissue as epithelial (as in the two cases in the present Exercise) establishes the metastatic nature of the tumour. The histological evidence, however, although identifying the lesion as a metastatic carcinoma, often fails to indicate the type of primary tumour involved. In some cases, nevertheless (as in Q2), the structure of the tumour is so characteristic that a more specific diagnosis can be made. This is particularly true in identifying metastases from carcinomas of kidney and thyroid. Metastatic melanoma often can be recognised by the identification of melanin pigment, or its precursors, in the tumour tissue. In the future the application of immunological methods from the identification of specific tumour antigens is likely to be of increasing importance in connection with the diagnosis of metastatic tumours.

The radiological changes in skeletal metastases are the result of bone formation and bone resorption in the affected areas. In most metastatic tumours there is histological evidence of both these processes, so accounting for the mixed pattern mentioned above, although one may predominate. Bone formation results from the activity of osteoblasts, which add bone to the surfaces of existing trabeculae or form new bony structures (Fig. 1.1). The mechanism of bone resorption in metastatic tumours is thought to be more complex. Osteoclasts, the normal agents of bone resorption, usually can be demonstrated (Fig. 1.2) and are clearly important, although it has been suggested that some types of tumour cell may themselves be able to resorb bone. The precise method by which tumour cells stimulate osteoblastic activity is not known. On the other hand it has been shown that some tumours produce an 'osteoclast activating factor' when grown in tissue culture. It has been suggested that this factor may induce resorption in bone metastases.

Treatment

The problems in the clinical management of patients with bone metastases are numerous and varied. They are related partly to the underlying malignant condition and partly to the clinical disabilities caused by the bone lesions.

With an isolated metastasis, it has become apparent that there are many indications for local surgical treatment, including ablation, internal fixation and even joint replacement. These measures, in association with radiotherapy and chemotherapy, particularly when applied to osteolytic lesions in weight-bearing bones, may help a patient to remain ambulant and independent and to avoid the occurrence of a pathological fracture. Antero-lateral decompression, coupled with internal fixation, may be indicated in patients with spinal cord compression due to vertebral collapse. These patients, however, invariably have a poor prognosis, because of widespread dissemination of the primary tumour.

Bone metastases may respond to radiotherapy or chemotherapy. Both cytotoxic drugs and hormones have their uses, the latter in the treatment of hormone-sensitive tumours of the prostate and breast.

A variety of palliative measures are available for the care of the terminal patient with advanced disseminated malignant disease.

References

Abrams HL (1950) Skeletal metastases in carcinoma. Radiology 55: 534–538

Drury RAB, Palmer PH, Highman WJ (1964) Carcinomatous metastasis to the vertebral bodies. J Clin Pathol 17: 448–457

Eildon G, Mundy GR (1978) Direct resorption of bone by human breast cancer cells *in vivo*. Nature 276: 726–728

Galasco SCB (1976) Mechanisms of bone destruction in the development of skeletal metastases. Nature 263: 507–508

Sissons HA (1980) Bone remodelling in relation to secondary tumors in the skeleton. In: Donath A, Courvoisier B (eds) Bone and tumours. Editions Médicine et Hygiene, Geneva

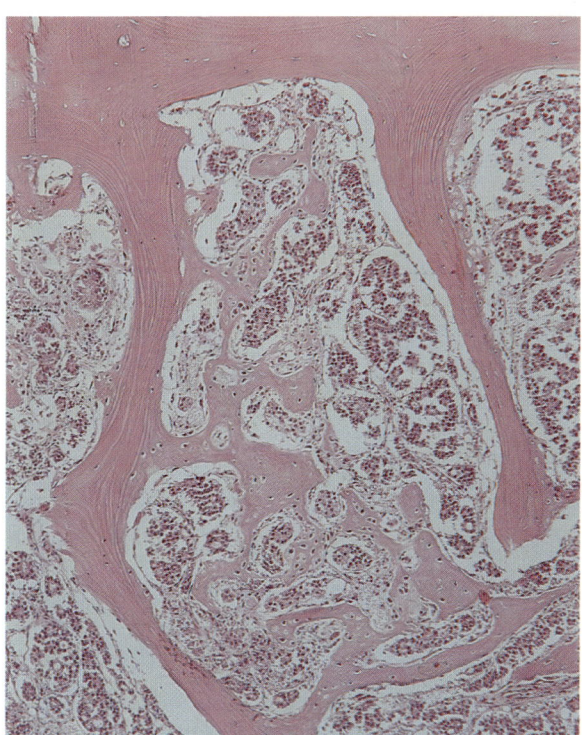

Fig. 1.1 Part of an osteosclerotic metastasis from a carcinoma of prostate, showing a network of newly formed bone trabeculae. The osteoblasts and osteocytes of the new bone are quite separate from the epithelial cells of the tumours. (×65)

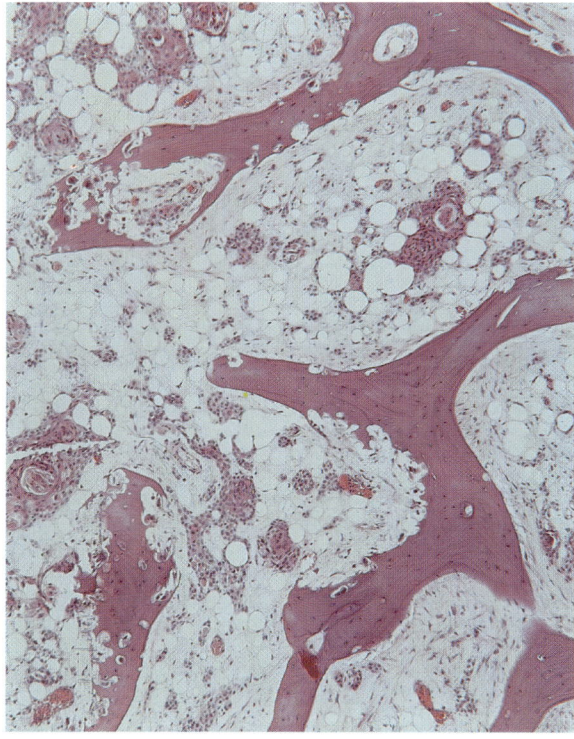

Fig. 1.2. The margin of an osteolytic metastasis (from a squamous carcinoma of lung) showing osteoclasts and resorption surfaces on the bone trabeculae. (×50)

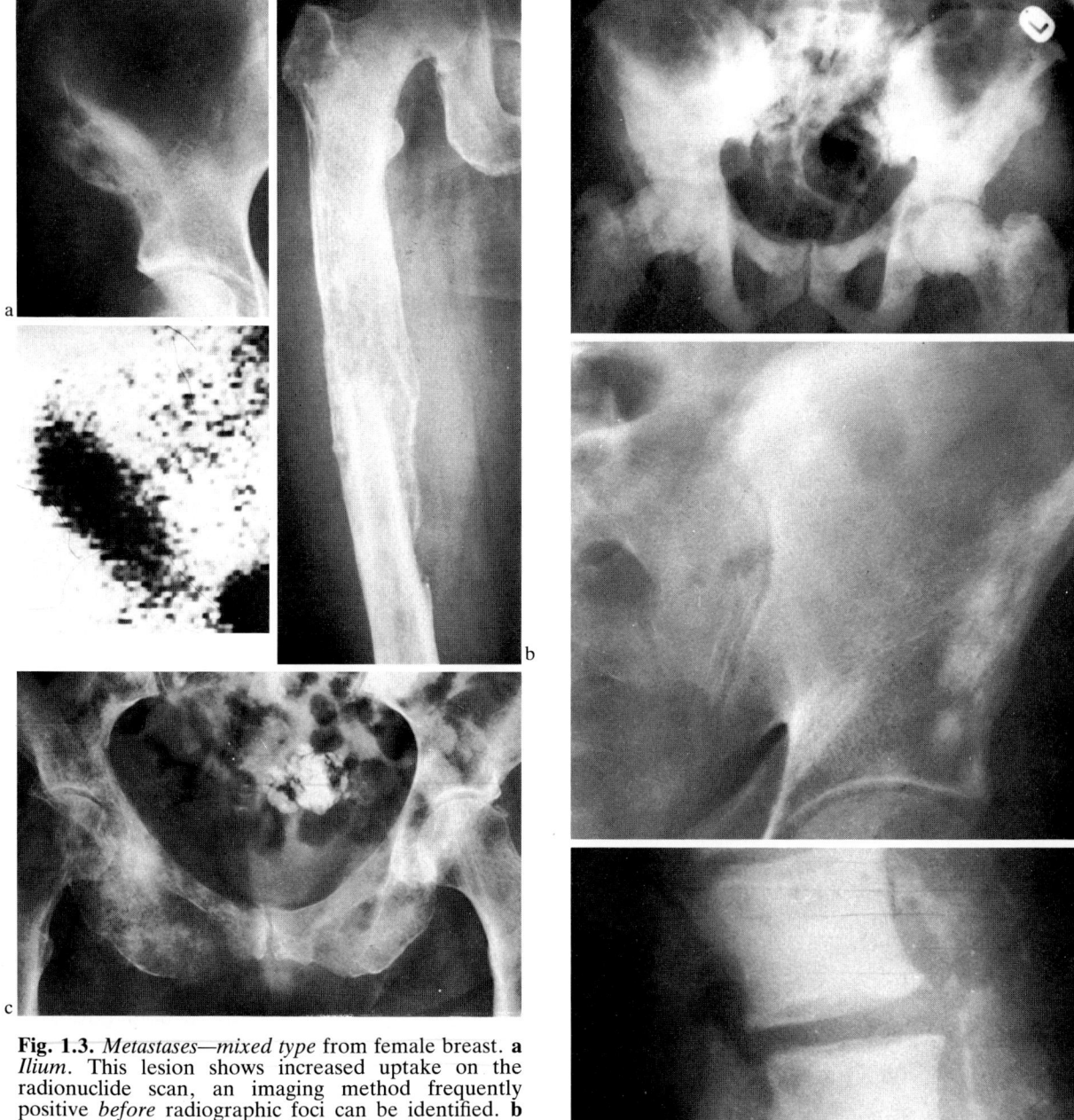

Fig. 1.3. *Metastases—mixed type* from female breast. **a** *Ilium.* This lesion shows increased uptake on the radionuclide scan, an imaging method frequently positive *before* radiographic foci can be identified. **b** *Femur.* This mixed metastasis, causing localised pain in a 65-year-old woman, was recognised 9 months after surgery for the primary neoplasm. **c** *Pelvis*—in this case bone destruction predominates. A calcified fibroid was demonstrated incidentally.

Fig. 1.4. *Metastases—multiple osteoblastic type* from: **a** *prostate*, much the most common—a pathological fracture of the left femur worsened the prognosis; **b** *bladder*—these metastases were widespread, but more commonly are lytic; **c** *stomach*, a relatively uncommon origin.

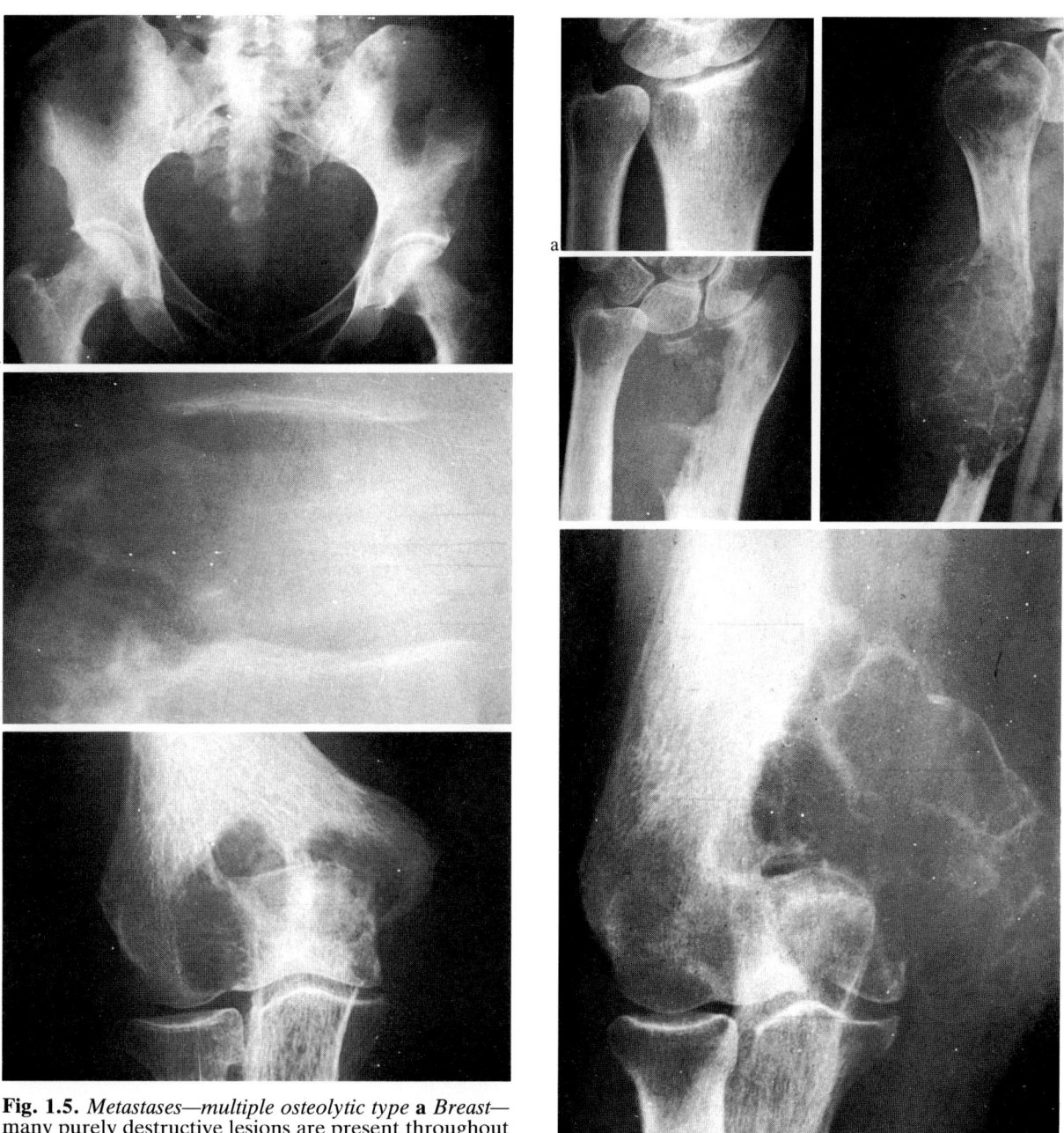

Fig. 1.5. *Metastases—multiple osteolytic type* **a** *Breast*—many purely destructive lesions are present throughout the pelvis and in the intertrochanteric portion of the left femur. **b** *Kidney*—body of L3 and distal end of humerus in a 55-year-old man. It is unusual to find more than six metastatic skeletal lesions from this primary tumour. In a younger patient the humeral deposit might have been interpreted as a giant-cell tumour.

Fig. 1.6. *Metastases—solitary lytic lesions* arise classically from primary tumours of lung, kidney and thyroid, frequently affecting the appendicular skeleton: **a** *Bronchus*, illustrating rapid growth in 6 months in the radius of a middle-aged man. **b** *Kidney*. This typically expanding and destructive lesion occurred in a middle-aged woman. **c** *Thyroid*. Another classically expansile lytic metastasis in a 73-year-old woman. Such lesions are relatively uncommon and may be found many years after resection of the primary tumour.

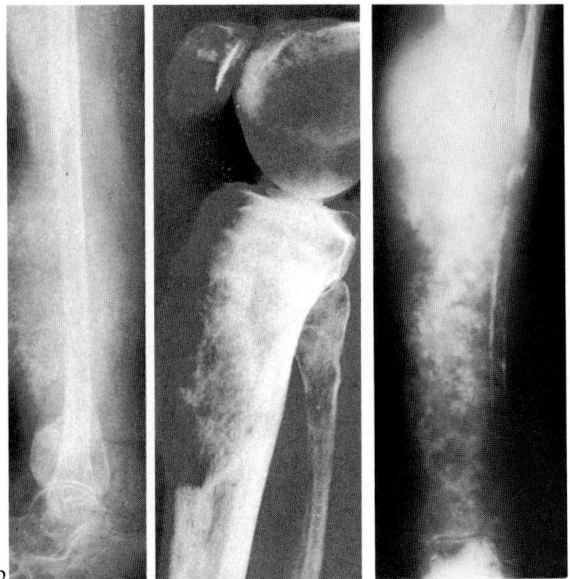

Fig. 1.7. *Metastases—tibial lesions.* Approximately half arise from primary tumours within the pelvis, causing localised pain and swelling. **a** *Bladder.* This lesion in a 76-year-old woman had been regarded as pyogenic osteomyelitis 5 months previously. **b** *Prostate* in a 72-year-old man. **c** *Prostate* with spread to fibula in an elderly man with remarkably mild pain.

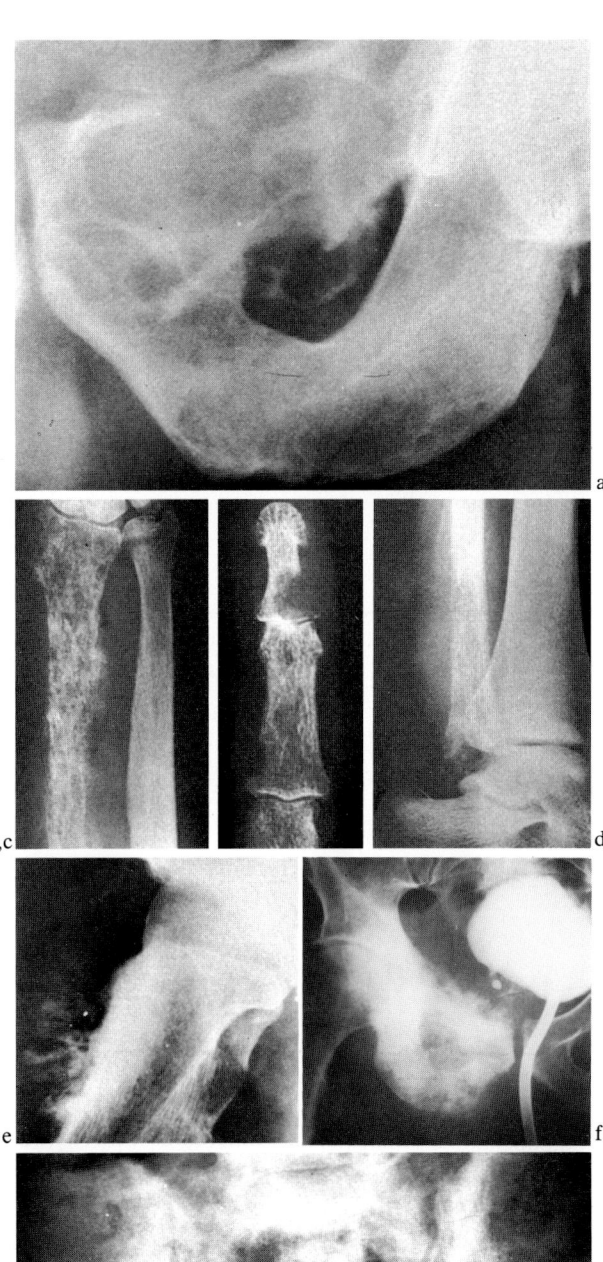

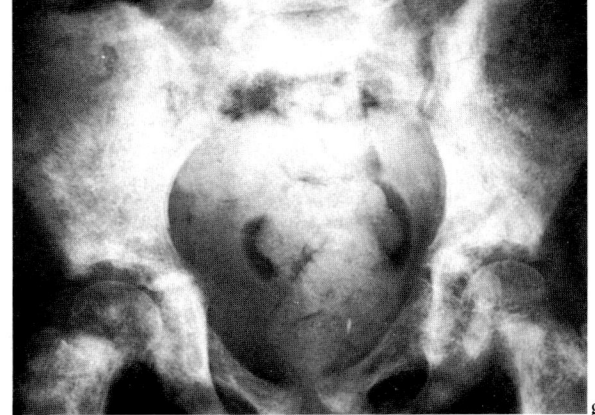

Fig. 1.8. *Metastases—unusual manifestations of origin, site and age.* Many of these lesions may be suspected initially of being primary neoplasms of bone. **a** This destructive pubic lesion was secondary to a *parotid tumour* resected 20 years previously. Only histologically was its nature established in this middle-aged woman. **b** The pattern of a reticulum cell sarcoma is simulated by this solitary infiltrating lesion of the radius from a *squamous cell carcinoma of the skin.* **c** These lytic phalangeal lesions were secondary to a *carcinoma of the lung*—a complication well recognised. **d** This infiltrating destruction in the distal end of the fibula in a 20-year-old woman, with mild pain and swelling of the ankle for a year, was regarded as a Ewing's tumour, but the biopsy showed it to be a metastasis from *lung*, then confirmed by examination of the chest. Such early metastases, especially from breast, carry a particularly sinister prognosis. This patient died within a few months. **e** Osteoblastic lesions resembling osteosarcoma in elderly patients with carcinoma of the *colon* and **f** *prostate*. **g** Secondary deposits in children are rare, with the exception of *neuroblastoma*, which was established in this 5-year-old girl. The infiltrating and widespread destructive lesions are difficult to differentiate from leukaemia, as indicated by the lucency of the right proximal femoral metaphysis. This child had presented with pain in the right hip and a limp, a generalised polyarthritis being suspected clinically.

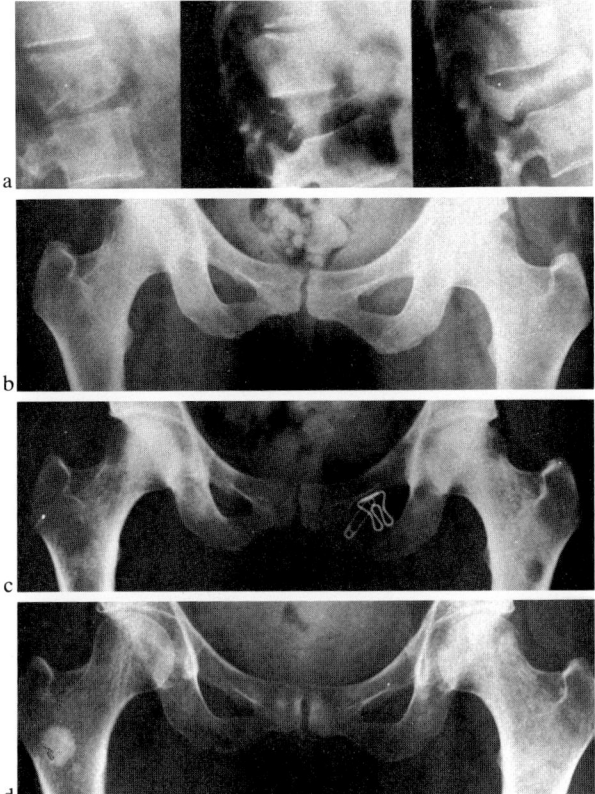

Fig. 1.9. *Metastasis from breast—response to treatment.* Destructive lesions in the body of L2 and proximal ends of the femora, in a 40-year-old woman with back pain, **a** on presentation, **b** 4 months after mastectomy, radiation therapy and cytotoxic drugs and, **c** 3 months later following bilateral oophorectomy. At first these aggressive and destructive metastases enlarged, but they showed a startling conversion latterly by an osteoblastic response **d**, making them extremely dense. The femoral metastases, initially indefinite, undoubtedly would have been shown at the time of the first examination by radionuclide scanning. This apparently satisfactory response had only short-lived success.

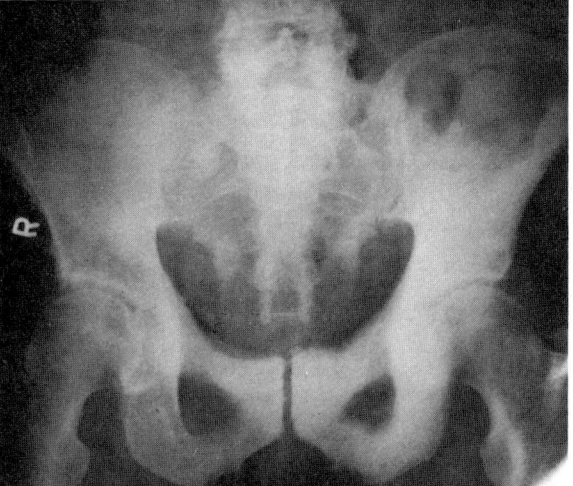

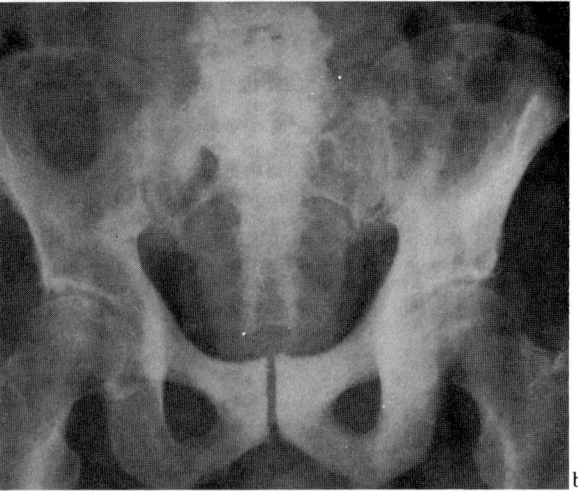

Fig. 1.10. *Metastases from prostate—response to treatment.* **a** This 74-year-old man showed diffuse sclerotic deposits throughout the skeleton. Extra-osseous extensions had resulted in peripheral densities around the ischial and pubic rami. Female hormone therapy was administered. **b** Five years later the patient was alive and well with no increase in size of the metastases and with regression of the peripheral densities.

Q1. This 74-year-old woman fell and injured her hip.

Clinically the hip was painful and passive movements were restricted in all directions. Marked shortening of the limb was evident. A fracture of the femoral neck was diagnosed.

Radiological examination confirmed the presence of subcapital fracture of the femur. All the bones were significantly demineralised with obvious cortical thinning, particularly in the femoral shaft.

Laboratory investigations:

Serum calcium	10.1 mg% (2.5 mmol/litre)
Serum inorganic phosphorus	5.0 mg% (1.7 mmol/litre)
Serum alkaline phosphatase	8 KA units (56 IU/litre)
Blood urea nitrogen	23.0 mg% (3.6 mmol/litre)
Sodium	150 mEq/litre (150 mmol/litre)
Urinary calcium	200 mg in 24 h (5 mmol in 24 h)

Twenty-four hours after the injury the femoral head was excised (Q1b) and replaced by a metallic prosthesis. In view of the radiological appearance an iliac biopsy was performed at the same time.

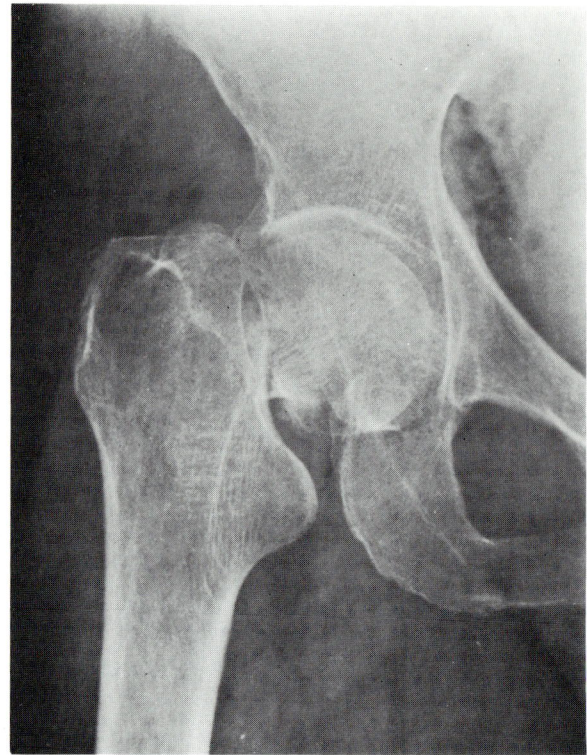

Q1a.

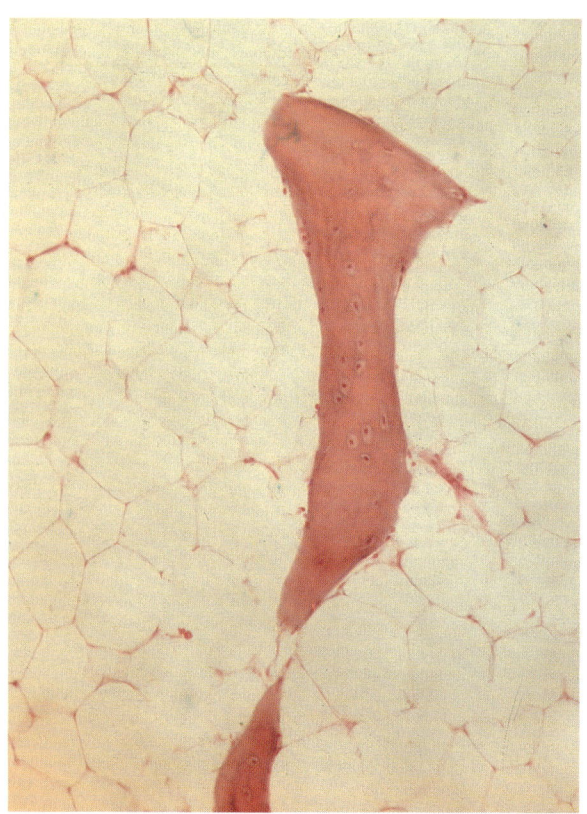

Q1b. (×138) femoral head

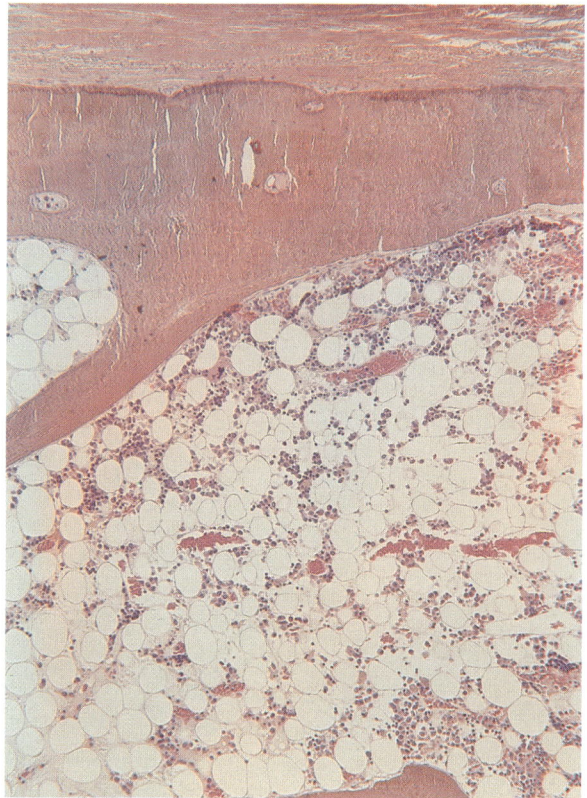

Q1c. (×54) iliac crest

Q2. The patient, a woman aged 31 years, had a history of recent pain in the right hip.

She had also complained of pain in the shoulders, feet and back for 2 years, following pregnancy.

Radiological examination showed a fracture of the neck of the right femur and generalised skeletal demineralisation. Further studies revealed healing fractures of the left 2nd, 3rd and 4th metatarsals.

Laboratory investigations:

Serum calcium	9.2 mg% (2.3 mmol/litre)
Serum inorganic phosphorus	1.4 mg% (0.45 mmol/litre)
Serum alkaline phosphatase	15 KA units (106 IU/litre)
Blood urea nitrogen	32 mg% (5.4 mmol/litre)
Sodium	137 mEq/litre (137 mmol/litre)
Urinary calcium	30 mg in 24 h (0.75 mmol in 24 h)
Faecal fat	3.8 g in 24 h (13.5 mmol in 24 h)

An iliac crest biopsy was carried out.

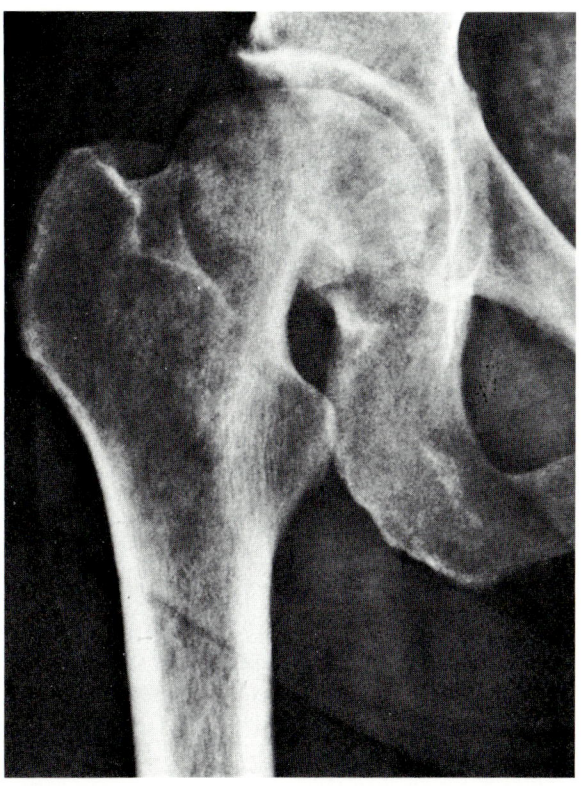

Q2a.

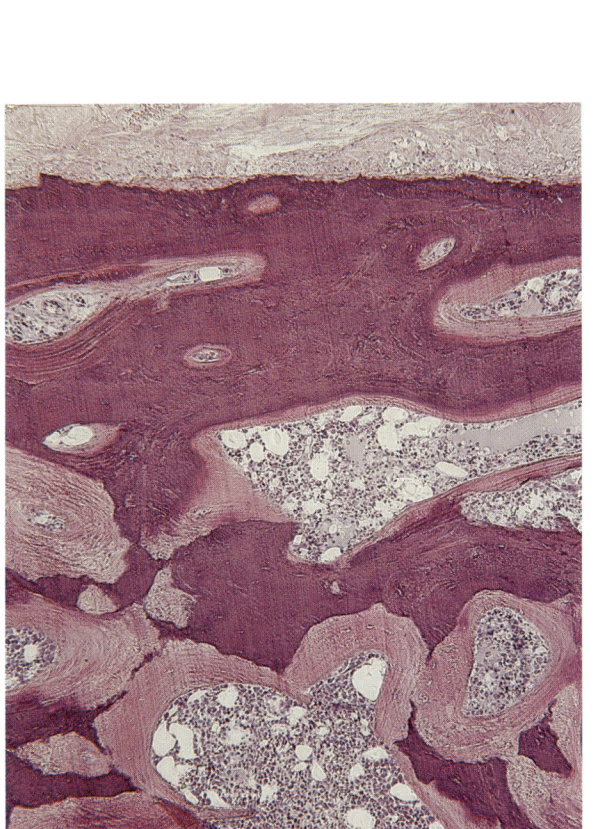

Q2b. (×54)

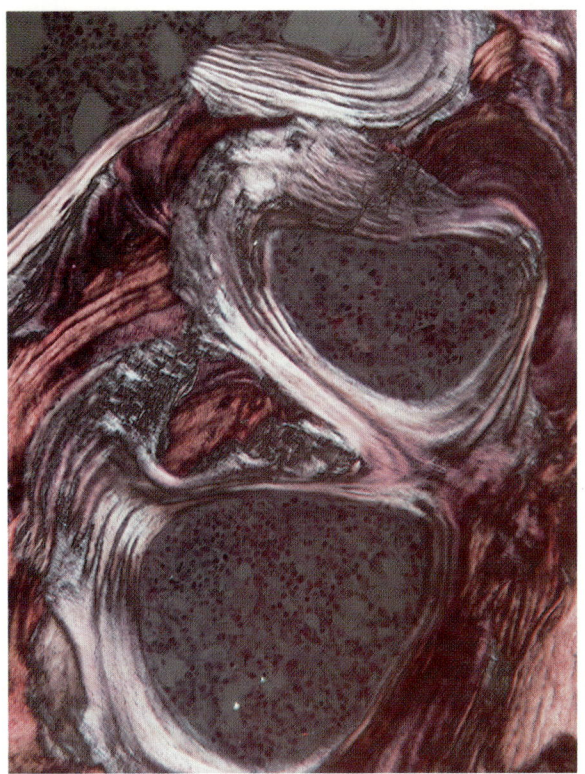

Q2c. (×112) Polarised light

A1. Osteoporosis with subcapital fracture of femoral neck

The marked rarefaction shown in the femoral shaft and pelvis also involved other parts of the skeleton. The normal biochemical findings indicate that this rarefaction is, in fact, osteoporosis (as opposed to osteomalacia or some other rarefying bone disease). The iliac crest biopsy enabled this diagnosis to be confirmed.

At operation, the femoral head was completely separated, and it was evident that its vascular supply was interrupted. Q1b shows the histological appearance of the bone and bone marrow in the femoral head. The outline of the fat cells in the marrow is normal, and the osteocyte lacunae contain normally staining cell nuclei. This is not surprising, despite the interruption of vascular supply, because of the short interval between the fracture and the removal of the femoral head. Carefully timed studies (Catto, 1965; Rosingh and James, 1969) have shown that some days must elapse before morphological changes can be recognised in routine histological sections. After that there is progressive loss of nuclear staining, and the necrotic bone tissue can be recognised by its empty lacunae. This is apparent in Fig. 1.1, from a femoral head removed 2 months after fracture.

Q1c shows the histological appearance of the iliac crest biopsy, as seen in a section of undecalcified bone stained with haematoxylin and eosin. The cortex is thin and bone trabeculae are few: this reduction in the amount of bone (osteoporosis) is the basis of the skeletal rarefaction that was evident radiologically. Osteomalacia can be excluded by the absence of osteoid tissue. The bone marrow, made up of fat cells and haemopoietic tissue, is normal. The iliac crest is frequently used for bone biopsies in cases of generalised bone disease because of its accessibility: the normal range of histological structure for this site is therefore well known (Byers, 1977).

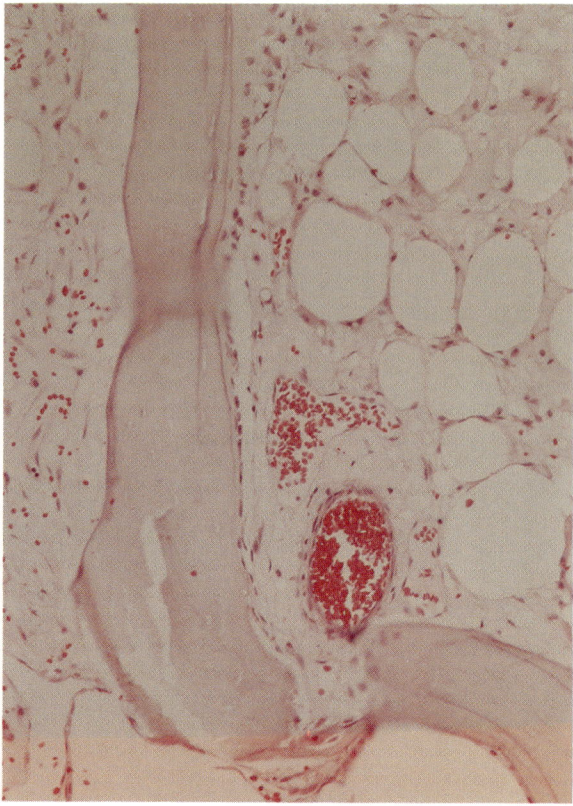

Fig. 1.1. From a femoral head removed 2 months after femoral neck fracture. Osteocyte lacunae are empty. The patent blood vessels indicate that revascularisation is occurring. (×138)

Osteoporosis

The term osteoporosis describes a group of conditions characterised by reduction in the amount of bone tissue present. It may be due, therefore, either to inadequate formation of bone or to accelerated resorption of bone. The physiological process of bone formation requires primarily an adequate supply of protein, calcium and phosphorus. Fundamental dietetic deficiencies of this type occur in *anorexia nervosa* or with *severe starvation*. Formation of osteoid from such protein demands normal osteoblastic function. Inherited failure of this function is believed to be responsible for the congenital disorder of *osteogenesis imperfecta*, an entity considered elsewhere in this work. Lack of vitamin C in the diet also impairs osteoblastic formation of osteoid, resulting in the essentially osteoporotic entity of *scurvy*. Endocrine factors play a major part in normal bone formation. Reduction of *sex hormones* as an involutional process in post-menopausal women is responsible for the increased incidence of osteoporosis in the female sex, but has been observed to develop also in males following castration. In contrast, excess activity of the thyroid gland, as in *thyrotoxicosis*, or of the adrenal and pituitary glands, causing *hypercorticism* (Cushing's syndrome), stimulates catabolism with accelerated resorption of bone, resulting again in osteoporosis. Another physiological requirement is *active use*, so that the permanently recumbent or paralysed patient inevitably develops orthostatic osteoporosis. In many cases, however, no definite explanation for generalised osteoporosis, as in Q1, can be established, so that these cases are termed *idiopathic*. Routine laboratory investigations are within normal limits.

Localised osteoporosis occurs with disuse, as in immobilisation of a limb in treatment of a fracture. Such changes may develop after a minor injury, or even spontaneously, and sometimes progress to such a degree that the condition is described as *reflex sympathetic dystrophy* or *Sudeck's atrophy*, invariably accompanied by pain, occasionally very severe. The cause of this disorder has never been established satisfactorily. The painful entity described more recently as *transient osteoporosis*, usually affecting a major joint such as the hip or the knee, is likely to be similar. Localised osteoporosis is a recognised complication of *radiation therapy* and is attributed to impaired vitality of the affected bones, which are liable to fracture easily.

Clinical Features

Idiopathic osteoporosis is common in elderly women. It is difficult to distinguish it from the 'normal' decrease in bone mass which occurs with increasing age and which is more pronounced in women than in men. Osteoporosis, by itself, produces no symptoms, but often comes to attention when it is complicated by fractures, usually involving the cancellous bone of the vertebral bodies or the femoral necks. Indeed, a subcapital fracture of the femur, so common in elderly women, is a frequent complication of idiopathic osteoporosis.

Dietetic deficiencies should be recognised by loss of weight. Scurvy, now excessively rare, is characterised in the child by painful swellings of the ends of long bones, spontaneous bleeding and anaemia. In the adult, bleeding from the gums, loss of teeth and muscular weakness due to chronic anaemia were classical signs of this disease.

Osteoporosis due to thyrotoxicosis is exceptional, even when the classical features of tremor, exophthalmos and thinning of the hair are obvious. On the other hand Cushing's syndrome is characterised by the triad of obesity, hypertension and depression of sexual function. Other important clinical features include diminution of pain sense and also impaired response to infections, due to the anti-inflammatory effect of cortisone and hydrocortisone. Symptoms caused by fractures or even an acute appendicitis may be masked. Cushing's syndrome due to pituitary or adrenal hyperplasia or neoplasms is rare, but the widespread therapeutic use of these hormones frequently causes iatrogenic symptoms and signs to develop. Of particular orthopaedic interest is disintegration of major joints due to a combination of osteoporosis, suppression of pain sense and mechanical stress, a particular complication of renal transplants. Similar changes have been attributed to prolonged analgesic therapy.

Localised osteoporosis of disuse, following immobilisation of a limb, normally regresses spontaneously after the fracture has repaired, particularly in young patients. The severe pain encountered with Sudeck's atrophy and transient osteoporosis, however, may persist for many months. In the latter condition migration of symptoms to other joints may take place.

Radiological Features

1. Site. In the *generalised* forms described above, the osteoporotic process involves the entire skeleton, but initially it tends to become apparent in the spine, particularly in its dorsal portion. An exception is juvenile scurvy, in which the abnormalities are evident around the affected joints and the anterior ends of the ribs.

Localised osteoporosis develops distal to a fracture or in an irradiated area of the skeleton. *Sudeck's atrophy* is confined to the bones of a hand or foot. *Transient osteoporosis* is observed around major joints, particularly the hip and the knee. Radionuclide scanning demonstrates increased uptake of the tracer and may show similar uptake around another major joint without symptoms but liable to become symptomatic at a later date because of the migrating pattern of this disease.

2. Appearance. Generalised osteoporosis. The reduction in bone mass results in decreased bone density in cancellous bone, with resorption first affecting the least important trabeculae, and cortical thinning, particularly on endosteal surfaces. These changes alone do not permit a radiological diagnosis other than osteopenia, a term meaning simply 'sparse bone', since a similar appearance may be caused by other diffuse disorders, such as osteomalacia, hyperparathyroidism and even, to some extent, widespread myelomatosis or metastatic disease. Nevertheless, the fractures of the spine and femoral neck, mentioned above, often provide a diagnostic clue. In the case of hypercorticism, a valuable diagnostic sign is provided by 'marginal vertebral condensation', a band of increased density, observed usually on the upper table of a partially compressed vertebral body. In addition fractures, frequently asymptomatic, may be detected in the ribs and pelvis. Occasionally an unsuspected focus of infection is identified. In scurvy in children the particularly osteoporotic areas are the zones of primary trabeculation adjacent to the metaphyses and the growth plates. These zones are fragile and fracture easily. Because absence of vitamin C also causes capillary fragility, bleeding follows such fractures, elevating the periosteum, loosely attached at this age, with the formation of subperiosteal haematomas, which often calcify and become dense. Continued deposition of the calcium phosphate complex into the sparse osteoid of the metaphyses produces the classical 'white line' of scurvy, which may be present also around the periphery of small growth centres (the Wimberger sign). Adults with scurvy show only diffuse osteoporosis.

Localised osteoporosis of disuse tends to be especially prominent in areas of high vascularity, such as the metaphyses in children and young adults. When the onset has been rapid the cortex, as well as the medullary bone, has been affected. Vertical and linear lucencies appear within the cortical bone, in contrast to generalised osteoporosis, in which cortical thinning occurs by slow but progressive absorption of the endosteal surfaces. In Sudeck's atrophy subarticular demineralisation is extensive, with preservation of the articular surfaces which are contrastingly prominent. Transient osteoporosis is characterised by diffuse peri-articular demineralisation of a major joint or by a partial area of resorption immediately adjacent to the articular surface. In both cases the radionuclide scan is positive.

Pathological Features

The reduction in the amount of bone tissue is apparent in histological sections of bones in osteoporosis, but the nature of the changes leading to the loss of bone is not so clear. The maintenance of a normal bone mass depends on a balance between bone formation by osteoblasts and bone destruction by osteoclasts, both of which are active throughout life. Osteoporosis can result from increased bone destruction or from decreased bone formation, or from a combination of the two. The cortex of an affected bone becomes thin and the trabeculae are slender and relatively few in number, supporting the radiological findings described above.

Treatment

Dietetic deficiencies should be corrected. Surgery may be necessary for thyrotoxicosis and Cushing's syndrome of natural origin. Caution is required in the use of steroid therapy.

For idiopathic osteoporosis many types of treatment (administration of calcium, oestrogens, fluoride, etc.) have been recommended, but good evidence of their effectiveness is elusive. Recent work, however, has indicated that prophylactic oestrogen therapy does reduce the incidence of post-menopausal osteoporosis. Localised osteoporosis, when painful, may be aided by physiotherapy. Both Sudeck's atrophy and transient osteoporosis resolve slowly, usually in about 1 year.

References

Avioli LV (1977) Osteoporosis: pathogenesis and therapy. In: Avioli LV, Krane SM (eds) Metabolic bone disease. Academic Press, New York

Byers PD (1977) The diagnostic value of bone biopsies. In: Avioli LV, Krane SM (eds) Metabolic bone disease. Academic Press, New York

Catto M (1965) A histological study of avascular necrosis of the femoral head after transcervical fracture. J Bone Jt Surg 47B: 749–776

Glimcher MJ, Kenzora JE (1979) The biology of osteonecrosis of the human femoral head and its clinical implications. Clin Orthop 138: 284–309; 139: 283–312; 140: 273–312

Lequesne M (1968) Transient osteoporosis of the hip—a non-traumatic variety of Sudeck's atrophy. Ann Rheum Dis 27: 463–471

Lequesne M et al. (1977) Partial transient osteoporosis. Skeletal Radiol 2: 1–9

Rosingh GE, James J (1969) Early phases of avascular necrosis of the femoral head in rabbits. J Bone Jt Surg 51B: 165–174

Sissons HA (1952) Osteoporosis and epiphyseal arrest in joint tuberculosis. J Bone Jt Surg 34B: 275–290

Stevenson FH (1952) The osteoporosis of immobilisation in recumbency. J Bone Jt Surg 34B: 256–265

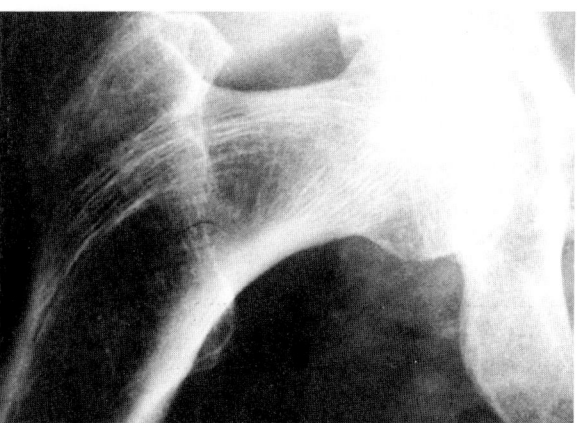

Fig. 1.2. *Senile osteoporosis*. Involutional changes in this 75-year-old woman had caused skeletal demineralisation. The least important weight-bearing trabeculae, however, are the first to be absorbed, thereby accentuating the remaining primary trabeculae.

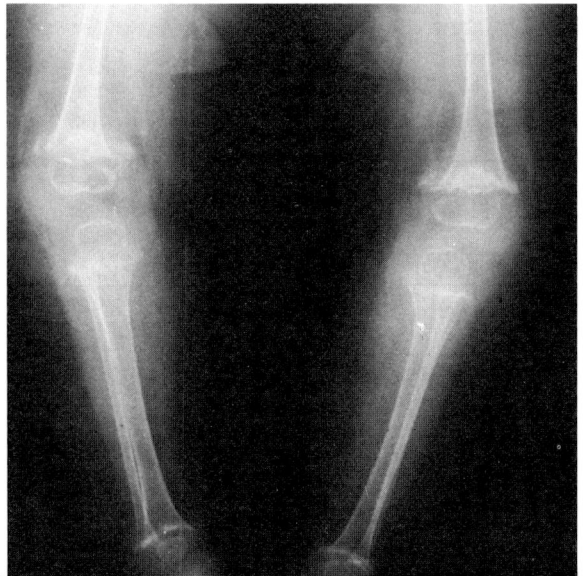
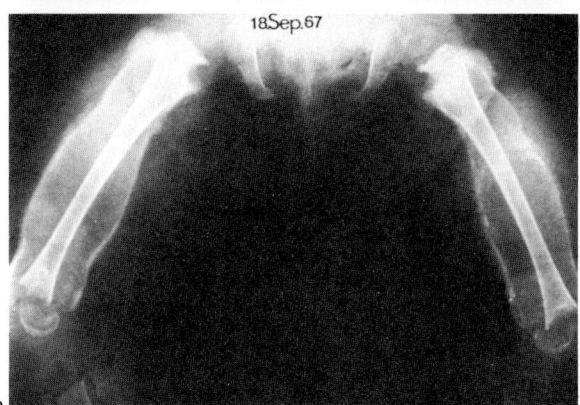
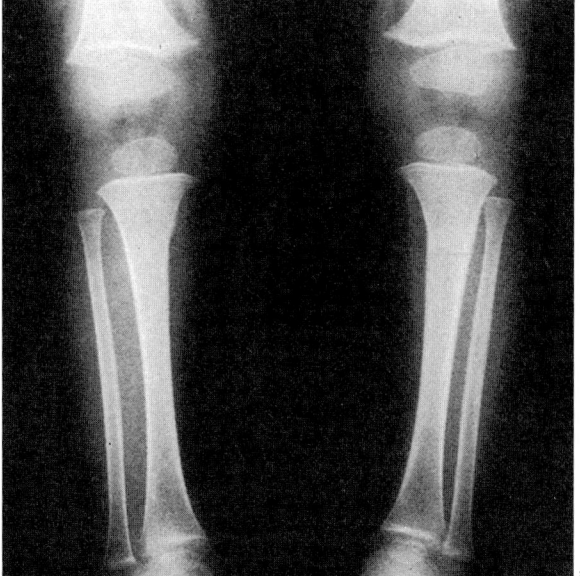
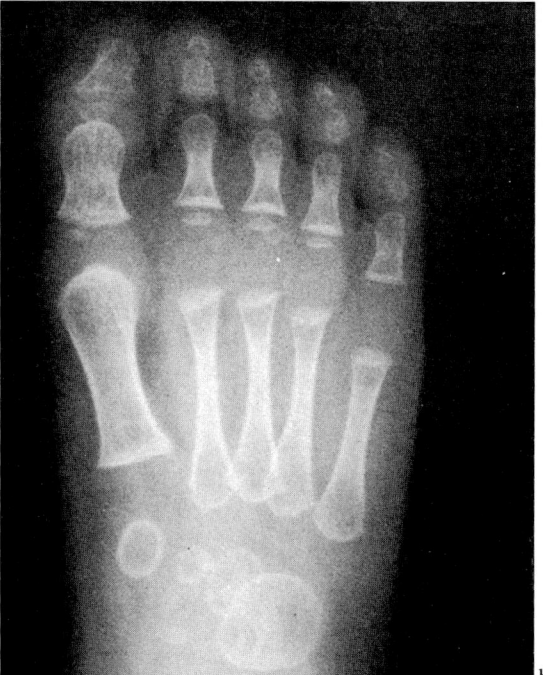

Fig. 1.3. *Scurvy.* **a** This 1-year-old baby girl was brought to hospital on account of progressive weakness, extreme irritability and marked tenderness of the legs. Generalised osteoporosis has affected particularly the zones of primary trabeculation on the diaphyseal sides of the metaphyses. These areas are so fragile that the majority have fractured, causing the bony projections described classically as 'beaks of Pelkan'. Continued deposition of calcium phosphate, within such osteoid as is present in the metaphyses, has resulted in the typical 'white lines' of the disease. Observe the same phenomenon causing peripheral densities around the epiphyseal centres, the classical Wimberger sign. This infant's diet had been virtually devoid of vitamin C. **b** Only a few weeks later huge subperiosteal haematomas had developed around each femur and had begun to calcify. The capillary fragility of the disease had resulted in excessive bleeding from the fractures, elevating the periosteum, which is loosely attached to its parent bone at this age. Not surprisingly, both distal femoral epiphyses fused prematurely as a consequence of these pathological fractures.

Fig. 1.4. *Scurvy—further examples.* **a** An earlier case in which the metaphyseal 'white lines' are particularly prominent, with generalised osteoporosis. These abnormalities were symmetrical. **b** 'White lines' and osteoporosis in the foot of this young child demonstrate exquisitely the Wimberger sign, especially around the periphery of the medial cuneiform. All the highly vascular metaphyseal areas are severely demineralised.

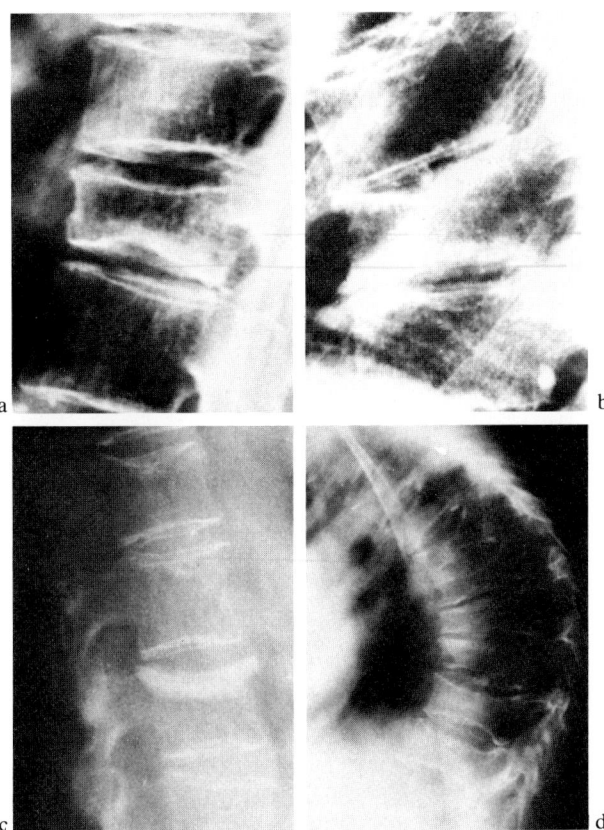

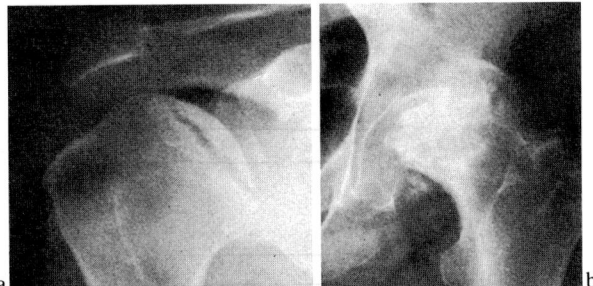

Fig. 1.6. *Cortisone arthropathy.* Disintegration of the heads of the right humerus and left femur occurred in this 58-year-old woman with widespread osteoporosis due to established Cushing's syndrome. The changes in the left hip were believed to have been accelerated by intra-articular injections of steroids. This 'crumbling hip' syndrome is encountered much more commonly as an iatrogenic complication, pain having been relieved by steroid therapy. Even more frequently such joint disintegration is associated with the prolonged use of analgesics, such as phenylbutazone or indomethacin.

Fig. 1.5. *Spinal osteoporosis—different causes.* **a** *Senile type* in an old woman with typical collapse of vertebral bodies. The stress-bearing vertical trabeculae which remain are prominent. **b** *Dietetic deficiency* in a 30-year-old woman with a 12-year history of anorexia nervosa caused a similar appearance at a much earlier stage. **c** *Metabolic disease.* Cushing's syndrome in an obese 32-year-old woman, with the helpful radiological sign of marginal vertebral condensation, due to excess steroid activity. Thyrotoxicosis also can cause osteoporosis. **d** *Idiopathic osteoporosis*, the rarest and unexplained type, resulted in multiple vertebral compression fractures and kyphosis in a young woman aged 23, with chronic backache. All investigations were negative.

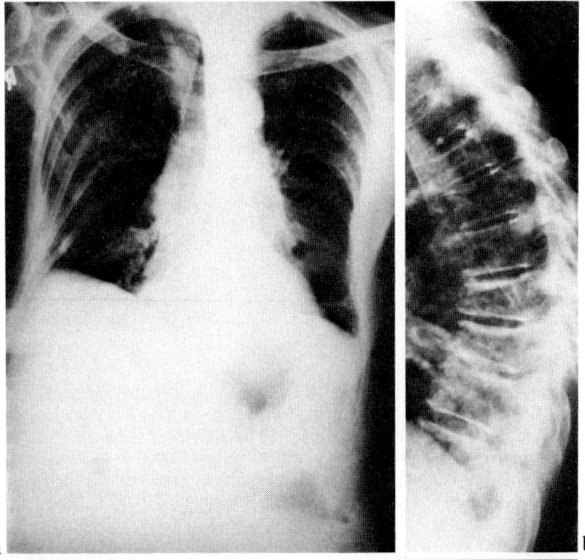

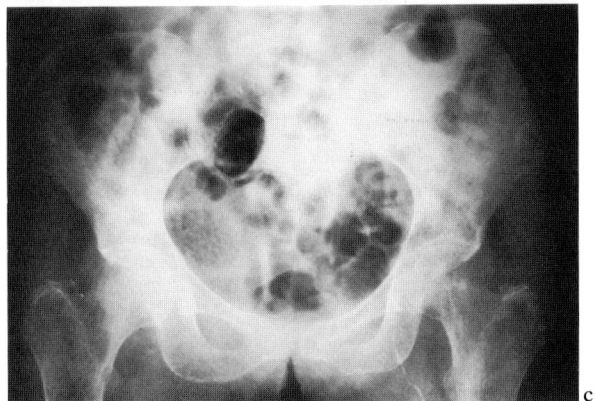

Fig. 1.7. *Iatrogenic Cushing's syndrome.* This 65-year-old woman developed rheumatoid arthritis 3 years earlier and had been treated continuously by steroid therapy. She had become obese and hypertensive. Radiological examination of **a** the chest revealed widespread osteoporosis with fractures of the ribs which were asymptomatic owing to suppression of pain sense by the adrenocortical hormones. The cavity in the left lower lobe was due to a staphylococcal abscess which had caused only minor symptoms and signs, illustrating the anti-inflammatory effect of steroids. **b** Osteoporosis in the spine was accompanied by numerous compression fractures of vertebral bodies, also asymptomatic. Observe again the virtually diagnostic sign of marginal vertebral condensation. **c** The pelvis was also osteoporotic, with a stress fracture in the left femoral neck.

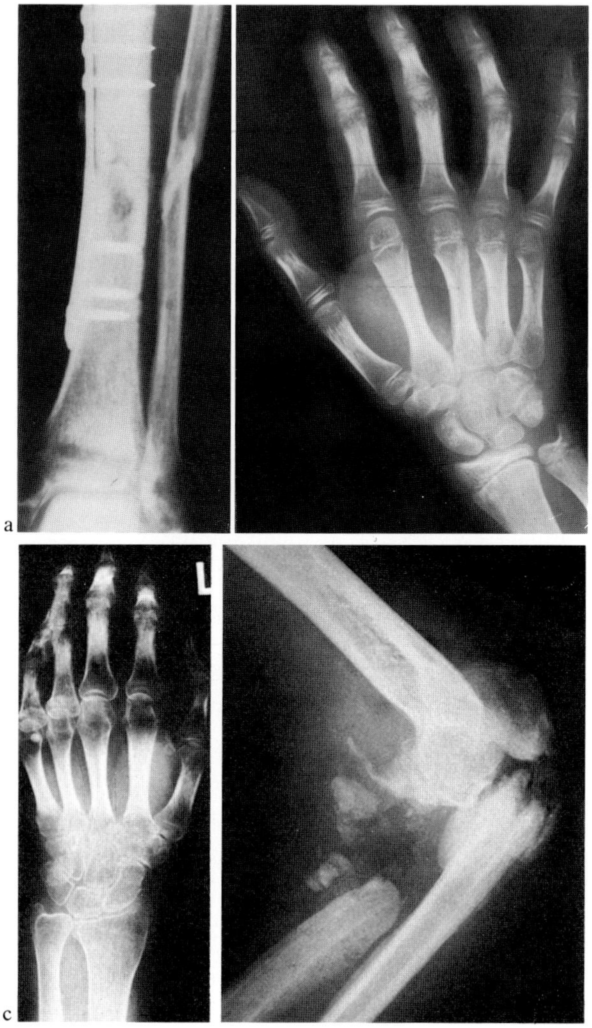

Fig. 1.8. *Osteoporosis due to disuse.* **a** *Distal to fractures* of the tibia and fibula, increased lucency being evident especially in the former metaphyseal areas. **b** *Hysterical paralysis* of the right hand in a 12-year-old boy caused this marked osteoporosis, again affecting particularly the highly vascular metaphyses. **c** *Sudeck's atrophy*—painful, post-traumatic osteoporosis of hand with etching of the articular surfaces, following a gun-shot wound of the elbow in a young man.

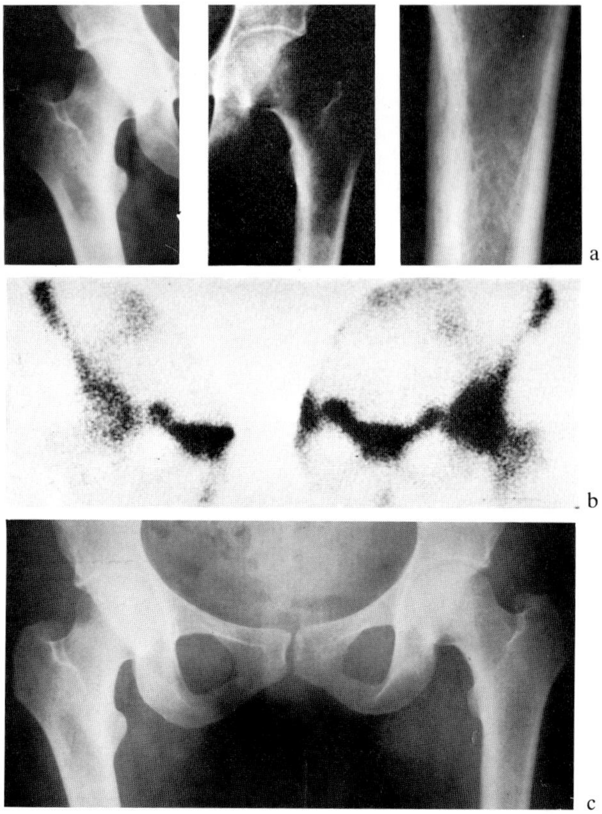

Fig. 1.9. *Transient osteoporosis of hip.* This 31-year-old woman developed pain in the left hip and leg during the last week of her first pregnancy. The pain persisted after a normal delivery. Six weeks later marked osteoporosis was evident in this area, its rapid onset being indicated by linear vertical lucencies within the cortex of the left femur (*see inset enlargement*). All investigations were normal except for an elevated alkaline phosphatase level. **b** Radionuclide scanning was positive. Without any definitive treatment, other than advice to avoid oral contraceptives, symptoms regressed slowly, as may be forecast with this unexplained entity. **c** A year later, when planning to have another child, the patient was free of symptoms and normal bone architecture had been restored. The relationship of this condition to pregnancy is undetermined. Most cases have affected men.

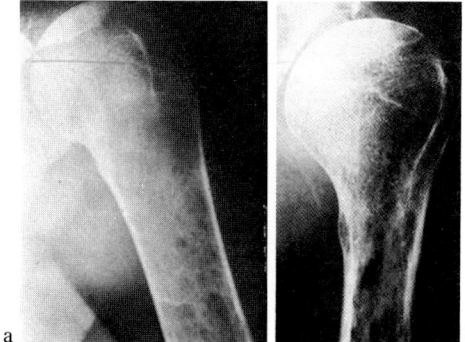

Fig. 1.10. *Post-radiation osteoporosis of humerus* in two women treated for carcinoma of the breast. (a) Mild. (b) Severe. The numerous lucencies should not be confused with metastases.

A.2 Osteomalacia

The biochemical findings (low serum calcium, moderate elevation of serum alkaline phosphatase and low urinary calcium, in the presence of a normal blood urea nitrogen and normal faecal fat), suggested a diagnosis of osteomalacia, which was supported by the history of generalised bone pain. Additional biochemical investigations failed to show evidence of intestinal malabsorption or renal disease, and a diagnosis of nutritional osteomalacia was established. The patient responded well to treatment with vitamin D.

The radiological pattern of diffuse osteopenia also suggested a metabolic disorder, but in this case the fracture of the femoral neck and those in the metatarsals (Fig. 2.1) provided further evidence of osteomalacia.

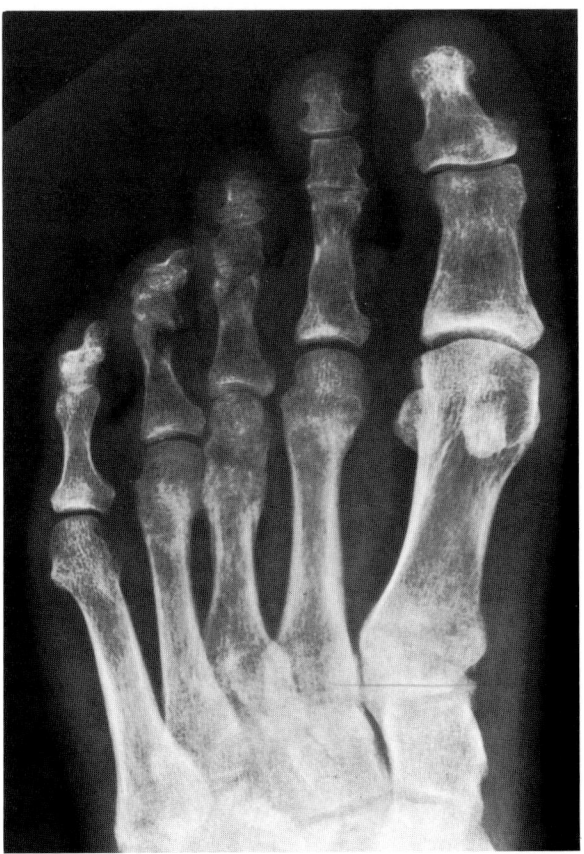

Fig. 2.1. The left foot of the patient in Q2 illustrates the gross generalised osteopenia which was present in this patient. The healing fractures of the 2nd, 3rd and 4th metatarsal necks are essentially repairing Looser zones.

The findings in the iliac crest biopsy confirm the diagnosis of osteomalacia. Q2b, from a section of undecalcified bone stained with haematoxylin and eosin, shows the large amount of pale-staining osteoid tissue (uncalcified bone) which covers the trabecular and cortical surfaces. Q2c shows a more magnified field of tissue from the same section as Q2b, viewed in polarized light. The osteoid tissue on the surfaces of the trabeculae shows the same lamellar arrangement as the deeper calcified tissue. The osteoid tissue lacks bone mineral, but its structure is otherwise that of normal lamellar bone.

Osteomalacia

The term osteomalacia (and rickets in children) describes a group of conditions in which there is a failure of calcification of bone tissue, indicated histologically by the presence of a large amount of osteoid tissue.

In the past, rickets and osteomalacia were frequently due to inadequate dietary intake of vitamin D, but improved dietary standards have reduced the incidence of nutritional osteomalacia and other causes, such as intestinal malabsorption (coeliac disease, pancreatic disorders, biliary obstruction, gastric surgery), renal failure or chronic liver disease, are now responsible for a greater proportion of cases of osteomalacia than formerly. Rickets or osteomalacia occurs also in a group of genetically determined renal tubular disorders (Fanconi syndrome, cystinosis, hypophosphataemia). Prolonged administration of certain drugs, as in anticonvulsant therapy for epilepsy, represents one of the many disorders which can cause osteomalacia. Some nutritional cases of osteomalacia still occur, particularly in elderly women. In Britain they are relatively numerous among the immigrant Asian population, where young individuals also can be affected.

Clinical Features

Adult patients with osteomalacia commonly complain of generalised bone pain, often in association with muscular weakness. The usual biochemical abnormality, in contrast to osteoporosis, where normal biochemistry is expected, is a low serum calcium and an increased serum alkaline phosphatase. These are the findings in the patient in Q2. Patients with renal tubular disorders show a normal serum calcium, a low serum phosphorus and a raised serum alkaline phosphatase.

Similar clinical and biochemical abnormalities are found in children with rickets, the juvenile form of osteomalacia. In the growing skeleton, however, other clinical features include weakness and failure to thrive leading to delayed development and a small stature. Swellings develop around growth plates and the costochondral junctions ('rachitic rosary'). Attention to the condition often is drawn by deformities, particularly genu valgum and genu varum.

Radiological Features

1. Site. This generalised bone disorder affects the entire skeleton, causing diffuse demineralisation. Areas of bone growth in children, particularly the metaphyses, are lucent owing to failure of calcification of osteoid.

2. Appearance. By itself the widespread osteopenia is not diagnostic, radiological recognition in the adult depending on the secondary signs of (a) *deformity*, especially in the pelvis, which may become trifoliate, and the spine, where central vertebral collapse is common, again affecting primarily the midthoracic area and (b) *Looser's zones* or *pseudofractures*, which take the form of bands of rarefaction in cortical bone, occupied by uncalcified or incompletely calcified callus-like tissue. They are often symmetrical, and occur in characteristic sites of skeletal weakness such as the femoral neck, pubic rami, ribs, the axillary border of the scapula, major long bones of the leg and metatarsals. In particular, any stress fracture of a femoral neck in an elderly patient, especially females, should cause the possibility of osteomalacia to be considered. These appearances may be complicated by changes of secondary hyperparathyroidism, a subject discussed in a later Exercise. In children the lucent metaphyses may be distorted and splayed and accompanied by obvious deformities, but pseudofractures are relatively uncommon.

Pathological Features

Osteomalacia is indicated by the presence of a large amount of osteoid tissue on the trabecular and other bony surfaces. In making a histological diagnosis of osteomalacia, care must be taken to exclude conditions, such as Paget's disease and fracture repair, where large areas of the bony surface can be covered by a layer—usually thinner than in osteomalacia—of osteoid tissue.

It is important to use sections of undecalcified bone for the identification of osteoid tissue: if the specimen is decalcified, the staining difference between osteoid tissue and calcified bone is lost. Technical procedures for the preparation of undecalcified bone sections are described by Page (1977).

Treatment

The primary essentials in nutritional osteomalacia are a satisfactory diet, containing an adequate amount of vitamin D, and exposure to sunlight. Osteomalacia due to other causes, such as vitamin D resistance, requires measures appropriate to the underlying abnormality, but in almost all cases high vitamin D dosage is necessary. Residual deformities of limbs may necessitate orthopaedic correction by osteotomy.

References

Chalmers J, Conacher WDA, Gardner DL, Scott PJ (1967) Osteomalacia—a common disease in elderly women. J Bone Jt Surg 49B: 403–423

Dent CE (1952) Rickets and osteomalacia from renal tubule defects. J Bone Jt Surg 34B: 266–274

Fourman P, Royer P (1968) Calcium metabolism and the bone. Blackwell Scientific Publications, Oxford Edinburgh

Page KM (1977) In: Bancroft JD, Stevens A (eds) Theory and practice of histological techniques. Churchill Livingstone, Edinburgh

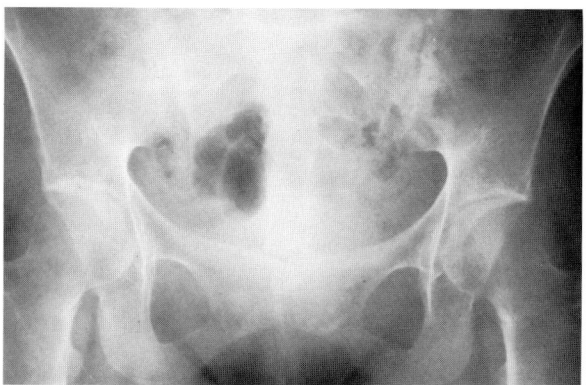

Fig. 2.2. *Dietetic osteomalacia—Looser zones.* This 21-year-old woman had complained of mild pain in the lower back and pelvis for 2 years. She was an Indian immigrant to Britain who had adhered to a strict vegetarian diet. In addition to widespread osteopenia, classical defects of Looser zones were evident symmetrically on the medial aspects of the femoral necks. These lesions responded promptly to treatment with an adequate diet and vitamin D supplements.

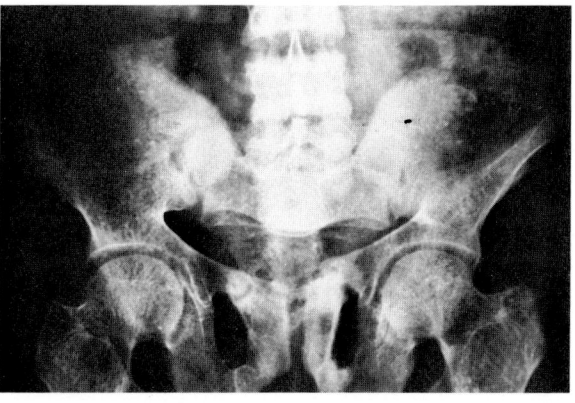

Fig. 2.4. *Osteomalacia.* Severe changes in the pelvis of this 28-year-old Indian woman, in a state of virtual starvation, include gross osteopenia, pseudofractures and deformity.

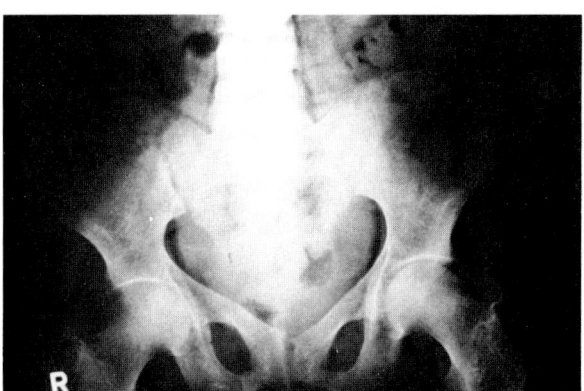

Fig. 2.3. *Osteomalacia due to steatorrhoea.* Generalised osteopenia in this middle-aged woman was accompanied by deformities of the obturator rings caused by pseudofractures, some of which have repaired. This case exemplifies one of the many causes of the disease which, radiologically, are indistinguishable.

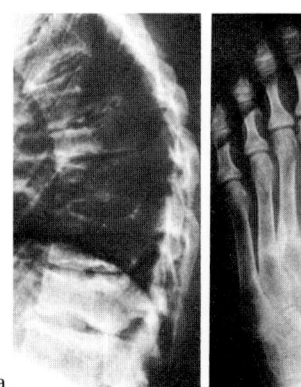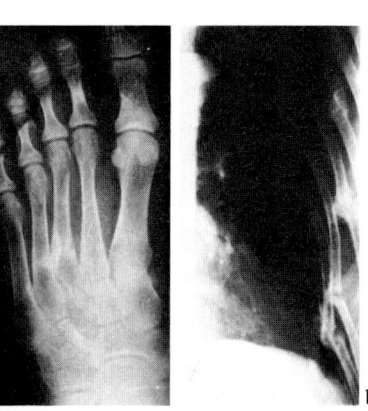

Fig. 2.5. *Osteomalacia—other sites of skeletal involvement.* **a** *Spine*, showing osteopenia with collapse of many vertebral bodies. **b** *Foot*, with Looser zones in the 3rd, 4th and 5th metatarsals. Foot pain from such lesions is a not uncommon cause of the condition presenting in an orthopaedic clinic. **c** *Ribs*, multiple fractures resulting from Looser zones. All these cases were due to intestinal malabsorption.

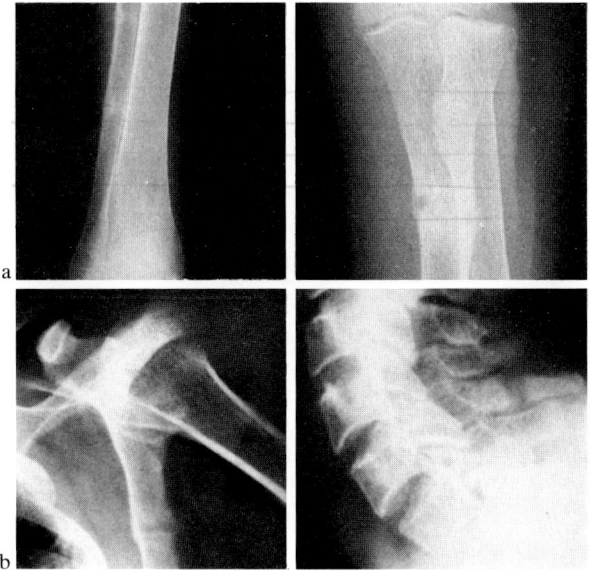

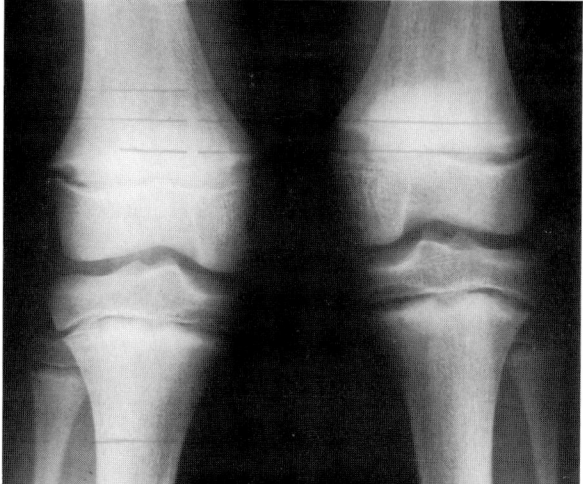

Fig. 2.6. *Osteomalacia—less common manifestations.* **a** *Long bones.* Typical Looser zones were present in the tibia, fibula and ulna of this middle-aged woman with idiopathic steatorrhoea, whose spine and foot are illustrated in Fig. 2.5a and b. Observe gross cortical thinning as part of the generalised osteopenia. **b** *Scapula.* The Looser zone shown in this patient has developed at a site uncommon, but well recognised. **c** *Cervical spine.* The Looser zone in this most unusual location, the spinous process of C6, was detected incidentally in routine survey of a 58-year-old woman with widespread skeletal stigmata of the disease, again associated with idiopathic steatorrhoea.

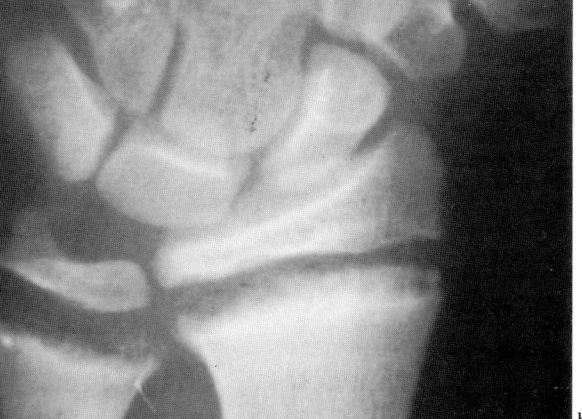

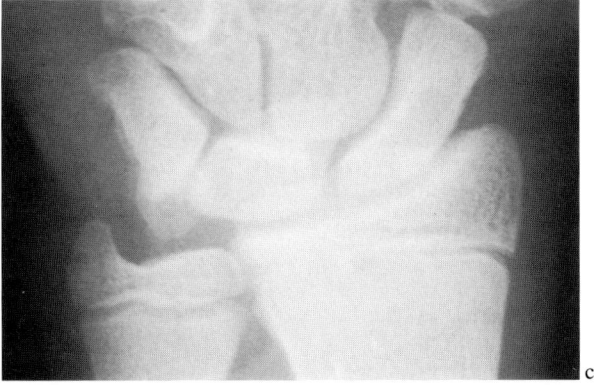

Fig. 2.7. *Dietetic rickets.* This 12-year-old boy developed a mild genu valgum deformity. Typical rachitic abnormalities were present **a** around the knees, where all the metaphyses were lucent and irregular due to failure of calcification of osteoid. Similar lesions were evident in other major metaphyses as illustrated **b** by the left wrist. All these abnormalities were cured by appropriate treatment as shown **c** by the normal appearance of the left wrist 18 months later.

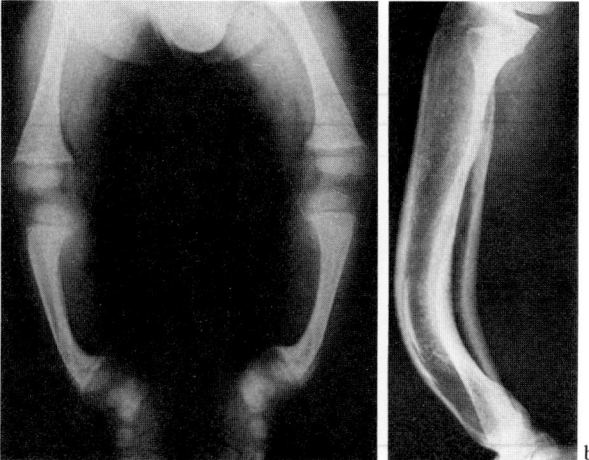

Fig. 2.8. *Advanced dietetic rickets.* **a** Gross manifestations of the disease are evident in this 3-year-old boy. In addition to classical metaphyseal lucencies, bowing deformities of the tibiae and fibulae are attributable to weight-bearing when the bone structure is pathologically weakened. Similar 'cupping' deformities may be apparent in the distal ends of the radius and ulna of a rachitic child, due to the stress of weight-bearing in the upper limbs incurred by crawling. **b** These bowing deformities of the tibia and fibula were symmetrical and were found in an elderly woman who had suffered from rickets in early childhood, long before the cause of the disease had been recognised in 1922. No adequate treatment had been provided.

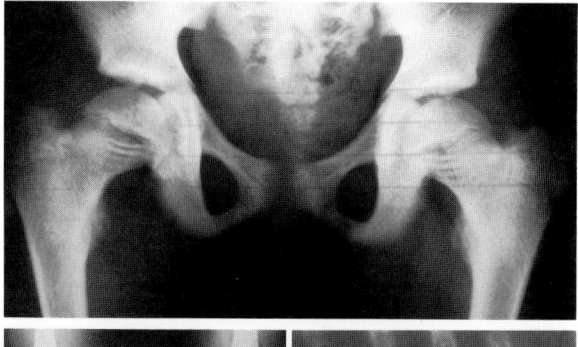

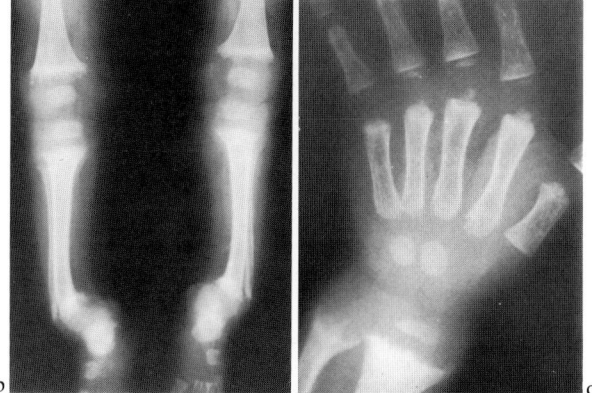

Fig. 2.10. *Rickets—some other causes*, all presenting similar radiological features. **a** *Vitamin D resistant type.* This has become relatively more common as the incidence of the dietetic type has declined. In this child all the major metaphyses were lucent. The numerous linear densities indicate repeated episodes of impairment of growth. **b** *Renal tubular dysfunction.* The gross rachitic changes in this 16-month-old boy were exceptionally severe. Failure of reabsorption of phosphates and some amino acids altered the serum calcium and phosphate levels, causing Fanconi's syndrome. **c** *Iatrogenic type.* This child had been treated with phenytoin for epilepsy. This drug has been shown to vitiate the effects of vitamin D so that rickets results. In this instance the abnormalities due to the disease were extensive, with particularly wide osteoid seams in the metaphyses. Observe the 'cupping' deformities of the distal ends of the radius and ulna.

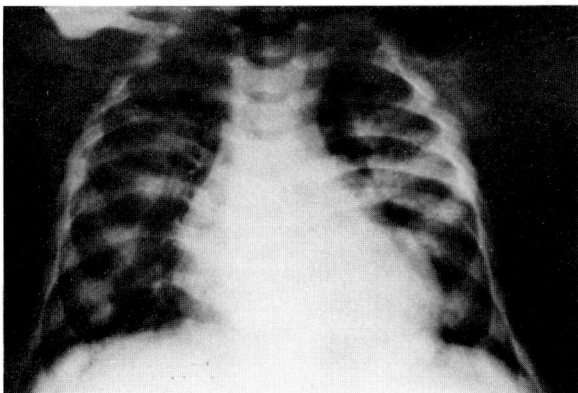

Fig. 2.9. *Rickets—the 'rachitic rosary'.* The anterior ends of the ribs represent further sites of endochondral ossification, comparable to the metaphyses, which are particularly susceptible to involvement by this metabolic disease. All the bones are osteopenic and the anterior ends of the ribs are swollen, lucent and disorganised. Clinical recognition of these swellings originated this descriptive term.

Q1. **The patient, a male aged 19 years, presented with a swelling of the upper calf, which had been present for many years and was increasing slowly in size.**

Clinical examination showed a hard mass, approximately 5 cm in diameter, deep to the calf muscles and attached firmly to the proximal end of the tibia. No other abnormality was found.

The radiograph showed a bony excrescence arising from the posterior surface of the tibia.

The lesion was excised.

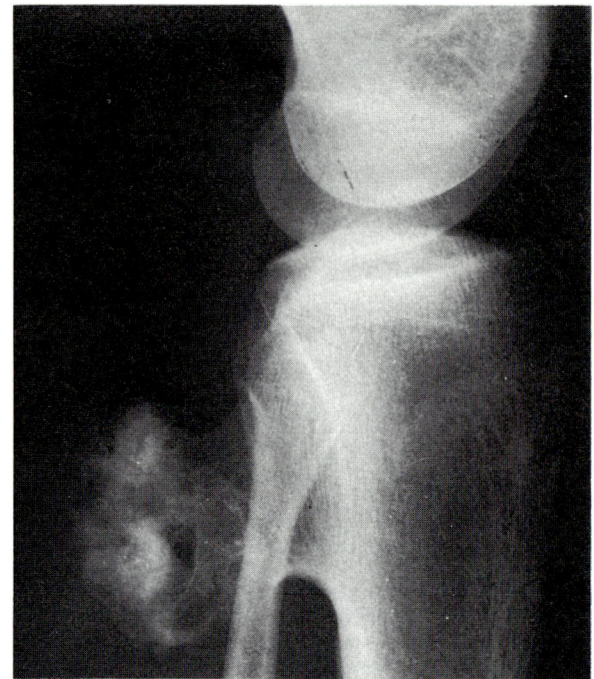

Q1a.

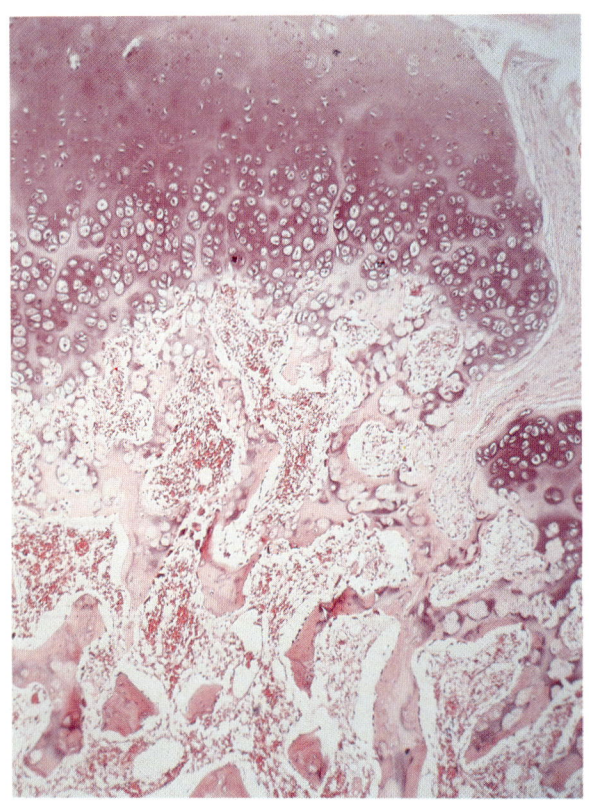

Q1b. (×44)

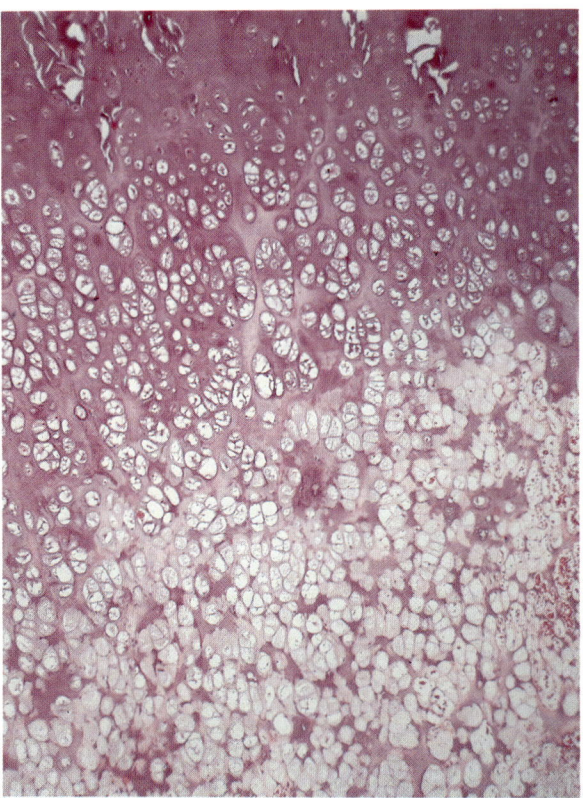

Q1c. (×52)

Exercise 4

Q2. This 24-year-old woman presented with a small painless swelling above the left knee. Four years later this swelling had enlarged and had become mildly painful.

Clinical examination confirmed the presence of a tender and fixed mass of bony consistency, apparently attached to the lateral femoral condyle.

Serial radiographs, Q2a, on presentation, and Q2b, 4 years later, did show the original bony mass to have increased in size and to have developed an irregular margin. Proximal to this lesion a satellite area of calcification was evident in the soft tissues.

Excision biopsy was performed.

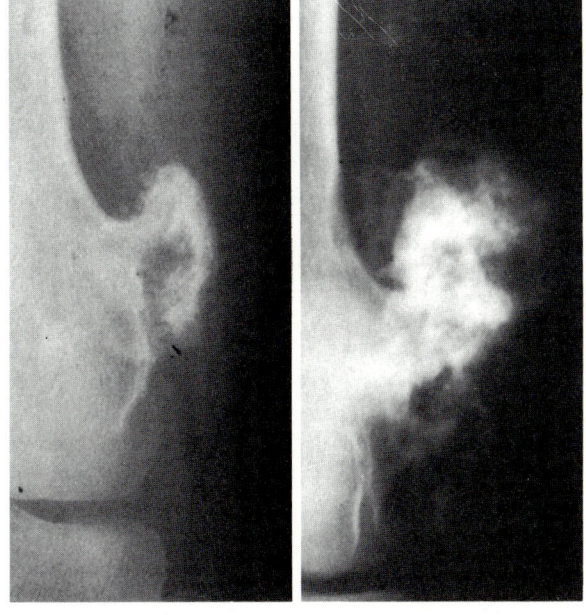

Q2a.   Q2b.

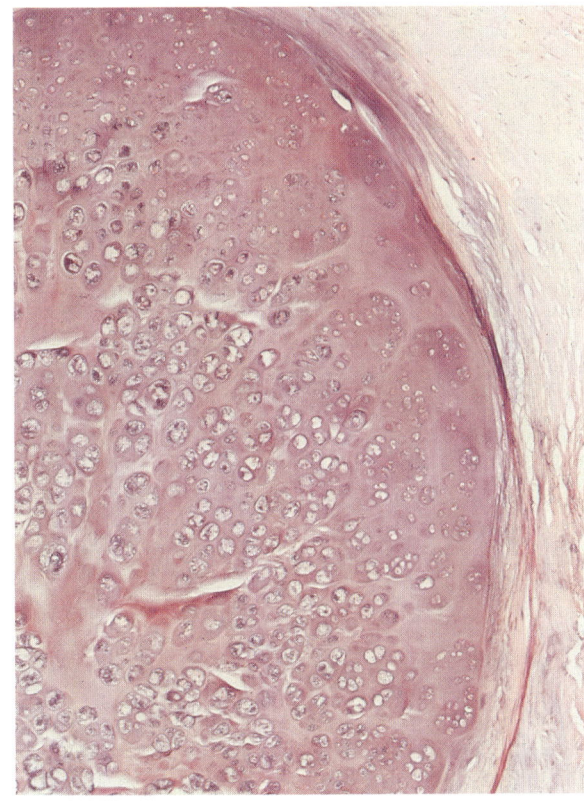

Q2c. (×49)

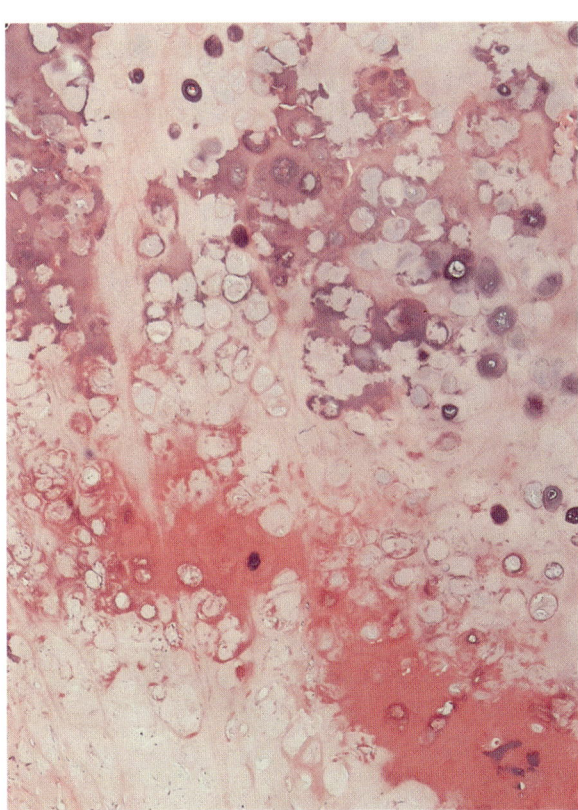

Q2d. (×43)

A1. Osteochondroma (exostosis) of tibia

The radiograph of this patient was diagnostic of an osteochondroma, the central trabecular structure merging with that of the medullary cavity of the tibia. The sharply defined margin of the tumour and absence of peripheral calcification indicated it to be benign.

Histologically, the lesion proved to be a typical osteochondroma. The illustrations (Q1b and c) are from the resection specimen, the appearance of which is shown in Figs. 1.1 and 1.2. Q1a shows the histological structure of the cartilage cap: this consists of mature cartilage which is undergoing calcification and endochondral ossification in a manner similar to the cartilage of a normal growth plate. The hypertrophic cartilage cells (Q1c) show some indication of an oriented columnar arrangement: calcification of the matrix is followed by disintegration of the cartilage cells and replacement of the tissue by cancellous bone. The tissue of the cartilage cap lacks the cellularity and cytological features of malignancy. The deeper part of the exostosis consists of cancellous bone which is continuous with the spongiosa of the upper part of the tibia.

No evidence of local recurrence had developed 8 years after the resection of the exostosis.

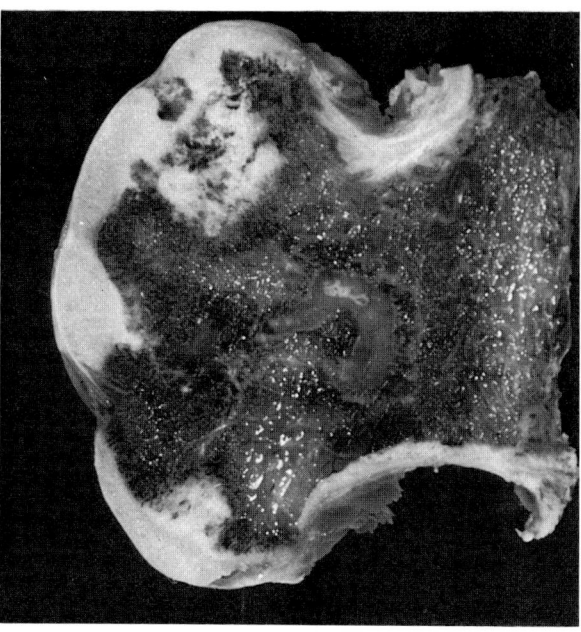

Fig. 1.1. This photograph of the resected specimen shows clearly the smooth cartilage cap of the osteochondroma and the confluence of its central trabeculae with those of the tibia.

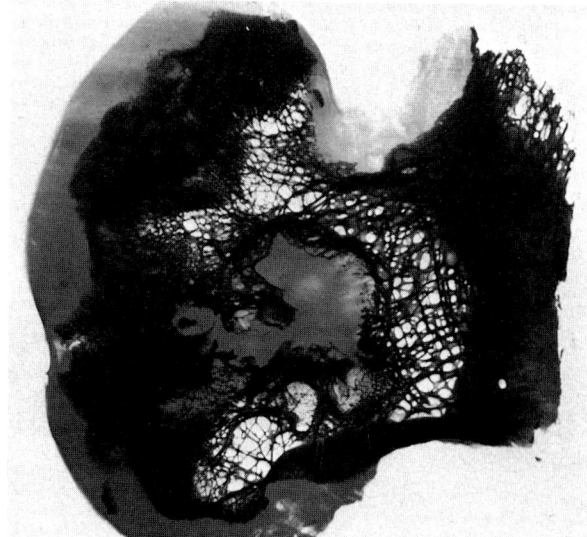

Fig. 1.2. The same features are evident in this radiograph of a slab of tissue from the specimen. Note the heavily calcified tissue adjacent to the cartilage cap and the cancellous bone in the deeper part of the specimen.

A2. Osteochondroma (exostosis) of femur

The lesion is clearly an osteochondroma. In this case, however, evidence of continued growth after skeletal maturity suggests the possibility of malignant change.

The histological illustrations (Q2c and d) are from the superficial part of the specimen, while Fig. 2.1 is a radiograph of a slab of tissue from it. As in Q1, the lesion is indeed an osteochondroma. Despite the radiological suggestion of chondrosarcoma, no histological evidence of malignancy was found. Although the cartilage cap is unusually thick, the degree of cellularity of the tissue is not great and the pleomorphic and binucleate cells, which would indicate a diagnosis of chondrosarcoma, are not present. Many sections from different parts of the lesion were studied carefully to exclude such a diagnosis. As in Q1, there is extensive calcification of cartilage, particularly in the deeper part of the lesion. Figure 2.2 shows the histological structure of an area where much of the cartilage has been replaced by mature cancellous bone and bone marrow, and where only a thin superficial layer of mature cartilage persists as a remnant of the cartilage cap.

The patient was alive and well, without evidence of local recurrence, 10 years after the resection of the lesion.

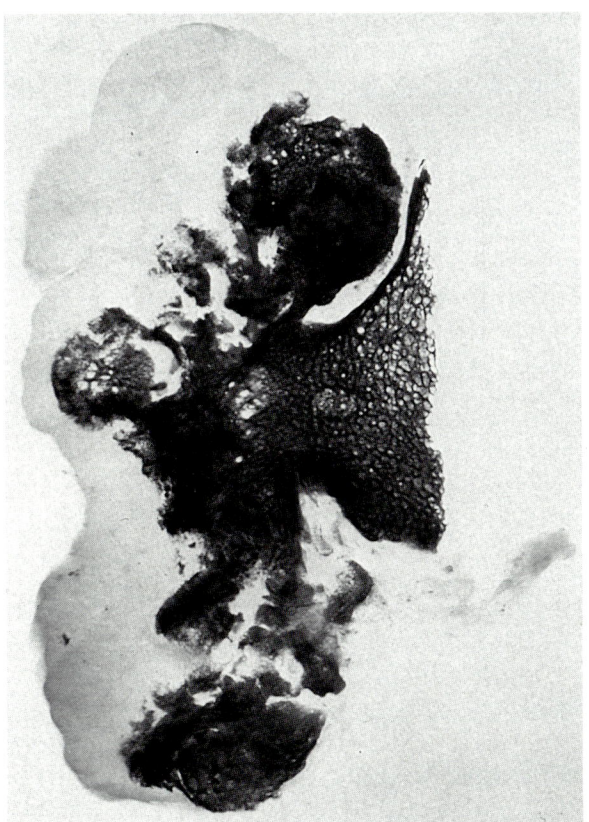

Fig. 2.1. Radiograph of slab of tissue from the resection specimen. As in Fig. 1.2, note the calcified tissue adjacent to the cartilage cap.

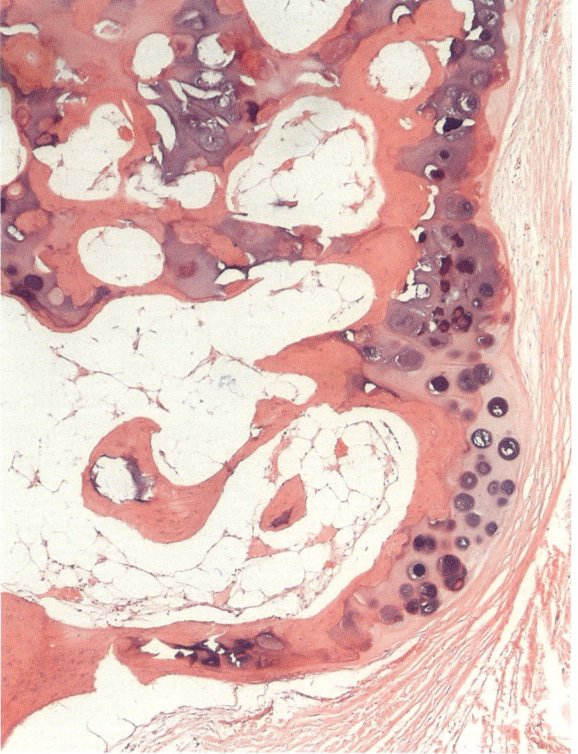

Fig. 2.2. Histological appearance of part of the lesion where much of the cartilage cap has been replaced by mature bone and bone marrow. (×43)

Osteochondroma (Cartilage-Capped Exostosis)

Exostoses may be solitary or multiple. They originate in bones which are preformed in cartilage, usually affecting the juxta-epiphyseal portions of the long bones, particularly in the region of the knee and the shoulder. In contrast to the solitary lesions, multiple exostoses are familial, being inherited as an autosomal dominant and affecting approximately half the offspring of an involved individual. Solitary exostoses are one of the commonest benign tumours of bone: they develop during the period of active skeletal growth, and their enlargement usually ceases with skeletal maturation.

Clinical Features

Many small lesions are asymptomatic and are discovered incidentally during radiological examination. A larger osteochondroma usually presents as a painless hard bony mass: symptoms are occasionally produced by pressure on nerves or vessels. Attention to the presence of such a tumour may be drawn by pain resulting from a fracture through a slender neck or by the formation of an overlying adventitious bursa. Bursae of this type may become infected and painful. Exostoses are particularly liable to produce symptoms when they lie between paired bones. A lesion, for example, between the distal ends of the radius and ulna may limit movement of the wrist, cause diastasis or even deform the adjacent bone by direct pressure.

In *multiple hereditary exostoses (diaphyseal aclasis)*, similar bony excrescences also develop during the growth period, but sometimes are accompanied by bowing or shortening of the affected bones as a result of interference with the normal growth and remodelling of the affected regions.

After skeletal maturity, the continued growth of a solitary exostosis, or of a lesion in multiple hereditary exostoses, should arouse suspicion of malignant change. This is very rare in solitary exostoses, but it has been reported in as many as 10% of patients with multiple lesions.

Radiological Features

1. Site. Any bone may be affected, but a predilection exists for the metaphyses of long bones.

2. Appearance. These bony masses originate from and merge with the cortex of the affected bone, with continuity of the central medullary bone. They project into and displace the adjacent soft tissues. The bony element is covered by a cartilage cap from which growth originates. Within this cap, as the cartilage matures, flecks of calcification often develop. The peripheral margin is usually clearly defined. The lesions may be *sessile* or *pedunculated*, the latter form occurring especially in the metaphyseal portions of long bones and being so orientated that the cartilage cap is directed away from the growing end of the bone.

In adult life, as the lesions mature, the cartilage cap decreases in thickness as it becomes replaced by bone. The deeper tissue undergoes progressive calcification and ossification. In addition to continued growth, radiological evidence of malignant change takes the form of enlargement of the cartilage cap, as recognised in serial studies by increase and spread of scattered calcifications.

Asymmetrical overgrowth of one or more epiphyseal centres, particularly in the ankle and knee, has been accepted as a non-hereditary dysplasia of unknown origin (*dysplasia epiphysealis hemimelica; Trevor's disease*).

Distinction should be made from *ivory osteoma*, an uncommon benign bony tumour, without a cartilage cap, arising only in the membrane bone of the skull and the paranasal sinuses. Such lesions in the frontal sinus may erode the cribriform plate to cause pneumocephalus.

Pathological Features

The pathological features of osteochondroma are illustrated well by the lesions shown in Q1 and Q2. The proliferating tissue of the lesion is the cap of uncalcified cartilage. As in a normal growth plate, the proliferating cartilage cells undergo great enlargement: the hypertrophic cells become arranged in irregular columns, and the calcified cartilage provides a scaffolding for the trabeculae of cancellous bone which replace it by a process of endochondral ossification. The deeper tissue of an osteochondroma consists largely of cancellous bone, but areas of calcified cartilage may persist and contribute to the radiological appearance of density.

In the rare cases where malignant change develops, it usually takes the form of activation of cartilage proliferation, as indicated by an increased degree of cellularity and by cytological features of chondrosarcoma; less often the malignant tumour takes the form of an osteosarcoma.

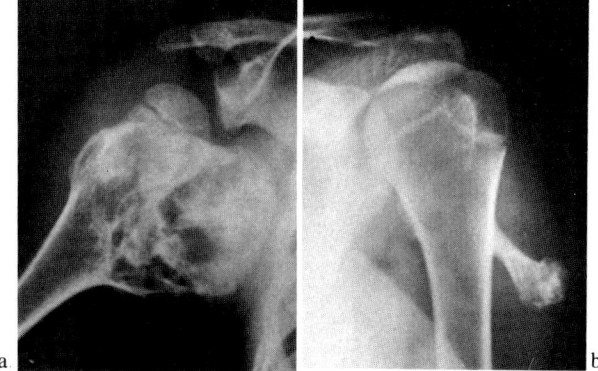

Fig. 1.3. *Osteochondroma.* Classical examples of these benign bone tumours in children, arising in the proximal end of the humerus—a typical juxta-epiphyseal site. **a** *Sessile type* with a broad base. **b** *Pedunculated type.* Observe that this exostosis is growing away from the end of the bone. The slender neck of a lesion of this type is liable to fracture.

Treatment

When an osteochondroma causes symptoms or produces functional disability, it should be excised. Suspicion of malignancy, in the form of enlargement of a previously quiescent exostosis, justifies removal for histological study. In the presence of a proven malignant tumour, more widespread radical excision, or even amputation, may be indicated.

References

Fairbank JT (1956) Dysplasia epiphysealis hemimelica. J Bone Jt Surg 38B: 237–257
Garrison RC, Unni KK, McLeod RA, Pritchard DJ, Dahlin DC (1982) Chondrosarcoma arising in osteochondroma. Cancer 49: 1890–1897
Jaffe HL (1943) Hereditary multiple exostosis. Arch Pathol 36: 335–357
Solomon L (1963) Hereditary multiple exostoses. J Bone Jt Surg 45B: 292–304

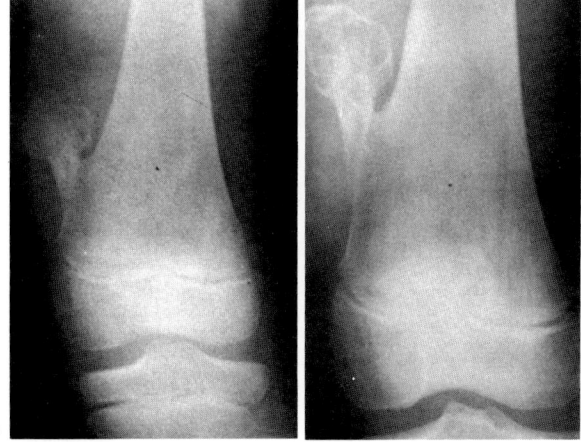

Fig. 1.4. *Pedunculated osteochondroma of femur.* These serial studies illustrate the potential rate of growth in childhood of these tumours. **a** A painless swelling found in this 9-year-old boy had **b** enlarged and become painful 2 years later.

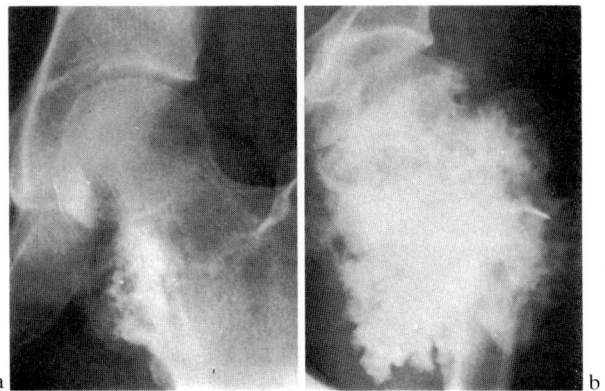

Fig. 1.5. *Osteochondroma.* More aggressive lesions in adults. **a** This sessile exostosis caused mild pain in a 36-year-old woman. It arose from the medial side of the femoral neck. Biopsy was undertaken to exclude malignancy. **b** This huge tumour surrounded the proximal end of the femur in a middle-aged nurse. Discomfort in the hip was probably attributable to slight lateral subluxation of the femoral head caused by another exostosis in the acetabulum. No evidence of malignancy was detected in many radiological studies and on biopsy. Disarticulation was performed at the request of the patient and complete examination of the specimen confirmed the tumour to be benign. The patient was alive and well 10 years later.

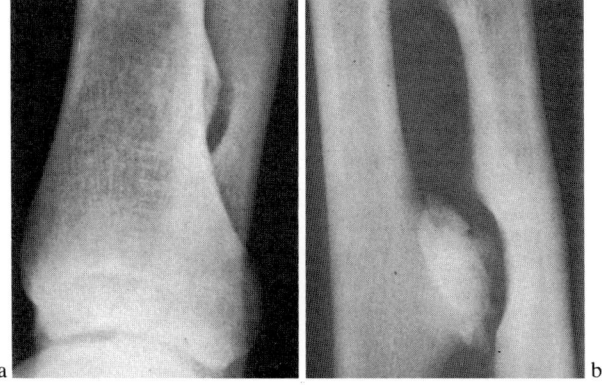

Fig. 1.6. *Osteochondroma eroding a paired bone.* **a** Tibial lesion affecting fibula. **b** Radial lesion affecting ulna.

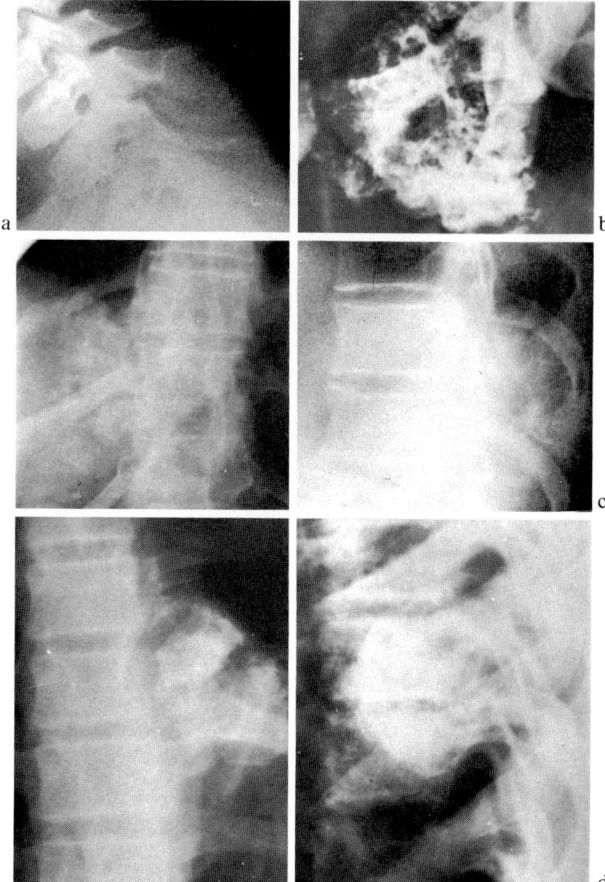

Fig. 1.7. *Osteochondroma—axial skeleton.* **a** *Spinous process of C7* in a 7-year-old girl with a painless swelling. Observe pressure erosion of the spinous process of T1. Over lesions like this adventitious bursae frequently form. **b** *Ischium.* This young man complained of a painless swelling in the groin. The irregular calcification made biopsy imperative to exclude malignancy. **c** *Neural arch of T11.* This patient was examined on account of the compression fracture of the body of T11, the tumour being discovered incidentally. Although the bony mass was palpable, it was painless. Biopsy was refused. **d** *Medial end of left 9th rib.* This mildly painful lesion had grown slowly for 2 years in a 14-year-old boy. In addition to scattered calcification, pressure erosion had developed on the left side of the body and neural arch of T9.

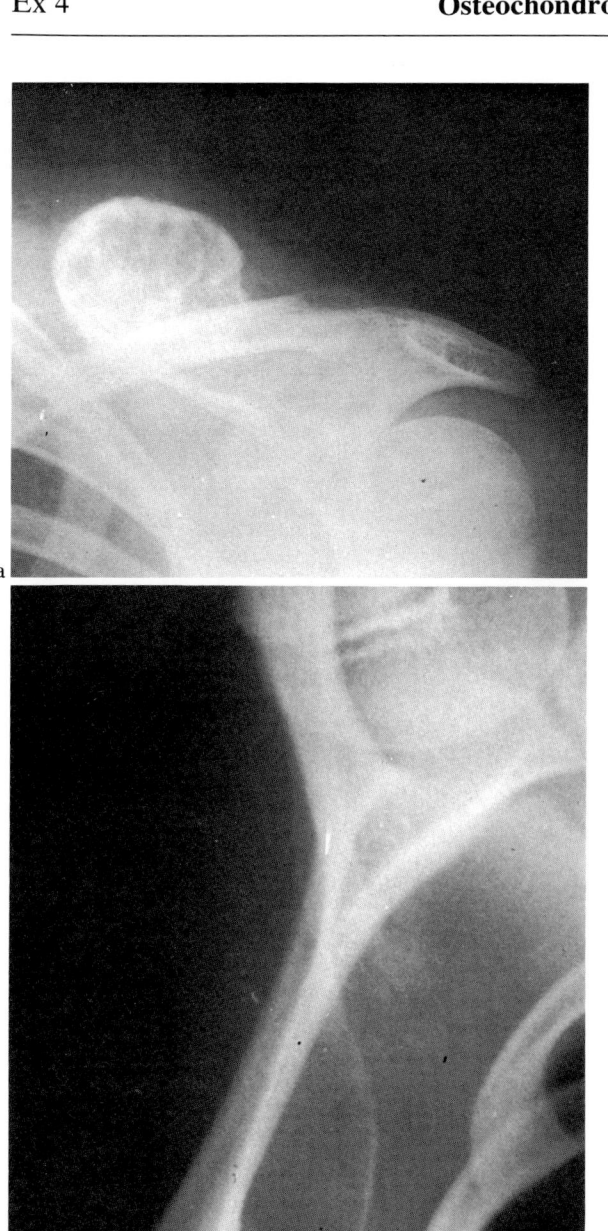
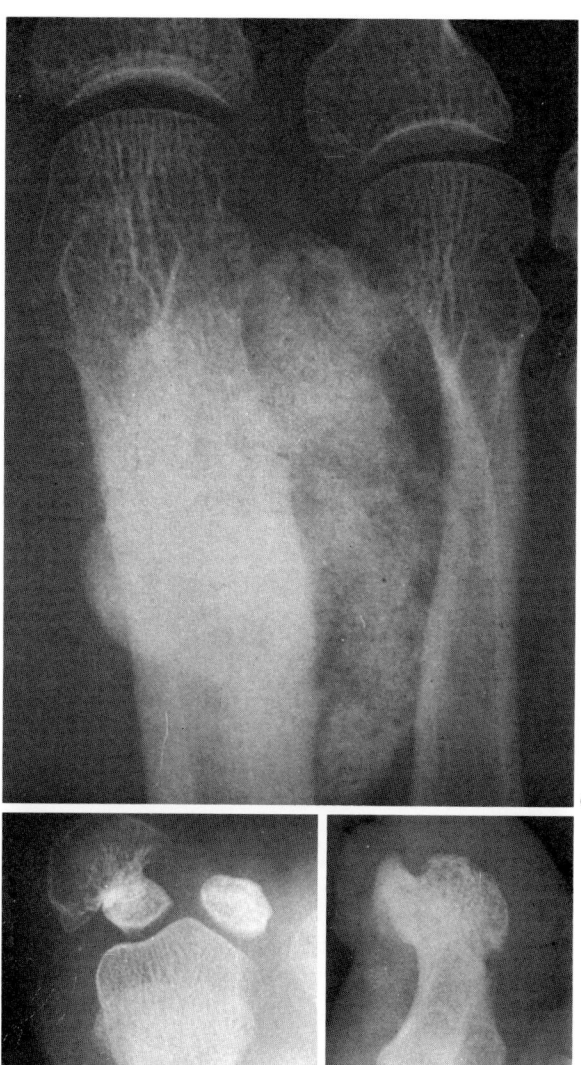

Fig. 1.8. *Osteochondroma—less common sites.* **a** *Upper border of scapula*, creating a cosmetic deformity. **b** *Medial side of scapula*—such lesions provoke painless but irritating crepitus by contact with the ribs. **c** *1st metatarsal shaft* with pressure erosion of the adjacent bone. Malignant change was excluded histologically. **d** *Medial sesamoid of hallux*, making footwear uncomfortable. **e** *Subungual exostosis of hallux*, raising the nail and causing pain.

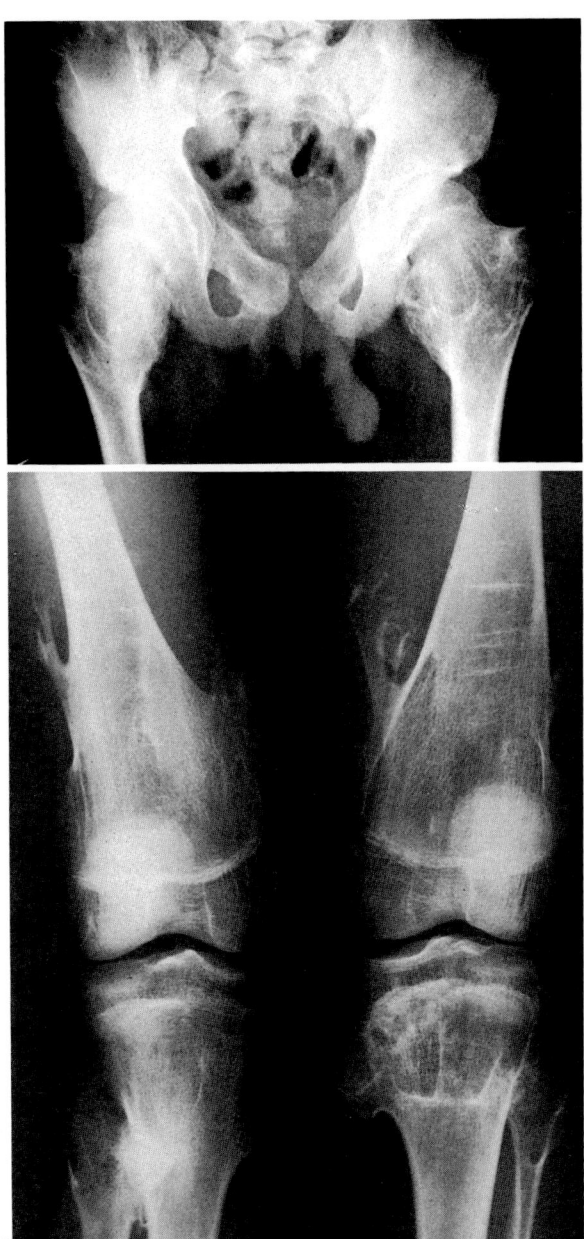
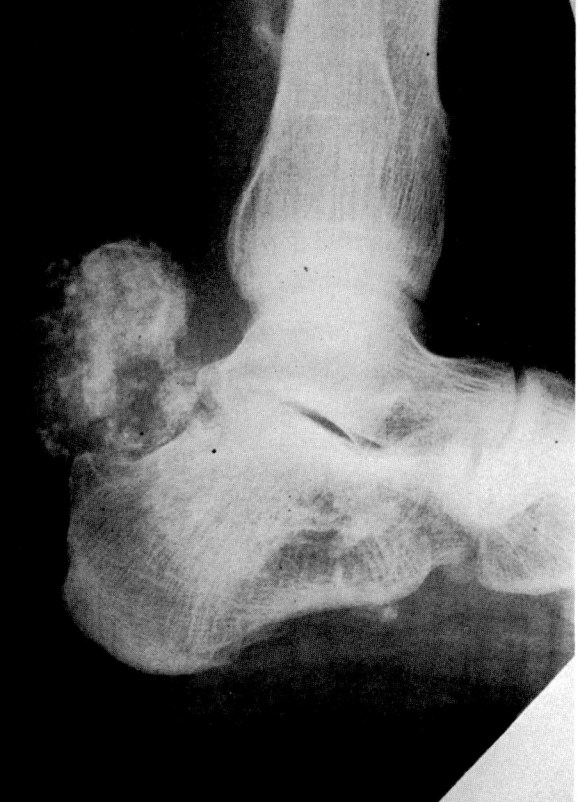
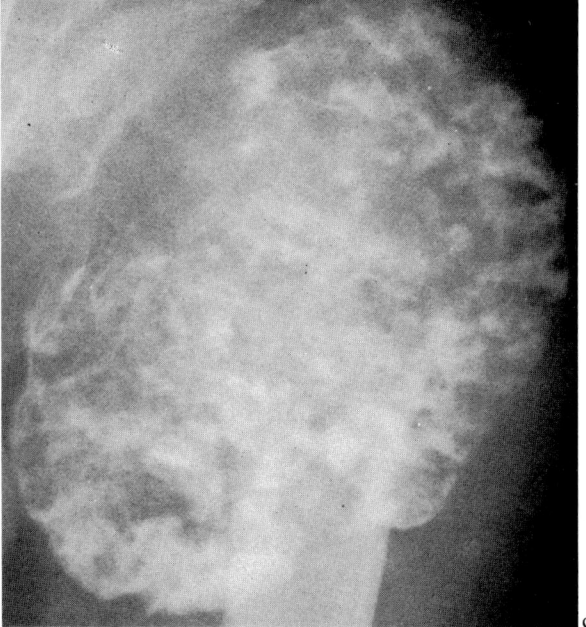

Fig. 1.9. *Diaphyseal aclasis (multiple hereditary cartilage-capped exostosis).* **a** Typical and symmetrical exostoses around the hips and knees of a youth whose mother had almost identical lesions. **b** This young man had been under observation since childhood with numerous exostoses. Several were excised, including this calcaneal lesion, because malignancy had been suspected, but never established histologically. The risk of this complication is much greater than in the case of a solitary exostosis. **c** In contrast, this femoral lesion, one of many exostoses, was found to be chondrosarcomatous in a 33-year-old man with localised and increasing pain. Metastases already had developed. Compare Fig. 1.5b in this Exercise. Radiological differentiation is impossible.

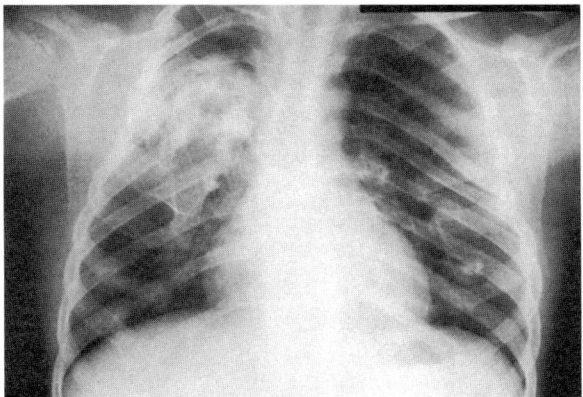

Fig. 1.10. *Diaphyseal aclasis.* Many tumours were present in this child. Those arising from the ribs on the right side were causing respiratory embarrassment and the largest lesion was excised.

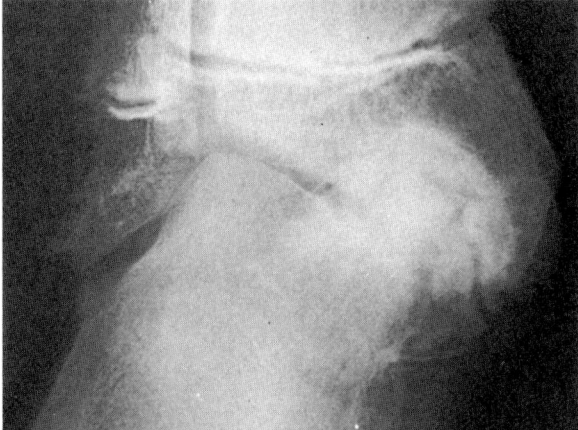

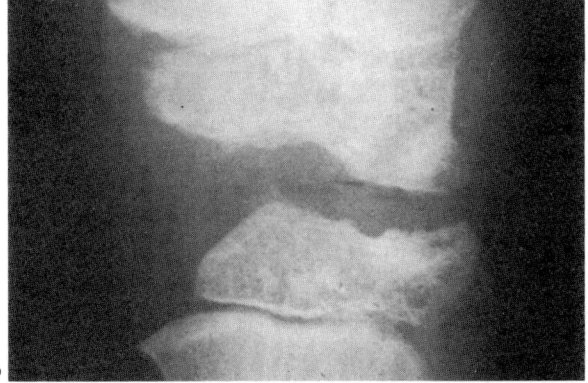

Fig. 1.11. *Dysplasia epiphysealis hemimelica (Trevor's disease).* Examples of this rare entity, which is of unknown origin and affects mainly the major joints of the leg, especially the ankle. These intra-articular osteochondromas are essentially confined to one side of the limb and cause considerable deformity. **a** *Ankle*—classical lesions of the medial aspects of the tibia and talus. **b** *Knee*—involvement of the lateral condyles of the femur and tibia.

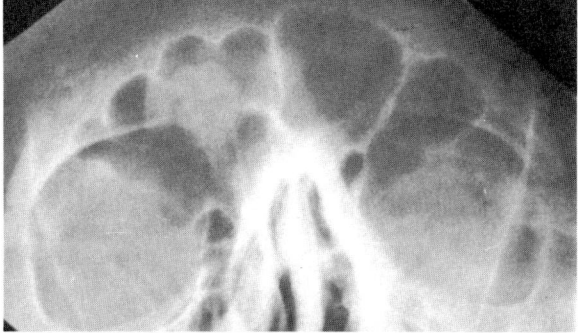

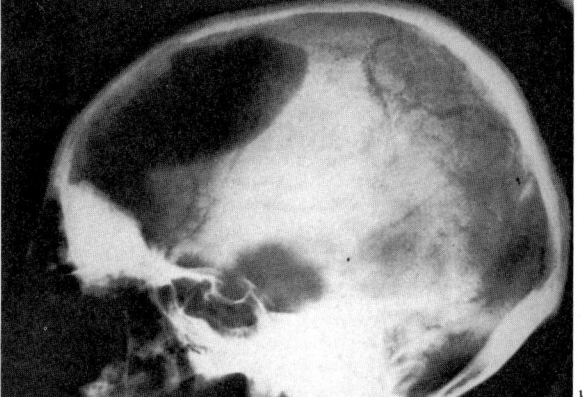

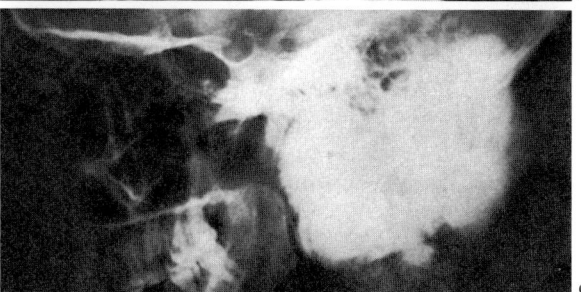

Fig. 1.12. *Osteoma.* The term osteoma is used to describe the rare, quiescent or slowly growing masses of mature bone tissue which occur usually in the frontal sinuses or on the external surface of the skull. Radiologically they exhibit extreme and diffuse density and have clearly defined margins. Histologically they consist of compact bone comparable to normal cortical bone. They are not covered by a cartilage cap. Although commonly regarded as benign tumours, their neoplastic nature has been questioned. Frequently they are asymptomatic or productive only of a painless swelling on the exterior of the skull. These examples show **a** a typical but asymptomatic lesion in the right frontal sinus, discovered incidentally following a head injury, **b** another osteoma of the frontal sinus in a 36-year-old man complaining of chronic headache—due to pressure erosion of the cribriform plate a pneumocephalus had developed—and **c** an exceptionally large osteoma arising from the occiput and causing only a cosmetic deformity.

Q1. This obese 77-year-old woman presented with increasing pain and stiffness of the right knee over a period of 13 years.

Her ability to walk was limited severely by pain. Clinical examination showed a mild genu varum deformity, attributed to laxity of the lateral collateral ligament. Flexion and extension of the right knee were reduced significantly. Routine laboratory investigations were normal.

Radiographs demonstrated marked narrowing of the medial compartment of the joint and of the patello-femoral articulation. Bony spurs were present on the medial side of the tibia, around the distal end of the femur and on the proximal pole of the patella. The subarticular bone in the medial tibial condyle was abnormally dense. Examination of other major joints, including the opposite knee, the hips and the shoulders, showed them to be affected similarly, but to a lesser degree.

Prosthetic replacement of the right knee was undertaken.

Histological preparations from the medial femoral condyle (Q1c) and the medial tibial condyle (Q1d) are illustrated below.

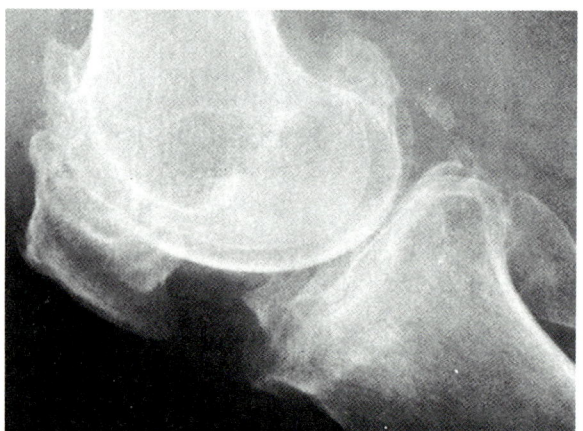

Q1a.

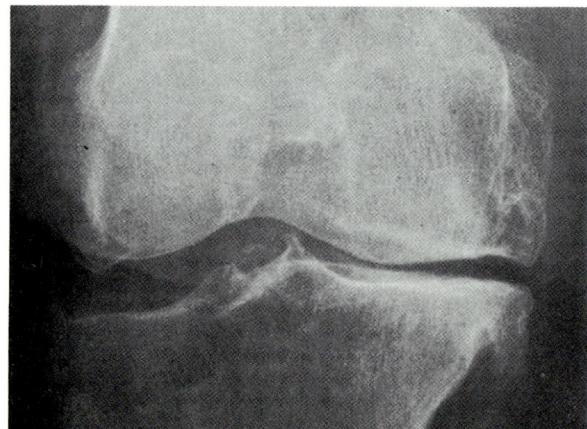

Q1b.

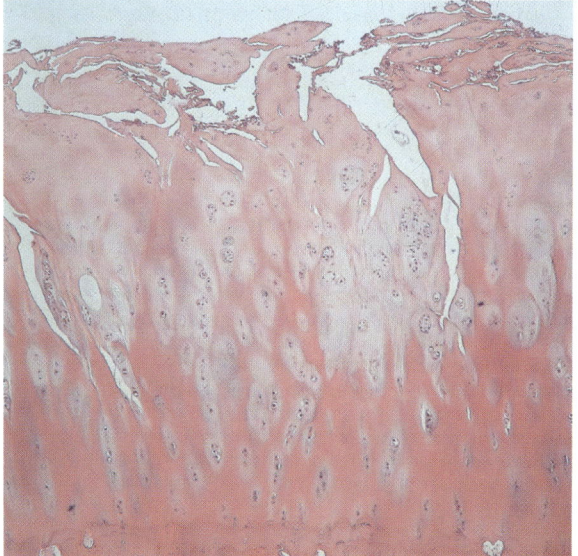

Q1c. (×27)

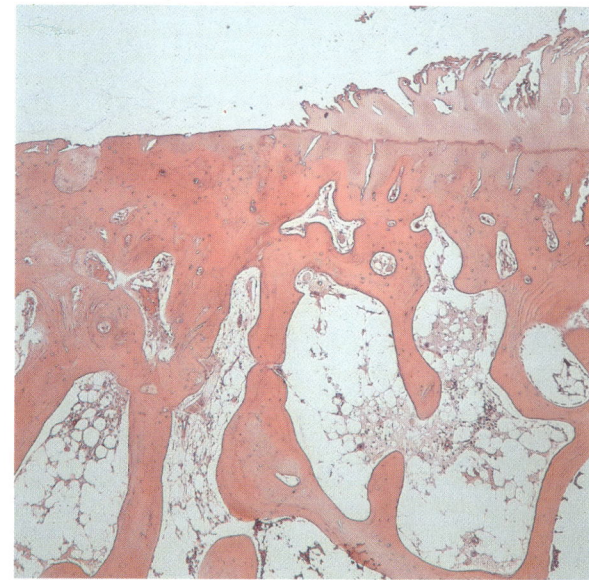

Q1d. (×27)

Q2. This 70-year-old woman had complained of intermittent pain in both hips for several years.

The right hip was affected more severely than the left. Walking was limited and required support with a cane. She was unable to put on her shoes or cut her toe-nails without assistance. On clinical examination, movement of both hips was found to be severely limited, apart from flexion, which was reduced to 60°. Laboratory investigations, including serological tests for rheumatoid arthritis, were negative.

Radiological examination showed the joint spaces of both hips to be significantly narrowed, with increased density of the subchondral bone. On the right side the femoral head had migrated medially to cause a protrusio acetabuli deformity and, on its margin, small bony spurs had formed. A small but well-circumscribed lucency was evident in the subarticular portion of the acetabulum. No other joints were affected.

The more symptomatic right hip was replaced by a prosthesis.

Q2b and c illustrate the histological appearances of different portions of the excised femoral head.

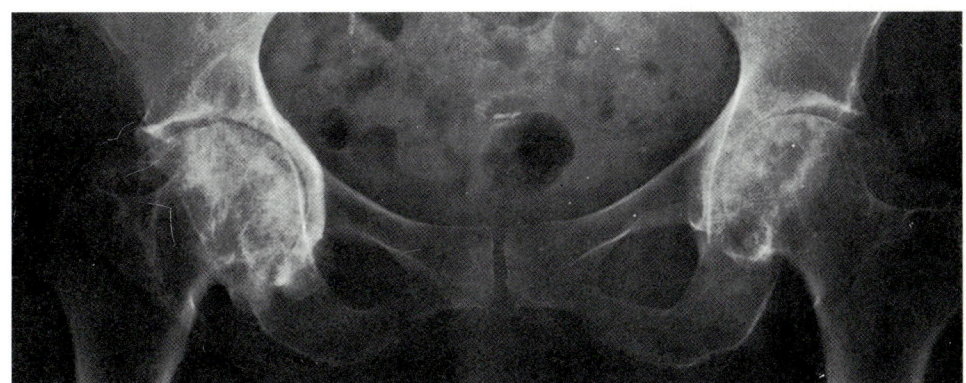

Q2a.

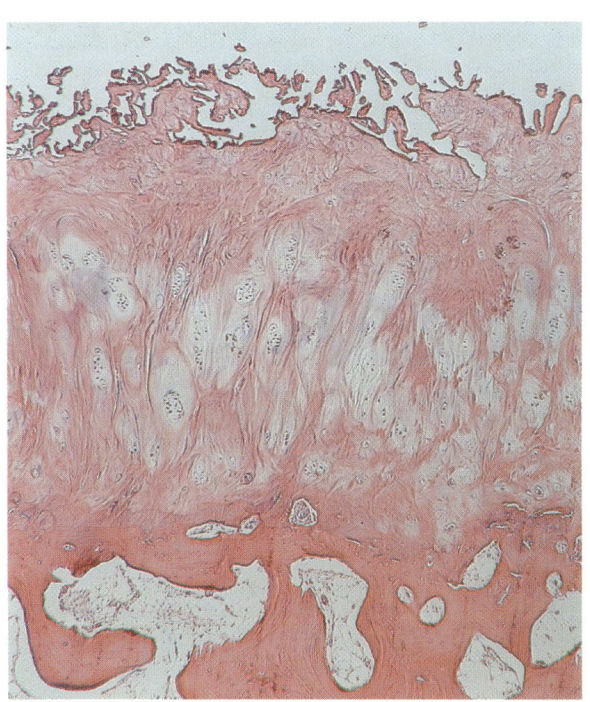

Q2b. (×30)

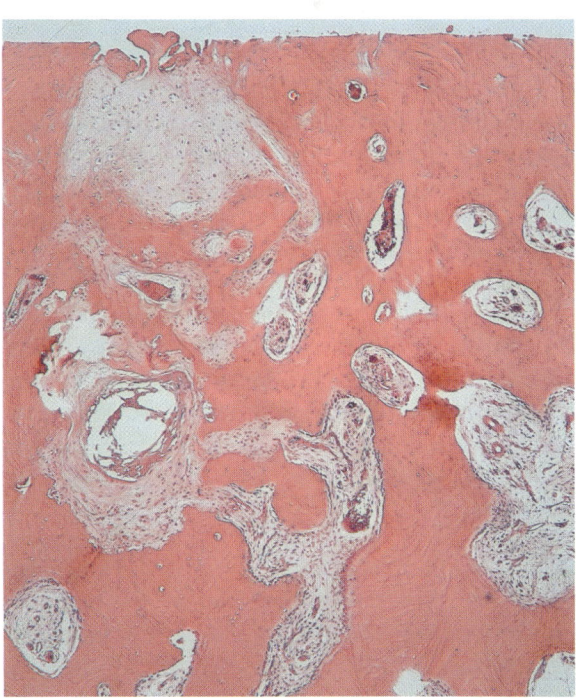

Q2c. (×30)

A1. Degenerative joint disease (osteoarthritis) of right knee—post-traumatic type

The clinical findings and the radiological appearance are typical of this extremely common cause of disability, often attributable, in weight-bearing joints, to the stresses induced by obesity. Narrowing of the medial compartment of the joint suggested destruction of at least the superficial layers of articular cartilage, although such an appearance may be observed also as a consequence of a meniscectomy. The bony spurs, or osteophytes, represent physiological responses to a disordered joint mechanism in an endeavour to achieve stability. Similarly, the increased density of the subchondral bone in the medial tibial condyle represents physiological thickening and strengthening of the trabeculae as a response to abnormal stress. Weakness of the lateral collateral ligament is indicated by widening of the lateral compartment of the joint, with secondary genu varum deformity. The latter features usually can be demonstrated more strikingly in films obtained in the erect position.

Q1c shows the articular cartilage of the medial femoral condyle to be decreased in thickness. Its surface, normally smooth, is deeply fibrillated and fissured. Much of the intercellular matrix of the cartilage has lost its normal staining characteristics and appears as zones of pale-staining tissue surrounding clusters of chondrocytes. These changes are characteristic of degenerative joint disease or osteoarthritis. They are regarded as part of a degenerative process. The clusters of chondrocytes, however, appear to result from a proliferative response, therefore representing a process of repair. In Q1d, from the medial tibial condyle, it is evident that the articular cartilage has undergone more extensive destruction, with only a tattered peripheral remnant. More laterally the surface consists of exposed bone. The subchondral trabeculae are thickened, accounting for the increased density observed radiographically. Figure 1.1, from the margin of the tibial articular surface, illustrates formation of an osteophyte, resulting from activation of endochondral ossification in the deep part of the remaining articular cartilage. It consists of a bony outgrowth covered by a layer of metaplastic cartilage, which is continuous with, and derived from, the pre-existing articular surface. The bone marrow of the osteophyte is fatty and haemopoietic cells are lacking. This structure bears a distinct resemblance to a small osteochondroma.

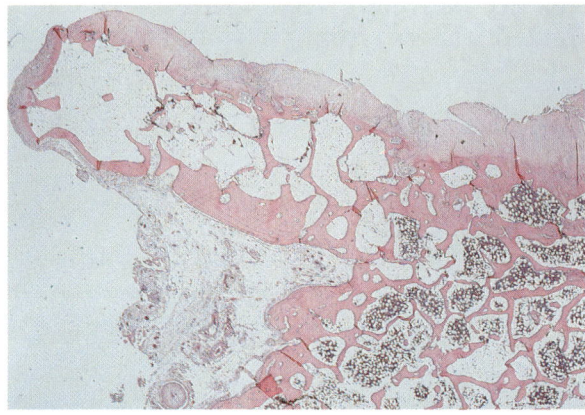

Fig. 1.1. An osteophyte from the margin of the articular surface of the tibia in the same patient, illustrating a bony outgrowth covered by metaplastic articular cartilage. (×10)

A2. Degenerative joint disease (osteoarthritis) of hips—post-inflammatory type

The clinical and radiological features in this patient typified degenerative changes of a classical type in both hips. The narrowing of the medial compartments of the joints and the presence of protrusio acetabuli on the right side suggested strongly an inflammatory origin. Abnormalities of this type are observed frequently as residues of former and overt rheumatoid arthritis. In the present case the lack of involvement of other joints and the negative serology make it impossible to offer a categorical and definitive diagnosis, evidence for an inflammatory background resting on the radiological appearances.

Q2b shows some of the remaining articular cartilage from a peripheral portion of the femoral head. Its thickness is decreased and the normally smooth surface is fibrillated and fissured. Once again the intercellular matrix has lost its normal staining characteristics. While some areas are relatively devoid of chondrocytes, others contain small clusters of these cells, surrounded by zones of pale-staining tissue. As in Q1, these abnormalities are characteristic of degenerative joint disease or osteoarthritis.

Q2c illustrates the appearance of the central, weight-bearing area of the femoral head. The articular cartilage has been destroyed completely and the surface of the exposed subchondral bone has been abraded by frictional contact with the acetabulum. The bone itself shows no sign of necrosis, but is sclerotic, with evidence of active remodelling on many of its trabecular surfaces, accounting again for the increased density of subchondral bone which was evident in the radiograph. The remaining marrow spaces are occupied by vascular fibrous tissue and by metaplastic fibrocartilage, some of which protrudes beyond the bony surface. At one point, breakdown of fibrous tissue is leading to the formation of a small subchondral 'cyst'. Such 'cysts' are characteristic of degenerative joint disease, being common in areas where destruction of articular cartilage has resulted in exposure of the underlying bone.

The extent of these changes, and their relationship to the radiological appearance of the joint, can be appreciated in Figs 2.1a and 2.1b, which show complete preparations from the femoral head. The loss of joint space clearly is the consequence of the extensive destruction of the articular cartilage. The projecting tongues of bone at the margins of the femoral head are parts of the circumferential marginal osteophyte which has developed as part of the osteoarthritic process. Such osteophytes are formed by activation of endochondral ossification in the deep part of the articular cartilage and change the contour to enlarge the extent of the articular surface—fundamentally a physiological response to a disordered joint mechanism.

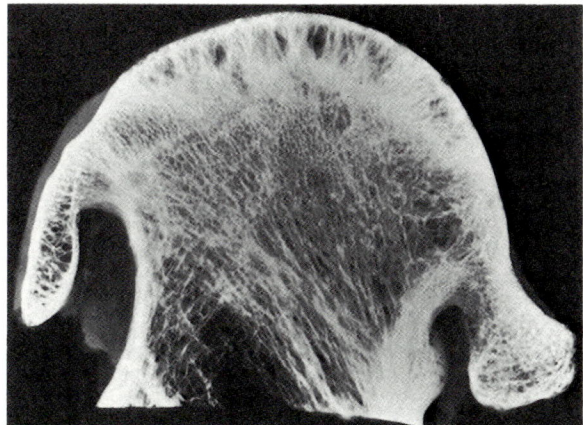

Fig. 2.1a. Radiograph of a slab section of bone from the resected femoral head. Note the altered structure of the subchondral bone, with increased density due to trabecular thickening, the numerous degenerative 'cysts' in the central weight-bearing area, which is denuded of articular cartilage, and the extensive marginal osteophytes associated with the remnants of articular cartilage.

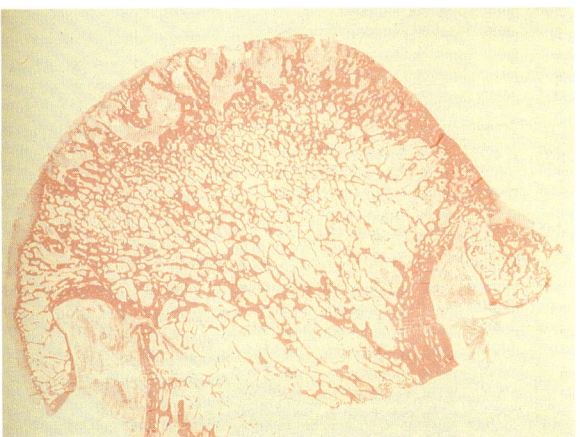

Fig. 2.1b. The histological preparation from the same specimen illustrates the morphological basis of the radiological abnormalities even more clearly. The thickened trabeculae, the subchondral 'cysts' and the marginal osteophytes are demonstrated in detail.

Degenerative Joint Disease (Osteoarthritis)

These terms are applied to progressive degenerative changes involving the articular surfaces of joints. This disorder is sometimes attributable to abnormal stresses caused by articular malalignment.

So-called secondary osteoarthritis is recognised to develop in the hip, for example, as a sequel to such orthopaedic conditions as congenital dislocation, acetabular dysplasia, Perthes' disease and slipped epiphysis. Secondary degenerative changes also may occur in the late stages of rheumatoid arthritis and may come to dominate the radiological features long after the clinical activity of the inflammatory process has subsided. Such secondary degenerative changes usually are recognised easily, on account of the clinical history and the radiological appearances.

The term 'primary' osteoarthritis, however, has been employed traditionally for those cases in which a precipitating factor cannot be identified, so that their origin cannot be diagnosed with certainty.

Clinical Features

Degenerative joint disease increases in incidence with advancing age. It involves different joints with varying frequencies. Different populations show differing patterns of joint involvement. Sometimes a single joint, or a pair of symmetrical joints, may be affected. In other cases the disorder may be widespread in many joints. Pain and stiffness of an affected joint are the main symptoms, both being more marked after periods of rest and relieved temporarily by movement. In major joints of the lower limbs these symptoms are accentuated by prolonged weight-bearing and may disturb sleep. Intra-articular effusions may develop and wasting of muscles occurs as a result of progressive restriction of movement.

The small joints of the hands and feet are involved commonly, specifically the 1st metatarso-phalangeal joint and the 1st carpo-metacarpal joint. Such lesions are responsible for relatively minor clinical disabilities, but may, as in the case of hallux valgus, require surgical intervention. On the other hand, degenerative joint disease involving the spine, hips and knees presents major clinical problems for which surgical management has become increasingly important. Successful prosthetic replacements of joints have restored a virtually normal life pattern to thousands of individuals who have been severely disabled.

Radiological Features

1. Site. As indicated above, any joint may be affected. Radiological examination, however, is requested most commonly for assessment of involvement of major joints, particularly the hips and knees, and the spine.

2. Appearance. Narrowing of a joint space, reflecting attrition of the superficial layers of articular cartilage, is the commonest early sign, sometimes requiring assessment of an opposite and normal joint for comparison. Subarticular lytic areas, 'cysts', may precede such narrowing, but usually develop later. Often single lesions of this type may become extremely large, especially if aggravated by trauma. When destruction of articular cartilage is very advanced, as in the case of burnt-out rheumatoid arthritis, these cystic subchondral lesions tend to be small and multiple. Physiological attempts at repair are represented by the development of subarticular sclerosis due to trabecular thickening and the formation of marginal osteophytes. The latter structures tend to stabilise an affected joint, a process particularly evident in their formation on the lateral side of a dysplastic acetabulum or on the concave side of a scoliotic curve. With total destruction of articular cartilage by a former inflammatory process, osteophyte formation is absent or insignificant, since the foundation tissue for their formation is no longer present. In certain joints, particularly the hip, characteristic radiological patterns may permit reasonably confident assessment of the factor precipitating the disorder.

Remarkable disintegration of major joints has been observed to occur as an effect of the relief of pain provided by prolonged exhibition of analgesics, such as phenylbutazone and indomethacin. Similar changes have been recognised as a complication of the presence of excess adrenocortical hormones, derived from either pituitary or adrenal causes, or as a result of steroid therapy, a finding discussed in greater detail elsewhere in this work.

Pathological Features

The earliest change appears to be a loss of proteoglycan from the intercellular matrix of the articular cartilage, with consequent loss of staining of this tissue. This is followed by fibrillation and fissuring of the superficial cartilage. The degenerating cartilage, particularly in weight-bearing joints, such as the hip and the knee, is destroyed progressively by mechanical abrasion. The exposed subchondral bone then undergoes progressive changes. It becomes sclerotic and the narrow spaces become occupied by fibrous tissue. Subchondral 'cysts' develop, probably as a result of degenerative change in areas of marrow fibrosis, although it has been suggested that entry of synovial fluid from the joint cavity may be concerned. Rarely, the subchondral bone may develop areas of infarction, which add to the severity of the destructive process.

The shape of the articular surfaces can become greatly altered, partly as a result of the mechanical attrition of the subchondral bone and partly through the remodelling activities associated with the formation of marginal osteophytes.

Repair of articular cartilage in degenerative joint disease is usually ineffective, probably because the unfavourable anatomical configuration of the eroded articular surfaces causes the cartilage damage to be self-perpetuating. Cartilage cells, however, do have the capacity for proliferation and for matrix synthesis. Under favourable circumstances re-establishment of a cartilaginous or a fibrocartilaginous surface can, in fact, take place.

In degenerative joint disease the synovial membrane of an involved joint usually shows a pronounced non-specific reaction, with numerous lymphocytes and plasma cells. It is essential that these features are not confused with the histological appearance of rheumatoid arthritis and other types of inflammatory joint disease.

Treatment

Conservative measures usually are adequate to obtain relief of the symptoms and signs due to degenerative joint disease. In many patients pain and discomfort are minimal or mild, in which case a satisfactory response to rest, using splints when appropriate, and the more efficient analgesics, may be expected. Diet should be controlled to combat obesity. Persistent pain ultimately may require surgical intervention. Arthroplasty is a common procedure in the treatment of such lesions as hallux rigidus and occasionally the provision of a stiff, but painless, joint by arthrodesis is acceptable. Surgical management, however, has polarised around the practice of prosthetic replacement of joints, except in younger individuals for whom osteotomy may be performed. This holding procedure, in the case of the hip for example, may relieve symptoms for as long as 10 years.

It is to be realised that the essential approach to the problem should be directed toward the prevention or, at least, the early detection of the primary disorder. Suitable management, at an early stage, then may prevent subsequent superimposition of degenerative joint disease. As an illustration it is salutary to remember that acceptance of malalignment in the treatment of a tibial fracture is likely to be followed ultimately by the development of degenerative changes in the knee or ankle.

References

Freeman MAR (1979) Adult articular cartilage, 2nd edn. Pitman, London
Law WA (1952) Osteoarthritis of the hip. Butterworth, London
Lawrence JS (1977) Rheumatism in populations. Heinemann Medical Books, London
Mankin HJ, Dorfman H, Lipiello L, Zarins A (1971) Biochemical and metabolic abnormalities in articular cartilage from osteoarthritic human hips. J Bone Jt Surg 53A: 523–537
Murray RO (1965) The aetiology of primary osteoarthritis of the hip. Br J Radiol 38: 810–824
Sokoloff L (1969) The biology of degenerative joint disease. University of Chicago Press, Chicago
Woods CG (1961) Subchondral bone cysts. J Bone Jt Surg 43B: 758–766

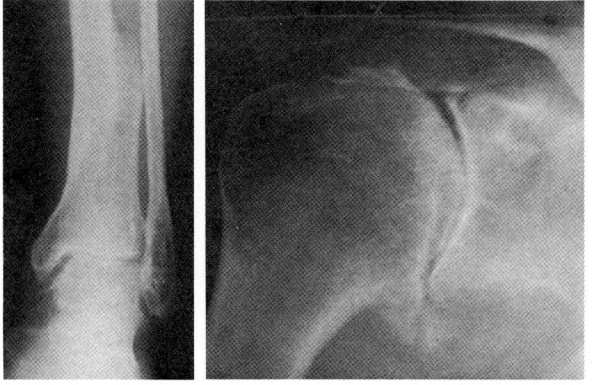

Fig. 1.3. *Degenerative joint disease (osteoarthritis)—effects of stress.* **a** Malunion of a tibial fracture incurred 10 years earlier caused persistent pain in the ankle of this 34-year-old woman. Observe lateral tilt of the talus, narrowing of the joint space and reactive subchondral sclerosis. Arthrodesis was required. **b** Degenerative changes in the shoulder are unusual. Narrowing of the joint space and osteophyte formation in this middle-aged man were due to the use of the right arm as a weight-bearing limb. Above-knee amputation had been performed 15 years earlier, necessitating constant use of a cane.

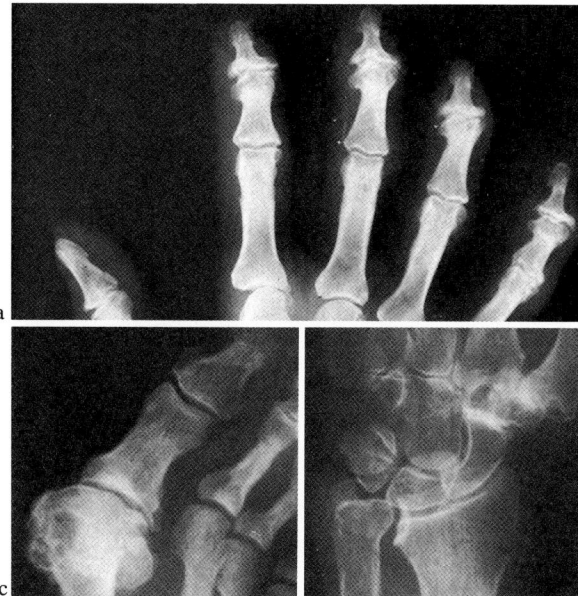

Fig. 1.2. *Degenerative joint disease (osteoarthritis)—common sites.* **a** The massive osteophytes around the terminal interphalangeal joints of the fingers are responsible for relatively painless swellings in elderly women and are known as Heberden's nodes. The term Bouchard's nodes is applied to similar lesions affecting the proximal interphalangeal joints. **b** This typical hallux valgus deformity caused chronic foot pain in an elderly man. The proximal phalanx has subluxated laterally. The 1st metatarso-phalangeal joints is narrowed and, in addition to marginal osteophytes, an exostosis has formed on the medial side of the 1st metatarsal head. **c** Severe degenerative change had affected the 1st carpo-metacarpal joint and the articulation between the trapezium, trapezoid and scaphoid—both very common sites of involvement—in this 78-year-old woman. Nevertheless, pain had been experienced for only 2 weeks, following a minor injury. Similar changes are evident in the distal radio-ulnar joint.

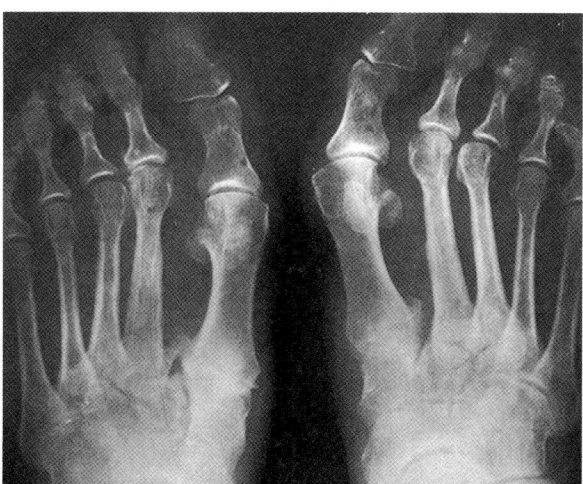

Fig. 1.4. *Degenerative joint disease (osteoarthritis)—occupational.* This 53-year-old woman, who was a professional ballet dancer, had complained of mild, but increasing, discomfort in the feet for several years. Degenerative changes, with prominent osteophyte formation, had affected the 1st and 2nd tarso-metatarsal joints, associated with lateral subluxations of the 2nd metatarsal bases. Observe, incidentally, stress thickening of the shafts of these bones. Despite these remarkable changes symptoms were insufficiently severe to interfere with her career.

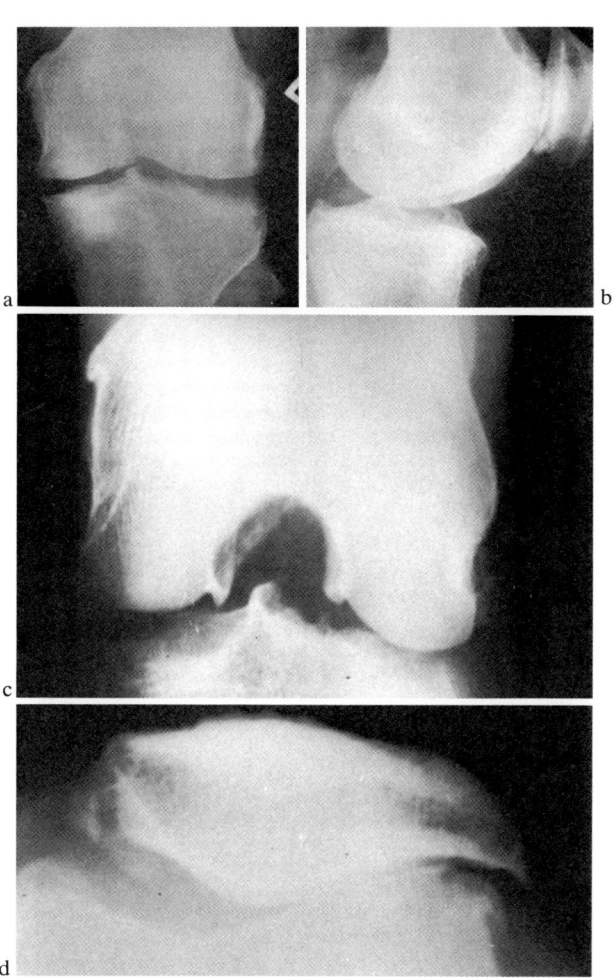

Fig. 1.5. *Degenerative joint disease (osteoarthritis)—due to athletic stress.* The knee is the joint particularly susceptible to trauma incurred by athletic activity. This 33-year-old man, an international squash champion, developed mild pain and instability of the left knee. The orthodox **a** frontal and **b** lateral projections showed narrowing of the femoro-tibial and patello-femoral articulations with marginal osteophyte formation. **c** The tunnel view, however, revealed further femoral osteophytes on each side of the intercondylar notch and slight prominence of the tibial spines, reflecting chronic stress at the cruciate ligament attachments. The patella is shown in the **d** axial projection to be subluxating laterally with an avulsive irregularity of its medial border. Observe, incidentally, ossification within the proximal portion of the medial collateral ligament—an appearance known as the Pellegrini-Stieda lesion and again the result of chronic stress. Adequate examination of the knee requires at least these four views.

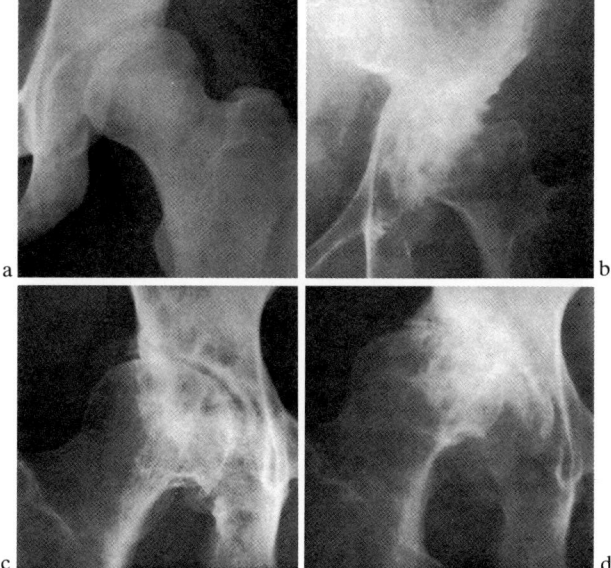

Fig. 1.6. *Degenerative joint disease of hip—secondary to acetabular dysplasia.* This developmental abnormality, often regarded as an incomplete form of congenital dislocation, exhibits the same sexual predominance and is a common cause of the disorder in women. **a** Gross acetabular dysplasia was virtually an incidental finding in this 17-year-old girl. The right hip was similarly affected. Subsequent development of degenerative change is likely, but not inevitable. **b** Frank degenerative changes, with obliteration of the joint space, subchondral sclerosis and osteophyte formation have been superimposed on an obviously dysplastic acetabulum in this 50-year-old woman. Symptoms had been present for only 2 years. Radionuclide scanning showed increased activity in this area. **c** This 51-year-old woman had complained of pain and stiffness of the left hip for 3 years. The outer portion of the joint space is narrowed, subchondral 'cysts' have formed and a retaining osteophyte has begun to develop on the lateral margin of the acetabulum. The femoral head is covered incompletely and a tendency to lateral subluxation is reflected by buttressing of the medial side of the femoral neck due to traction on the capsular attachment. The acetabulum is shallow. **d** Four years later all these features had been accentuated. More lateral displacement of the femoral head is evident. Increased subchondral sclerosis and enlargement of the acetabular osteophyte, despite eburnation of the articular surfaces, represent physiological responses. Such cases are described frequently as 'primary' or 'idiopathic', but the radiological appearance of acetabular dysplasia establishes completely the cause of the condition.

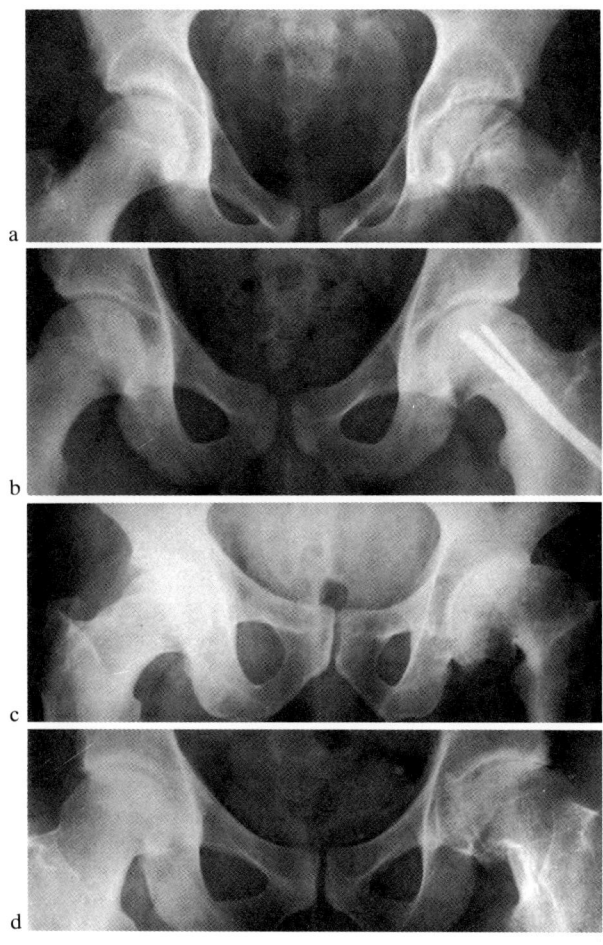

Fig. 1.7. *Degenerative joint disease (osteoarthritis) of hip—secondary to slipped epiphysis.* The oblique plane of the proximal growth plate of the femur renders it peculiarly susceptible to stresses and strains, particularly during the adolescent years, occasionally causing frank epiphysiolysis or slipping of the epiphysis. Even with prompt treatment a residual varus deformity of the femoral head may alter the anatomical structure of the hip joint, rendering it liable to undergo degenerative changes later in life. Slipped epiphysis is more common in boys, particularly if they are obese or unusually tall and slender. The latter features have caused an endocrine basis for the disorder to be postulated. **a** This 14-year-old boy had been limping for 2 months and complaining of pain in the left knee, which he attributed to a fall 6 months earlier. Classical medial tilt of the left femoral head is evident, with marked metaphyseal lucency. Although the entity may be recognised first by a sudden exacerbation of pain, the history of this youth is more typical. Symptoms may be very mild. It is important to appreciate that, when they are referred to the knee in an adolescent, they may originate, in fact, from the hip. The displaced epiphysis was stabilised surgically by pinning. **b** Three years later the boy was asymptomatic and both proximal femoral growth plates had fused. The residual varus deformity of the left femoral head, however, had caused slight secondary remodelling of the left acetabulum to simulate primary acetabular dysplasia. **c** This 67-year-old man had developed pain in the left hip during the preceding 8 years. No history of a previous injury or of symptoms in adolescence could be obtained, but the varus deformity of the left femoral head was considered to be attributable only to a former slipped epiphysis with secondary acetabular dysplasia. Degenerative changes had narrowed the joint space and stimulated subchondral sclerosis. **d** Lesser abnormalities of the same type were present in the left hip of a 43-year-old man. He had been an active footballer, but recalled limping after games when adolescent 30 years before. Painful symptoms in the left hip had been present for only 3 months. The radiological appearance is entirely consistent with an old slipped epiphysis, although this pattern of disease also is described frequently as 'primary' or 'idiopathic'.

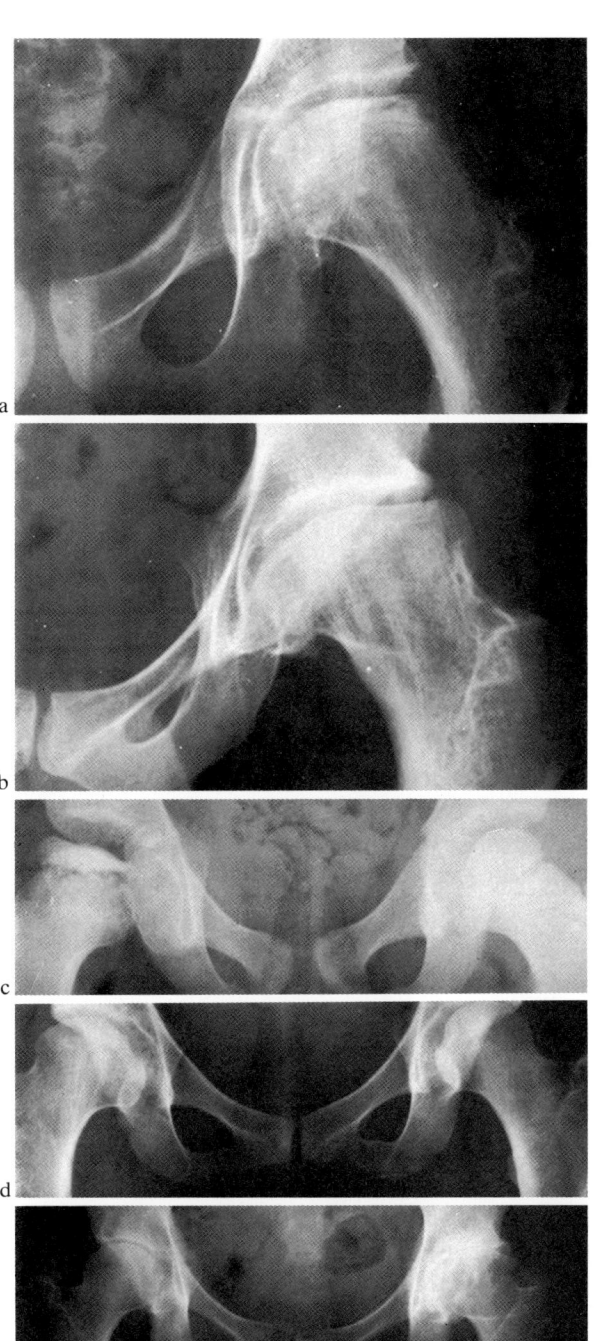

Fig. 1.8. *Degenerative joint disease (osteoarthritis) of hip—secondary to Perthes' disease.* Perthes' disease, characterised by avascular necrosis of the femoral head in children, is described in more detail elsewhere in this work. The residual deformity which may follow the disorder, however, represents another malformation of the hip which may precipitate degenerative changes later in life. Although with successful treatment this sequence of events is unusual, it must be appreciated that the occasional case may be asymptomatic and recognised only by chance. It is therefore possible for yet another type of 'primary' or 'idiopathic' osteoarthritis of the hip to be diagnosed on account of its radiological appearance. **a** After several years of treatment the left femoral head of this child with Perthes' disease was flattened, but fragmentation had been repaired largely by consolidation. The acetabulum had become mildly dysplastic. **b** Nineteen years later the femoral head was flattened and deformed further, with marked widening and shortening of the femoral neck. Such a joint clearly is liable to subsequent degenerative changes. **c** Another typical case of Perthes' disease of the right hip in a 6-year-old girl with classical flattening and condensation of the epiphysis and lucencies in the metaphysis was followed 18 years later **d** by a typical residual abnormality. At this time the patient was asymptomatic. The right femoral head is larger than its counterpart, as a result of hyperaemia, which has induced also premature fusion of the growth plate. The femoral neck is therefore short and wide. Observe again the development of mild secondary acetabular dysplasia. **e** Degenerative changes in the painful left hip of this 58-year-old woman are typified by narrowing of the joint space, cyst formation in the femoral head, subchondral sclerosis and marginal osteophytes. The enlargement of the left femoral head and the short femoral neck conform to the radiological pattern observed to follow Perthes' disease. No relevant history of an illness in childhood was obtained.

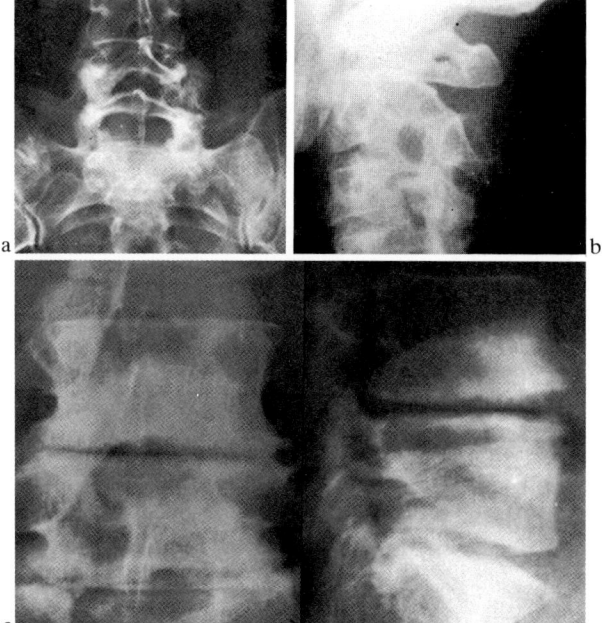

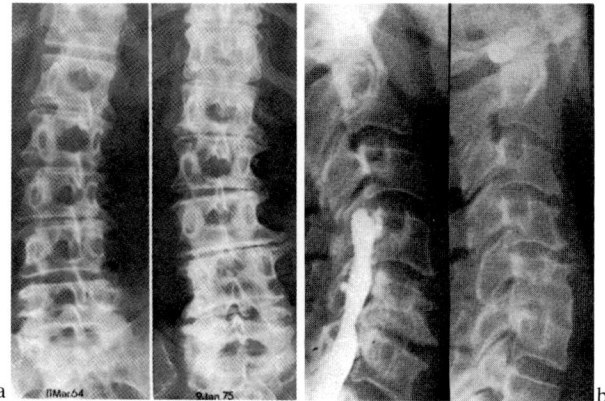

Fig. 1.10. *Degenerative joint disease (osteoarthritis)—role of the osteophyte.* **a** This 68-year-old woman presented with low back pain. Several degenerative disc lesions were associated with a scoliosis. Osteophytes had formed on the left, or concave, side of the scoliotic curve. Eleven years later the patient was asymptomatic and growth of the osteophytes had stabilised the scoliosis. **b** Osteophytes on the posterior side of this C5/6 degenerative disc lesion had indented the opaque column during myelography. The patient was a 54-year-old woman. This painful lesion was treated by anterior cervical fusion with an excellent result. Four years later the posterior osteophytes, by Woolf's law being required no longer, had been resorbed. These cases illustrate the physiologically reparative role of osteophytes.

Fig. 1.9. *Degenerative joint disease (osteoarthritis)—spinal lesions.* The posterior intervertebral joints are true diarthrodial articulations and often develop degenerative changes comparable to those described above. No true joints, however, are present between the vertebral bodies, where the shock-absorbing mechanism of the semi-fluid nucleus pulposus is contained within the strong annulus fibrosus. Prolapse of an intervertebral disc is possibly the most common of orthopaedic ailments. The narrowed disc space, which commonly results, does develop localised osteophytes and subchondral sclerosis, so that the difference is somewhat academic. On the other hand instability at the level of a disc derangement, demonstrated best by comparison of lateral films in flexion and extension, may be accompanied by the formation of small bony excrescences remote from the cartilage covering the vertebral end-plate. These 'traction spurs' are the result of stress at the attachments of the anterior common ligament.
a Chronic low backache in a 65-year-old woman, without nerve root symptoms, was attributed to degenerative change in the left L4/5 posterior intervertebral joint with massive osteophyte formation. Lesions of this type usually are demonstrated more clearly in oblique projections, as in **b**, a case of a 62-year-old man with chronic pain radiating from the neck into the left arm. Degenerative change in the left C3/4 posterior joint had led to the formation of large osteophytes which encroached on the exit foramen. Diminution of the space for this nerve root was probably increased by radiolucent cartilaginous caps on these osteophytes. Radiological examination of the cervical spine after an injury 3 years earlier had revealed no abnormality. **c** This typical L4/5 degenerative disc lesion was found in a 54-year-old woman who had complained of intermittent back pain and sciatica for 9 years. In addition to the narrowed disc space, localised osteophyte formation and subchondral sclerosis are evident. In such cases differentiation from an old and inactive infective discitis may be difficult.

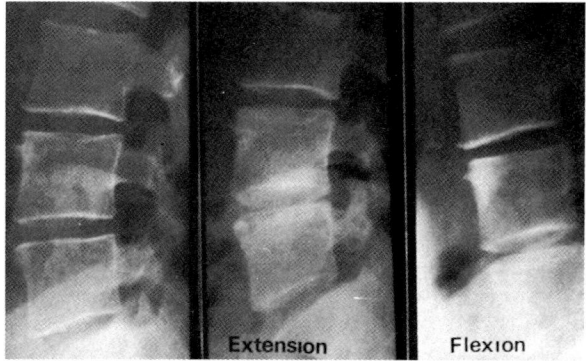

Fig. 1.11. *Derangement of L3/4 intervertebral disc with 'traction spur'.* This 46-year-old woman with sciatica for 2 months was found to have a narrowed L3/4 disc space. In addition the osseous excrescence on the anterior aspect of the body of L4 was remote from the disc space and represented a 'traction spur' at the attachment of the anterior common ligament. Such abnormalities usually indicate instability, as is demonstrated by comparison of the studies in extension and flexion. Although frank degenerative changes have not yet developed in relation to this lesion, some subchondral sclerosis is evident in the antero-superior portion of the body of L4.

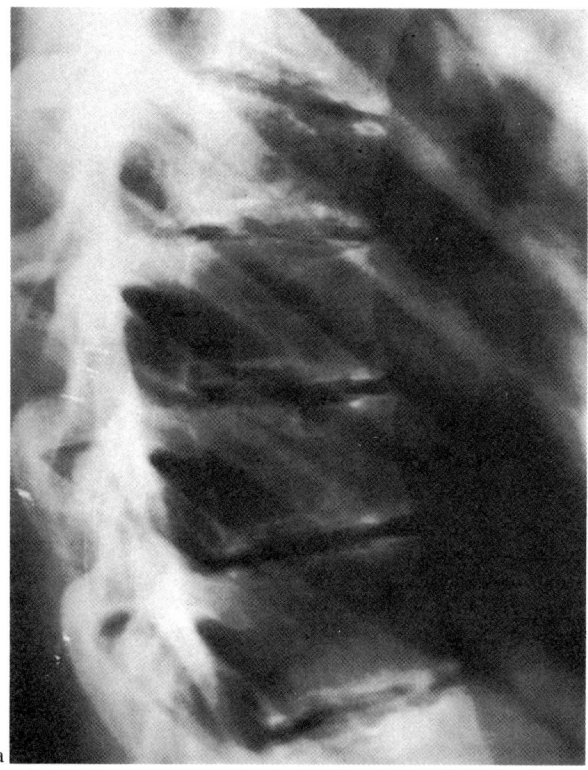 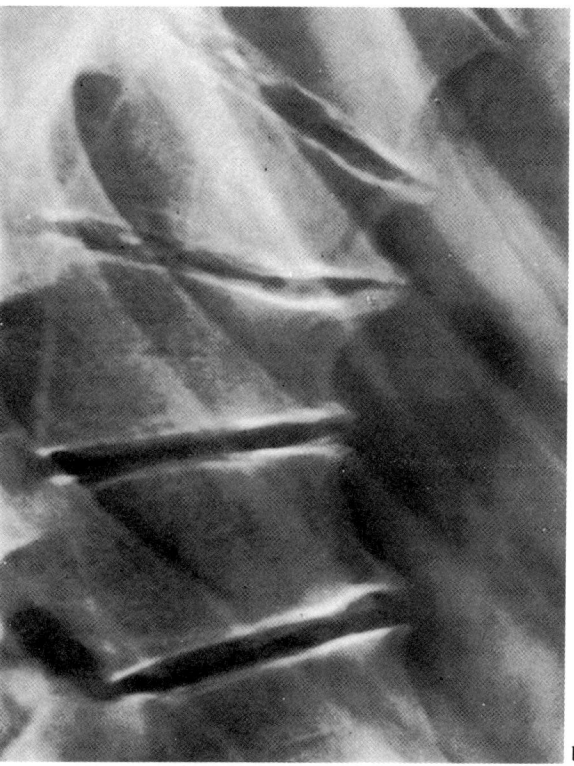

Fig. 1.12. *Scheuermann's disease.* This common disorder often is responsible for mild pain, especially affecting the dorsal spine, in adolescents. Boys are affected more than girls. A traumatic origin is generally accepted, as the condition has been recognised to be associated with such activities as trampolining and water-skiing. Herniation of the nucleus pulposus through a vertebral end-plate causes a Schmorl's node. In Scheuermann's disease such lesions are multiple and frequently cause anterior wedging of vertebral bodies. **a** Multiple disc herniations in this adolescent boy illustrate a typical example of the disorder. **b** The residual deformities in this young adult man have resulted in marked kyphosis, secondary degenerative changes having stimulated prominent osteophyte formation.

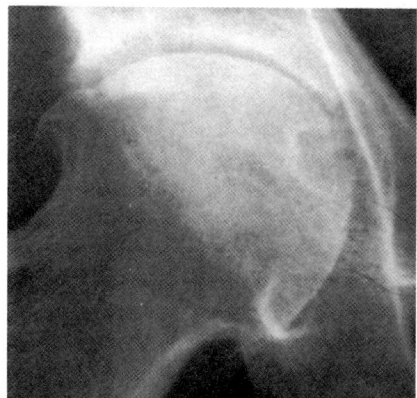 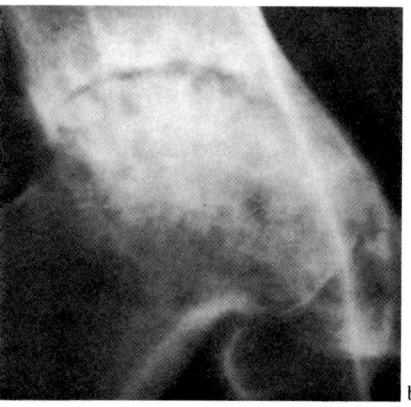

Fig. 2.2. *Iatrogenic arthropathy of hip.* This 63-year-old woman had complained of increasing discomfort and pain in the right hip for 2 years. **a** Narrowing of the medial compartment of the joint and the presence of a marginal circumferential osteophyte were interpreted as manifestations of degenerative joint disease. Observe similarity to Q2a. Symptoms were relieved for many months by analgesics of the phenylbutazone type. More severe pain and disability prompted further examination 5 years later. **b** By this time extreme disintegration of the acetabulum and femoral head had taken place, with protrusio acetabuli deformity and actual destruction of the original osteophyte. Further clinical and radiological studies disclosed evidence not only of rheumatoid arthritis, but also of psoriasis, emphasising the post-inflammatory type of degenerative joint disease which was evident in the original film. These inflammatory arthritides are discussed elsewhere in this work.

Q1. A 12-year-old girl complained of an ache above the left ankle for many months. Its onset had been insidious and no history of trauma could be elicited. More recently frank pain had developed.

Clinical examination revealed slight swelling of the distal end of the tibia with localised tenderness in this area. Movements of the ankle were full and painless.

A well-circumscribed lucency was demonstrated radiologically in the area of clinical suspicion. The endosteal margins were clearly defined by a thin sclerotic border showing a very narrow zone of transition. The overlying cortex was attenuated and slightly expanded.

Surgical exploration of the lesion was undertaken.

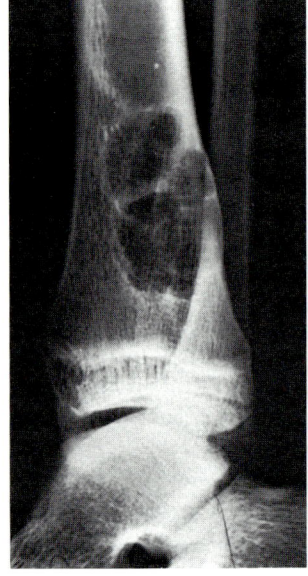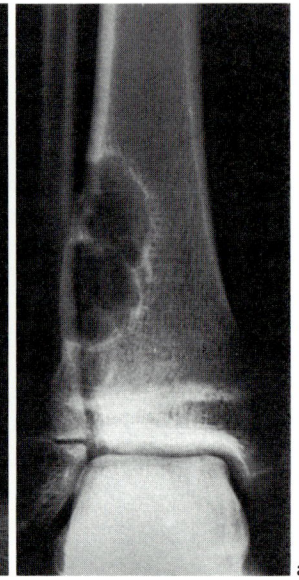

Q1a.

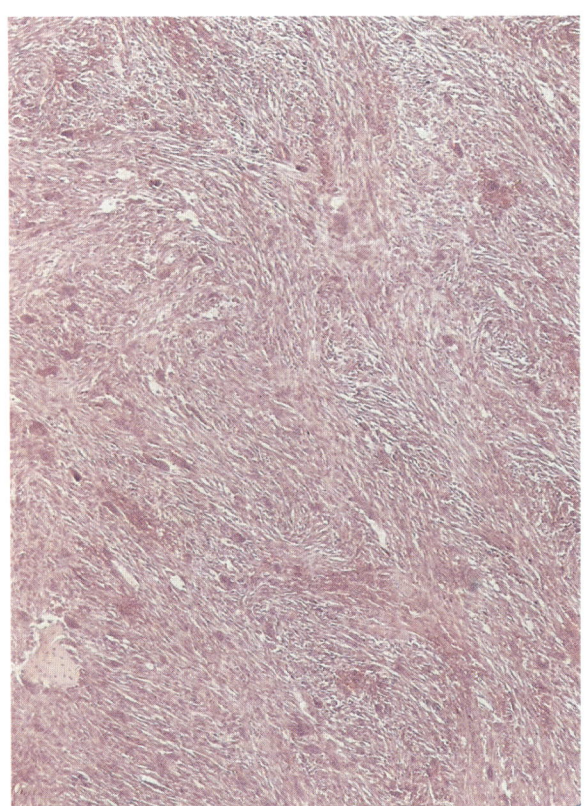

Q1b. (×50)

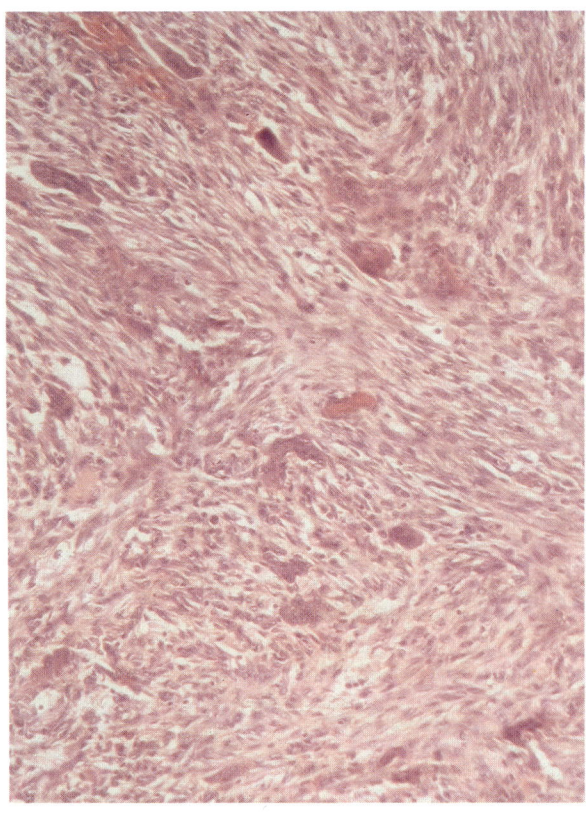

Q1c. (×140)

Exercise 6

Q2. This girl, aged 14, presented with a history of mild pain in the left hip of 1 month's duration.

No abnormality was detected clinically.

Radiological examination showed a loculated lytic area affecting the entire width of the femur. The cortex overlying this area had become abnormally thin and, on the medial aspect, was minimally expanded. A minute infraction was, almost certainly, the cause of the recent pain. As in the previous case, the endosteal margin was sclerotic, with a narrow zone of transition.

The lesion was explored surgically.

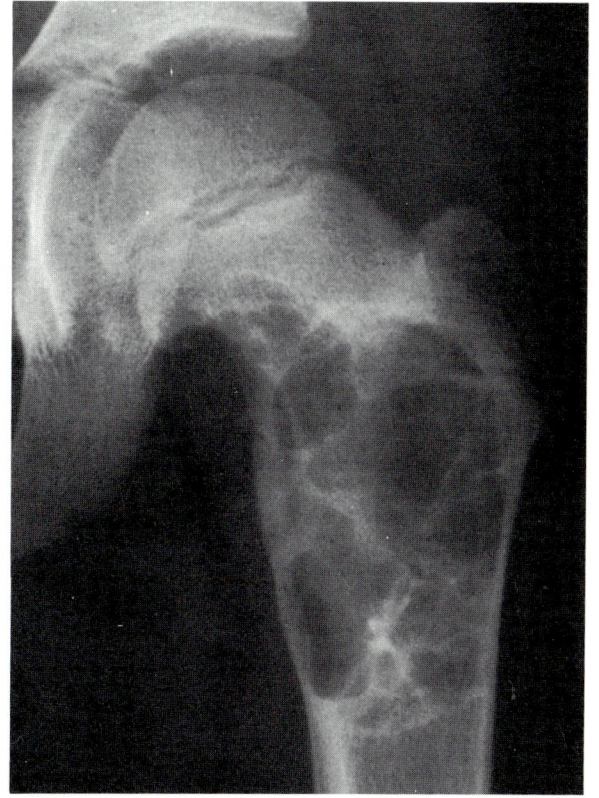

Q2a.

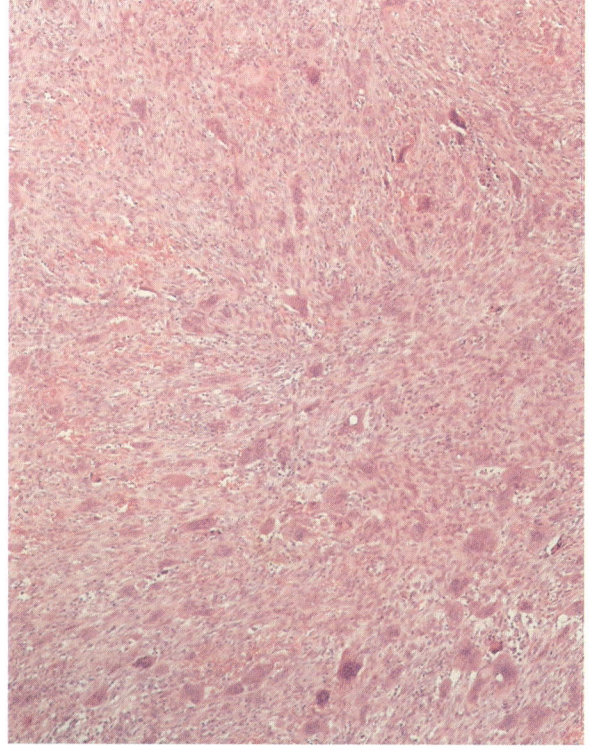

Q2b. (×50)

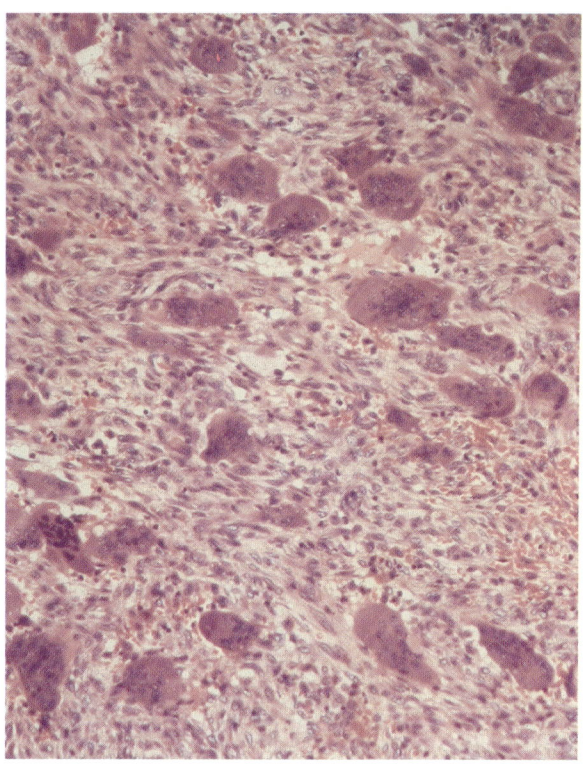

Q2c. (×140)

A1. Non-ossifying fibroma (fibrous cortical defect) of tibia

The radiological appearance of the lesion is characteristic of non-ossifying fibroma. At operation, the lesion was found to consist of solid tissue, soft and friable in consistency and yellowish-brown in colour. It was curetted and packed with bone chips. Histologically (Q1b and c) the material consists of spindle-celled fibrous tissue with scattered giant cells. Collections of lipid-containing foam cells are also present (Fig. 1.1) and, with haemosiderin pigment (Fig. 1.2), are responsible for the yellowish-brown colour of the lesion. These findings, too, are characteristic of non-ossifying fibroma.

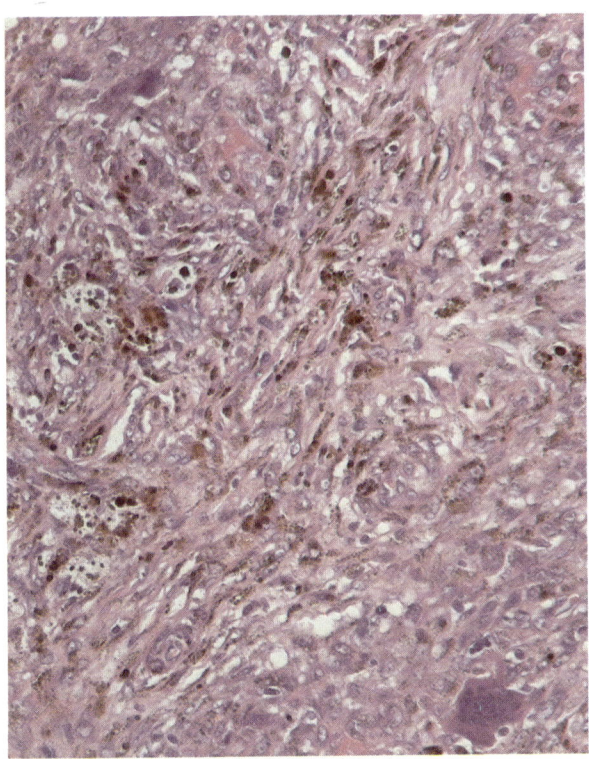

Fig. 1.2. An area of more cellular tissue from the same lesion, with dark granules of haemosiderin pigment, much of which has been phagocytosed by histiocytes. (×235)

A2. Non-ossifying fibroma of femur

In this case the site of the lesion, together with the clinical and radiological findings, suggested a diagnosis of simple (unicameral) bone cyst, but this was not substantiated by the pathological findings. Operation revealed that the lesion was not a cyst, but a circumscribed mass of solid pale fleshy tissue. It was curetted and packed with bone chips.

Histologically (Q2b and c) this lesion, like the previous one, consists of spindle-celled fibrous tissue with scattered giant cells. The giant cells show, more than in the previous case, the typical morphological appearance of osteoclasts and their number might even suggest a diagnosis of giant-cell tumour. Such a diagnosis can be excluded, however, not only because of the age of the patient and the site of the lesion, but also because of the microscopic appearance of the 'stromal' tissue between the giant cells, particularly its fibrous appearance.

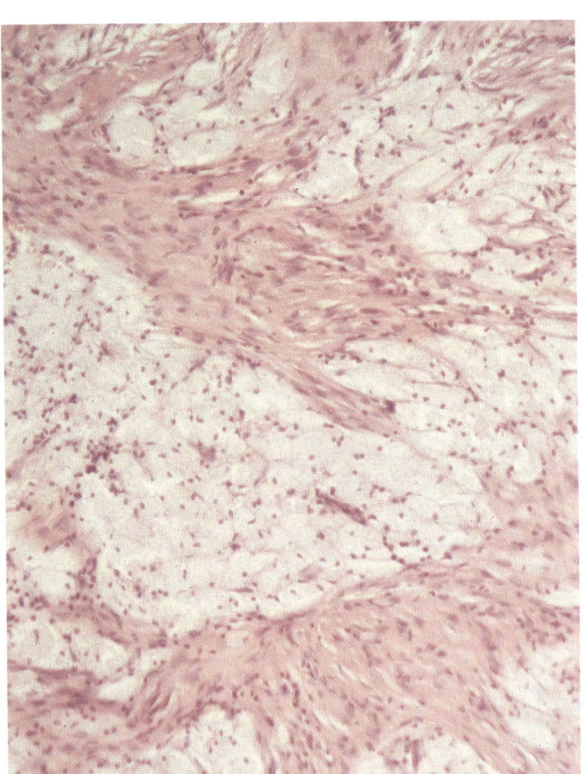

Fig. 1.1. Spindle-celled tissue with conspicuous collections of lipid-containing foam cells in the same patient. (×140)

Non-ossifying Fibroma (Fibrous Cortical Defect)

Fibrous cortical defects represent a common anomaly of bone growth, occurring in as many as 30% of children, most commonly between the ages of 5 and 8 years. Two males are affected for every female. These lesions are usually discovered as an incidental radiological finding and tend to regress spontaneously. Some, however, do enlarge and are detected in the later years of adolescence and even in adult life, when they are known as non-ossifying fibromas.

Clinical Features

The radiological demonstration of these essentially asymptomatic lesions usually follows examination to exclude a bone injury. Rarely, an actual pathological fracture may be found, but otherwise symptoms are lacking.

Radiological Features

1. Site. These lesions originate in the metaphyses of long bones, particularly around the knee. The frequency of their observation at this site may reflect simply the frequency of radiographic examination of this area.

2. Appearance. Eccentric, oval, lytic defects occur in long bones, with slight expansion and thinning of the overlying cortex. The endosteal margin is serpiginous and sclerotic, with a narrow zone of transition. Some become sufficiently large to extend across the affected shaft, therefore being liable to sustain a pathological fracture, particularly in such a slender structure as the fibula. Differential diagnosis rarely presents difficulty, but, as in Q2, a large non-ossifying fibroma may simulate a bone cyst or other benign fibrous lesions, such as fibrous dysplasia, especially in the uncommon situation of the abnormality persisting into adult life. Serial studies more usually show complete regression or, occasionally, a residual area of sclerosis.

Pathological Features

As shown in Q1 and Q2, these lesions consist of spindle-celled fibrous tissue, with scattered giant cells, sometimes with deposits of haemosiderin pigment and collections of lipid-containing foam cells. Non-ossifying fibroma formerly was regarded as a giant-cell tumour 'variant', but it is now accepted as a separate entity with an entirely different pattern of age incidence, radiographic appearance and histological structure. Sometimes, as in Q2, a histological resemblance to giant cell tumour may be observed, but the fibrous nature of the stromal tissue, as well as the absence of large numbers of giant cells—when an adequate sample of tissue is studied—allows the histological distinction to be made without too much difficulty. Large lesions of non-ossifying fibroma can sometimes be confused, histologically, with malignant fibrous histiocytoma, an entity discussed in another Exercise. Broder has made the tentative suggestion that, on occasion, non-ossifying fibromas may be precursors of unicameral bone cysts.

Treatment

In general, surgical intervention for asymptomatic fibrous cortical defects is unwarranted, although biopsy may be justified if the diagnosis is in doubt. Larger non-ossifying fibromas, particularly following fracture, require more active treatment; this is usually curettage or local excision followed by packing with bone chips or insertion of a protective inlay graft.

References

Broder HM (1968) Possible precursor of unicameral bone cysts. J Bone Jt Surg 50A: 503–507
Caffey J (1955) On fibrous defects in cortical walls of growing tubular bones. Adv Pediatr. 7: 13–51
Campbell CJ, Harkness J (1957) Fibrous metaphyseal defect of bone. Surg Gynecol Obstet 104: 329–336
Hatcher CH (1945) The pathogenesis of localised fibrous lesions in the metaphyses of long bones. Ann Surg 122: 1016–1030
Jaffe HL, Lichtenstein L (1942) Non-osteogenic fibroma of bone. Am J Pathol 18: 205–221

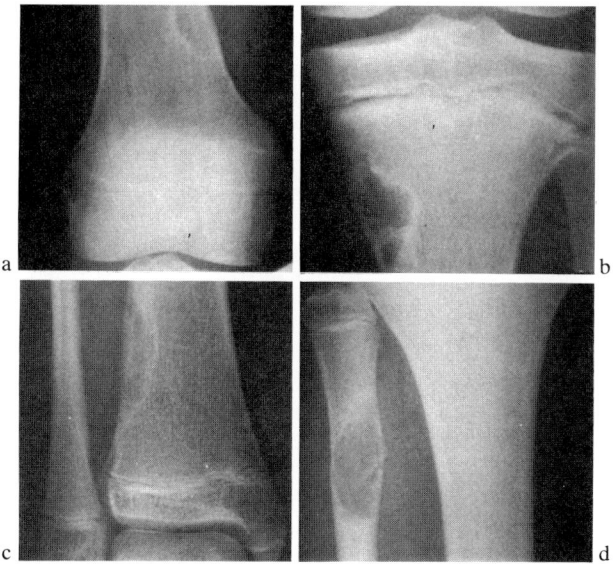

Fig. 1.3. *Non-ossifying fibroma—typical appearances in children*, showing a narrow, serpiginous endosteal margin, with slight thinning and expansion of the overlying cortex. **a** *Femur*. **b** *Tibia*—proximal end. **c** *Tibia*—distal end. All these lesions were discovered incidentally in children. **d** *Fibula*. An infraction had caused pain in this case.

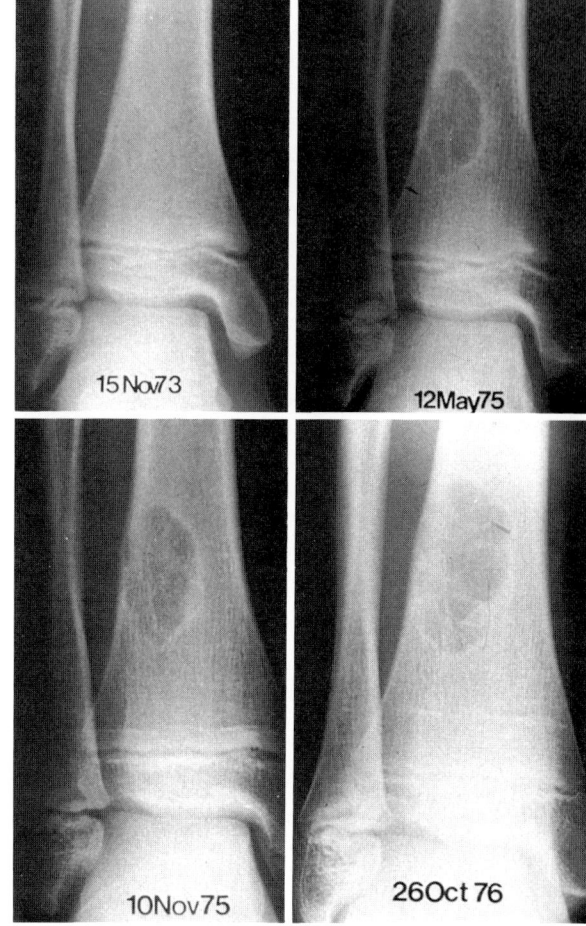

Fig. 1.5. *Non-ossifying fibroma of tibia*. At the age of 13 this boy also was examined to exclude a fracture. Serial studies showed the lesion to enlarge. The patient was aware of the possibility of a fracture and complained of a mild ache, particularly when playing football. After curettage and packing with bone chips the diagnosis was confirmed histologically.

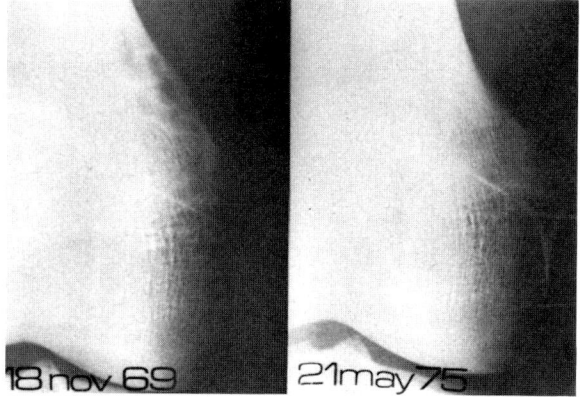

Fig. 1.4. *Non-ossifying fibroma of femur*. Another incidental finding in a 15-year-old boy who was examined to exclude a fracture. Six years later almost complete replacement by normal bone had taken place, with only minimal residual sclerosis. No biopsy was performed.

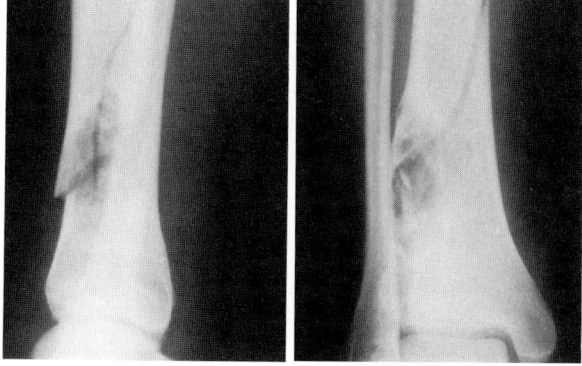

Fig. 1.6. *Non-ossifying fibroma of tibia*. This pathological fracture occurred through a typical tumour in a 17-year-old girl, previously asymptomatic, who fell while skating.

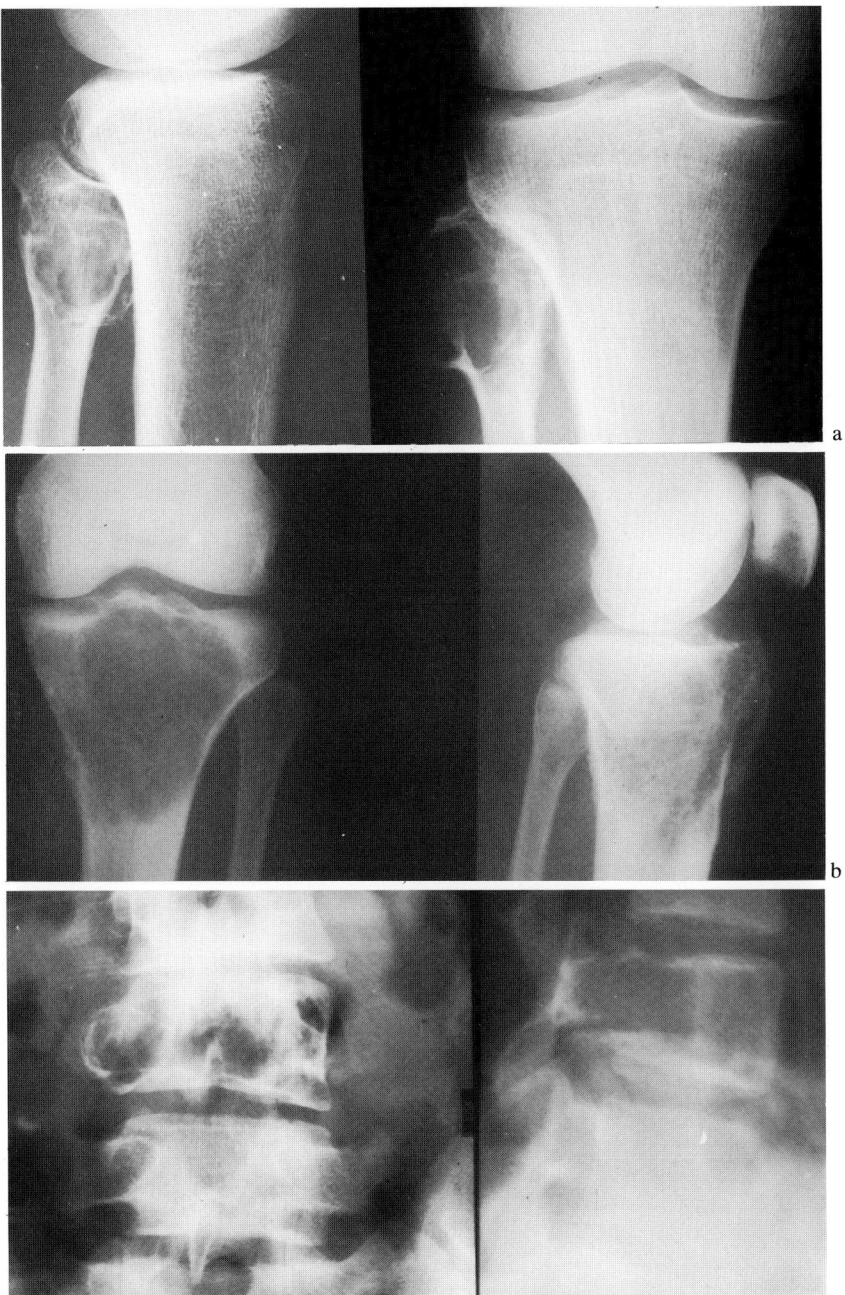

Fig. 1.7. *Benign fibrous lesions in adults.* All these lesions were considered pre-operatively to have other diagnoses, but in each case a *non-ossifying fibroma* was established histologically. **a** This expanding tumour of the head of the fibula had caused a swelling with mild pain of several months duration in this 45-year-old man. A diagnosis of aneurysmal bone cyst was preferred pre-operatively to giant cell tumour in view of the clear definition of the endosteal margin. At operation solid fibrous tissue was found. **b** This 36-year-old man had complained of mild pain in the knee for 6 weeks. The aggressive appearance of the subarticular tibial lesion was alarming and was interpreted as a giant-cell tumour, but again the macroscopic and histological appearances were diagnostic. **c** This lytic lesion in the L4 vertebral body in a young woman with low back pain also caused diagnostic difficulty, the possibilities being considered pre-operatively including aneurysmal bone cyst, chondroma and fibrous dysplasia.

These cases illustrate the radiological difficulty which may arise with these lesions in adults, as opposed to their easy recognition in young patients, when biopsy may be avoided.

Q1. This 44-year-old man complained of persistent pain and stiffness in the left hip.

A fracture of the left femoral neck, sustained 7 years before, had been treated by closed reduction and immobilisation.

On clinical examination a fixed adduction deformity was demonstrated and flexion of the hip was limited to 70°.

Radiological examination revealed a transverse band of density in the subcapital portion of the femoral neck consistent with sound union of the former fracture. Within the femoral head itself mixed areas of density and lucency were evident, with a step defect in the articular margin. The joint space was abnormally narrow and a bony spur was present on the lateral aspect of the head of the femur.

The femoral head was excised and replaced by a prosthesis.

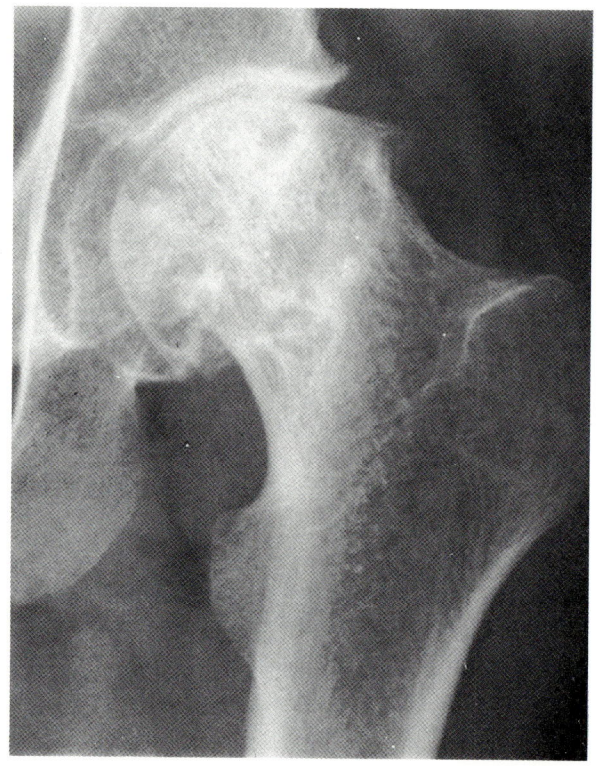

Q1a.

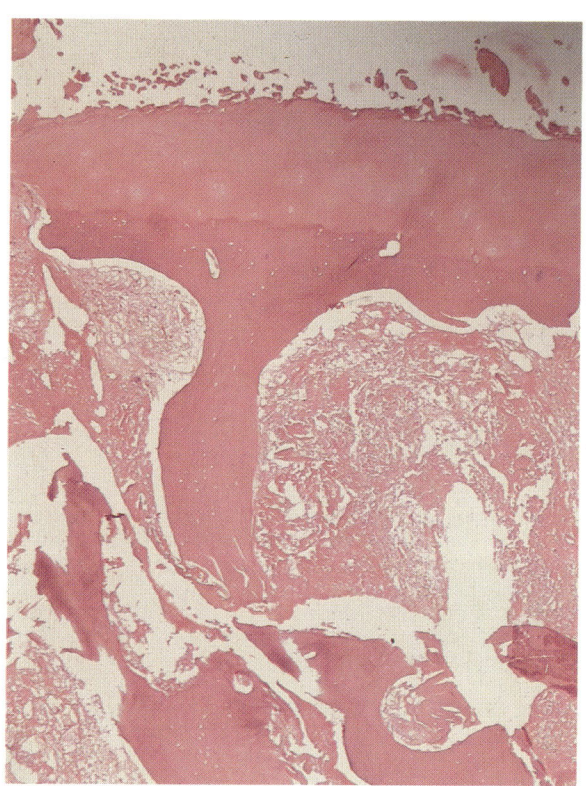

Q1b. (×36)

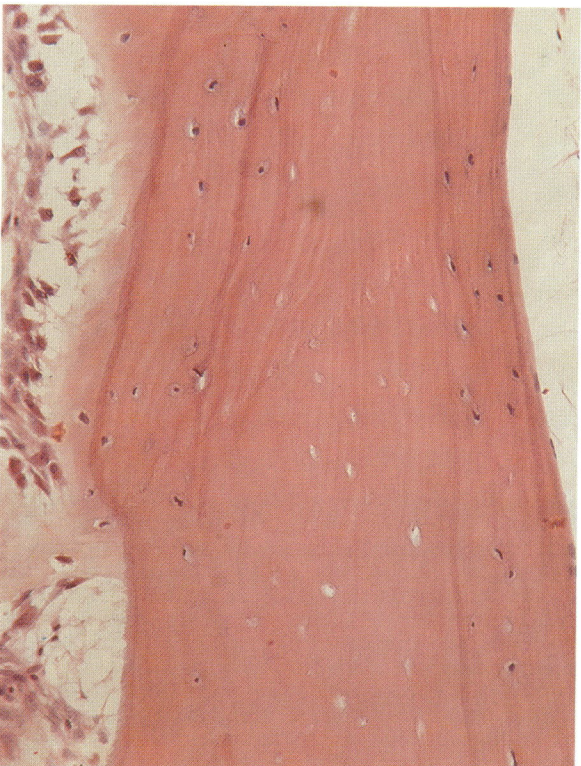

Q1c. (×168)

Exercise 7

Q2. This 39-year-old man had complained of chronic pain in the right hip for nearly 2 years.

Clinical examination disclosed generalised limitation of movement of the hip, with absence of internal rotation.

On radiological examination a large osteolytic lesion was evident in the femoral head, with a well-defined sclerotic margin. The superior part of the head had undergone a mild degree of collapse, which was particularly apparent in the tomogram.

In this case also, prosthetic replacement of the hip was performed.

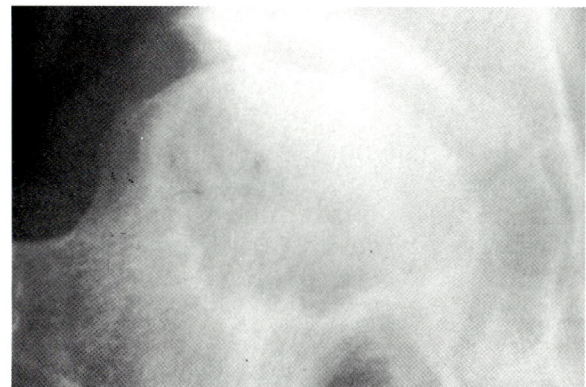

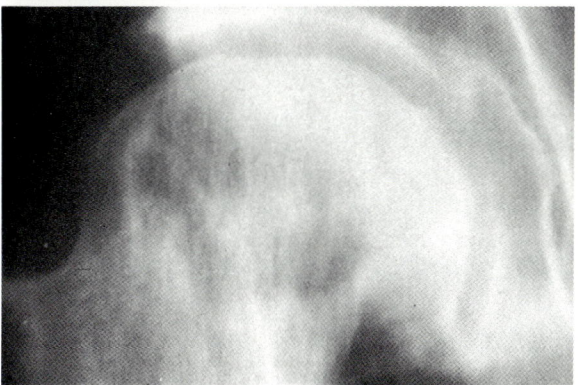

Q2a.

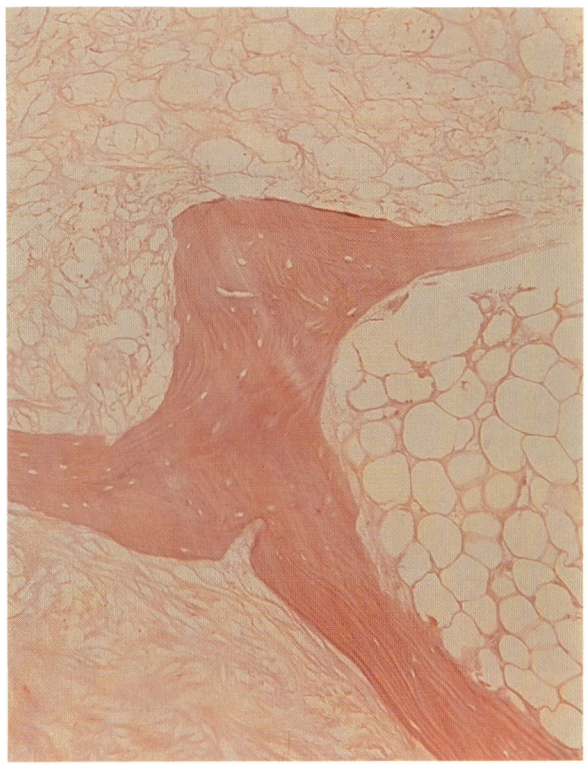

Q2b. (×94)

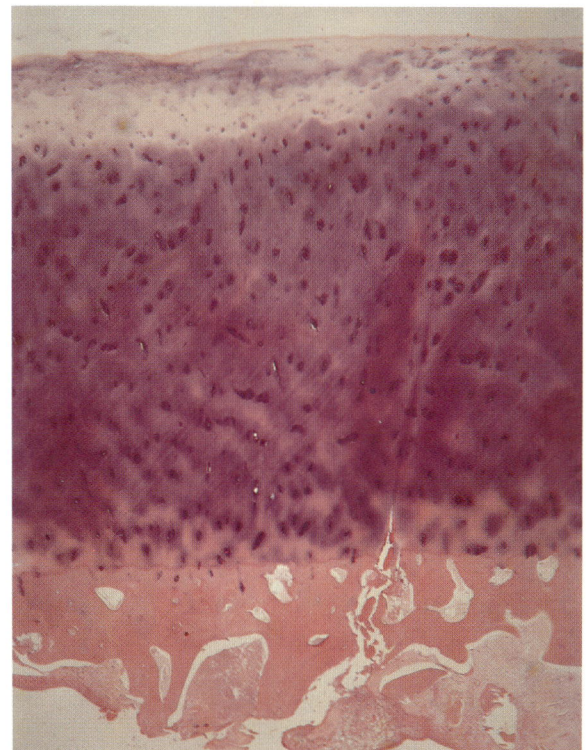

Q2c. (×25)

A1. Post-traumatic necrosis—femoral head

The radiological appearance typifies necrosis of the femoral head. The former fracture had consolidated soundly, but the vascular supply to the femoral head had been impaired. The weakened subchondral bone has suffered more recent infraction, causing the interruption in the outline of the articular surface. The narrowing of the joint space and the early marginal osteophyte indicate the presence of secondary degenerative joint disease (osteoarthritis).

On pathological examination the resected femoral head exhibits classical evidence of necrosis of bone and bone marrow, with revascularisation and remodelling. In a radiograph of a slab of tissue from the femoral head (Fig. 1.1) the area of infarction (necrosis), which involves the proximal portion of the femoral head, is marked by a patchy alteration in trabecular pattern and bone density. The site of the femoral neck fracture is apparent as a poorly outlined transverse zone towards the cut surface of the specimen. In the subchondral region, this slab radiograph shows more bony collapse than is apparent in the pre-operative radiograph. Q1b shows necrotic bone trabeculae with empty osteocyte lacunae. These bone trabeculae have remained unchanged, except for fragmentation and collapse, since the onset of bone necrosis at the time of the fracture. In this part of the femoral head the bone marrow also is necrotic. Q1c, from a revascularised part of the femoral head, shows evidence of previous necrosis in the form of empty osteocyte lacunae within the central part of the trabecula illustrated. In contrast, the superficial layers contain nucleated osteocytes and represent viable bone tissue which has been formed following revascularisation. This tissue is covered by many active osteoblasts which are evident on the left side of the illustration. This new bone is responsible, at least in part, for the appearance of patchy increase in bone density in the slab radiograph. In some parts of the infarct (Fig. 1.2) the necrotic bone marrow has undergone fibrosis and calcification, the latter process contributing to the appearance of increased bone density.

Outside the area of residual infarction, the bone and bone marrow of the femoral head, as a result of revascularisation, show a more normal histological structure (Fig. 1.3). All the bone tissue contains viable osteocytes, and patent capillary blood vessels are present in the marrow. Many of the bone trabeculae, including that illustrated in Fig. 1.3, are reduced in thickness. This feature is responsible for the patchy rarefaction of the bone of the femoral head which is evident in both the pre-operative and slab radiographs. (Q1a, Fig. 1.1).

Following total prosthetic replacement excellent restoration of pain-free function was obtained.

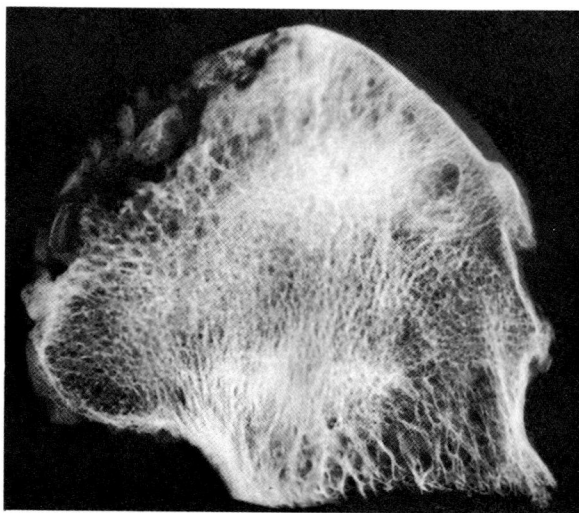

Fig. 1.1. Radiograph of a slab of tissue from the femoral head. Note the patchy alterations in bone density in the area of infarction involving the upper part of the head. Collapse of the subchondral bone is accompanied by a break in the continuity of the articular surface.

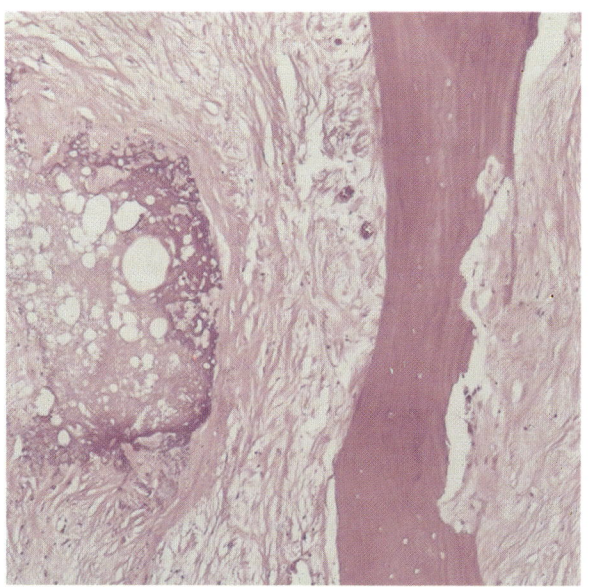

Fig. 1.2. Part of the infarcted area, showing marrow fibrosis and calcification. On the right side of this dead trabecula, osteoclastic resorption is evident. (×73)

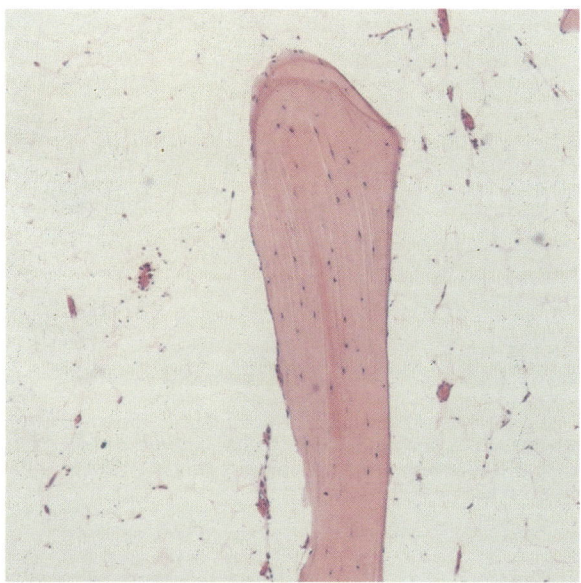

Fig. 1.3. Part of the femoral head remote from the infarcted area, showing viable bone and bone marrow. (×73)

A2. Systemic necrosis—femoral head (Dysbaric osteonecrosis: Caisson disease)

This patient, a tunnel worker for 20 years, had been involved in compression chamber work for 11 years. During this period he had suffered from 'the bends' on numerous occasions, with pain involving the shoulders, elbows and wrists, and the hips, knees and ankles.

Again, the radiological appearances are characteristic of infarction of the femoral head, with partial collapse of the subchondral bone. The dense margin of the lesion indicates the presence of a front of revascularisation. Similar areas of infarction were present in other bones. The infarct in the right femoral head had been detected radiologically (Fig. 2.1) during a routine survey approximately 2 years earlier, at which time the patient had no symptoms and collapse of the articular surface had not occurred. (Prophylactic surveys of this type are usual in individuals exposed to this occupational hazard).

Most of the femoral head was involved by a large area of infarction, but the abnormalities are demonstrated at an earlier stage than in Q1. Figures 2.2 and 2.3 show the appearance of the resected femoral head in a specimen photograph and the corresponding slab radiograph. The area of infarction can be identified in the photograph as the pale central area; the slab radiograph shows the line of reactive bone sclerosis which corresponds to a narrow zone of revascularisation at the margin of the lesion. A subchondral fracture is evident. The necrotic bone deep to the articular cartilage has been destroyed, perhaps by mechanical abrasion, altering the contour of the femoral head and leaving the articular cartilage as a loose covering shell.

The corresponding histological changes are illustrated in Q2b, where the presence of bone necrosis is confirmed by the empty osteocyte lacunae. The marrow, too, is necrotic. The outline of fat cells is preserved, but no cell nuclei can be identified. Q2c shows the tissue separated by the subchondral fracture. In this case the articular cartilage, which receives its nutrition by diffusion from the synovial fluid, remains viable.

Bone Necrosis

Bone death occurs when the vascular supply to a particular skeletal segment suffers transient or permanent interruption. The condition is usually the result of a major or even a minor injury (*post-traumatic necrosis*), but may be a sequel to a variety of other disorders involving the bony structures (*systemic necrosis*). In both instances, as in the case of other tissue systems, infarction develops.

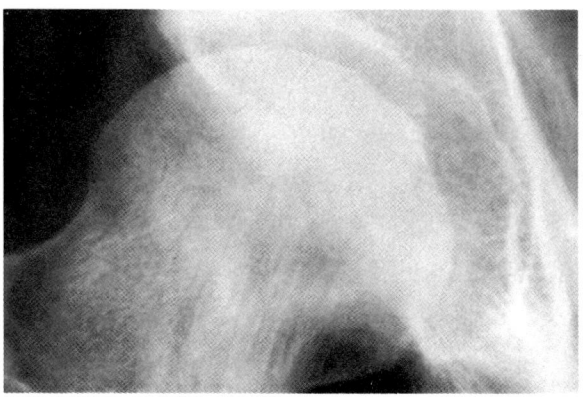

Fig. 2.1. This radiograph, obtained nearly 2 years earlier when the patient was asymptomatic, already showed the area of infarction to be outlined by the sclerotic margin of a revascularisation front.

Post-traumatic Necrosis

Clinical Features

Initially the infarcts by themselves produce no clinical signs or symptoms, pain resulting only at a later stage when the affected and consequently weakened bone fractures. Such fractures frequently involve articular surfaces, consequently causing arthralgia in the affected joint, with limitation of movement. In the immature skeleton necrosis of the femoral head is a constant feature of Perthes' disease, possibly resulting from the transient interruption of the blood flow as a result of intracapsular tamponade following trauma, and may be encountered also as a sequel to the shearing injury to the proximal femoral growth plate associated with slipping of the upper femoral epiphysis.

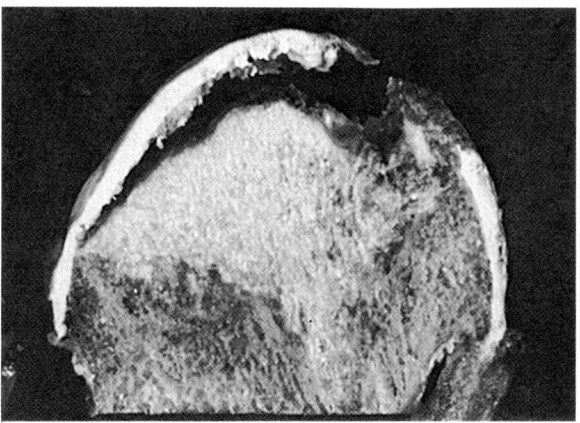

Fig. 2.2. Photograph of the resected femoral head, demonstrating the infarct and the subchondral fracture.

Radiological Features

Devitalised bone does not in itself produce radiological abnormalities. An affected segment may remain avascular for many months in children or even years in adults without developing an abnormal radiological appearance. During such periods, however, radionuclide studies show decreased uptake of the tracer. Those changes which ultimately are observed are due either to repair during the process of revascularisation or the effects of mechanical stress, especially weight-bearing, on bone which has been rendered brittle by its pathological state.

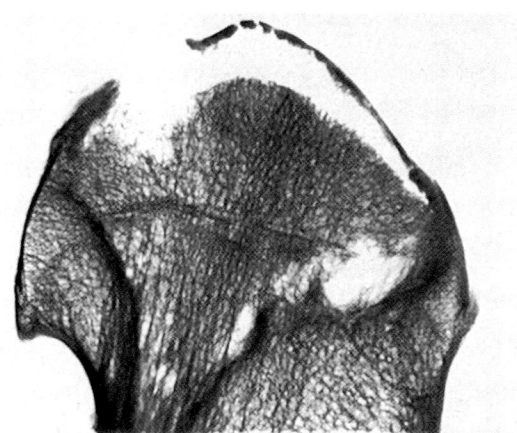

Fig. 2.3. The slab radiograph of the resected specimen shows the dense zone of marginal sclerosis around the infarct and the residual shell of separated subarticular bone.

1. Site. Owing to the anatomical arrangement of the vasculature, a peculiar affinity exists for this complication to affect the femoral head, the proximal pole of the scaphoid and the body of the talus. Necrosis may develop also in certain small bones, such as the lunate and navicular, in growing epiphyseal centres and in fragments detached from convex articular surfaces, frequently in the absence of a frank history of trauma. Lesions of this type, known historically by the terms 'osteochondritis' and 'osteochondritis dissecans', are discussed in another Exercise.

2. Appearance. Revascularisation of an intact area of bone necrosis usually results in diffuse increase of density. The margin of the revascularisation front often is particularly dense, as illustrated in Fig. 2.1. If mechanical stress is avoided, complete remodelling and a normal appearance finally develops. The earliest evidence of damage to a necrotic femoral head may be a thin line of rarefaction in the subchondral bone—the 'crescent' sign. Much more commonly, as in Q1 and Q2, some degree of disintegration of the area of dead bone ensues, so that a mixed pattern of density and lucency is observed, together with frank disruption of articular margins or even gross fractures.

Pathological Features

The histological features of necrosis of bone are similar, whatever the cause. At an early stage, the area of infarction is recognised simply by the death of marrow cells and the disappearance of normally staining cells from the osteocyte lacunae of bony structures. Later, the appearance of the tissue is complicated by a number of secondary factors. Revascularisation of the necrotic tissue occurs, but this is usually a slow process and months or years may elapse before the infarcted area returns to normal, if ever it does so. Revascularisation usually leads to the replacement of the necrotic bone marrow by fibrous tissue, and is accompanied by cellular remodelling of the bone itself. Osteoclasts erode the surfaces of some necrotic trabeculae, while osteoblasts form bone on other parts of the surface. This remodelling results in variations in the radiographic density of the revascularised area. Predominance of osteoclastic function is reflected by increased lucency, whereas the new bone laid down by osteoblasts on the scaffolding of intact, but dead, trabeculae is responsible for zones of sclerotic density. Rarely, impaction of fragmented bone trabeculae in the marrow spaces also may cause an increase in radiological density. The 'relative density', however, of an infarcted area of bone is due usually to disuse osteoporosis of the surrounding bone tissue, and may occur before revascularisation enables any cellular changes to occur in the dead bone. Degenerative calcification of the fibrotic bone marrow present in a bone infarct (Q1c) can occur also, usually at a late stage.

Treatment

Treatment of avascular necrosis is essentially preventative where this is practical, for example, in dysbaric osteonecrosis and radiation necrosis.

Unfortunately the majority of these lesions do not present clinically before the condition has become established.

The most critical areas of involvement are those occurring in weight-bearing joints, particularly the hip. The broad principle of treatment of such lesions is the relief of weight-bearing, either by the use of appropriate splints or calipers, or by surgery when containment of an affected area is obtained by varus osteotomy of the femur or even pelvic osteotomy. In the older patient, where such procedures may be impractical, prosthetic replacement of an affected joint may be indicated.

Systemic Necrosis

Necrosis of bone may result from causes other than trauma, including the following:

1. Dysbaric osteonecrosis (Caisson disease) is attributed to the impaction of liberated nitrogen bubbles in the lumen of capillaries as a result of over-rapid decompression. This occupational disorder is a well-recognised hazard in deep-sea divers, workers in compressed air and, rarely, aviators. The humeral and, less commonly, the femoral heads are affected, as in Q2. A history of episodes of acute bone pain (the 'bends') usually is obtained. Medullary infarcts in major long bones are common, being marked radiologically by zones of lucency surrounded by a thin margin of density reflecting reactive sclerosis. Histologically the same pattern of empty osteolacunae is demonstrated, with thickening of the peripheral and viable trabeculae and fibrosis of the intervening trabeculae. Very rarely, the wall of a medullary infarct undergoes malignant change.

2. Post-radiation necrosis has been recognised for many years as an iatrogenic complication of radiotherapy, but is extremely uncommon in the present era. Following irradiation, the bone becomes osteoporotic. Although subsequent repair may manifest limited new bone formation, bones weakened by this process are susceptible to fractures, which often fail to unite, and to actual disintegration. The fields of irradiation which are particularly liable to develop such changes include those for breast cancer, the upper ribs and the proximal end of the humerus, and for gynaecological and prostatic cancer, the pelvis and proximal end of the femur. The even rarer complication of post-radiation sarcoma is discussed in another Exercise.

3. Blood disorders, such as sickle cell disease, Gaucher's disease and, very rarely, polycythaemia vera, may give rise to skeletal infarctions, not only in subarticular locations, but also in medullary cavities.

4. Thermal injuries causing bone necrosis include frostbite (pernio), affecting digits in particular, and electrical burns due to direct heat from high voltage currents. Furnace workers in the steel industry may be at risk of these injuries.

5. Chronic alcoholism frequently provokes chronic pancreatitis, which in consequence results in fat emboli causing infarcts. These are liable to be observed especially in the medullary cavities of major long bones and in the femoral head.

6. Poisoning by various toxic substances may produce bone necrosis. Radium salts have long been recognised to cause diffuse areas of bone destruction. Initial osteoporosis may or may not be followed by diffuse areas of sclerosis, believed to represent attempted repair.

7. Idiopathic infarcts, for which no valid explanation can be offered, are encountered occasionally. In recent years such enigmatic lesions have been reported in the femoral heads of young women during or shortly after pregnancy.

Some of these entities are considered further in their appropriate context elsewhere in this volume.

References

Catto M (1965) A histological study of avascular necrosis of the femoral head after transcervical fracture. J Bone Jt Surg 47B: 749–776

Catto M (1976) Pathology of aseptic bone necrosis. In: Davidson JK (ed) Aseptic necrosis of bone. Excerpta Medica, Amsterdam

Davidson JK et al. (1977) The significance of bone islands, cystic areas and sclerotic areas in dysbaric osteonecrosis. Clin Radiol 28: 381–393

Glimcher MJ, Kenzora JE (1979) The biology of osteonecrosis of the human femoral head and its clinical implications. Clin Orthop 138: 284–309; 139: 283–312; 140: 273–312

Kay NRM, Park WM, Bark M (1972) The relationship between pregnancy and femoral head necrosis. Br J Radiol 45: 828–831

Norman A, Bullough P (1963) The radiolucent crescent line. An early diagnostic sign in avascular necrosis of the femoral head. Bull Hosp Joint Dis 24: 99–104

Ratliff AHC (1962) Fractures of the neck of the femur in children. J Bone Jt Surg 44B: 528–542

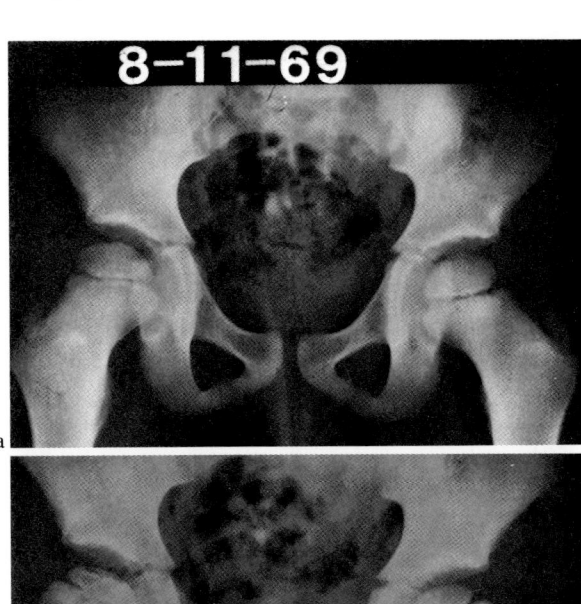
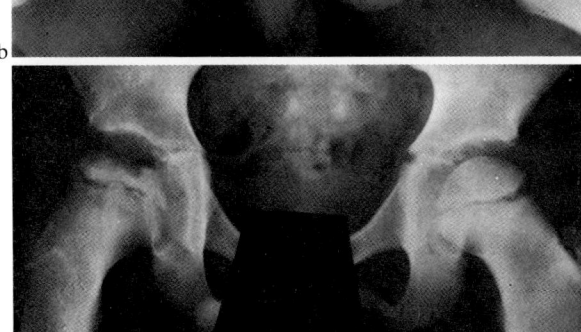
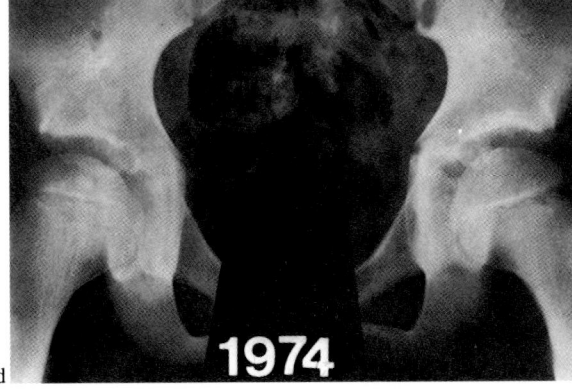

Fig. 1.4. *Post-traumatic necrosis—Perthes' disease.* **a** Characteristic early changes of this entity are illustrated in an 8-year-old boy presenting with a mildly painful limp of several weeks' duration. The joint space is apparently widened due to arrested growth of the epiphyseal nucleus. Such widening is observed also in the 'irritable hip syndrome', which is due to a traumatic effusion and which usually resolves with bed rest. In addition the curvilinear subchondral lucency shown in the oblique projection **b** indicates that the bone is necrotic and that an infraction of the weakened subchondral bone has occurred. **c** Despite immediate protection by relief of weight-bearing in a caliper, extensive necrosis had developed a year later. Symptoms resolved and after a further 4 years an almost normal appearance **d** had been restored, the ossification centre for the femoral head being only minimally flatter than its counterpart.

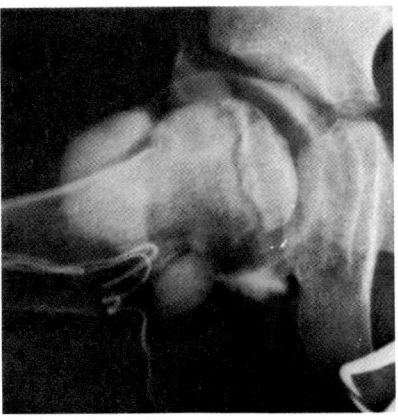
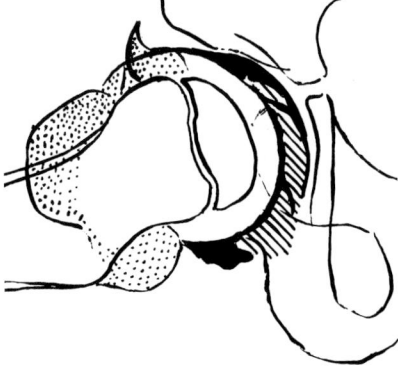

Fig. 1.5. *Post-traumatic necrosis—Perthes' disease.* This more severely necrotic femoral head is shown by the arthrogram still to be surrounded by spherical cartilage, a good prognostic sign. Hypertrophy of the soft tissues of the acetabular notch, shown as a filling defect (*hatched area in the tracing*), causes persistent displacement. Changes in this condition are considered to be due to a traumatic effusion transiently obstructing the venous return, leading to avascular necrosis and growth arrest. Hypertrophy of the capsule and soft tissues are thought to result from the secondary hyperaemia.

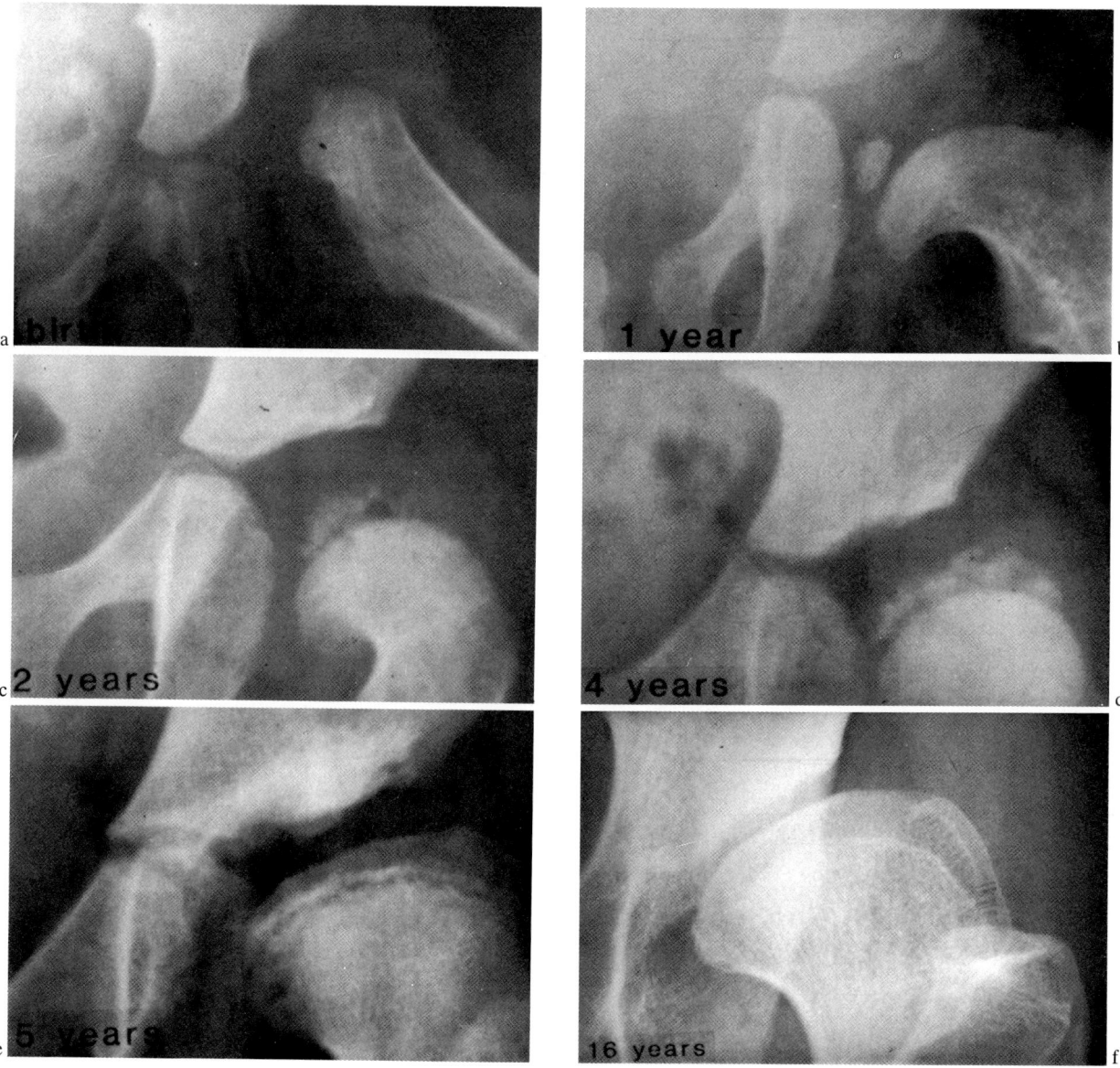

Fig. 1.6. *Post-traumatic necrosis—complicating congenital dislocation of the hip.* The blood supply of the femoral head in congenital dislocation may be compromised either by overforceful manipulation or by immobilisation in wide abduction and rotation. In consequence the femoral head may become necrotic and undergo changes comparable to those observed in severe cases of Perthes' disease. This series illustrates the effects of this iatrogenic disaster, now relatively rarely encountered, from birth to the age of 16 years.

The child, typically, was a girl. The occurrence of congenital dislocation of the hip in boys is much less common. Observe fragmentation of the ossification centre, with marked residual flattening. The acetabulum finally is grossly dysplastic and covers the deformed femoral head incompletely. Such a joint is extremely liable to develop premature degenerative changes (see Exercise 5). Nevertheless the clinical result was satisfactory at this time, the patient walking well with no obvious limp.

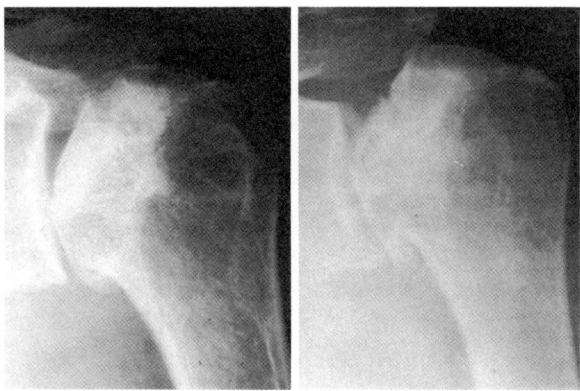

Fig. 2.4. *Systemic necrosis—caisson disease.* This 44-year-old man, with pain in both shoulders and 90° limitation of abduction, presented first in 1965, having been employed as a tunnel worker from 1953 to 1959. During that time he had suffered five attacks of the 'bends' requiring recompression. The dense infarct in the head of the humerus disintegrated further during the subsequent 4 years. These changes were symmetrical. The head of the humerus is more often affected than the head of the femur in this condition.

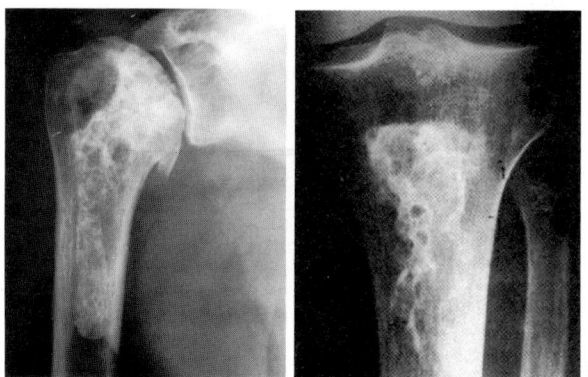

Fig. 2.5. *Systemic necrosis—medullary infarcts.* **a** Another tunnel worker with similar irregularity of the articular surface of the head of the humerus, due to disintegration of a dense subchondral infarct. In this instance the infarct extends into the medullary cavity. Such infarcts may be detected, usually symmetrically, without joint involvement and do not cause symptoms. The left humerus of this patient was similarly affected. **b** These infarcts in the tibia and fibula also were symmetrical and similar lesions were found in each femur of this 54-year-old man undergoing routine investigation for chronic alcoholism. Infarcts of similar appearance may be encountered with no explanation for their presence.

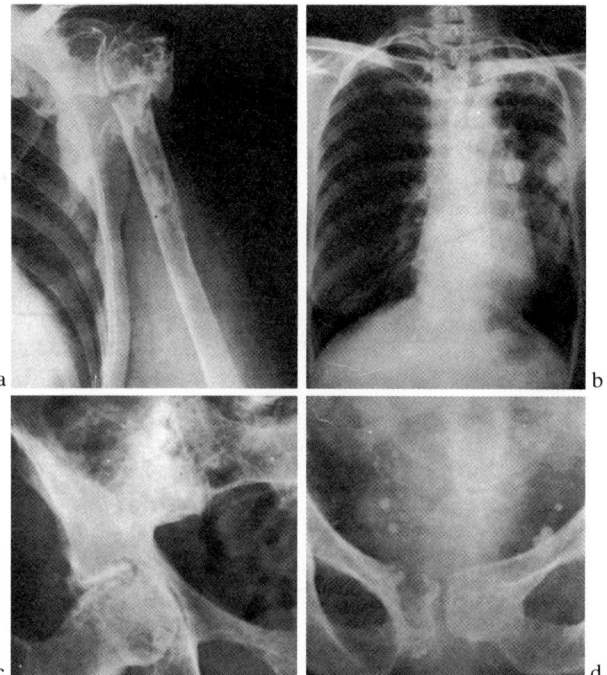

Fig. 2.6. *Systemic necrosis—effects of radiation therapy.* **a** *Humerus* with pathological fracture. Lesser changes of the same type had affected the scapula. Observe also lymphoedema of the arm as a result of surgical clearance of the axillary lymph nodes. **b** *Ribs* with multiple fractures. Note the left mastectomy. Both these patients had been treated for breast cancer approximately 10 years before. **c** *Femoral head and ilium*, with irregular areas of sclerosis, pain developing 5 years after irradiation for cervical cancer in this 63-year-old woman. **d** *Pubis*. The pathological fracture through this lytic area causing chronic groin pain in a 71-year-old woman was due to necrosis following radiation for gynaecological cancer 4 years previously.

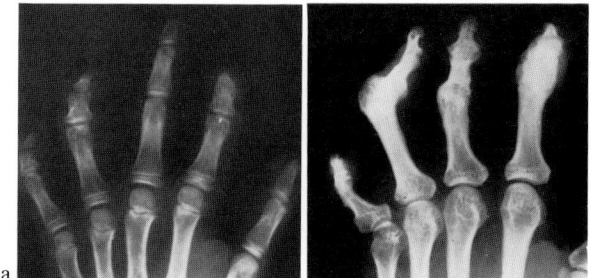

Fig. 2.7. *Systemic necrosis—thermal injuries.* **a** *Frost-bite (pernio).* This 10-year-old Canadian boy lost a mitten while skiing. During the subsequent phase of acute swelling the vascular supply to several phalanges was compromised, resulting in abnormal bony texture and shortening due to premature fusion of the affected growth plates. **b** *Burns—late deformity.* This 32-year-old woman, examined to exclude a fracture, had gross flexion deformities of the fingers of both hands due to severe burns incurred in childhood. Several phalanges are atrophic and shortened by premature epiphyseal fusion.

Exercise 8

Q1. This 56-year-old man had complained of pain in the wrist and forearm for 2 years.

Clinical examination showed prominence of the distal end of the ulna, with slight radial deviation of the hand and wrist. No other abnormality was detected.

Radiological examination of the forearm revealed thickening and increased density of the entire ulna, with almost complete obliteration of the medullary cavity. This bone was bowed and increased in length, so that the distal radio-ulnar joint was dislocated.

In order to correct the orthopaedic deformity the distal end of the ulna was excised and the specimen was submitted for histological examination.

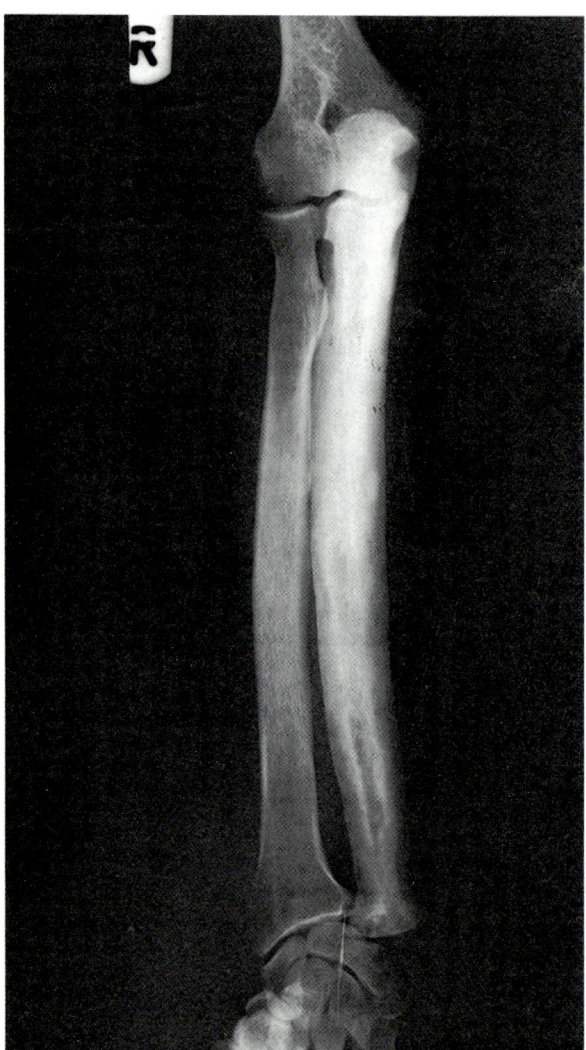

Q1a.

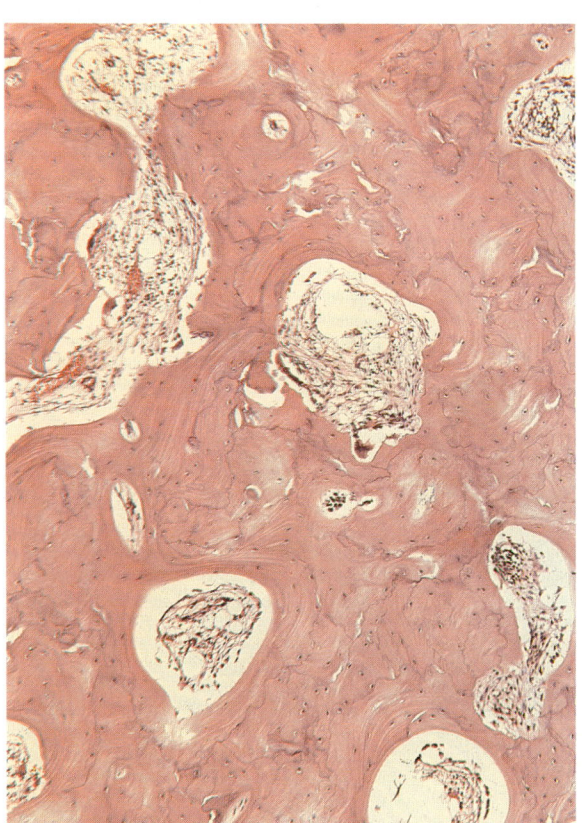

Q1b. (×64)

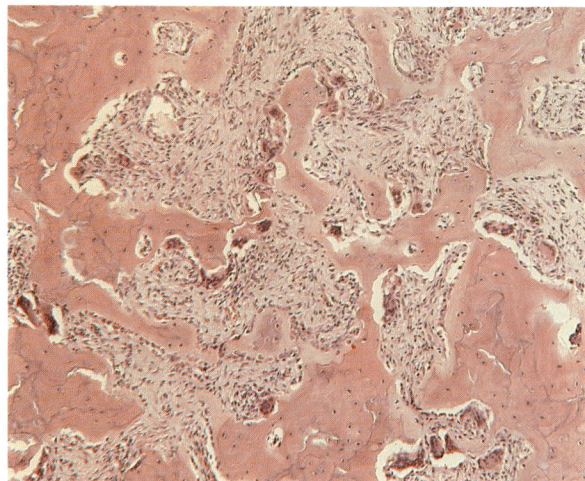

Q1c. (×64)

Q2. This patient, a woman aged 57 years, presented with a history of pain in the leg for 3 months.

Clinical examination revealed anterior bowing of the tibia, which was associated with an area of warmth and localised tenderness over the proximal portion of the subcutaneous surface of the bone.

Radiological examination showed that the anterior tibial bowing coincided with an abnormal texture of the bone extending over almost half its length and confined largely to its anterior aspect. The proximal and distal ends of the tibia appeared normal. In the frontal projection particularly an oval lytic zone was evident.

A biopsy was performed.

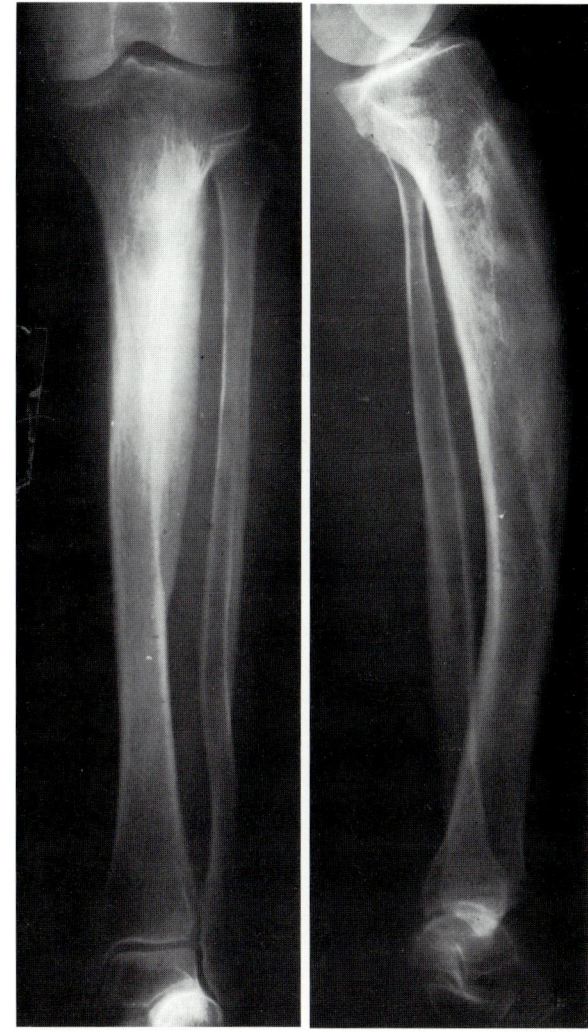

Q2a.

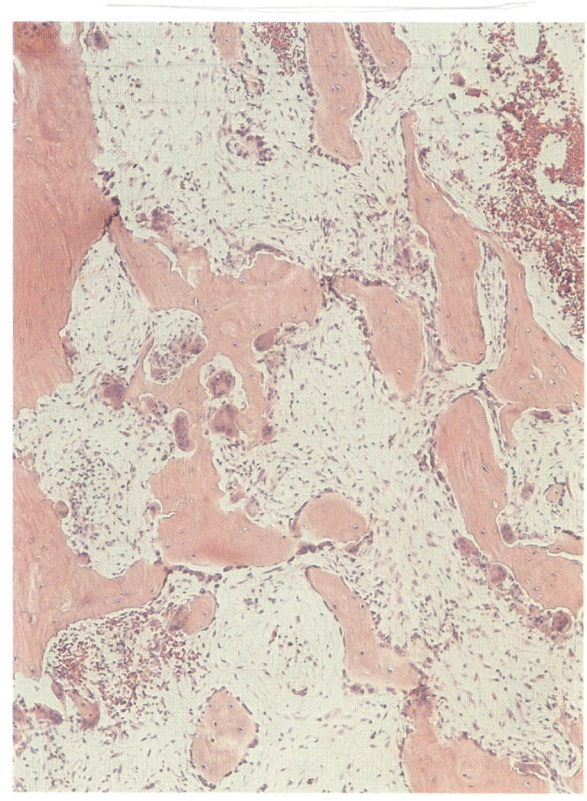

Q2b. (×56)

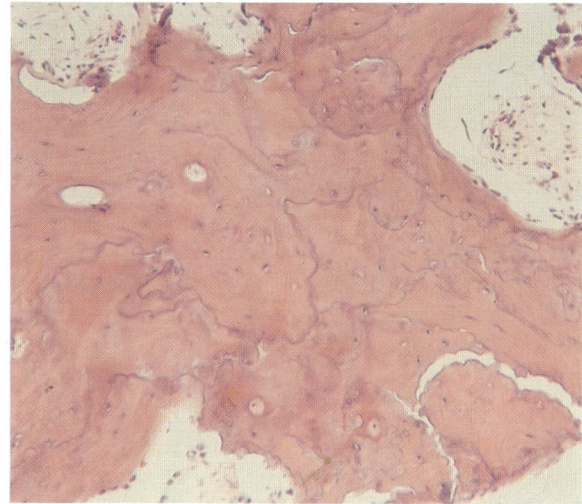

Q2c. (×82)

A1. Paget's disease of ulna

The radiological changes in Paget's disease, in the vast majority of cases, are virtually pathognomonic, so that opportunities for histological study of excised or biopsy specimens are infrequent. In this instance the overgrowth of the affected bone, both in length and in width, is characteristic, especially when coupled with extreme cortical thickening, narrowing of the medullary cavity and a coarse trabecular pattern.

The histological findings confirm the diagnosis of Paget's disease. Q1b shows the thickened bone trabeculae which are responsible for the radiological appearance of coarse trabeculation and increased density. These structures also present the mosaic pattern of cement lines which is characteristic of this disorder. The numerous cement lines indicate abnormally active bone remodelling. Q1c illustrates the active osteoclasts and osteoblasts which are responsible for this process. The spaces between the bony structures are occupied by fibrous tissue.

A2. Paget's disease of tibia

Pre-operatively several possible diagnoses were considered in this case, including fibrous dysplasia, sarcomatous change in a benign fibrous lesion and hyperparathyroidism. The last was excluded by normal serum calcium and phosphorus estimations, but a clue to the correct diagnosis was provided by a serum alkaline phosphatase value of 80 KA units (575 IU/litre), the increased value indicating an increased rate of bone formation. This radiological appearance in Paget's disease is distinctly unusual, as involvement of bone in this disease is almost always subarticular in location. Nevertheless, since 1967, when this case was originally studied, the authors have observed similar patterns in a small number of patients (tibia 6, fibula 1 and humerus 1).

The histological findings were most instructive. The biopsy material showed clearly the histological changes of Paget's disease. Q2b, from an area of altered cancellous bone from the deep part of the lesion, shows newly formed bone trabeculae whose surfaces are covered with osteoblasts and osteoclasts, the latter situated in eroded Howship's lacunae. The space between the trabeculae, normally filled with fatty or haemopoietic marrow, is occupied by spindle-celled fibrous tissue. Q2c is from an area of denser bone in the region of the original cortex. It shows the mosaic pattern of cement lines which is characteristic of Paget's disease. Each irregular cement line marks the site of a previous resorption surface where osteoclastic activity has been followed by osteoblastic bone formation. The number, and the arrangement, of the cement lines is a reflection of the activity of bone remodelling in Paget's disease.

Paget's Disease

Paget's disease is a condition of unknown aetiology, occurring almost exclusively in individuals over 40 years of age and characterised by enlargement and deformity of various bones. The incidence of Paget's disease varies greatly in different parts of the world. For example, the highest incidence in Britain is in a small area around Manchester. Relatively few cases have been reported in African or Asian populations. In Britain, radiological evidence of Paget's disease is encountered, often incidentally, in about 2% of people over the age of 55 years. In some cases only a single bone is affected; in others, many bones are involved.

Clinical Features

The disease is frequently diagnosed as an incidental radiological finding in the complete absence of clinical symptoms and signs. Less frequently deformity, such as bowing of the legs or, classically, enlargement of the skull, draws attention to the condition. These deformities are due essentially to relative softening of bone due to the remodelling process. They include protrusio acetabuli, engendering degenerative hip disease; basilar impression of the skull, causing cranial nerve pressure symptoms; vertebral collapse, producing spinal root pressure symptoms; and, even, occasionally paraplegia. From such lesions pain caused by pressure on nerves is common, but pain may be due to the bone disease itself, being constant, unremittent and worse at night. Fractures of the weakened bone, often spontaneous and unexpected, represent another cause of recognition of the disorder. They may be complete, incomplete or of an avulsion type at sites of muscular attachment. The innumerable microscopic arteriovenous shunts, in the presence of widespread skeletal involvement, are reputed to precipitate high output cardiac failure, but in practice this complication is distinctly unusual.

Paget's disease is an important precancerous condition, being associated with an increased incidence of primary malignant tumours of bone. Paget's sarcoma is discussed in another Exercise. It is a rare complication of Paget's disease, affecting fewer than 1% of symptomatic cases.

Radiological Features

1. Site. Any bone can be affected. The axial skeleton, including the vertebrae, the pelvis and particularly the sacrum are involved most commonly; other sites include the skull and major long bones, especially the tibia and the femur. Anterior bowing of the tibia and antero-lateral bowing of the femur are characteristic features of the fully developed form of the disease. Such bowing of the long bones of the lower limbs is probably attributable to the effect of weight-bearing on bones of reduced strength. Isolated lesions may be observed occasionally in the small bones of the hands and feet.

2. Appearance. These features depend on the phase of the disorder at the time of the initial presentation. In the earlier, or 'active' phase an expansile area of lucency is evident, often causing enlargement of the affected bone. As the years pass the development of appositional bone produces the much more common 'mixed' or 'combined' phase in which the bone texture is abnormally coarse. The appearance, ultimately, is that of widespread and dense sclerosis, representing the 'amorphous' phase of the disease. Serial studies over many years can show slow extension of the lesion and transition from the active to the combined or amorphous phase.

In long bones, particularly, Paget's disease is almost invariably subarticular in location, extending along the shaft to terminate in a sharply demarcated 'flame-shaped' margin. Only a few exceptions to this rule, largely involving lesions of the mid-shaft of the tibia, as in Q2, have been observed. These features, coupled with overgrowth of the affected area, usually permit a confident radiological diagnosis. The abnormal bones are brittle. Increment fractures often develop on the convex aspects of bowing deformities and complete fractures may occur spontaneously and are characteristically transverse in type.

In the axial skeleton, the pelvis and vertebrae are frequently involved. In a single vertebra a lesion in the active phase may simulate closely the coarse vertical striation of a *haemangioma*, but even then some overgrowth usually provides a diagnostic clue. In the mixed phase a typical 'picture-frame' of density constitutes one of the classical appearances. The complications of protrusio acetabuli, compression of vertebral bodies and basilar invagination of the skull, all due to the fragility of the pathological bone, have been noted. The clearly defined osteolytic lesions in the skull, designated as *osteoporosis circumscripta*, represent the active phase of the disease. In this instance, too, slow progression to the mixed phase, with focal areas of sclerosis and marked overgrowth of the vault, may be observed. The sclerotic phase in elderly men may evoke difficulty in differentiation from prostatic metastases. The latter, however, are usually multiple and do not cause bony enlargement. A vertebral lesion of this type usually can be distinguished from a metastasis or Hodgkin's disease in the same way.

Pathological Features

Histologically, the lesions of Paget's disease show disordered and extremely active bone remodelling. The basic abnormality appears to be an increase in osteoclastic resorption, which is followed by active osteoblastic bone formation, and these two processes continue while the lesion remains active. The bone, initially porotic, becomes increasingly dense and develops the mosaic pattern of cement lines which is pathognomonic of the condition. The bone marrow in the affected areas becomes replaced by vascular fibrous tissue. Some lesions, which may be presumed to have reached a quiescent stage, have plentiful mosaic areas, but lack active remodelling.

When the distinctive pattern of cement lines, recognised in 1932 by Schmorl, is present, a specific histological diagnosis of Paget's disease can be made. A somewhat similar pattern of cement lines sometimes may be produced by a local disturbance of remodelling in other conditions, such as osteomyelitis or osteoarthritis, but the number and the irregularity of the cement lines in these conditions is not usually so great. In lesions of undoubted Paget's disease, however, one not infrequently encounters areas, as in Q2b, where the typical pattern is not present. This is because the abnormal trabeculae have not yet undergone enough alternating cycles of resorption and formation to produce the characteristic pattern. On a purely histological level, particularly in a limited biopsy specimen, difficulty can arise sometimes in distinguishing between the changes of Paget's disease and hyperparathyroidism (discussed elsewhere in this volume), but radiological and biochemical investigations usually help to make the diagnosis clear.

The increased activity of skeletal remodelling in Paget's disease is reflected in a high rate of skeletal accretion of calcium, and the lesions consequently appear active with radionuclide scanning. Serum alkaline phosphatase values are elevated, indicating increased osteoblastic function, while serum calcium and phosphate levels are normal. The urinary excretion of hydroxyproline, derived from the breakdown of collagen, is increased. The finding, on electron microscopy, of virus-like inclusions in the nuclei of osteoclasts in Paget's disease has prompted interest in the possibility of an infective basis for this fascinating disorder, for which the aetiology still remains to be established. It is, indeed, of interest to recall that the pathological report in the first case reported by Sir James Paget in 1877 stated 'The whole microscopical architecture of the bone has been altered; the structure appears to have been almost entirely removed and laid down afresh on a different plan and in a larger mould', a statement which is still valid.

Treatment

Treatment is essentially conservative. Pain in Paget's disease is the principal indication for therapy. In the past, medical treatment has been protean.

At the present time, three drugs are utilised in an attempt to suppress osteoclastic bone resorption and to prevent excessive and uncontrolled osteoblastic bone formation. These are calcitonin, diphosphonates and mithramycin.

The calcitonins are polypeptides produced by the parafollicular or C cells of mammalian and human thyroids and by the ultimobranchial bodies in the fish. A synthetic salmon calcitonin is most commonly used. It is effective in relieving pain within the first 6 weeks of subcuticular or intramuscular injections. Radiological and histological improvement is reported as a sequel to long-term therapy (Bijvoet et al.). The dose varies between 100 i.v. daily and 50–100 i.v. three times a week. Adverse effects include nausea, flushing, peripheral paraesthesia and occasional diarrhoea.

Diphosphonates are analogues of pyrophosphate; resistant to naturally occurring enzymes, they are essentially bone crystal poisons. They also inhibit bone turnover and disorganised bone remodelling. Presently, sodium etidronate (EHDP) is used at a dosage of 5–10 mg/kg body weight. Dichloromethylene diphosphonate (Cl_2MDP) and 3-amino-1-hydroxypropylidene-1, 1-diphosphonate (APD) are still the subjects of clinical trials.

Mithramycin is a cytotoxic antibiotic which is used experimentally because it has a rapid biochemical effect and reduces severe pain; it has still to be authorised for general use.

Calcitonin and diphosphonate, in particular, can be monitored by the early fall in the excretion of urinary hydroxyproline and the subsequent suppression of the raised alkaline phosphate level.

In general, the younger the age of onset the more rapid the progression of the disease. For this reason, disease which causes symptoms in the young individual requires vigorous treatment.

Paget's disease and cardiac failure in the elderly are common and usually unrelated. Both calcitonin and EHDP reduce the cardiac output when this is raised and, further, calcitonin accelerates sodium loss.

Chemotherapy is indicated in patients with cranial nerve compression and paraparesis, but because its efficacy remains to be established, neurosurgical decompression should not be delayed.

Healing of pathological fractures may be normal or delayed. Because of the effects of calcitonin and diphosphonates there are theoretical reasons for withholding these medications if fractures occur, although, in practice, calcitonin injections are usually continued.

The value of orthopaedic, surgical intervention remains to be established. Techniques directed toward the correction of deformities occurring in this disease may or may not be successful. Results appear to be related to the degree of activity of the disease in the affected bone and the rate of bone turnover. The outcome of surgical procedures may be prejudged in relation to the level of activity indicated by isotope scanning. Joint replacement relieves pain when secondary osteoarthritis has occurred. Depending on the extent of the disease in individual bones, it may be necessary to use either extended or custom built prostheses.

References

Barker DJP, Clough PWL, Guyer PB, Gardner MJ (1977) Paget's disease of bone in 14 British towns. Br Med J 1: 1181–1183

Bijvoet OLM, Hosking DJ, Herman HPJ, Reitsma PH, Frijlink (1978) In: Copp DH, Talmage RV (eds) Endocrinology of calcium metabolism. Excerpta Medica, Amsterdam Oxford

Deuxchaisnes CN de, Krane SM (1964) Paget's disease of bone: clinical and metabolic observations. Medicine (Balt): 43: 233–266

Hamdy RC (1981) Paget's disease of bone. Assessment and management. Praeger, Norwich

Meunier P, Edouard C, Bernard J (1974) Histologie quantitative et dynamique de l'os pagetique. Acta Orthop Belg 40: 351–362

Paget J (1877) On a form of chronic inflammation of bones (osteitis deformans). Trans R Med Clin Soc Lond 60: 37–64

Rebel A, Malkani K, Basale M, Bregon C (1976) Osteoclast ultrastructure in Paget's disease. Calcif Tissue Res 20: 187–199

Schmorl G (1932) Über Ostitis deformans Paget. Virchows Arch 283: 694–751

Singer FR (1977) Human calcitonin treatment of Paget's disease of bone. Clin Orthop 127: 86–93

Univ. York (5–7 April 1981) Diphosphonates and Paget's disease of bone. Symposium published in Metabolic Bone Disease and Related Research, 3, nos. 4 and 5, pp 217–335

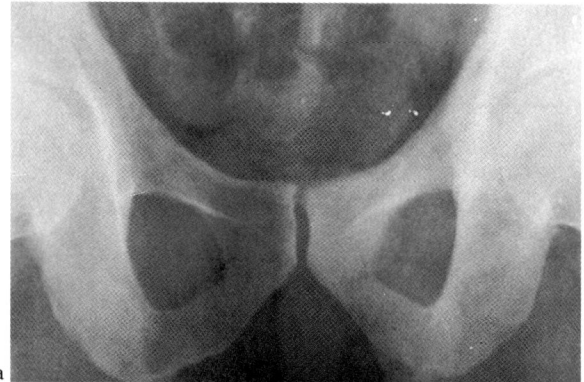
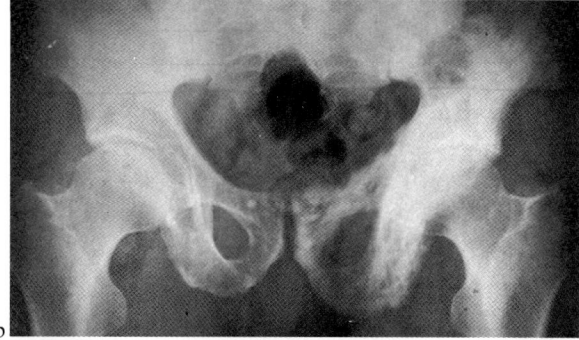
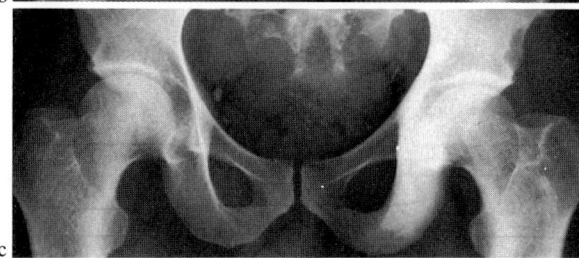

Fig. 1.1. *Paget's disease—various forms.* **a** *Active (early) phase.* Incidental findings in a 48-year-old man with backache. The left ischium is enlarged with some coarsening of texture. Thickening of the left iliopectineal line provides an early and diagnostic sign of the disease. **b** *Mixed (combined) phase.* This 64-year-old man had complained of pain in the left hip for 1 year. The entire left innominate bone is larger than its counterpart, with a very coarse trabecular pattern. Softening of the bone has resulted in an early protrusio acetabuli deformity and thickening of the iliopectineal line is evident again. **c** *Amorphous (sclerotic) phase.* The enlargement and diffuse increase of density of the left ischium was detected in an elderly man with backache attributed to a similar lesion in the body of L4. Hodgkin's disease or prostatic metastases were suspected, but histologically Paget's disease was established. In our experience transition from the mixed phase to the amorphous phase is observed very rarely.

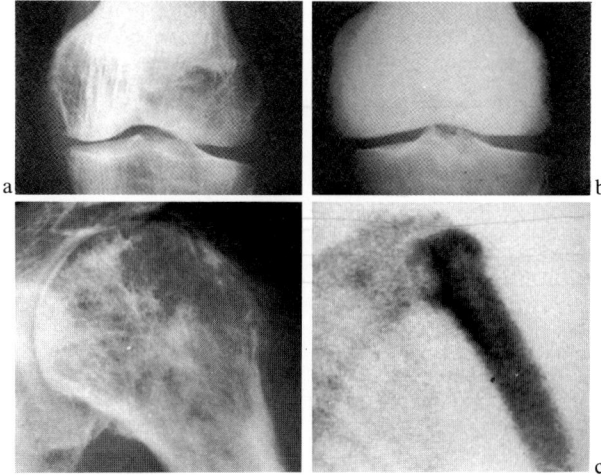

Fig. 1.2. *Paget's disease.* **a** *Distal end of femur. Active form* with coarse trabeculation and **b** *amorphous form* with extreme increase of density—a much rarer manifestation. In each case the lesions are subarticular. **c** *Humerus. Mixed form* with typical increase of uptake on radionuclide scanning.

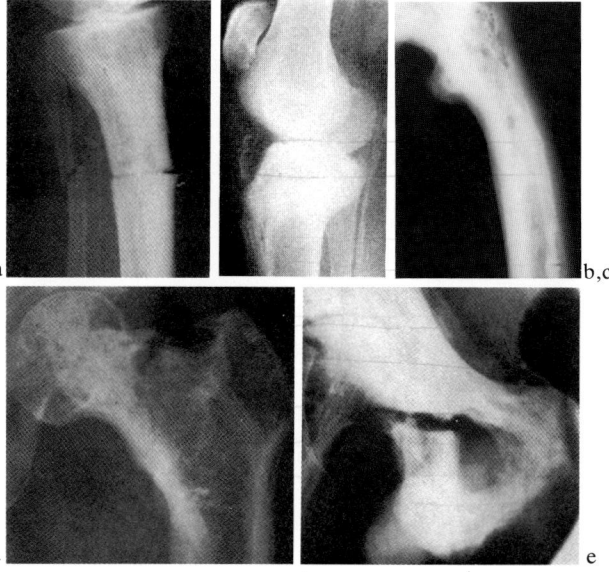

Fig. 1.3. *Injuries to the brittle bone of Paget's disease*—often a cause of clinical presentation. **a** Typical and spontaneous *transverse ('banana') fracture* of tibia. Contrast the oblique fracture through the normal bone of the fibula. **b** *Avulsion injury* of tibial tuberosity. Observe 'flame-shaped' demarcation of the abnormal bone. **c** *Increment fractures* on the convex aspect of a femur bowed by the disease. **d** *Stress fracture* of femoral neck. **e** *Transverse fracture* of ischium. This fracture occurred in an elderly man while tying a shoelace and was the first indication of Paget's disease.

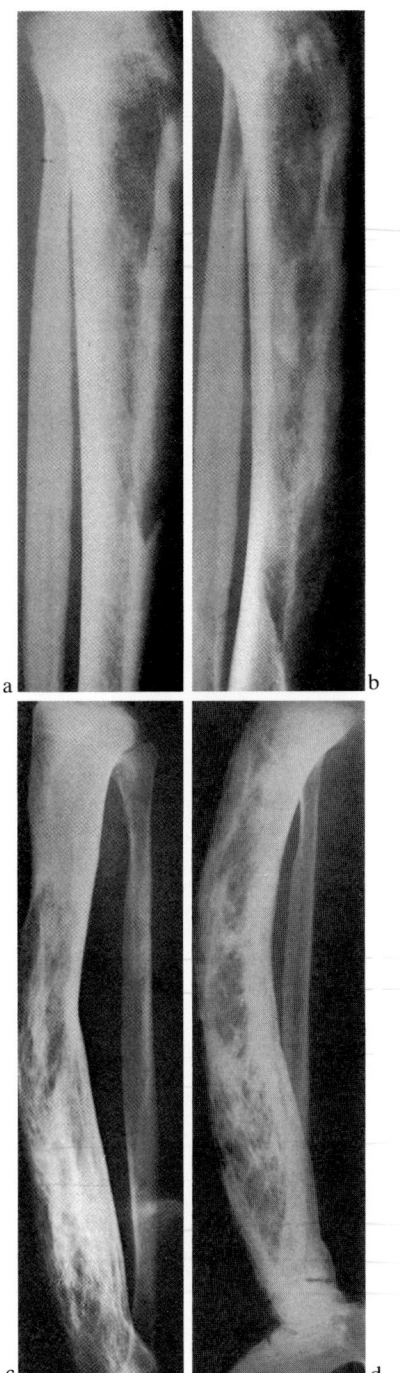

Fig. 1.4. *Paget's disease of tibia.* These characteristic examples of expansion of the affected bone, with coarse trabeculation and typical 'flame-shaped' margins of demarcation, illustrate progession of the disease: **a** 49-year-old woman; **b** same woman 7 years later; **c** 28-year-old man (the disease is extremely rare at this age); **d** same man 10 years later when typical bowing had developed. Much more often follow-up studies indicate the disease to be static.

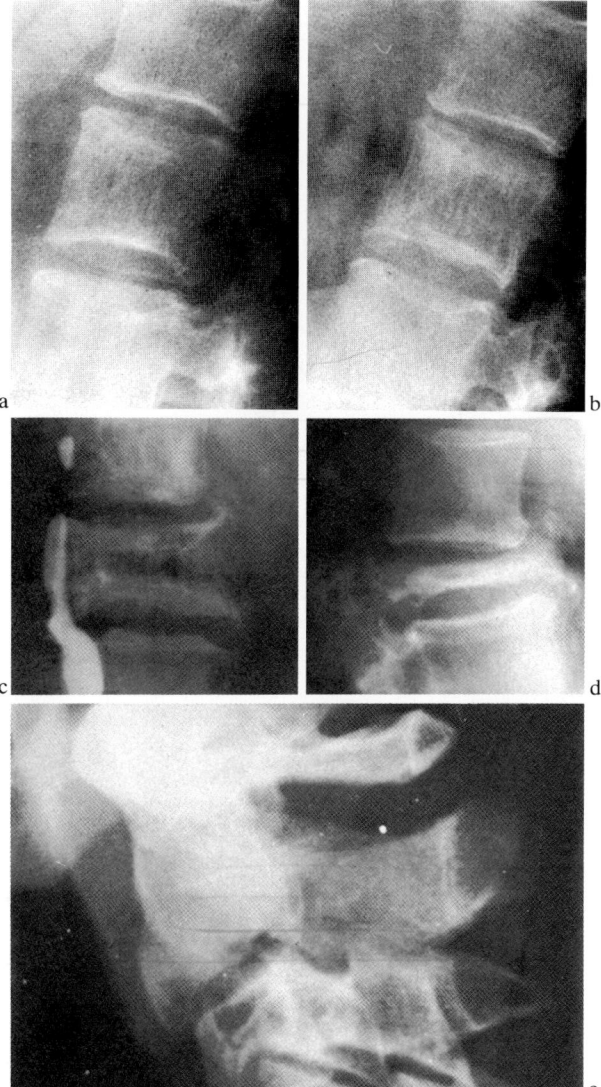

Fig. 1.5. *Paget's disease—spinal lesions.* **a, b** Another unusual example of progression from the early active phase to the mixed phase. This 52-year-old woman's back pain had subsided at the time of the examination 6 years later, when the classical enlargement and 'picture-frame' appearance had developed. Initially the changes simulated a haemangioma of L3. **c** Gross involvement of L3 in this 58-year-old man with back pain for 7 years had caused encroachment on the spinal canal. **d** Marked vertebra plana deformity of L2 due to more severe collapse of softened bone in a 47-year-old woman with back pain for 1 year. The coarse pattern of the disease extended into the neural arch. The body of T11 was affected similarly in this patient. **e** A less common example of the amorphous form affecting and enlarging the body of C2 in a 38-year-old man with pain in the neck. The diagnosis was established histologically.

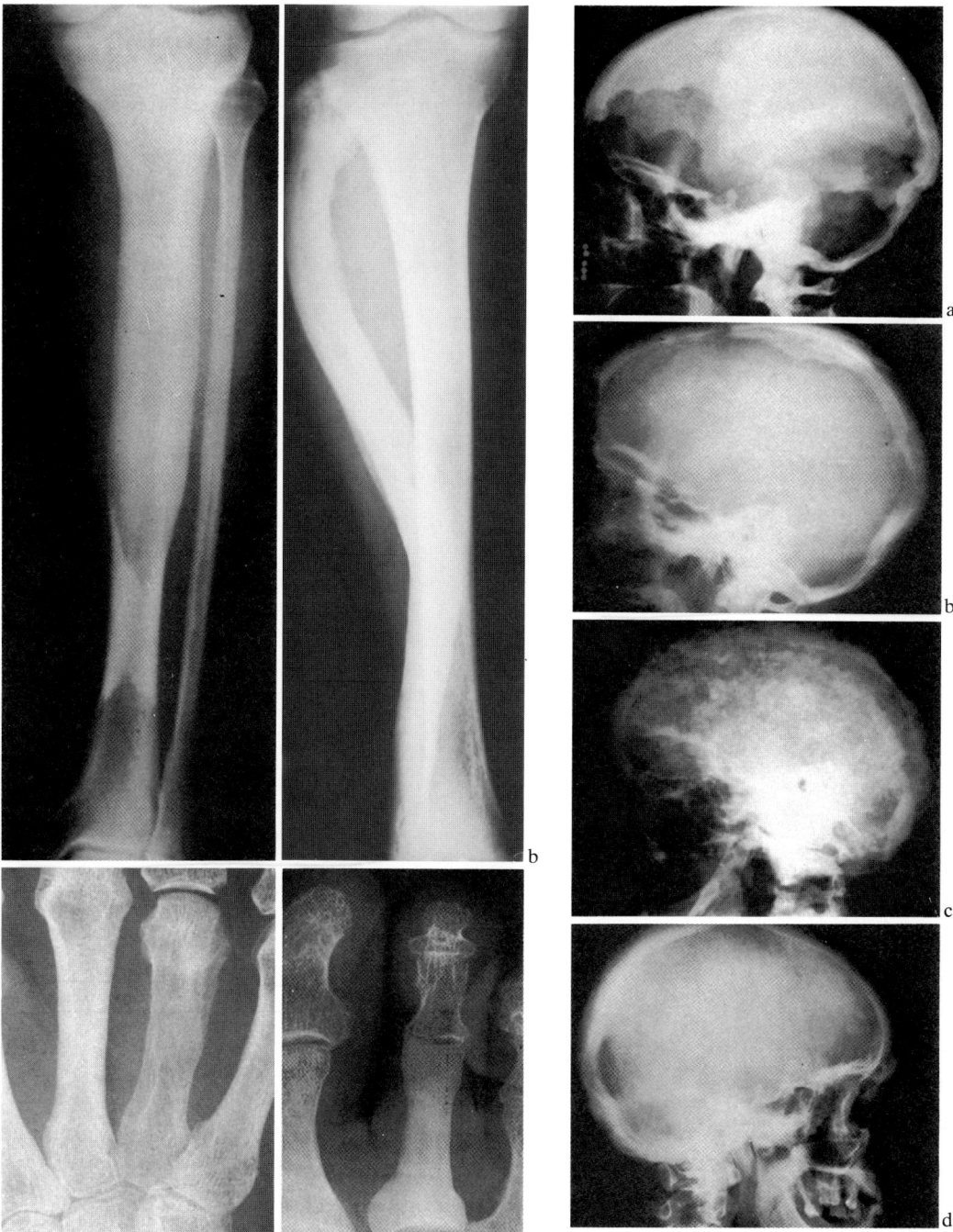

Fig. 1.6. *Paget's disease—unusual manifestations and sites.* **a** *Tibia*, with involvement of both ends of the bone by the active phase and well-demarcated 'flame-shaped' margins of the areas of disease. **b** *Fibula*, with deformity of this paired bone due to overgrowth in relation to the tibia. **c** *4th metacarpal*—active phase in a 50-year-old woman with localised pain. **d** *Proximal phalanx of 2nd toe*—an incidental finding of the amorphous form in an elderly woman. Observe bony enlargement in each of these examples of the disease. *Any* bone can be affected.

Fig. 1.7. *Paget's disease—skull.* **a, b** Progression of the *active* phase—*osteoporosis circumscripta*—over 10 years in a 68-year-old woman presenting with headache. **c** *Mixed* form with some degree of basilar impression. **d** *Amorphous* form in an elderly patient with widespread disease.

Exercise 9

Q1. This 67-year-old man presented on account of a swelling in the right popliteal fossa. This swelling had been present for many years and had enlarged slowly. It had caused no significant pain except on forced flexion of the knee.

On clinical examination the swelling was found to be hard and slightly mobile, but was not significantly tender. Flexion of the affected knee was limited to 90°, but no crepitus was elicited. No other clinical abnormality was detected. All routine investigations were negative.

Radiographs showed the swelling to be bilobular, clearly defined and to contain a multitude of calcific densities.

Surgical excision of the lesion was undertaken.

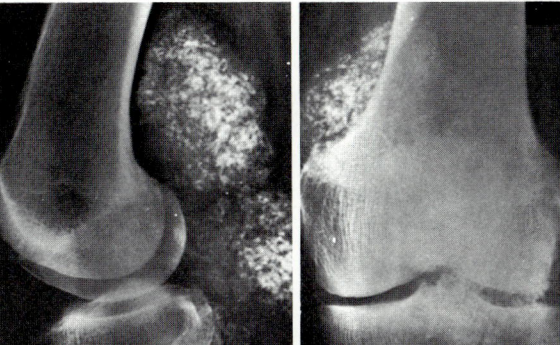

Q1a.

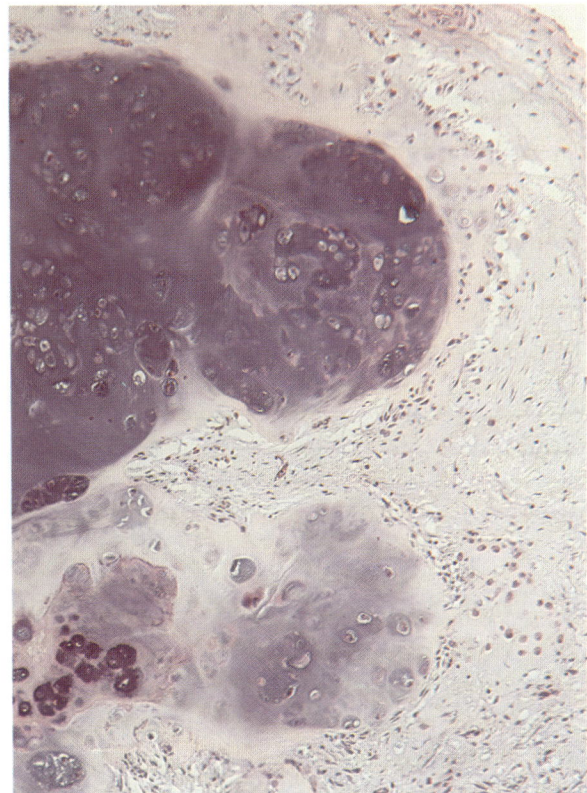

Q1b. (×100)

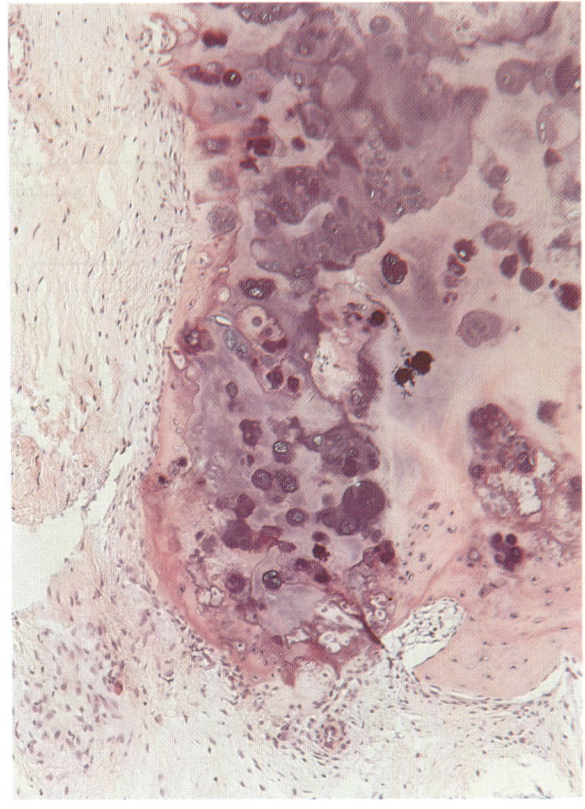

Q1c. (×90)

A1. Synovial chondromatosis in semimembranosus (Baker's) cyst

The relatively minor symptoms and signs caused by the swelling, coupled with the long history of its existence, suggested a benign lesion. The numerous opacities demonstrated radiologically were similar in size and were situated outside the joint. The bilobular pattern indicated them to be contained within a semimembranosus or adventitious bursa. The diagnosis of synovial chondromatosis confined to such a synovial structure was confirmed macroscopically at operation, when the entire cyst was dissected and excised without difficulty. On division of the mass, numerous nodules of bluish cartilaginous tissue of firm consistency were found within its wall, but many had separated to become loose.

The histological appearance also was characteristic of synovial chondromatosis. Small nodules of cartilage were separated by fibrous tissue and some synovially lined spaces could be identified. Many of the cartilaginous nodules were calcified, staining a deep blue colour, while others, without calcification, stained a lighter blue (Q1b). In some, however, as in Q1c, evidence was present not only of calcification, but also of endochondral ossification. The appearance of some of the intervening strands of fibrous tissue suggests conversion of fibroblasts to cartilage cells, indicating true cartilaginous metaplasia. Although these features are evident in Q1b, they are demonstrated even more clearly in Fig. 1.1.

Synovial Chondromatosis

This unusual disorder of synovial tissue, regarded by some as a benign neoplasm, is characterised by the development of multiple cartilaginous bodies arising from metaplasia of the subserous layer of the internal surface of a joint capsule or other synovially lined cavities, such as bursae and tendon sheaths. Although the majority of these nodules remain attached to the synovial surface and may form large masses of solid tissue, some may separate to form loose bodies. Young and middle-aged adults particularly are affected, with an especial affinity for males.

Malignant degeneration is excessively rare, but a small number of cases of this complication have been reported.

Clinical Features

The condition tends to be indolent and virtually always is solitary. Mild and long-standing discomfort in an affected joint is the usual presenting complaint, with slowly increasing limitation of movement and the development of a localised, tender swelling. Crepitus may be elicited, especially when the

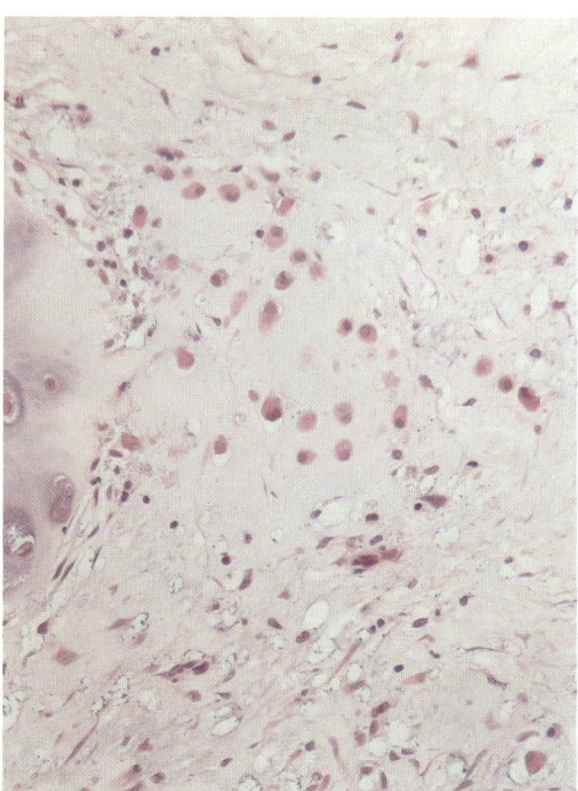

Fig. 1.1. A more enlarged field from Q1a, showing the transition from spindle-celled fibroblasts to rounded cartilage cells surrounded by cartilage matrix (cartilaginous metaplasia). (×255)

disease is sufficiently advanced for loose bodies to be present. Episodes of locking then may be reported.

Radiological Features

1. Site. Established lesions have been observed most commonly in the knee and, less often, the hip. Other major joints liable to be involved include, in decreasing order of frequency, the shoulder, elbow, ankle and wrist. Affection of small joints, bursae and tendon sheaths is distinctly unusual.

2. Appearance. The most characteristic appearance in the affected joint is the presence of small calcified opacities, related mainly to the surrounding synovium, but also within the joint itself. Such a pattern, however, is evident only in established disease. In earlier stages, accompanying the initial symptoms, diffuse peri-articular osteoporosis is likely to represent the only radiological abnormality. In cases of this type, preservation of the joint space and the articular surfaces tends to exclude an infection, but may cause the rare entity of transient osteoporosis to be considered (see Exercise 3). The cartilaginous masses which form become visible only when they calcify. Even before this stage some may have separated into the joint as loose bodies, when they may be demonstrated arthrographically as multiple filling defects. These uncalcified cartilaginous nodules may cause para-articular pressure erosions, recognisable in plain films and strongly suggestive of a synovial disorder. Pigmented villonodular synovitis then may enter the differential diagnosis.

Occasionally confusion with a chondrosarcoma has arisen, CT studies then having proved to be of considerable diagnostic value. Symptoms, however, are usually so prolonged that these synovial and intra-articular masses at least have begun to calcify when the initial radiological examination is undertaken. Faint stippled densities are then apparent, developing into rounded opacities of pathognomonic appearance. Their number may vary from a dozen to many hundreds. A diagnostic feature is their tendency to be of the same size and rarely to become larger than 2 cm in diameter, offering marked contrast to the loose bodies of degenerative joint disease. It will be recalled that the latter have an entirely different origin, developing from cartilaginous fragments separated by trauma from articular surfaces (see Exercise 5).

Pathological Features

At an early stage the synovial membrane of the affected joint may show microscopic foci of cartilaginous metaplasia. Later, rounded nodules of established cartilage are present and may continue to enlarge. These cartilaginous nodules may be located within, or attached to, the synovial membrane. Some may be loose within the joint cavity. The cartilage may undergo calcification. In nodules with a vascular attachment this calcification may be followed by endochondral bone replacement.

The cartilaginous tissue in synovial chondromatosis may be markedly cellular, so that occasionally the appearance has been regarded mistakenly as a chondrosarcoma. It lacks, however, the cellular and nuclear pleomorphism to be expected in a malignant tumour. The distinct separation of cartilaginous nodules in synovial chondromatosis contrasts with the more diffusely lobular pattern of a true cartilage tumour.

Treatment

Total synovectomy is the ideal treatment of choice, but technical difficulties often prevent the procedure from being complete, so that recurrences are not infrequent. When symptoms are mild an expectant attitude may be adopted, and simple arthrotomy and removal of offending loose bodies may permit procrastination for long periods. In some cases prosthetic replacement of the affected joint may be advisable.

References

Ginaldi S (1980) Computed tomography feature of synovial osteochondromatosis. Skeletal Radiol 5: 219–222

Kaiser TE, Ivins JC, Unni KK (1980) Malignant transformation of extra-articular synovial chondromatosis: report of a case. Skeletal Radiol 5: 223–226

Lequesne MD et al (1981) Capsular constriction of the hip: arthrographic and clinical considerations. Skeletal Radiol 6: 1–10

Milgram JW (1977) Synovial osteochondromatosis. A histopathological study of thirty cases. J Bone Jt Surg 59A: 792–801

Murphy FP, Dahlin DC, Sullivan CR (1962) Articular synovial chondromatosis. J Bone Jt Surg 44A: 77–86

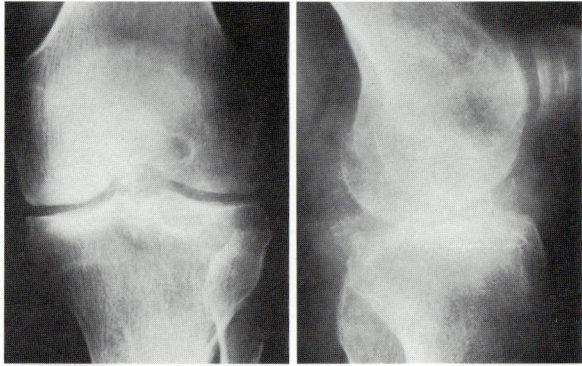
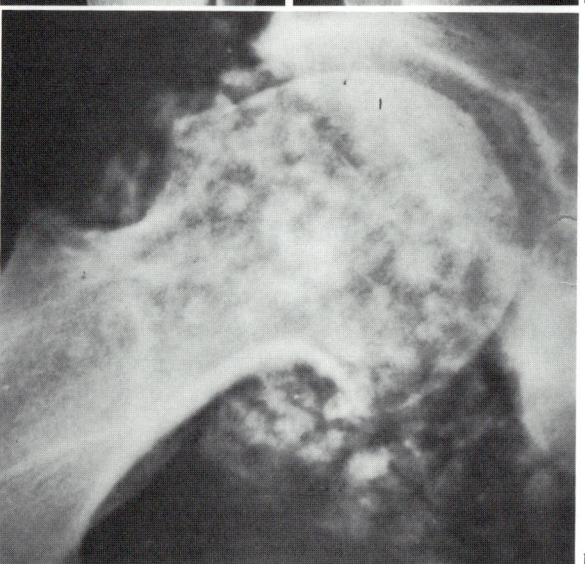

Fig. 1.3. *Synovial chondromatosis—established lesions.* **a** The knee is the most common site for this rare synovial disease. This 66-year-old man had complained of increasing pain and stiffness of the left knee for 3 years. Faint calcific densities are present within a swollen joint with a thickened capsule. Many clearly defined para-articular erosions are evident, particularly around the intercondylar notch of the femur. Extensive synovectomy relieved pain, but a fixed flexion deformity persisted. **b** The calcified densities around this painful hip in a middle-aged man represent more advanced disease. Observe their almost uniform size. The articular surfaces and the joint space, however, are well preserved.

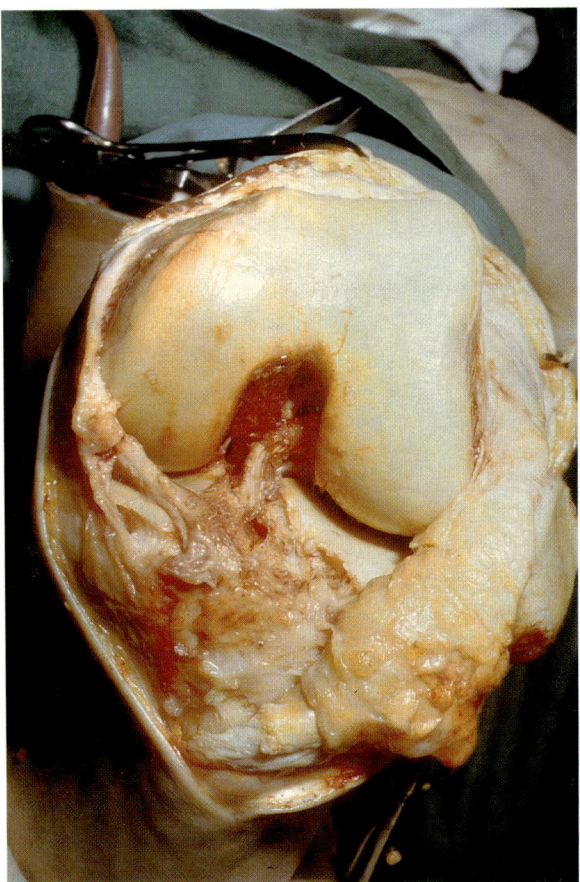

Fig. 1.2. *Synovial chondromatosis.* This knee at operation shows the destruction that can occur in a joint due to the presence of multiple loose bodies. In this instance the anterior aspect of the lateral tibial condyle and the intercondylar notch of the femur are eroded. Cartilaginous nodules are present in the thickened synovium.

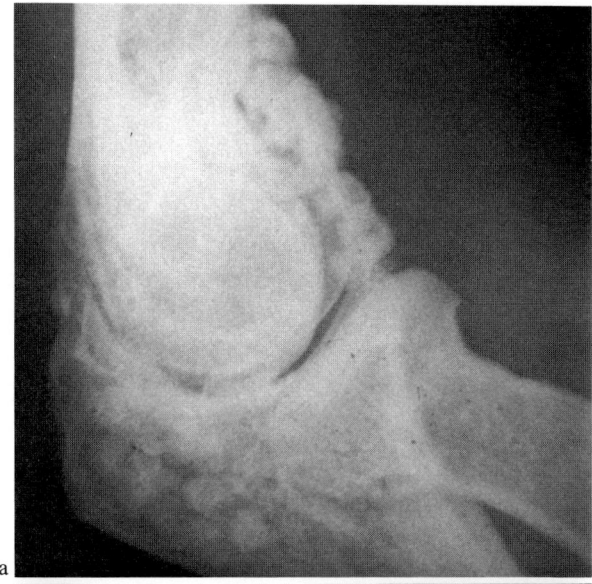
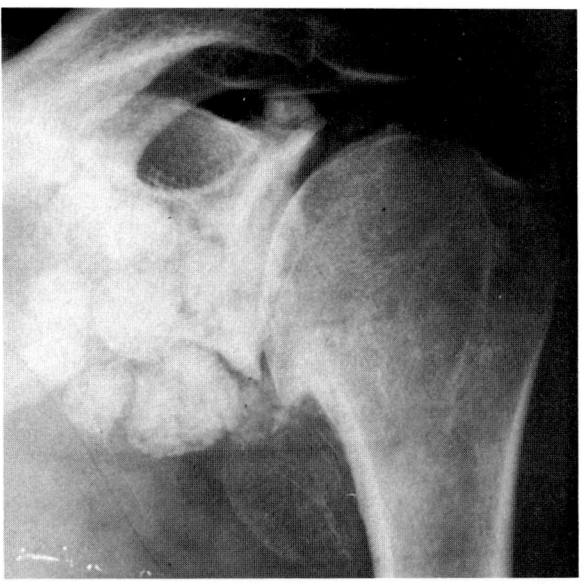

Fig. 1.4. *Synovial chondromatosis—other major joints* involved less commonly include **a** the elbow and **b** the ankle. In both these young adult men symptoms of increasing pain and stiffness had developed over many months. Operative confirmation of the diagnosis was obtained. Observe again the similarity in size of the calcified opacities. **c** Loose bodies ('joint mice') caused the same symptoms and signs in the shoulder of this 36-year-old man.

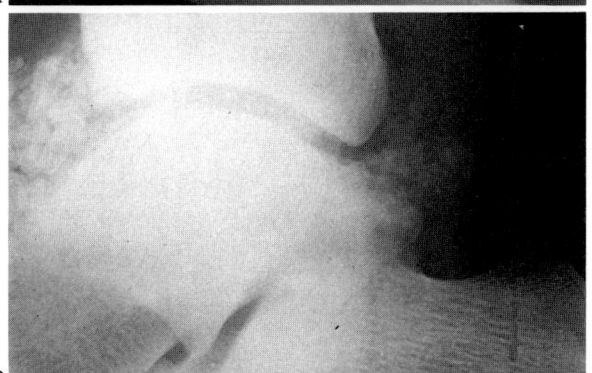

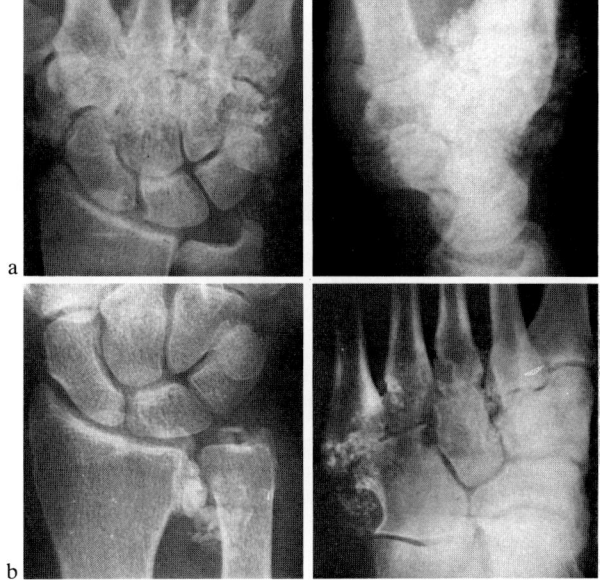

Fig. 1.5. *Synovial chondromatosis—unusual sites and manifestations.* **a** This 31-year-old man, with mild pain and stiffness of the left wrist for 3 years, responded initially to synovectomy, but a recurrence took place within a few years. Following further synovectomy he was still a competent golfer 20 years later. The multiple calcified densities are typical of the disease. **b** In this 48-year-old woman with a similar history, classical radiological features of synovial chondromatosis were confined to the right distal radio-ulnar joint. In this instance excision of the distal end of the ulna permitted synovectomy to be complete and recurrence was avoided. **c** Mild discomfort in the left foot of this young man had been present for only 6 months, but the typical multiple densities and clearly defined para-articular erosions around the tarso-metatarsal joints already presented a diagnostic radiological appearance.

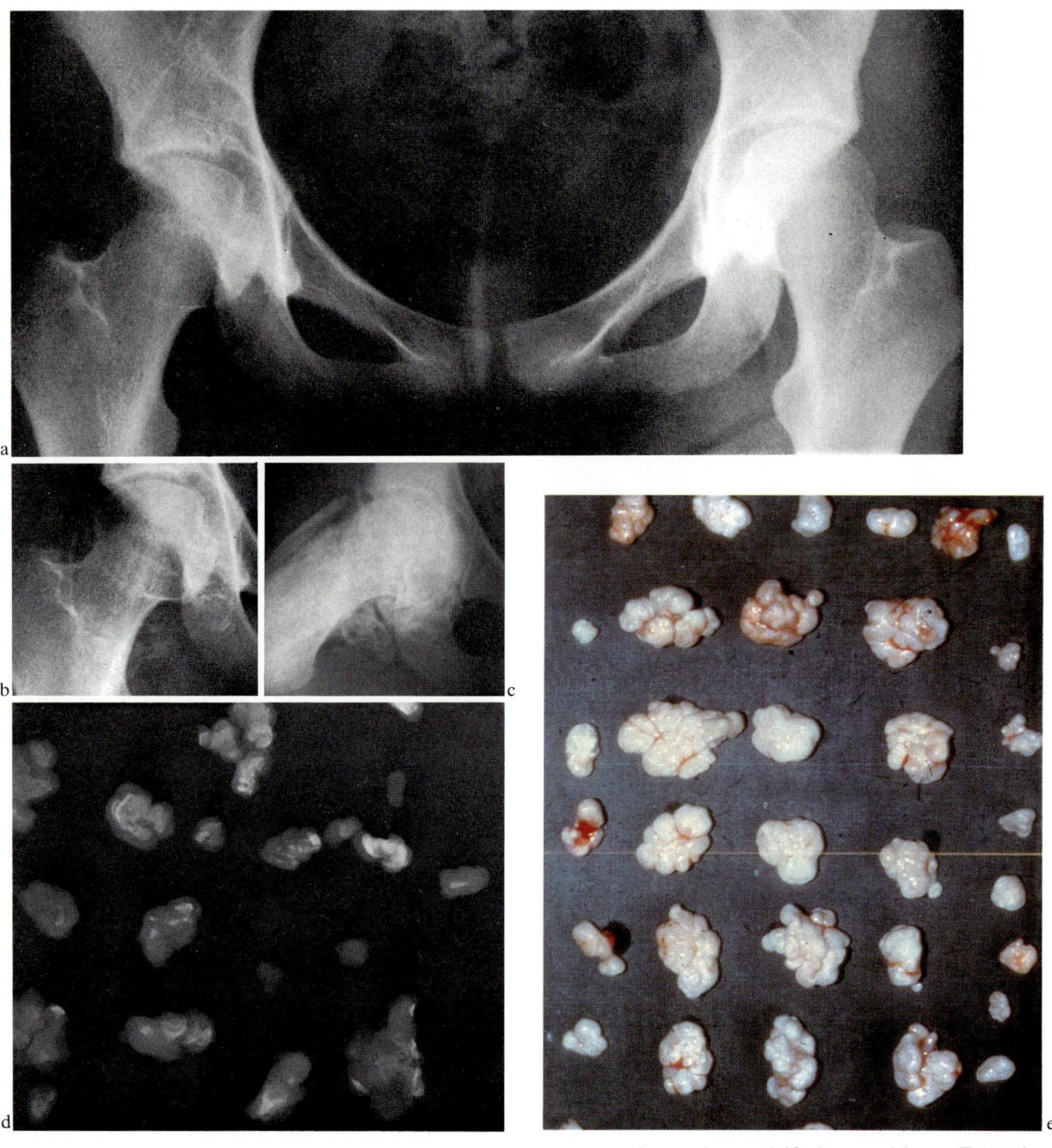

Fig. 1.6. *Synovial chondromatosis—insidious onset.* This 23-year-old woman had complained of a mild ache in the right hip for a year. The initial radiograph revealed no abnormality, but further examination on account of persistent pain 3 months later **a** showed significant demineralisation in this area. At this time the appearance was interpreted as transient osteoporosis and no specific treatment was offered. Symptoms continued and limitation of movement developed during the subsequent 18 months, when **b** typical calcification had become evident around the joint. An arthrogram **c** indicated many filling defects to be present and to be larger than the calcified opacities. Extensive synovectomy was performed with an excellent clinical result. No recurrence had taken place within the following 6 years. **d, e** The radiograph and photograph of the excised loose bodies show them to have varied considerably in size, some being approximately 2 cm in diameter. The smallest consist of uncalcified cartilage, while others of greater age contain some calcification or even endochondral ossification. The radiographic appearance of the opacities being of similar size therefore may be misleading.

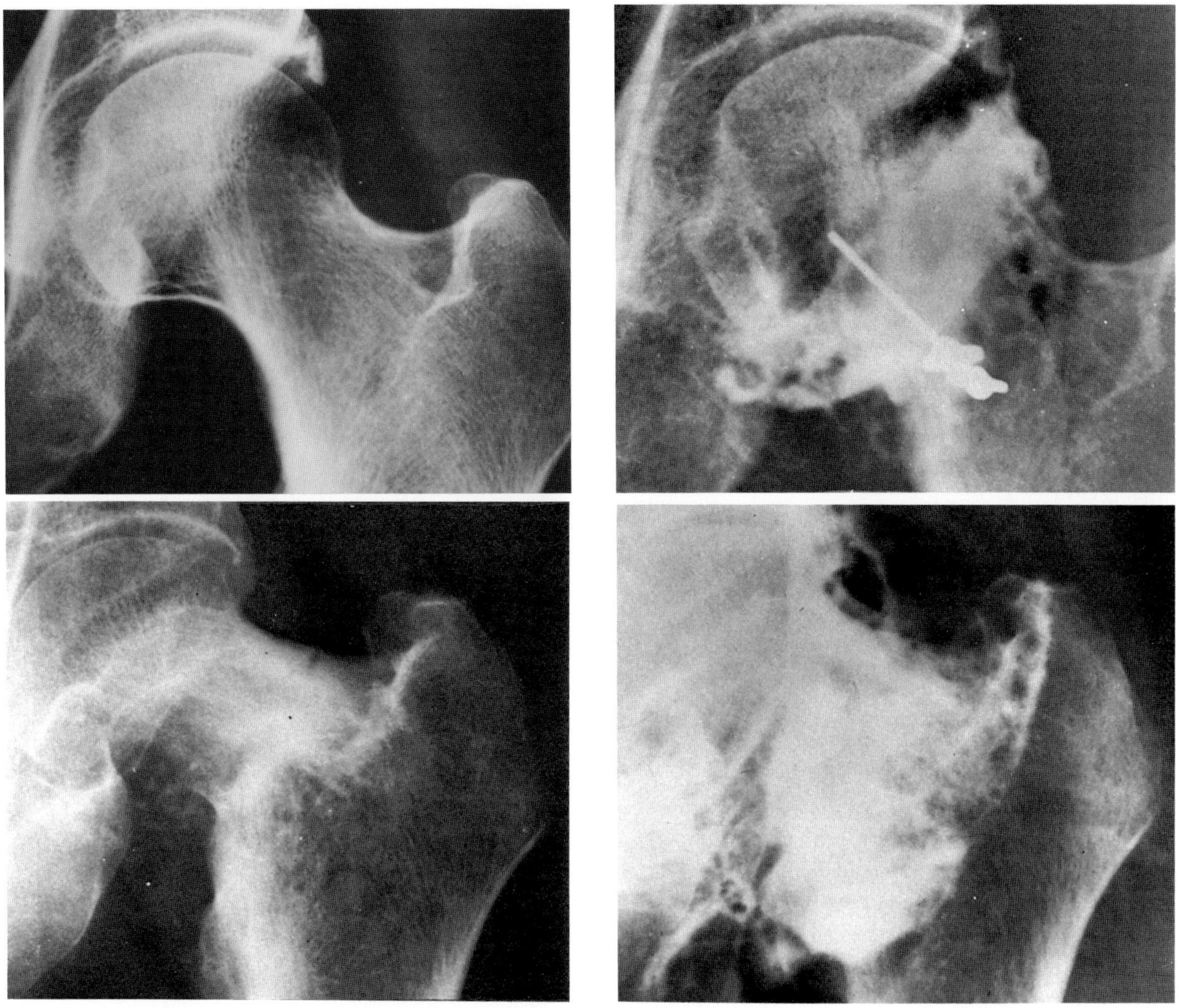

Fig. 1.7. *Synovial chondromatosis—value of arthrography.* These examples emphasise the value of this investigation. **a** This 51-year-old woman had complained of intermittent pain in the left hip for 12 years, but clinical examination revealed only slight limitation of movement. Plain films were normal, but the arthrogram showed numerous filling defects with a reduced capacity of the joint due to constriction of the capsule. **b** A constant ache around the left hip of this 48-year-old woman had been present for several years and had been exacerbated during the previous few weeks. Although the exacerbation was attributed to an obvious stress fracture of the femoral neck, the erosion on the medial side of this structure, coupled with flecks of calcification in the adjacent soft tissues, aroused clinical suspicion of a chondrosarcoma. Radiologically, however, the appearance was more suggestive of synovial chondromatosis, a diagnosis confirmed by the arthrogram. This study revealed a large number of filling defects both in the capsule and within the joint. Prosthetic replacement was performed with a satisfactory clinical result.

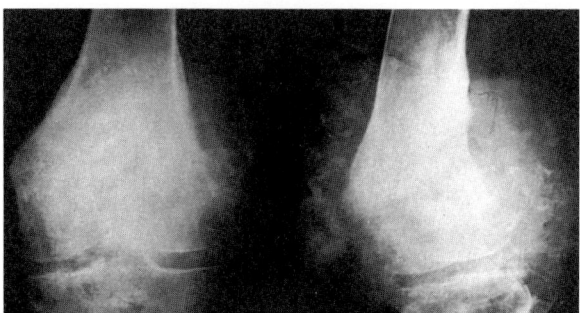

Fig. 1.8. *Synovial chondromatosis—chondrosarcomatous degeneration.* This middle-aged man developed a large and painful swelling of the left knee, superimposed on a long history of discomfort in this joint. Synovial biopsy established the chondrosarcomatous nature of the lesion. No previous radiographs had been obtained, but the presence of multiple calcified opacities and the long history of discomfort led to the belief that this case was an example of this exceedingly rare complication of synovial chondromatosis.

Q1 A 59-year-old man presented with pain and swelling of the left forearm, present for 2 weeks and increasing in severity. He had felt unwell for several weeks, following a severe cold complicated by sinusitis.

Clinical examination showed a diffuse swelling of the forearm, exquisitely tender over the mid-shaft of the ulna. Extremes of movement were painful. The clinical findings otherwise were unremarkable.

Radiologically a diffuse area of medullary osteolysis was observed in the mid-shaft of the ulna, with a wide zone of transition between normal and abnormal bone. The overlying cortex had been eroded and a pathological fracture had occurred, with separation of a bony fragment. Marked, but diffuse, swelling of the surrounding soft tissues was present, as is apparent in the soft tissue radiograph on the right.

The lesion was explored.

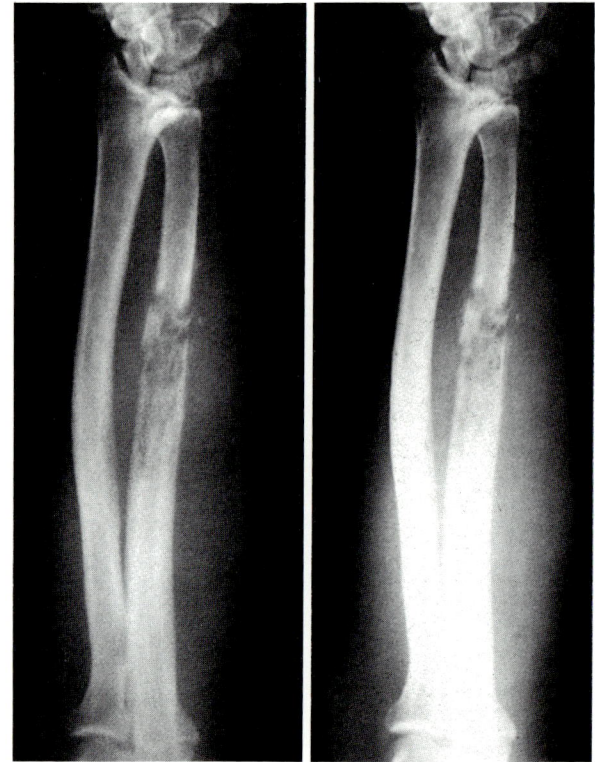

Q1a.

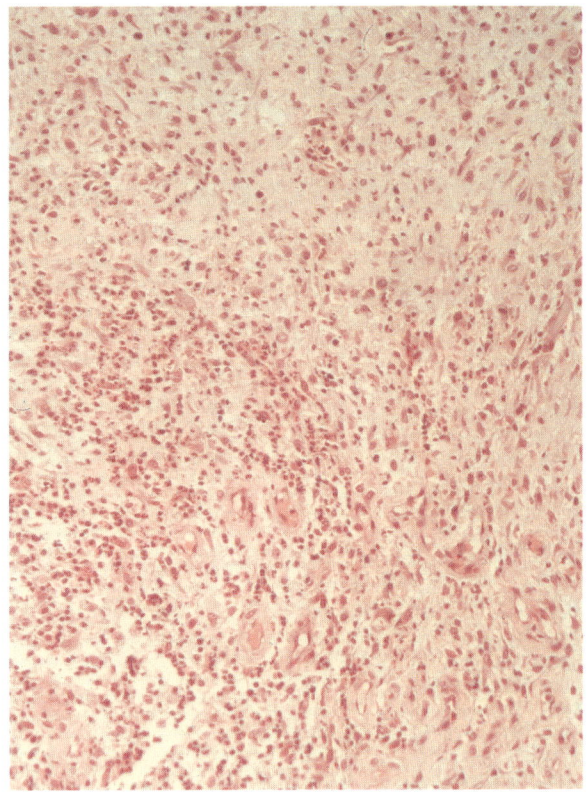

Q1b. (×140)

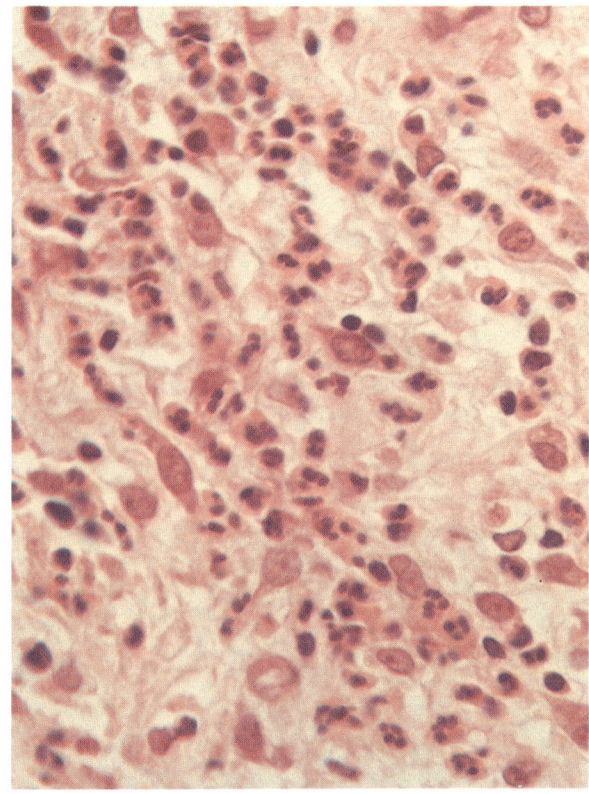

Q1c. (×560)

Exercise 10

Q2. This 36-year-old man had complained of intermittent pain around the right knee for several weeks.

On clinical examination the knee was found to be swollen and tender. Movements of the joint were limited by pain and the quadriceps muscles were wasted.

Radiologically no abnormality was detected in the knee joint itself, apart from the presence of an effusion, but a periosteal reaction was evident on the distal end of the femoral shaft, with a suggestion of diffuse medullary osteolysis in this area.

The knee joint was explored and sections from the synovium are illustrated below.

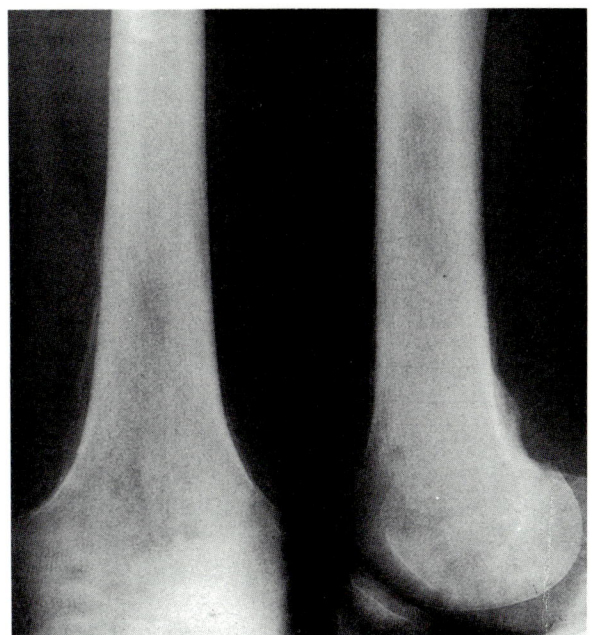

Q2a.

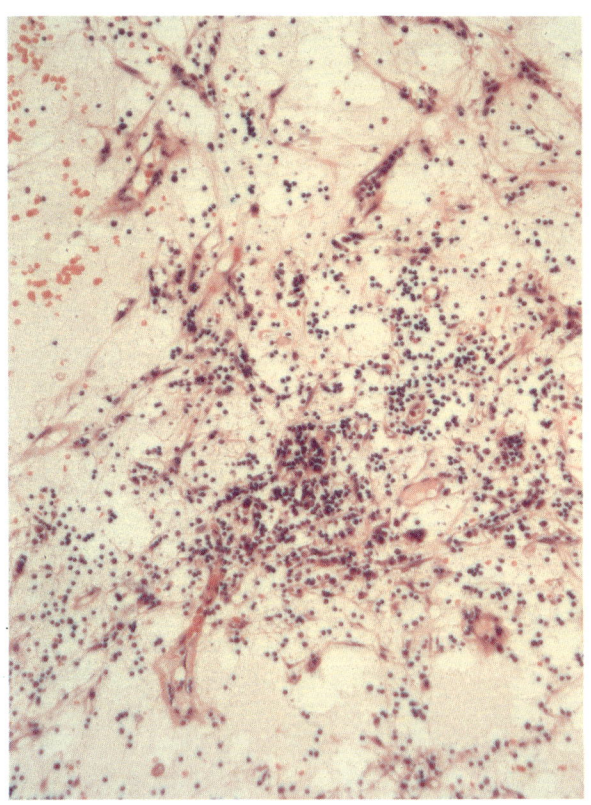

Q2b. (×140)

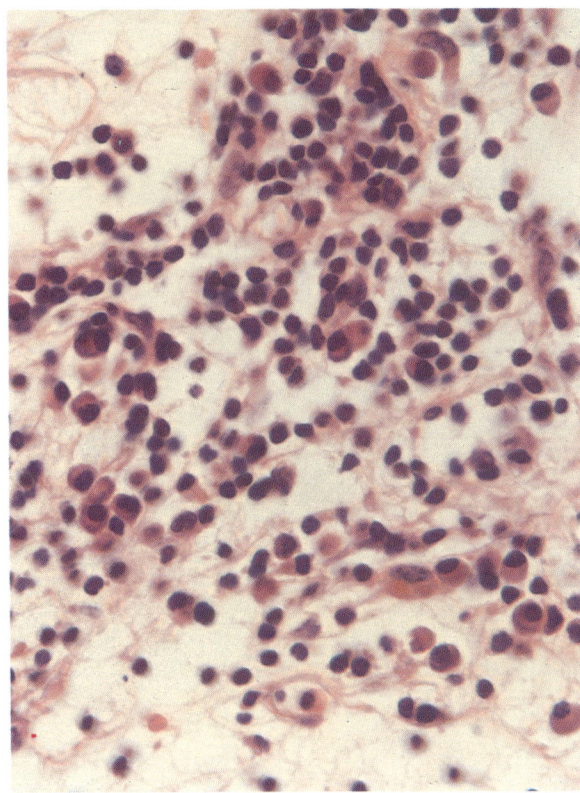

Q2c. (×560)

A1. Pyogenic osteomyelitis

The clinical and radiological features are those of an acute inflammatory lesion progressing to a chronic stage. The history of recent sinusitis is of significance with regard to the route of infection, namely haematogenous spread.

Although the patient was not febrile, his leucocyte count was 18 500 per mm^3 (80% neutrophils).

The radiographic pattern of an infiltrating medullary lesion might suggest a malignant neoplasm, but the presence of a sequestrum in relation to the pathological fracture is strongly in favour of infection. Of even more importance is the *diffuse* soft tissue swelling, which indicates the presence of extensive inflammatory oedema. Extensions of skeletal tumours into adjacent soft tissues usually have, in contrast, a clearly circumscribed peripheral margin.

The lesion was explored to obtain bacteriological confirmation of the diagnosis and to remove infected and necrotic tissue. Gram-positive cocci were identified in a stained smear from the lesion and *Staphylococcus aureus* was grown on culture. Histological examination of the tissue removed at operation shows the features of an acute inflammatory process. The abnormal tissue consists of blood vessels and inflammatory cells (Q1b). Most of the cells can be recognised by their darkly staining multilobular nuclei as polymorphs (polymorphonuclear leucocytes), although the larger nuclei of fibroblasts and endothelial cells are also evident (Q1c). In addition, lymphocytes and plasma cells are present (Fig. 1.1), the latter appearing as round mononuclear cells with well-defined basophilic cytoplasm and a paler area adjacent to the nucleus. The presence of these cells indicates that the infection already has reached a subacute or chronic stage.

Pyogenic Osteomyelitis

Suppurative (pyogenic) osteomyelitis is a frequent and important type of bone infection. It usually commences as an acute process, and in the days before specific chemotherapy was available it often continued as a long-standing chronic infection. This sequence is uncommon today, although the emergence of resistant organisms makes it an ever-present threat to the patient.

Pyogenic osteomyelitis is usually the result of haematogenous dissemination of bacteria from another lesion or portal of entry, not necessarily conspicuous. It can be caused also by the extension of a soft tissue infection to an adjacent bone or by the direct introduction of bacteria from outside the body, as in a compound fracture or a surgical procedure.

Clinical Features

Acute haematogenous osteomyelitis can occur at any age, but is most frequent in young children. In a young patient, the typical clinical features are those of an acute febrile illness, together with local pain, later accompanied by redness and swelling. Malaise, fever and leucocytosis are present. In adults these generalised symptoms and signs may be less pronounced.

The diagnosis depends ultimately on the identification of the infecting organism. This is usually the result of direct culture from the bone lesion, although blood culture may be used to provide diagnostic information in the early acute febrile stage of osteomyelitis.

In infantile septic arthritis the portal of entry of the infection is either the umbilical stump or consequent to a transfusion. Devastating destruction of the hip and, less commonly, the shoulder or other major joints, may ensue.

In children osteomyelitis favours especially the highly vascular metaphyses of long bones. By this age, the growth plate is established and provides a barrier to the spread of infection towards an adjacent epiphysis; at this stage, septic arthritis is therefore a relatively rare complication with the notable exception of the hip joint. More commonly the infection, if uncontrolled, tends to spread along the marrow cavity. It may eventually involve the whole shaft of the bone, with impairment of the blood supply and consequent necrosis. Alternatively, either with or without treatment, the infection may subside, often forming a residual localised (Brodie's) abscess. These abscesses may harbour the infecting organism during prolonged periods of quiescence lasting many years. Occasionally such infections may reactivate and become painful.

In adults axial lesions are more common, usually having their inception in an intervertebral disc. They are discussed elsewhere in this work.

It is important to appreciate that steroid therapy, by suppressing pain and leucocytic response, may be associated with silent and often severe spread of infections.

Radiological Features

1. Site. Any bone may be affected, but a predilection exists, as mentioned above, for the metaphyses of long bones in children and for the spine in adults. Pyogenic infection of joints is much less common than tuberculous infection.

2. Appearance. Acute lesions are usually associated with diffuse soft tissue swelling and obliteration of soft tissue planes. Although radionuclide scanning is positive at a very early stage, actual radiological abnormality of bone is unlikely to become evident for 7–14 days, when poorly defined medullary osteolysis and non-specific periosteal reaction may develop, frequently regressing rapidly following appropriate antibiotic therapy. In a localised lesion, a peripheral sclerotic reaction, together with an overlying maturing periosteal reaction, may indicate the formation of a Brodie's abscess. The shape of such an abscess tends to be oval or round, with finger-like projections—a valuable diagnostic sign described as 'tunnelling' and best demonstrated by tomography. The internal margin of the abscess has a clearly defined sclerotic edge. In more severe cases necrosis is followed by the formation of sequestra; these maintain their original mineral content and thus appear dense in relation to the rarefied appearance of the surrounding bone. The sequestra vary in size from small bony fragments to the entire diaphysis. In such instances massive hypertrophy of the surrounding periosteum forms an involucrum through which a transverse defect, or cloaca, may provide a channel for discharge of pus ultimately through a draining sinus.

Pathological Features

The commonest infecting organism is *Staphylococcus aureus*, although a variety of other organisms, including streptococci, *B. proteus*, *E. coli* and various salmonellae, also can be responsible. In recent years, osteomyelitis has been increasingly encountered in drug addicts, when it is often caused by *Pseudomonas aeruginosa*. Infections with organisms of the salmonella group occasionally occur in children with sickle-cell disease. Osteomyelitis may occur in infants and children with the rare 'chronic granulomatous disease', and in other conditions in which the polymorphonuclear response is impaired.

Histologically, the lesions of suppurative osteomyelitis are characterised, in the acute stage, by an abundance of neutrophil polymorphs; as the process becomes more chronic, other types of inflammatory cells, particularly lymphocytes and plasma cells, accumulate (Fig. 1.1). Necrotic bone may be present (Fig. 1.2) and is recognised by the presence of empty osteocyte lacunae (see Exercise 7). There may be evidence of osteoclastic resorption of bone (Fig. 1.2) and of osteoblastic bone formation (Fig. 1.3). It is usually easy to identify biopsy material from suppurative osteomyelitis as inflammatory; conditions such as eosinophil granuloma are sometimes mistaken, on histological examination, for inflammatory lesions.

Other Types of Osteomyelitis. Tuberculous osteomyelitis (which is discussed elsewhere in this work) is another important form of inflammatory bone disease with a distinctive pattern of histological reaction which includes caseation and the formation of tuberculous granulation tissue. Bone lesions do occur, although rarely, in a variety of other infective processes, including fungal infections and syphilis.

Treatment

Treatment, in the acute stage, is by parenteral administration of an appropriate antibiotic, together with the surgical release of pus and the excision of necrotic and infected tissue. With a *Staphylococcus aureus* infection, either known or suspected, a broad spectrum penicillinase-resistant drug can be administered until the specific antibiotic sensitivities of the infecting organism are known. Areas of known, or even unsuspected, activity may be recognised easily by radionuclide scanning. Confusion may arise in sickle-cell disease in differentiating an infarct from infection.

References

Clawson DK, Dunn AW (1967) Management of common bacterial infections of bones and joints. J Bone Jt Surg 49A: 164–182

Kemp HBS, Lloyd-Roberts GC (1974) Acute necrosis of the capital epiphysis following osteomyelitis of the proximal femoral metaphysis. J Bone Jt Surg 56B: 688–697

Specht EE (1971) Hemoglobinopathic Salmonella osteomyelitis. Clin Orthop 79: 110–118

Trueta J (1959) The three types of acute haematogenous osteomyelitis. J Bone Jt Surg 41B: 671–680

Waldvogel FA, Medoff G, Swartz MN (1970) Osteomyelitis: a review of clinical features, therapeutic considerations and unusual aspects. N Engl J Med 282: 198, 260, 316

Wolfson JJ, Kane WJ, Laxdal SD, Good RA, Quie PG (1969) Bone findings in chronic granulomatous disease of childhood. J Bone Jt Surg 51A: 1573–1583

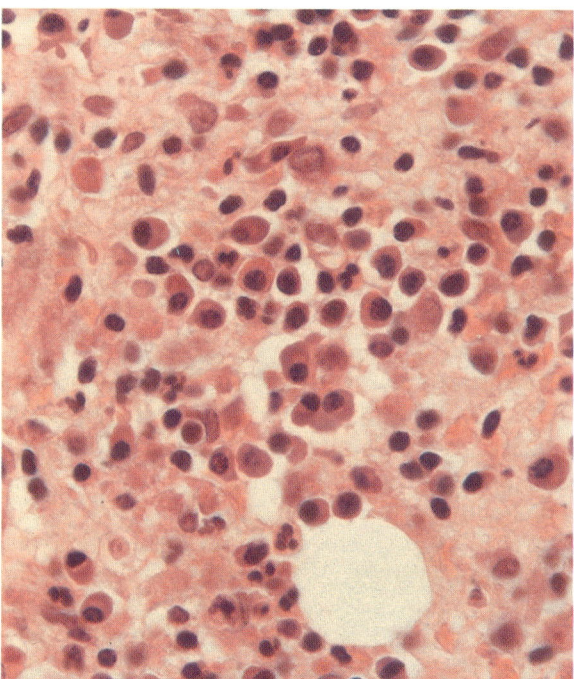

Fig. 1.1. Chronic inflammatory cells (lymphocytes and plasma cells) in tissue from the lesion in Q1. (×560)

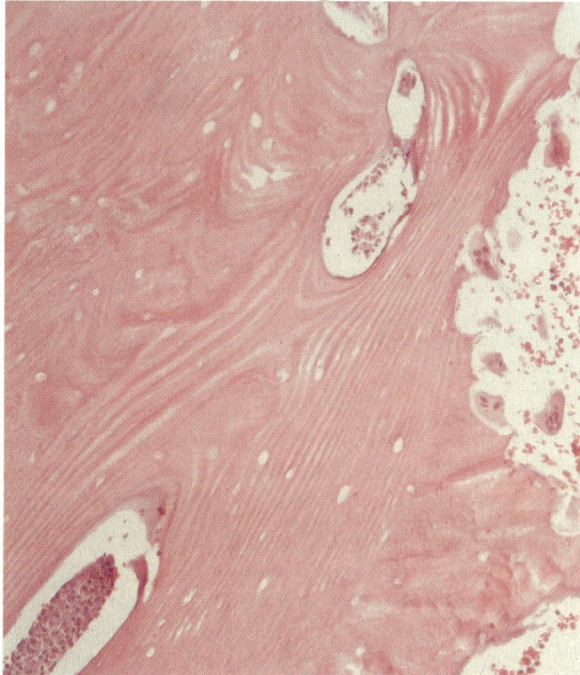

Fig. 1.2. Necrotic bone from a lesion of suppurative osteomyelitis. Osteocyte lacunae are devoid of cell nuclei. Osteoclasts are resorbing the dead bone. (×125)

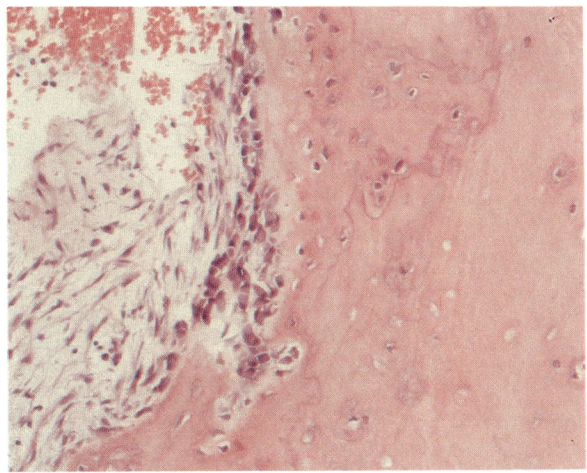

Fig. 1.3. Osteoblastic bone formation from another lesion of suppurative osteomyelitis. An area of newly formed viable bone is present between the layer of osteoblasts and the deeper necrotic bone. (×125)

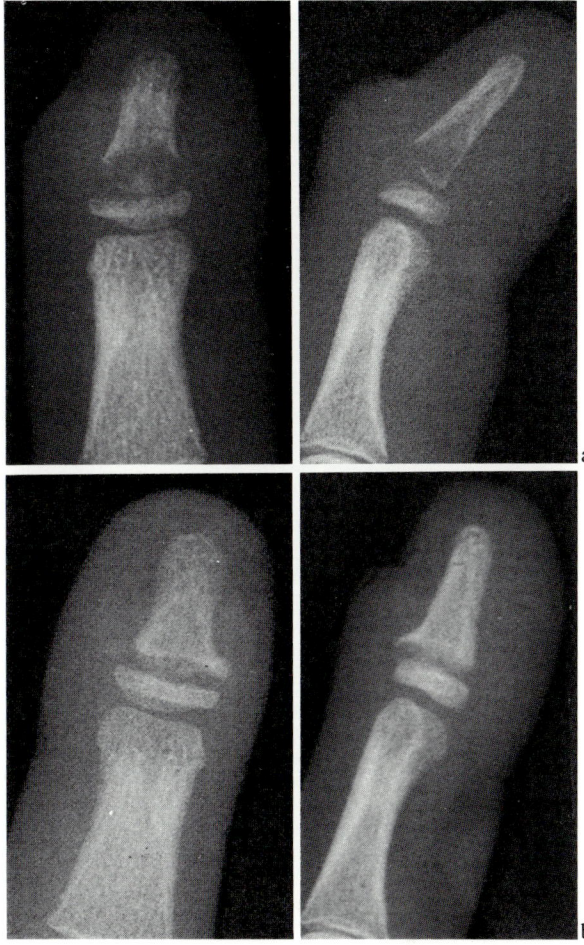

Fig. 1.5. *Acute osteomyelitis of terminal phalanx.* **a** Similar metaphyseal destruction, without spread to the epiphysis, and soft tissue swelling are evident in a 9-year-old girl with a history of an injury 2 weeks before. The same pattern may be observed with whitlows. **b** Six weeks later, following removal of the nail and antibiotic treatment, the metaphyseal lesion has repaired, but the soft tissue swelling has not resolved completely.

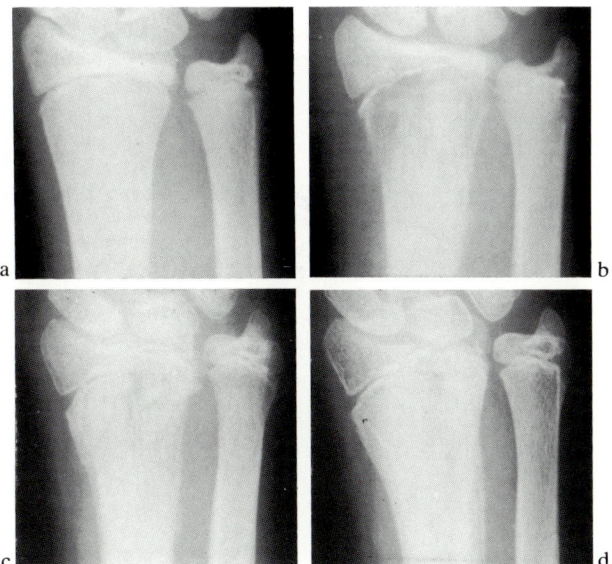

Fig. 1.4. *Acute osteomyelitis of distal radial metaphysis* in a 12-year-old girl with acute pain in the right wrist. **a** On presentation, no radiological abnormality is demonstrated, but a radionuclide scan at the time would have been positive. Even at this time surgical drilling could well have released pus and relieved pain. **b** Eight days later *diffuse* soft tissue swelling is evident and poorly defined medullary and cortical destruction has developed. Spread of the infection towards the joint has been arrested by the barrier of the growth plate. **c** One month later, following surgical intervention and antibiotic therapy, the lesion is sclerosing and the soft tissue swelling has regressed. **d** Two months later activity had subsided completely, with more sclerosis and organised periosteal reactions.

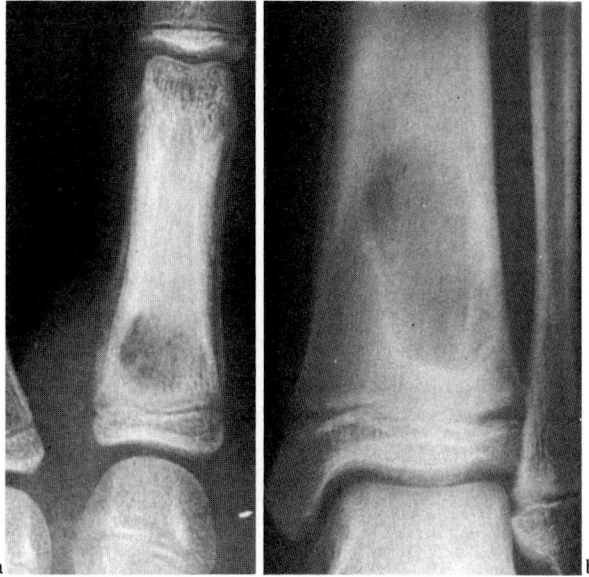

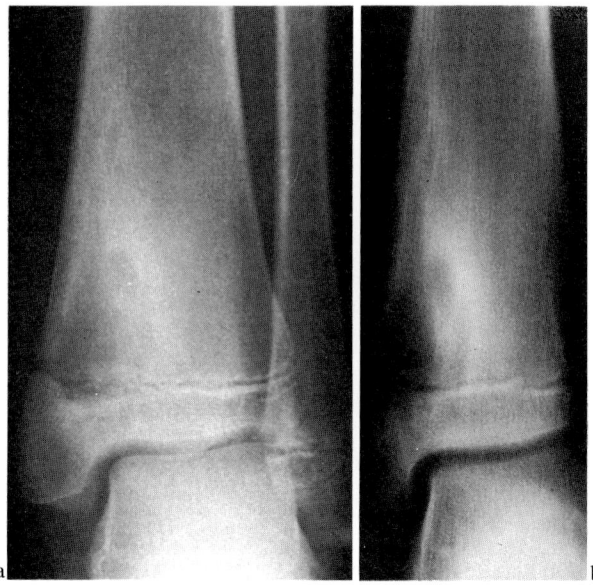

Fig. 1.6. *Subacute osteomyelitis.* **a** *Proximal phalanx.* This adolescent developed chronic pain and swelling following an infected abrasion to the knuckle incurred in a fight. In addition to diffuse soft tissue swelling a periosteal reaction surrounds the diaphysis and a Brodie's abscess is forming in the metaphysis. Observe integrity of the growth plate. **b** *Distal tibial metaphysis.* This 8-year-old girl had complained of pain in the left ankle for many months. The lytic lesion in the distal end of the tibia represents a more completely formed Brodie's abscess, but an overlying periosteal reaction persists.

Fig. 1.8. *Chronic osteomyelitis of tibia.* **a** This Brodie's abscess was detected in a 10-year-old boy with a chronic ache in the left ankle. The abscess is surrounded by a well-defined sclerotic reaction. At the proximal end of the lesion a classical 'tunnel' is shown which is outlined well in **b** the tomogram. Rather unusually, some peripheral encroachment on the growth plate is evident.

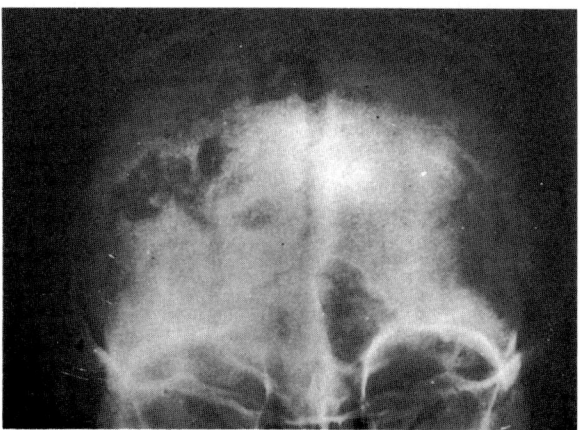

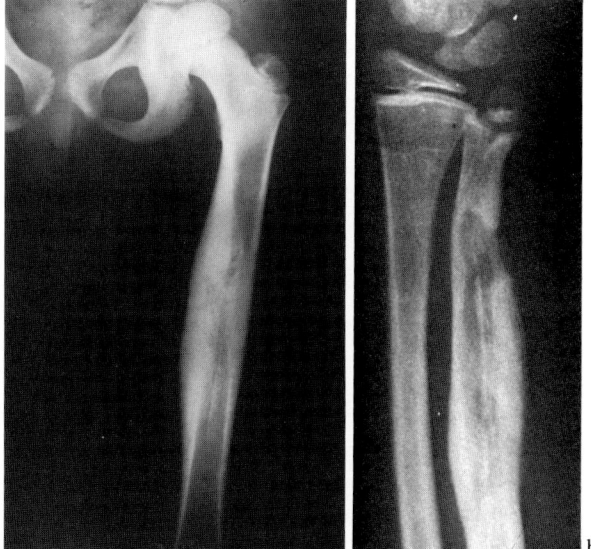

Fig. 1.7. *Subacute osteomyelitis of frontal bone.* This youth contracted infection of the right frontal sinus, which is opaque due to mucosal thickening. From this portal of infection extensive destruction followed, the finger-like lucencies illustrating the diagnostic sign of 'tunnelling'.

Fig. 1.9. *Chronic osteomyelitis.* **a** *Femur,* showing gross thickening of the medial cortex, with a lucent cloaca, and sclerotic narrowing of the medullary cavity. This appearance is known by the classical term 'Garré's sclerosing osteomyelitis'. **b** *Ulna,* again with cortical thickening and a cloaca, but containing a dense linear sequestrum. Involvement of the distal growth plate has caused the bone to be shortened.

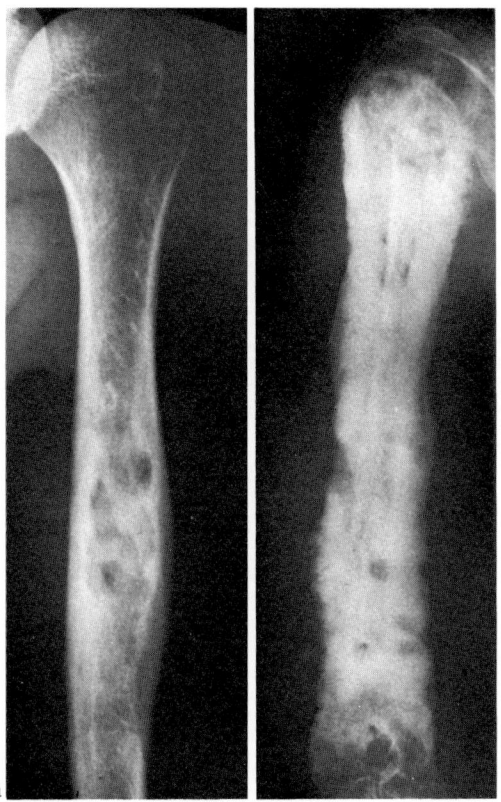

Fig. 1.10. *Chronic osteomyelitis.* **a** *Humerus.* This osteolytic expanding lesion in the mid-shaft of the humerus was found in a 45-year-old man with pain in the arm of 2 months' duration. The endosteal margin is sclerosed and clearly defined with a distal 'tunnelling' extension. Fusiform cortical thickening represented a long-standing and organised periosteal reaction. The appearance is typical of a Brodie's abscess, but a chondrosarcoma was suggested pre-operatively. Greenish pus was found at operation and subsequently it was found that the patient had a history of osteomyelitis of the tibia in childhood. Such examples of late reactivation of osteomyelitis are not very rare. **b** *Humerus in a child.* The entire diaphysis has sequestrated and is surrounded by an enormous involucrum. This case dates from the pre-antibiotic era and such cases are unlikely to be encountered now in developed parts of the world.

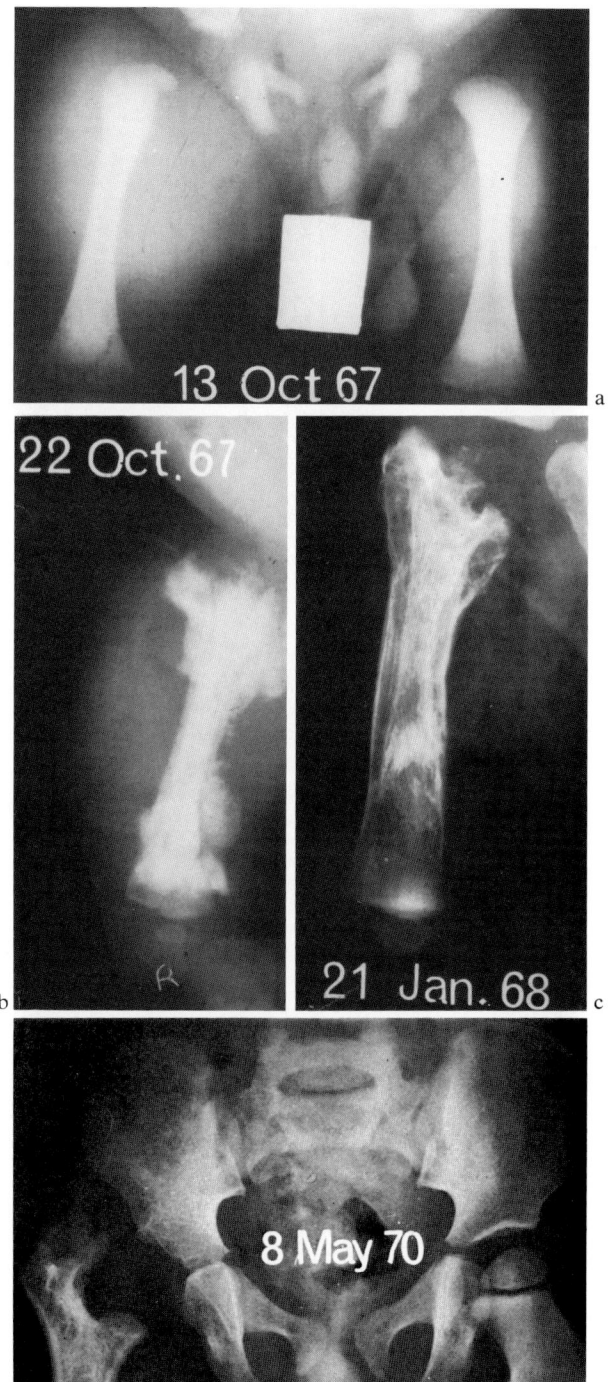

Fig. 1.11. *Infantile septic arthritis—evolution.* **a** This 3-month-old infant with a large and painful swelling of the right thigh, was pyrexial and had a white blood cell count of 22 600. Early changes of osteomyelitis in the proximal end of the femur were present, with metaphyseal destruction and periosteal reaction. The joint space of the hip was abnormally wide. An unexplained fracture of the distal femoral metaphysis was noted. **b** Within 9 days an exuberant periosteal reaction had developed to form **c** an involucrum surrounding the sequestrated and necrotic femoral shaft. Impairment of growth of the femoral head had already begun and **d** 2 years later its absence was accompanied by shortening of the limb and dislocation of the hip. Such an appearance in a child is virtually diagnostic of a former infection of this type.

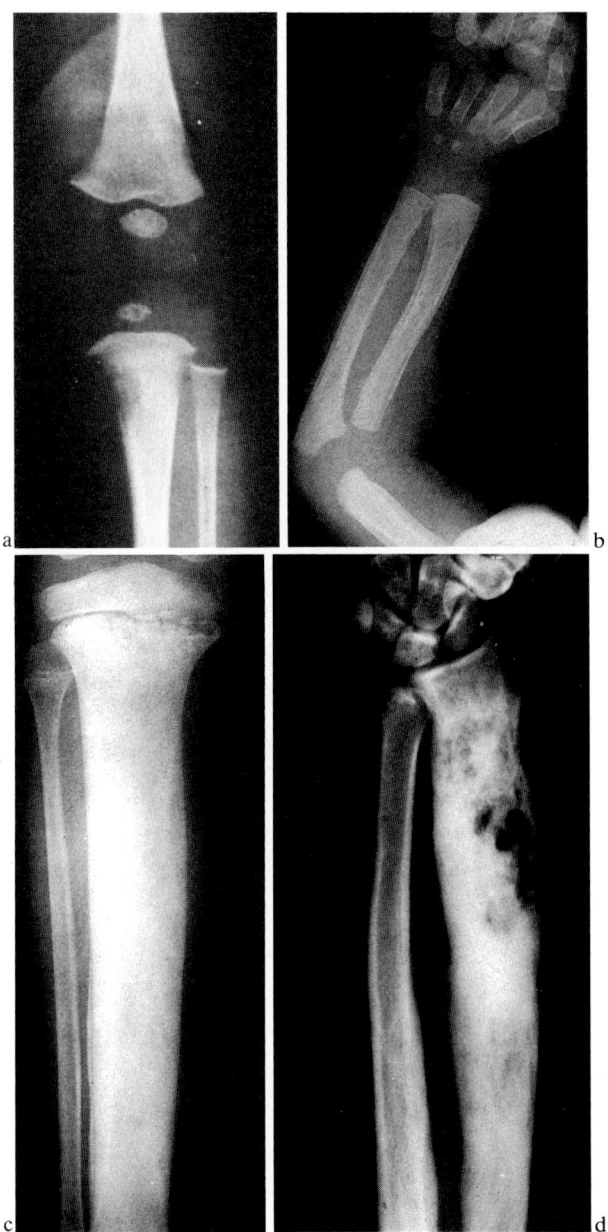

Fig. 1.12. *Osseous syphilis* is now distinctly unusual, but may be encountered still in underdeveloped countries. Histological studies are rarely undertaken, but the bone lesions show a combination of periosteal new bone formation and gummatous inflammatory tissue. These radiological examples of this chronic infection illustrate *congenital lesions*. **a** Granulomatous erosion of the medial sides of the proximal tibial and the distal femoral metaphysis in an infant. These erosions were symmetrical and represent the classical Wimberger sign. **b** Diffuse periosteal reactions and **c** organised periosteal reactions with metaphyseal destruction in older children. **d** The combination of destruction and sclerotic reaction which characterises bone involvement by *acquired syphilis* in adults. This diagnosis was established serologically.

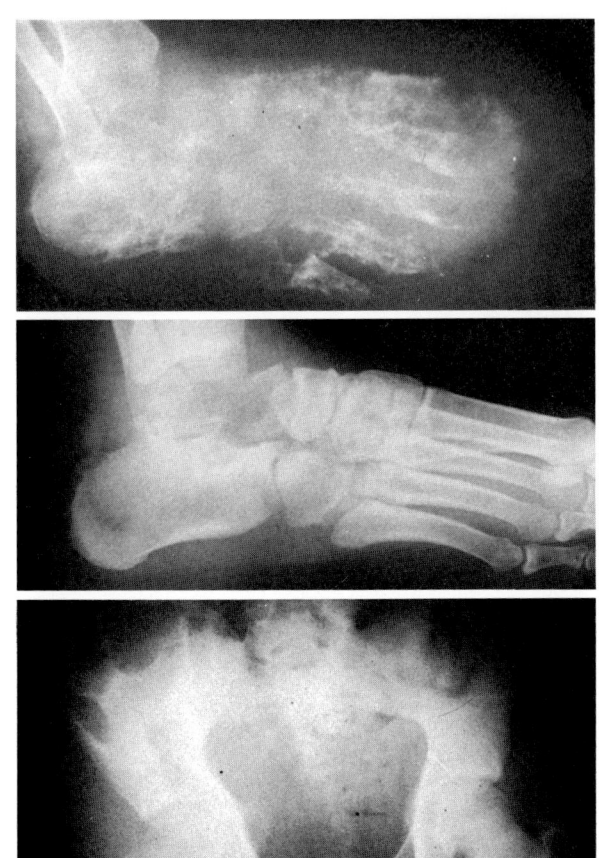

Fig. 1.13. *Fungus infections*, of which various types are endemic in certain geographical areas, particularly subtropical and tropical regions, often cause destructive lesions. In the earlier stages the radiological appearance may not be specific, but later some characteristic patterns emerge. Only a few can be illustrated here: **a** *Mycetoma of foot* with widespread destruction in a Sudanese patient. This is the most common site to be affected, but such areas as the hand and skull may be involved. **b** *Blastomycosis of talus*, in a 32-year-old Brazilian man, caused this non-specific destructive lesion. **c** *Coccidioidomycosis of right ilium* in a young adult living in the San Joaquin valley in California. A large destructive lesion in the right ilium is associated with an abscess. Many of these fungus infections cause ulceration and are complicated by the entry of secondary pyogenic organisms.

A2. Reticulum-cell sarcoma of femur with secondary synovitis of knee

This case is illustrated to emphasise the importance of close collaboration between clinician, radiologist and pathologist. The radiological report, describing the lytic area and the periosteal reaction and suggesting the possibility of a malignant tumour, was disregarded, or never read, by the clinician. The initial clinical diagnosis was monarticular rheumatoid arthritis, which can, indeed, stimulate an adjacent diaphyseal periosteal reaction. At operation the presence of an effusion was confirmed and the thickened synovial membrane was biopsied. Q2b and c, from this biopsy, show non-specific chronic inflammatory changes. The tissue is oedematous as indicated by the pink-staining fluid distending its interstices. Numerous capillary blood vessels are present and are surrounded by collections of lymphocytes and plasma cells. No tumour tissue is present.

The patient's symptoms became more severe. The significance of the periosteal reaction was appreciated ultimately and a biopsy of the distal end of the femur was performed. This specimen showed the presence of tumour tissue (Figs. 2.1, 2.2). The tumour is made up of rounded and spindle-shaped cells with considerable nuclear pleomorphism. More detailed histological studies established a diagnosis of reticulum-cell sarcoma.

An amputation was carried out, and Fig. 2.3 shows the gross appearance of the tumour: it involves the whole of the distal part of the femur, with extension to soft tissues anteriorly and posteriorly. There was no evidence of lymph node involvement, indicating that the tumour was primary in bone. The patient died 5 years after surgery, with evidence of pulmonary metastases.

Reticulum-cell sarcoma and other round-cell tumours of bone are discussed elsewhere in this work.

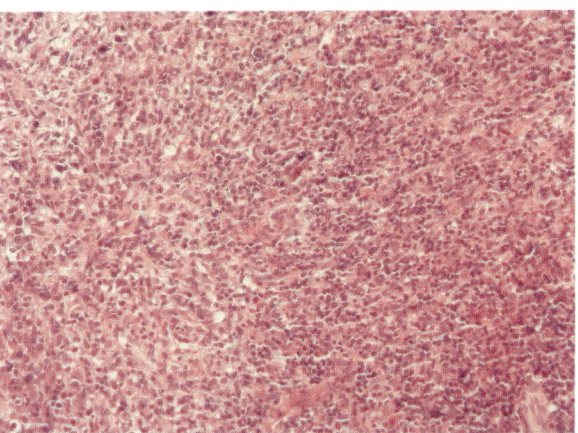

Fig. 2.1. Tumour tissue from lower femur in Q1. The field consists of a mass of rounded and ovoid cells.

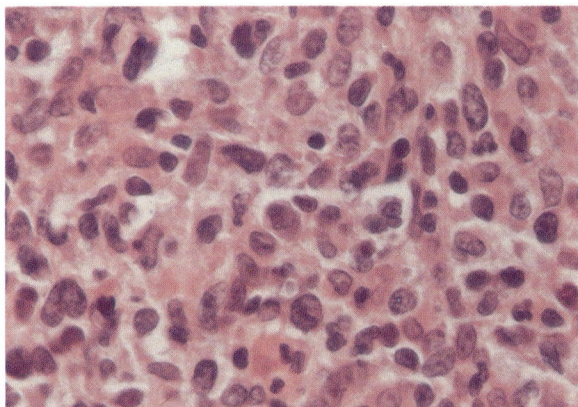

Fig. 2.2. More magnified view of tissue in Fig. 2.1 showing the features of a malignant tumour (reticulum-cell sarcoma). The cell outlines are indistinct: there is a considerable degree of nuclear pleomorphism.

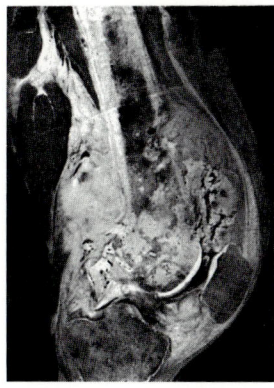

Fig. 2.3. Gross appearance of the tumour in the amputation specimen. The bone marrow is replaced by pale tumour tissue which extends to form a soft tissue mass anteriorly and posteriorly.

Q1. This 61-year-old man had complained of chronic pain in the left knee for a year. This pain was aggravated by exercise.

A large effusion within the joint was detected clinically, with restriction of movement and wasting of the muscles of the thigh. The patient was febrile. The erythrocyte sedimentation test (ESR) was 85 mm/h.

Radiological examination confirmed the presence of an effusion and showed narrowing of the joint space, peri-articular demineralisation, a periosteal reaction on the femoral shaft and para-articular erosions on the medial tibial condyle and the posterior aspect of the tibia.

Surgical exploration was undertaken.

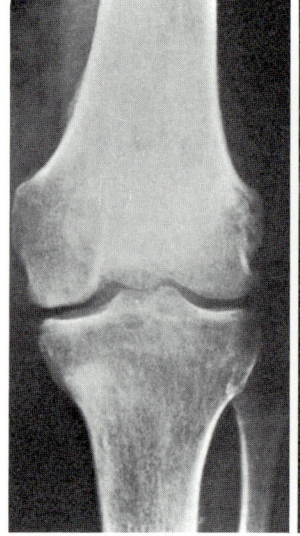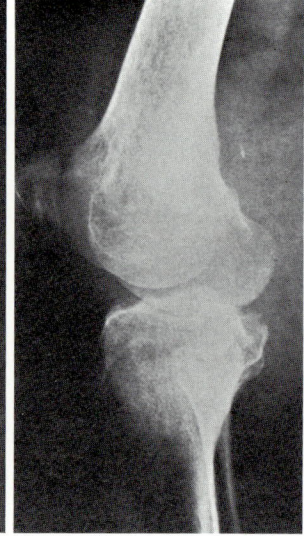

Q1a.

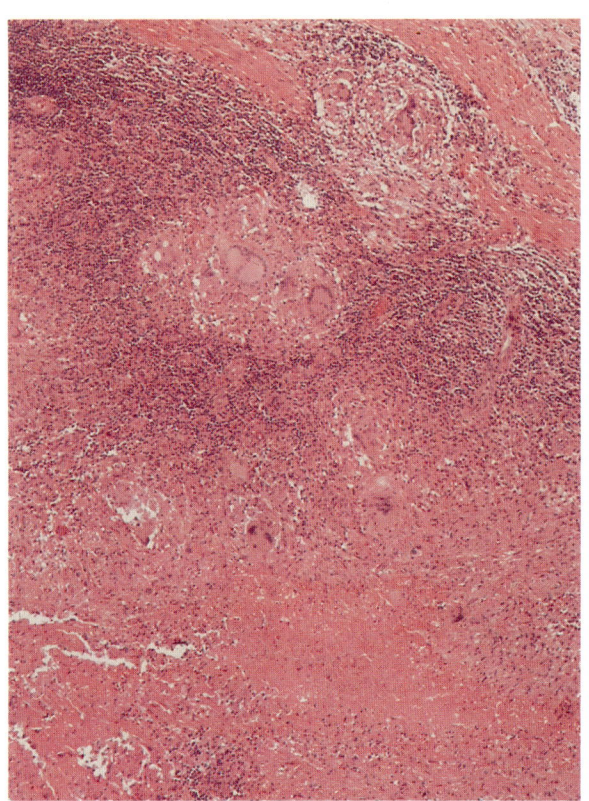

Q1b. (×54)

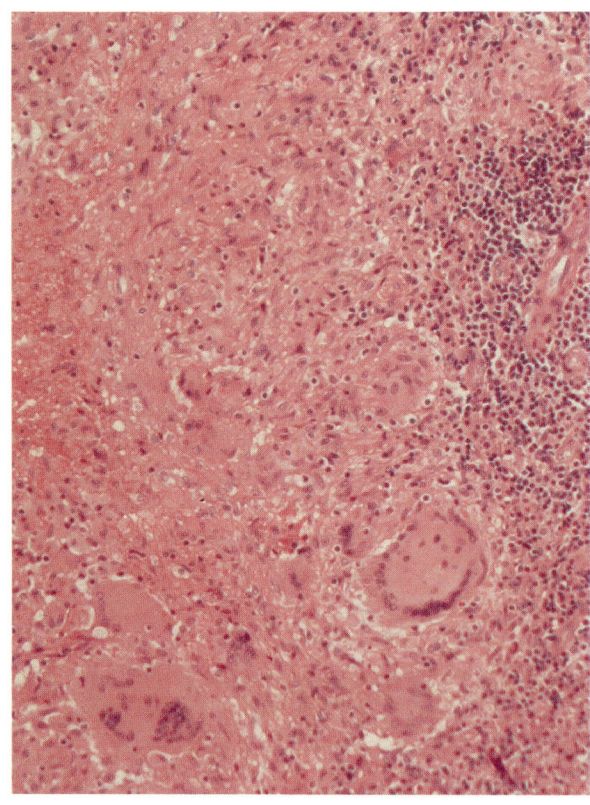

Q1c. (×140)

Q2. This 44-year-old clergyman complained of increasing stiffness of the right shoulder for 18 months.

Recently he had observed a swelling in the deltoid region, evident clinically with some erythema of the overlying skin. All movements of the shoulder were limited, but pain was elicited only with abduction. A history of 'sarcoidosis' 8 years before was obtained.

The radiograph shows extensive erosion of the gleno-humeral articular surfaces, lucencies in the humeral head, generalised osteoporosis and diffuse swelling of the surrounding soft tissues. A film of the chest demonstrated the presence of calcification in the right upper lobe.

Laboratory investigations: ESR 9 mm/h, Hb 15.0 g, WBC 6000 per mm^3

Surgical exploration was undertaken.

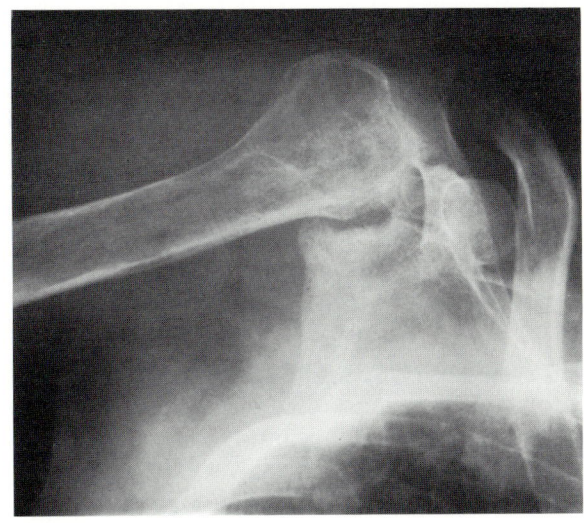

Q2a.

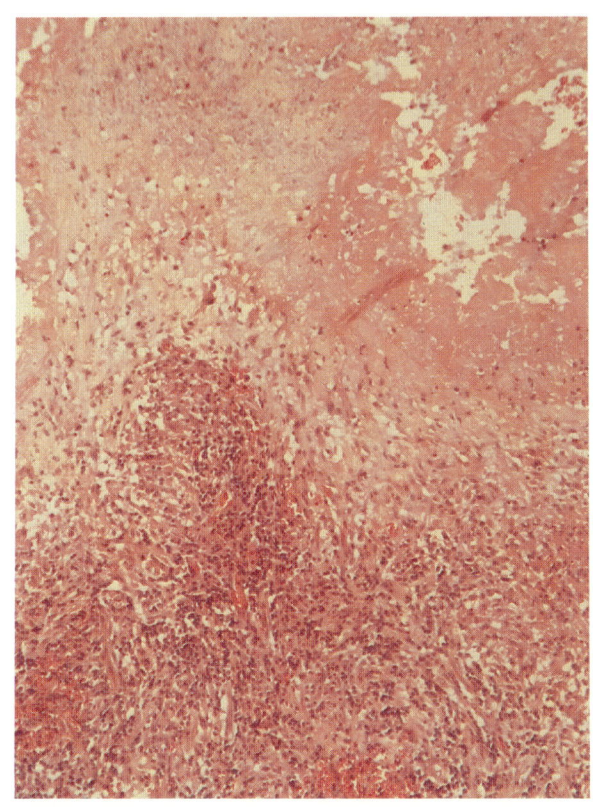

Q2b. (×100)

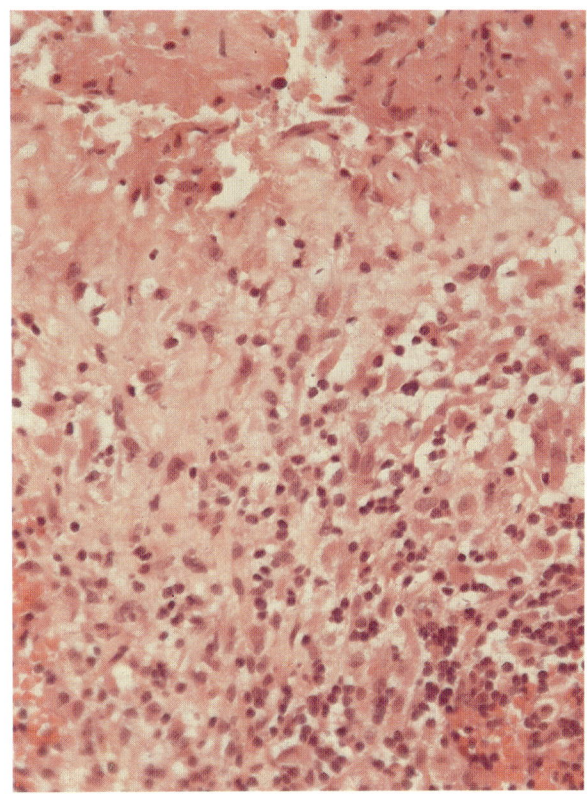

Q2c. (×275)

A1. Tuberculous arthritis of knee

The clinical findings, suggesting a chronic low-grade infective arthritis, were supported by the radiological appearance. The diffuse peri-articular demineralisation indicated chronic hyperaemia. The erosions at the capsular attachments incriminated synovium.

The histological appearances, in the tissue removed from the joint, are characteristic of tuberculosis (Q1b). The synovial membrane is replaced by a mass of chronic inflammatory granulation tissue containing typical tubercles and areas of caseous necrosis. The tubercles, from which the condition takes its name, are nodular aggregates of epithelioid cells and fibroblasts, and contain characteristic multinucleated giant cells (Q1c). These, in contrast to the giant cells found in other conditions (foreign body giant cells, osteoclasts, giant cells of giant-cell tumour) have their nuclei situated at the periphery of the cell. The epithelioid cells are mononuclear inflammatory cells (macrophages); numerous lymphocytes and occasional plasma cells are also present.

In addition to extensive changes in the synovial membrane, the present case shows evidence of bone involvement (Figs. 1.1a and b). Bone trabeculae in a circumscribed area of subchondral bone are necrotic, and tuberculous granulation tissue, with tubercles and giant cells, is extending in the marrow spaces at the margin. The small size of the area of bone involvement suggests that it is a recent extension from the joint, and not an antecedent lesion.

Acid-fast organisms were identified in sections stained by the Ziehl-Neelsen method, and the diagnosis of tuberculosis was confirmed further by culture.

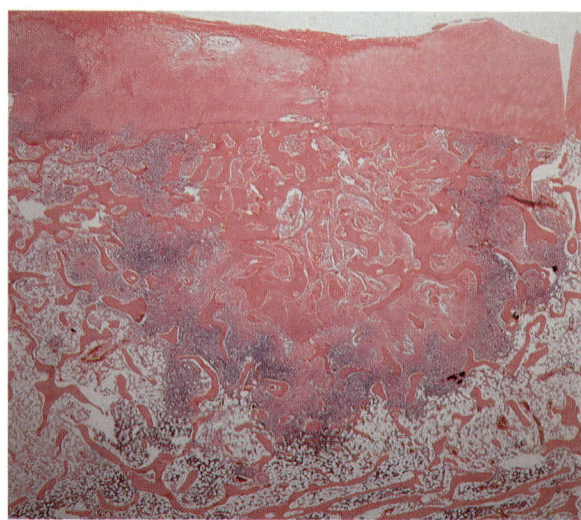

Fig. 1.1a. A focal area of involvement of subchondral bone is present in the resected patella. (×8)

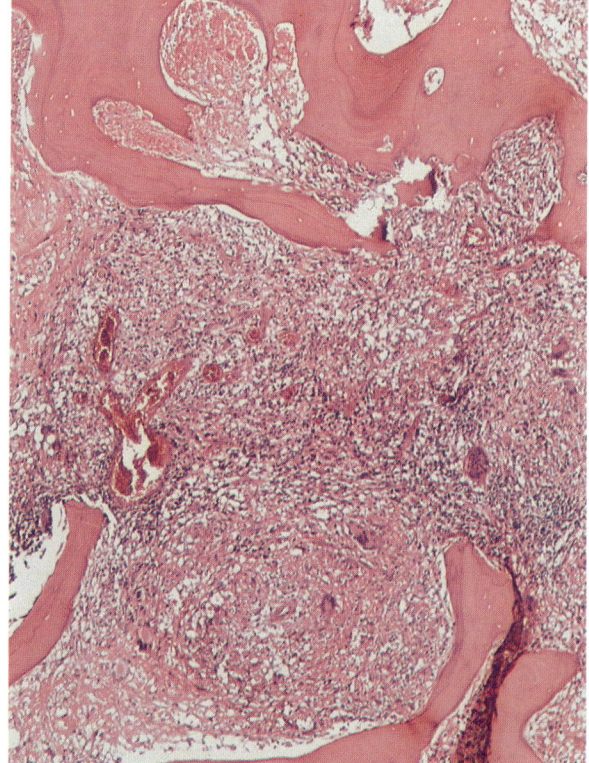

Fig. 1.1b. Greater magnification of the same field shows necrotic bone trabeculae with empty osteocyte lacunae. The marrow spaces are occupied by tuberculous tissue with scattered giant cells. (×54)

A2. Tuberculous arthritis of shoulder

This case is important in illustrating how insidious, both clinically and radiologically, may be the progress of such infections. As indicated below, even the histological findings were not entirely specific and the diagnosis in this middle-aged man with a misleading clinical history was established ultimately only by culture of the organism from the thick tuberculous pus which was found at operation. This pre-operative diagnosis, however, had been made clinically, lack of significant leucocytes and elevation of the ESR being by no means unusual in such lesions. Nevertheless, the formation of an abscess around a tuberculous shoulder was unusual, relative lack of pus being responsible for the common descriptive term of *caries sicca*.

Moreover, the radiological pattern is typical of a chronic inflammatory arthritis. Its indolent nature is characterised by absence of reactive sclerosis, aiding differentiation from pyogenic infection.

In this case the histological changes are less specific, although, as in the previous case, acid-fast bacilli could be identified in material from the joint. The biopsy (Q2a and b) shows chronic inflammatory granulation tissue with lymphocytes and epithelioid cells, but without recognisable tubercles or tuberculous giant cells. Necrosis is evident.

This lack of diagnostic histological features is quite frequent in joint tuberculosis.

The cavity in the humeral head was curetted and treatment with streptomycin, para-aminosalicylic acid and isoniazid was instituted with an excellent clinical result.

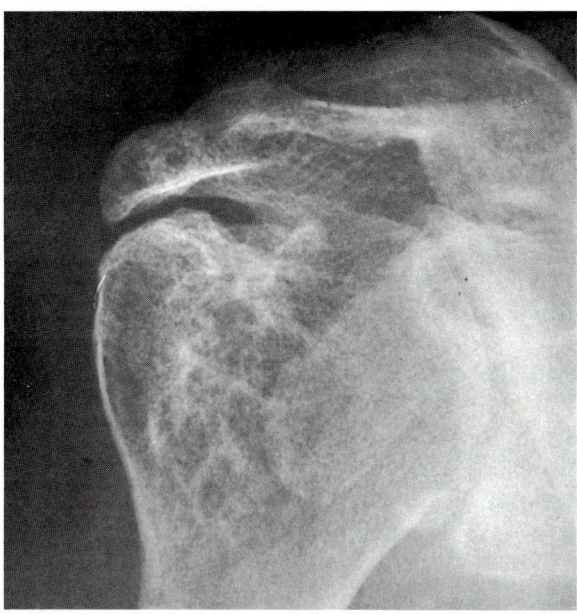

Fig. 2.1. Three years later the lesion in the humeral head had sclerosed and the articular surfaces had become more clearly defined, with only minor residual irregularity. The joint space was narrowed, but across it no bony fusion had occurred. All these features indicated the infection to be inactive. Nevertheless, mild, but persistent, discomfort in an essentially fibrous ankylosis was treated successfully by arthrodesis.

Tuberculous Arthritis

Tuberculous infections of joints, as in the case of the remainder of the skeleton, are distinctly less common than in the past. This improvement is largely the result of improved public health measures, preventive medicine and the introduction of antituberculous drugs. This disease, nevertheless, is encountered still in areas of economic deprivation and in immigrants from such areas to the Western world. Joint lesions of this type are exceeded in frequency only by tuberculous osteomyelitis of the spine, an entity considered elsewhere in this work.

Clinical Features

The usual causes of presentation are mild pain, swelling and restriction of movement of a single joint, usually in childhood, although people of any age may be affected. Enlarged regional lymph nodes may be palpable, but, apart from slight pyrexia in the evenings, evidence of a florid infection is commonly lacking. The process is essentially indolent until the initial synovial involvement spreads to the adjacent bone. The ESR is elevated and the tuberculin test (Mantoux reaction; PPD reaction) is usually positive. The complication of sinus formation with secondary infection is much rarer than it was in the pre-antibiotic era.

Radiological Features

1. Site. The hip and knee are the joints most commonly involved, followed by other major joints, including the carpus and tarsus.

2. Appearance. Early. Soft tissue swelling is accompanied by increasing osteoporosis with, in the immature skeleton, accelerated maturation of growth centres and premature epiphyseal fusion, all these features reflecting hyperaemia. Similar and indistinguishable changes may be observed in multiple joints in juvenile rheumatoid arthritis and haemophilia. Minor periosteal reactions may be apparent adjacent to the affected joint.

Late. Erosions develop at capsular attachments and eventually on peripheral portions of articular surfaces, with consequent reduction in the width of the joint space. In the stage of healing these persistent irregularities develop marginal sclerosis and the soft tissue swellings regress. Fibrous ankylosis may occur, but, in the absence of secondary infection, bony ankylosis is rare.

Pathological Features

Tuberculous arthritis may originate in the synovial membrane or may develop from an adjacent focus of tuberculous osteomyelitis. In either case the disease is secondary to a primary focus in the lungs, although this has usually resolved, clinically and radiologically, by the time the joint involvement develops. In former times milk-borne bovine tuberculosis, with a primary focus in the tonsil and secondary spread to the cervical chain or the Peyer's patches in the ileum and then to the mesenteric lymph nodes, sometimes was concerned, but is now rarely, if ever, encountered. Involvement of a joint commonly develops during childhood and the primary focus often has healed before the skeletal lesion becomes evident.

In tuberculous arthritis, histological sections of the synovial membrane usually show, as in Q1, a combination of caseous necrosis and typical tuberculous tissue. In some cases tubercles are few, and much of the tissue shows only non-specific inflammatory changes. A limited biopsy then, as in Q2, may fail to establish that the lesion is tuberculous. Biopsy of the synovial membrane, or of a regional lymph node, is the accepted procedure for diagnosis. The biopsy material should be examined both histologically and bacteriologically. *Mycobacterium tuberculosis*, the causative organism, an 'acid-fast' bacillus, sometimes can be identified, in stained preparations or by culture, in synovial fluid.

Treatment

When the infection is largely confined to the synovium, the patient is treated by bed rest, splintage and light traction when a weight-bearing joint is involved. Non-weight-bearing joints only require immobilisation by splintage. Concurrent chemotherapy consists of the use of antituberculous drugs, a combination of rifampicin, para-aminosalicylic acid and isoniazid administered for a minimum period of 9 months. Alternative antituberculous drugs, for example, streptomycin and ethambutol, are also used if the tubercle grown from biopsy material subsequently exhibits drug resistance or if the patient fails to respond clinically.

Synovectomy, originally widely practised, now is indicated rarely. When it is employed, active mobilisation of the affected joint post-operatively is essential.

Advanced disease leads to destruction of subchondral bone, resulting in a painful fibrous ankylosis. Such lesions are treated either by arthrodesis or by joint replacement, as exemplified by A2 in this Exercise.

Reference

Boldero JL, Kemp HS (1960) The early bone and joint changes in haemophilia and similar blood dyscrasias. Br. J Radiol 39: 172–180

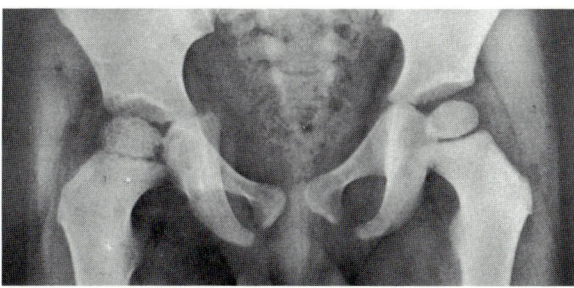

Fig. 1.2. *Tuberculous arthritis of right hip* in a 6-year-old girl with a limp and pain of several months' duration. Increased lucency of the whole area and enlargement of the right femoral head reflect the chronic hyperaemia induced by this infection. The bony articular margin is already slightly irregular and the growth plate is narrower than its counterpart, indicating it to be tending to fuse prematurely.

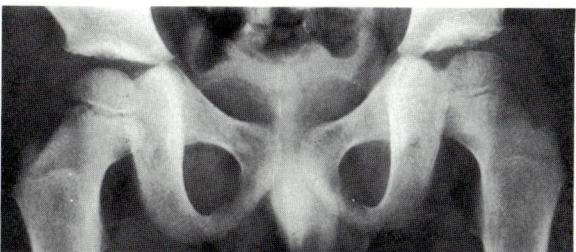
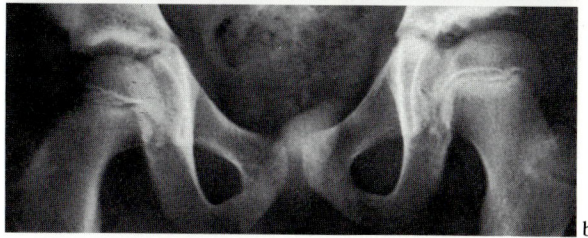

Fig. 1.3. *Tuberculous arthritis of left hip*. This 4-year-old boy presented with a limp and slight pain in the left hip. **a** Chronic hyperaemia due to the infection had caused this femoral head also to be more osteoporotic and larger than its counterpart. **b** Five years later, following prolonged recumbency and streptomycin therapy, activity had subsided and a normal bone texture had been restored. The enlarged femoral head, however, was covered incompletely by an acetabulum which had developed secondary dysplasia—the typical appearance of the classical *coxa valga magna luxans*. Coxa valga is often attributable to lack of the physiological stress of weight-bearing.

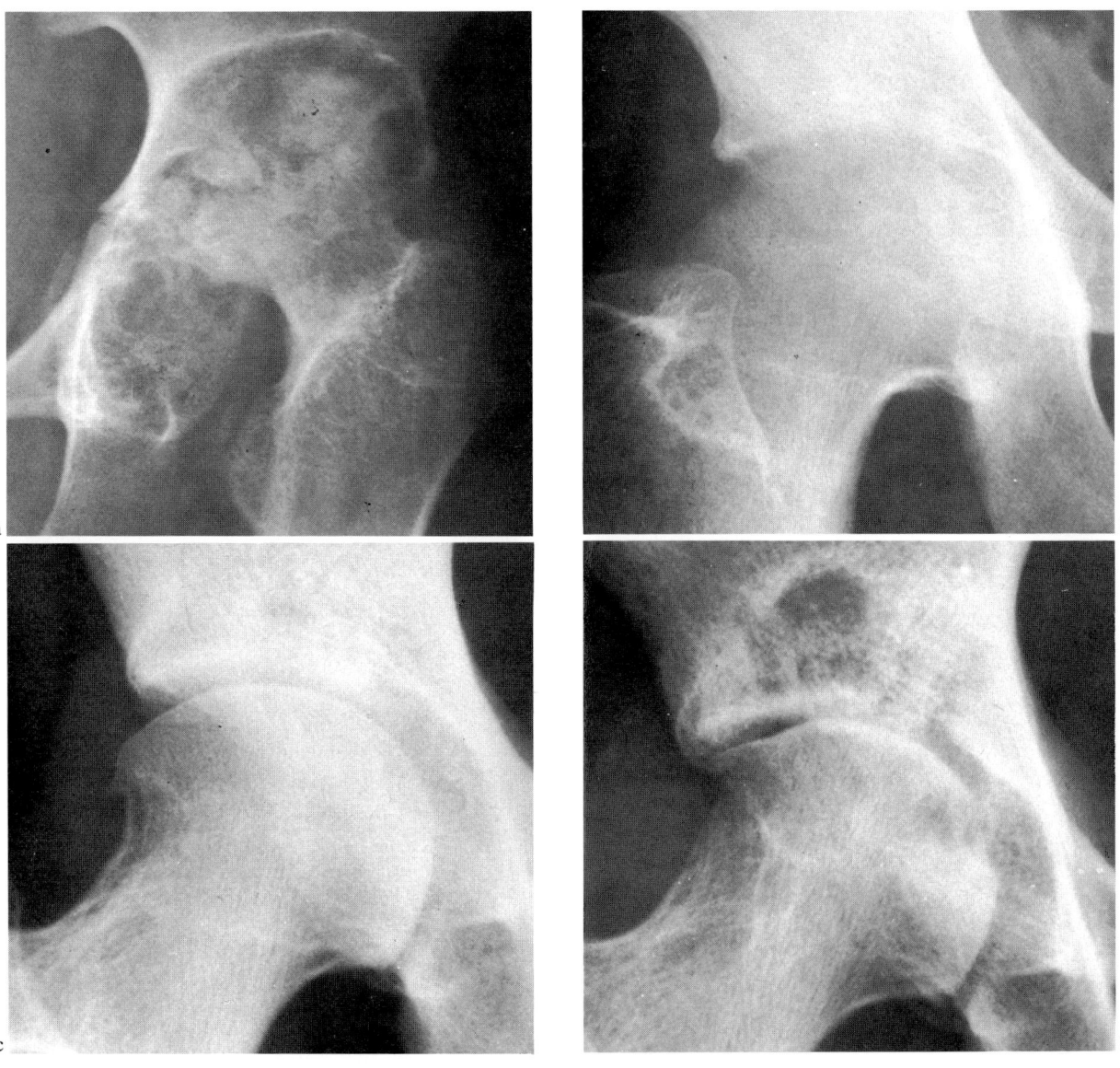

Fig. 1.4. *Tuberculous arthritis of hip—further examples.*
a *Late effects.* Extreme destruction in an 8-year-old boy treated in the pre-antibiotic era. Quiescence is indicated by marginal sclerosis and flecks of calcification in a former abscess, a feature rare since the introduction of antituberculous drugs. **b** *Active lesion* in a 22-year-old man. Observe hazy definition of an osteoporotic femoral head. **c** *Synovial erosions* at the capsular attachments on the femoral neck of this young woman were disregarded. **d** Two years later symptoms persisted and the acetabular lytic lesion was confirmed to be tuberculous. This appearance is unusual and comparable to *caries sicca* in the shoulder.

All these patients had presented with mild pain and a limp of several months' duration.

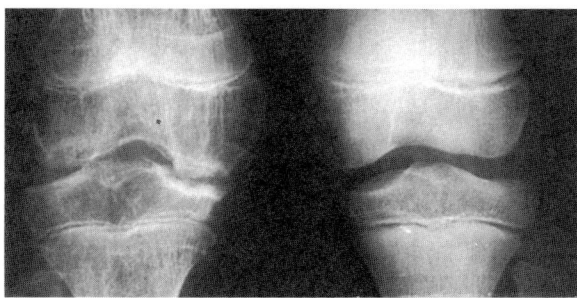

Fig. 1.5. *Tuberculous arthritis of right knee* in an 8-year-old boy. The same features of osteoporosis and epiphyseal overgrowth, due to chronic hyperaemia, are evident. The articular surfaces of the medial femoral and tibial condyles have been eroded.

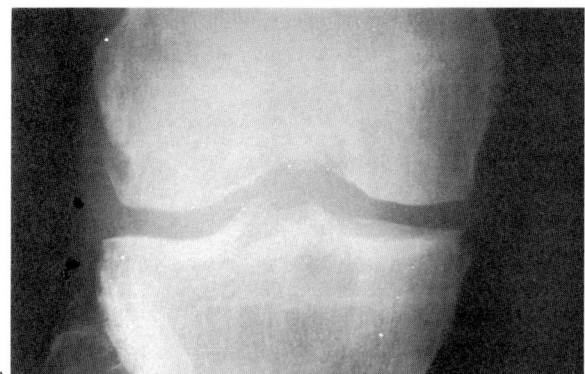
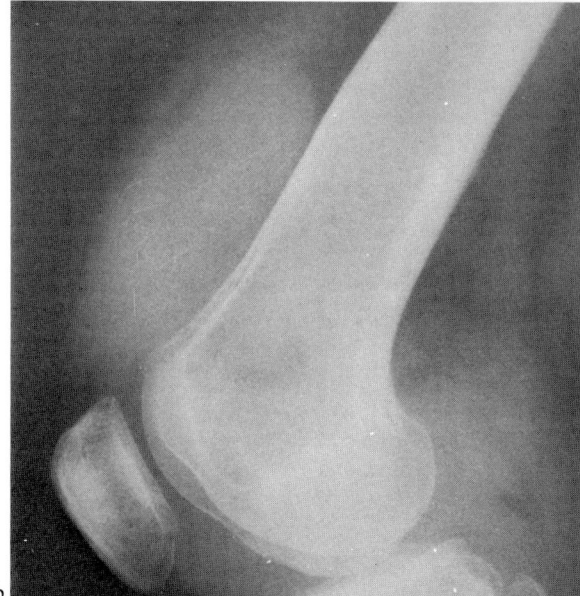

Fig. 1.6. *Synovial tuberculosis of knee.* In this 32-year-old woman with a chronically painful knee the joint space is distended, particularly in the suprapatellar pouch. Para-articular osteoporosis was evident, with erosions on the capsular attachments on the tibia.

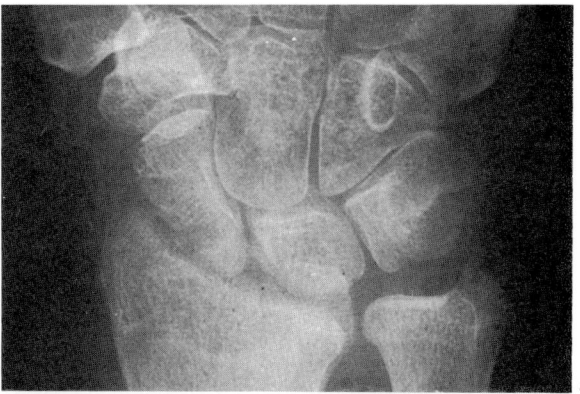
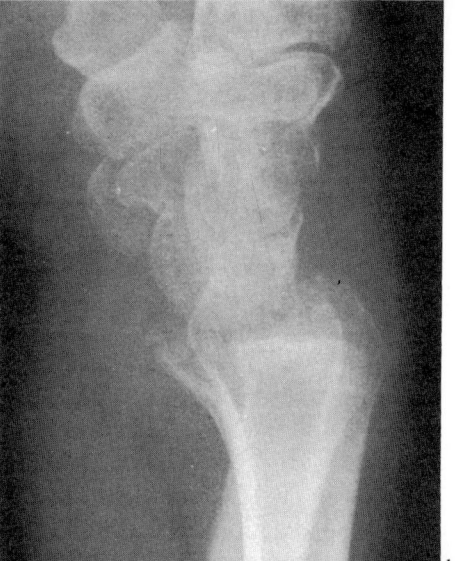
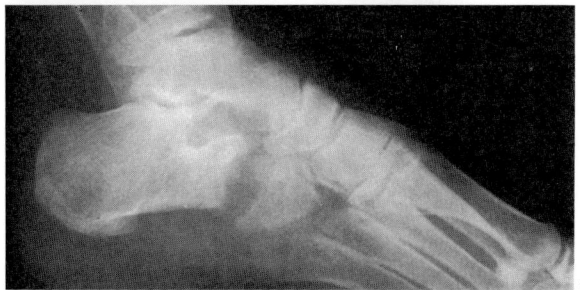

Fig. 1.7. *Tuberculous arthritis—less common sites.* **a,b** Wrist in a 28-year-old man with chronic pain and swelling. All the articular margins lack precise definition and diffuse osteoporosis is accompanied by soft tissue swelling. A faint periosteal reaction is present on the ulnar aspect of the radial shaft. **c** This 25-year-old woman had been under treatment for 8 years for this lesion of the tarsus in the pre-antibiotic era. The articular margins are eroded extensively, particularly in the calcaneo-cuboid joint. Diffuse hyperaemic para-articular osteoporosis is evident. Amputation ultimately was necessary.

Q1. This 24-year-old woman injured her little finger in a fall.

On clinical examination a fracture of the proximal phalanx was suspected, but, in addition, a hard swelling was felt on the palmar aspect of the finger; this swelling caused limitation of movement. The patient had been aware of this swelling since the age of 9 years and had noticed it to enlarge slowly, but without pain.

Radiological examination confirmed a transverse fracture through a well-defined lucent area in the base of the proximal phalanx and showed also further lucent and expanding lesions in the distal end of this phalanx and in the middle phalanx. The remainder of the skeleton appeared normal.

The finger was amputated.

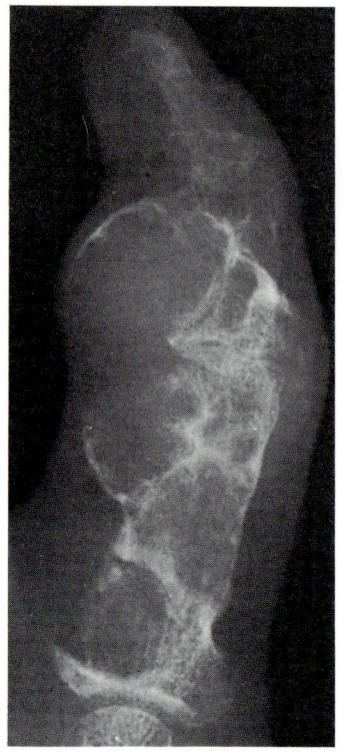

Q1a.

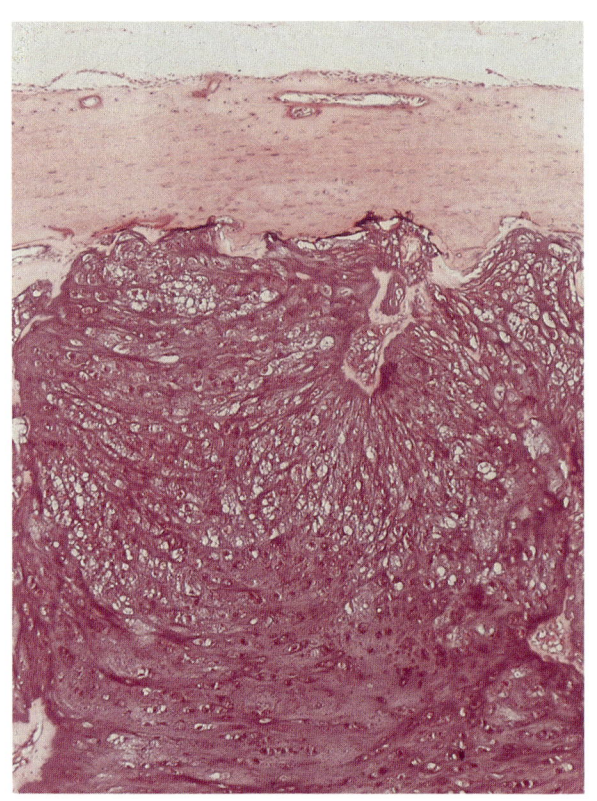

Q1b. (×54)

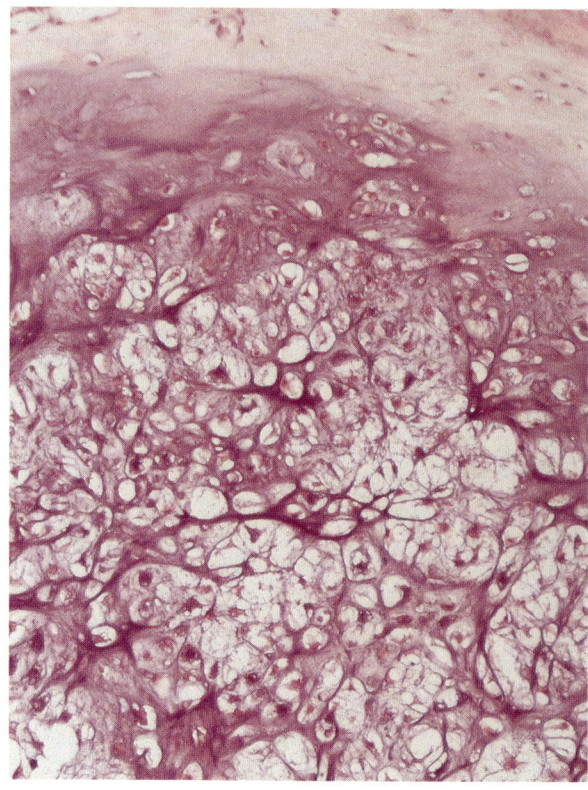

Q1c. (×140)

Q2. This 23-year-old woman complained of mild pain in the left forearm. The pain had begun following a minor injury a year previously, when she had been moving furniture. Since that time a constant ache had persisted.

On clinical examination slight tenderness was elicited on palpation of the middle of the forearm, but no other abnormality was detected.

A radiograph of the forearm revealed a large osteolytic area in the distal third of the radius with marked attenuation of the lateral cortex. More proximally in the same bone, further lucent areas of an expansile nature were present, within which irregular densities were evident. Skeletal survey disclosed a similar appearance in the proximal end of the left humerus, with endosteal cortical erosions, but no other bony abnormality was detected.

Both lesions were explored.

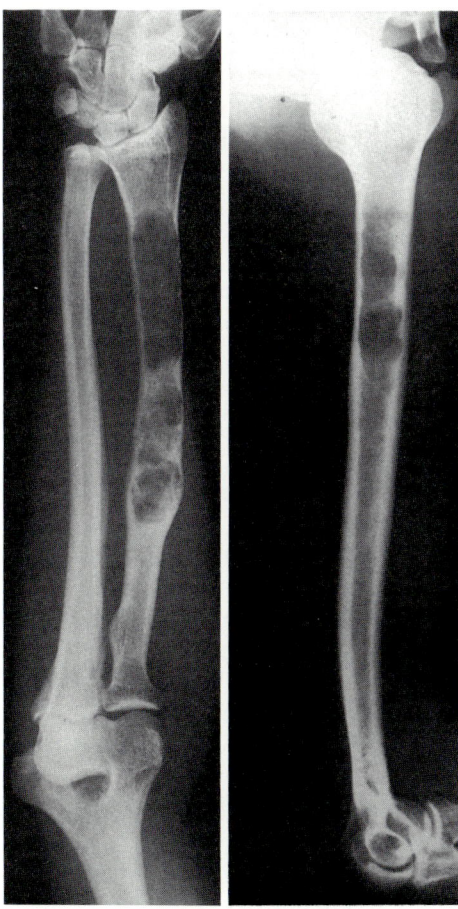

Q2a.

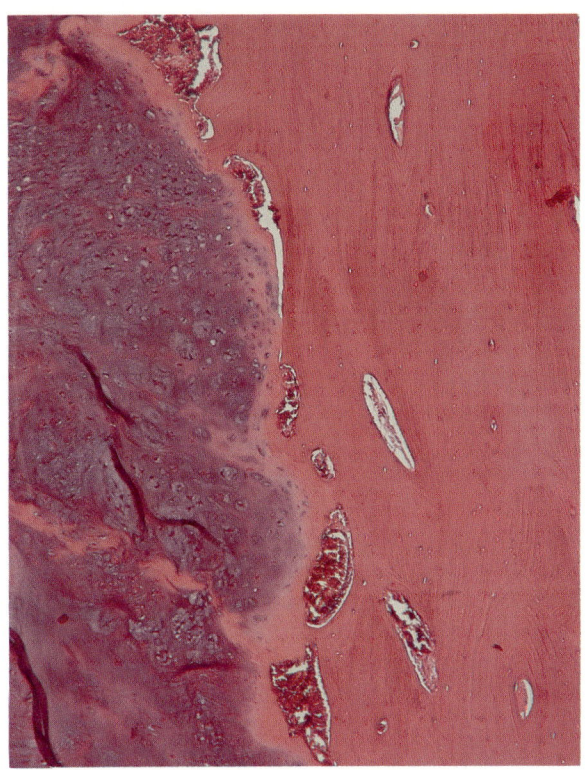

Q2b. (×45)

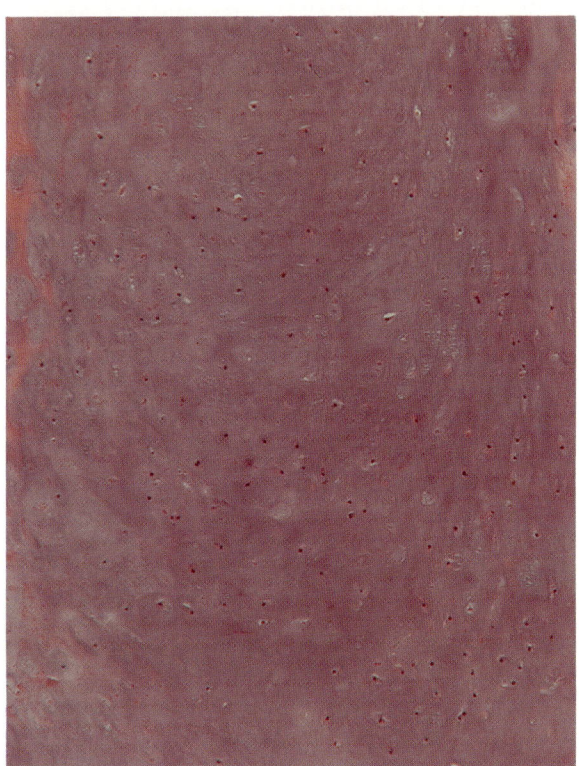

Q2c. (×90)

A1. Multiple enchondromas of phalanges of little finger

These lytic, expanding lesions, containing flecks of calcification, are typical of these cartilaginous neoplasms. Their sharply defined and sclerotic margins suggested them to be benign, but in view of the history of progressive enlargement of the swelling, it would have been unwise to exclude malignant chondrosarcomatous degeneration, even though such a complication is very rare in these tumours occurring in the hands and feet.

In the amputated specimen portions of the middle and proximal phalanges had been replaced by hyaline cartilage, which had extended into the palmar soft tissues. Q1b and c show the appearance of this cartilaginous tissue, which is expanding and eroding the overlying cortical bone (Q1b). The tumour tissue is highly cellular and somewhat pleomorphic, but hyperchromatic nuclei, binucleate cells and mitotic figures are not present. Experience has shown that this degree of cellularity, which might indicate malignancy in a cartilaginous tumour arising in a major long bone or in the axial skeleton, may be observed in benign enchondromas in the small bones of the hands and feet, especially when the lesions are multiple.

A2. Multiple enchondromas of radius and humerus

The history given by the patient and the clinical findings made radiological examination essential. The resulting appearance was surprising and unexpected, particularly in view of the totally asymptomatic lesions in the left humerus. The expansile lucencies in the middle third of the radius and in the humerus presented a pattern characteristic of benign enchondromas, a diagnosis supported by the irregular opacities consistent with calcification in cartilaginous neoplasms. Doubt, however, was cast on the more aggressive appearance of the osteolytic lesion in the distal third of the radius, so that exclusion of chondrosarcomatous degeneration was considered necessary. For this reason surgical exploration of the affected bones was undertaken.

The histological illustrations are from the lesion of the distal third of the radius. Material from the lesion of the humerus showed essentially the same appearance. Q2b and c show poorly cellular mature cartilage without any atypical features. The cells are small and regular. Pleomorphism and mitotic activity are absent. As in Q1, the tumour tissue is eroding the endosteal surface of the cortex, but the histological appearance is that of a slowly growing, almost quiescent enchondroma, with no evidence of malignancy.

Enchondroma

These benign cartilaginous tumours are extremely common, representing approximately 10% of all skeletal neoplasms. The sex incidence is equal. They are observed usually in children and young adults.

Clinical Features

Most enchondromas are recognised either as the result of a pathological fracture, particularly in small bones, as in the present Q1, or on account of a cosmetic deformity due to a bony-hard swelling. They may be detected incidentally by radiological examination. Actual pain rarely is caused by a benign enchondroma, unless it is produced by pressure on a nerve. When pain does develop it is essential to consider the possibility, especially in lesions of long bones and the axial skeleton, of chondrosarcomatous degeneration. This complication is more common when the lesions are multiple.

If multiple enchondromas are widespread throughout the skeleton the diagnosis becomes that of the generalised bone disorder of dyschondroplasia (enchondromatosis; Ollier's disease). This entity resembles multiple exostoses (see Exercise 4) in being a generalised disturbance of cartilage growth, but does not show a familial pattern of occurrence. Dyschondroplasia may be complicated by association with haemangiomas of skin and soft tissue (Maffucci's syndrome), in which case the incidence of chondrosarcomatous change is distinctly higher.

Radiological Features

1. Site. Of enchondromas, 50% arise in the hands and feet, with a marked predilection for the hands. The remainder occur mainly in major long bones, such as the ribs, sternum, scapula and pelvis. In children, metaphyseal involvement is common. A few of these tumours have a periosteal (parosteal) location.

2. Appearance. The typical lesion is shown as a well-defined translucency within a medullary cavity, with a sclerotic margin and a narrow zone of transition. As they grow slowly, the overlying cortex becomes thinned and expanded, the endosteal aspect developing smooth scalloped erosions. Periosteal reaction usually is lacking unless a pathological fracture has occurred, in which case the pattern may be complicated by callus formation. As the cartilage matures, calcification develops within it, varying from 'snowflakes' to massive irregular densities of the 'popcorn' type. In children with dyschondroplasia, lucent columns of cartilage often extend into the shafts of the long bones from the growth plates. Associated haemangiomas are recognised by soft tissue masses containing numerous calcified phleboliths. Alteration, particularly in long bones, of the appearance of an enchondroma in serial studies, together with the development of pain, provides a warning of the possibility of malignancy. Organised periosteal reactions then produce fusiform expansion of the affected area.

Pathological Features

Enchondromas consist essentially of mature cartilage. They take the form of rounded or nodular masses, usually in the medullary cavity of the affected bone, although periosteal lesions also can occur. The cartilage is poorly cellular. The cells are small and the pleomorphism of a malignant tumour is not present. The histological recognition and evaluation of malignancy in cartilage tumours is notoriously difficult, but a high degree of cellularity and the presence of binucleate or mitotic cells may suggest a diagnosis of chondrosarcoma, particularly in a growing lesion in a major long bone in an adult. As already noted, lesions in multiple enchondromata may show marked cellularity, and even mitotic activity, in the absence of malignant change.

Treatment

In many cases no special treatment is required, other than orthodox measures for fractures, which usually heal without complications. Curettage and packing with bone chips may be performed and large cosmetic deformities may be improved by excision, often incomplete, of the offending mass. A peripheral chondrosarcoma often will require amputation, but some may be suitable for prosthetic replacement, particularly in the proximal end of the femur, an especially common site.

References

Rockwell MA, Saiter ET, Enneking WF (1972) Periosteal chondroma. J Bone Jt Surg 54A:102–108.

Spjut HJ, Dorfman HJ, Fechner RE, Ackerman LV (1971) Tumours of bone and cartilage. Atlas of tumor pathology, 2nd series, Fasc. 5. Washington: Armed Forces Institute of Pathology

Takigawa K (1971) Chondroma of the bones of the hand: a review of 110 cases. J Bone Jt Surg 53A: 1591–1600

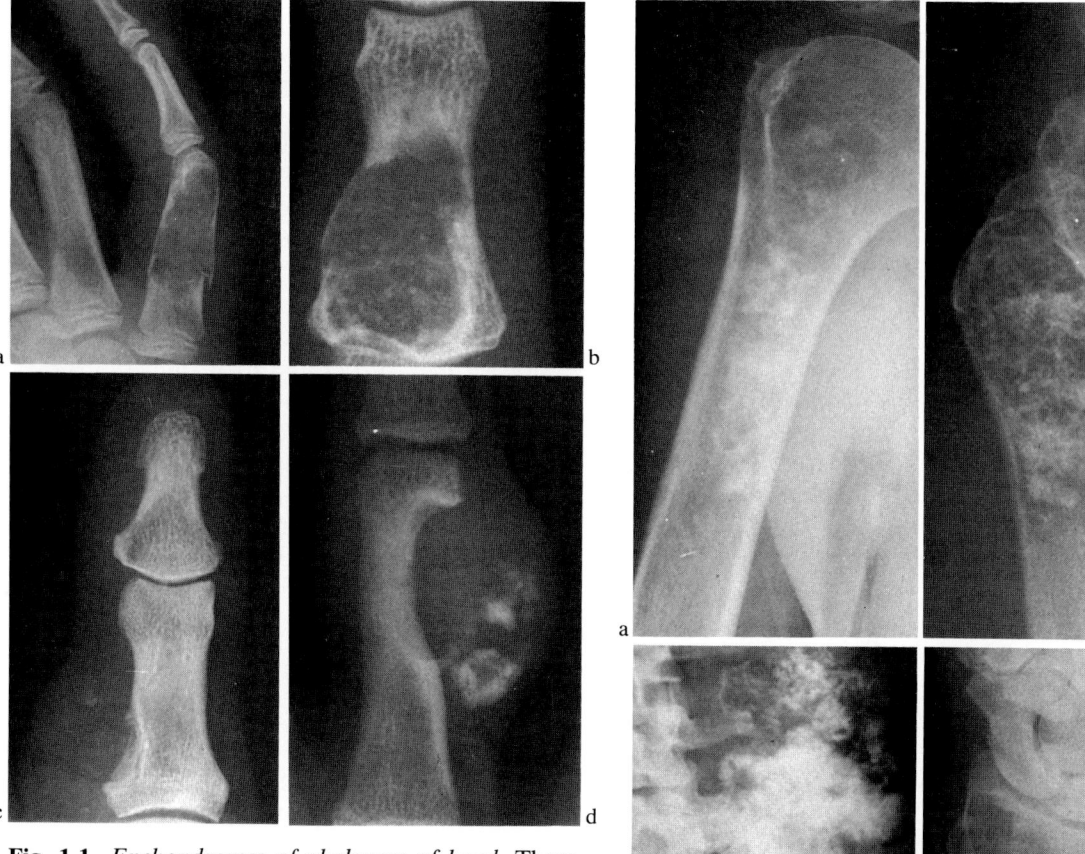

Fig. 1.1. *Enchondromas of phalanges of hand.* These tumours are very common. **a** A pathological fracture drew attention to this typically osteolytic lesion in an 8-year-old girl. Endosteal erosion and thinning of the overlying cortex had occurred, but the tumour was insufficiently mature to have developed significant evidence of calcification. **b** This characteristic enchondroma in a young woman caused the cosmetic deformity of a hard painless swelling. The endosteal margin has a narrow and sclerotic zone of transition and punctate calcifications have appeared within the cartilaginous mass. **c** In this instance the tumour has arisen in a parosteal location, causing a smoothly outlined cortical erosion and a soft tissue extension which contains flecks of calcification resembling snowflakes. **d** This parosteal chondroma in a 15-year-old girl is even more prominent and is calcified more extensively.

Fig. 1.2. *Benign cartilaginous tumours in adults.* In all these cases malignancy was suspected, the diagnosis only being established finally by histological assessment after biopsy. **a** *Humerus.* The nodular or 'popcorn' medullary calcification in this patient lay within a poorly defined lucent lesion. **b** *Head of fibula.* This tumour caused significant expansion of the bone, evident clinically as a painless swelling. Similar calcification had developed. Attention to its presence was drawn by symptoms arising from pressure on the lateral popliteal nerve. **c** *Ilium.* The large swelling produced by this huge expansile mass was palpable clinically. Although extensively calcified, two areas of lucency were suspected to be malignant. **d** *Radius.* In contrast no calcification was evident in this lytic area in a 60-year-old man who complained of mild pain in the wrist. Biopsy was performed to exclude a metastasis, but only benign cartilaginous tissue was present.

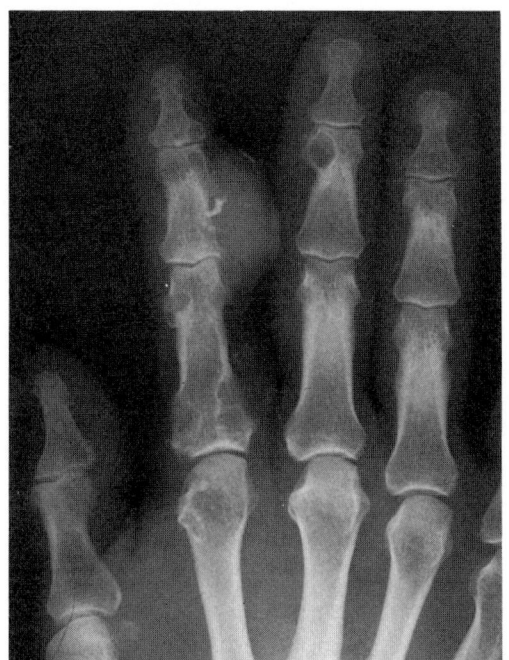

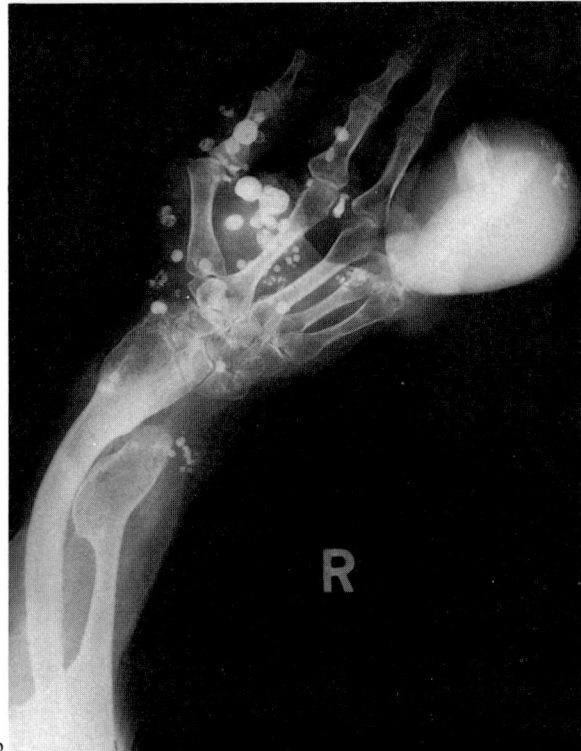

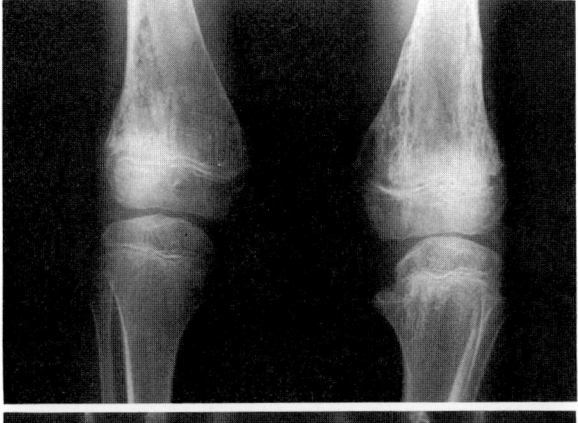

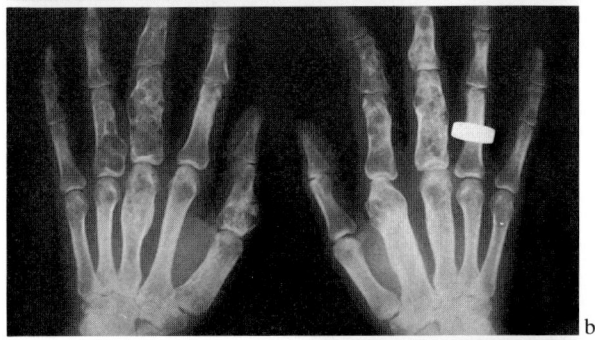

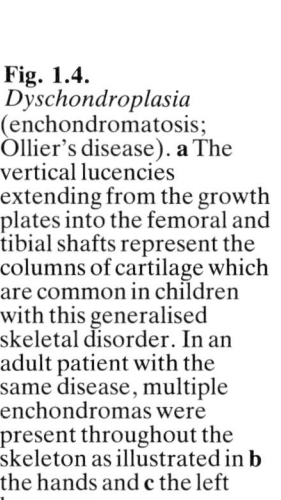

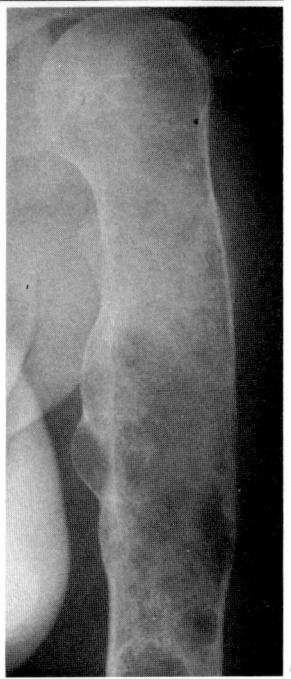

Fig. 1.3. *Multiple enchondromas.* **a** Typical lesions were present in the hand of this 61-year-old man. He had been aware of the swelling of his index finger for 40 years. He believed it not to have changed for at least 10 years. **b** *Maffucci's syndrome.* In this patient multiple enchondromas had caused the modelling abnormalties of the radius and ulna. They were associated with many soft tissue haemangiomas, characterised by the presence of numerous phleboliths.

Fig. 1.4. *Dyschondroplasia* (enchondromatosis; Ollier's disease). **a** The vertical lucencies extending from the growth plates into the femoral and tibial shafts represent the columns of cartilage which are common in children with this generalised skeletal disorder. In an adult patient with the same disease, multiple enchondromas were present throughout the skeleton as illustrated in **b** the hands and **c** the left humerus.

Q1. This 45-year-old man, an Indian immigrant from East Africa, presented with persistent back pain of 1 year's duration.

Anorexia and lassitude had resulted in mild cachexia. On clinical examination the only abnormality detected was localised tenderness over T11.

Radiographs revealed a destructive process in the body of T11, causing anterior and right lateral wedging. Partial loss of definition of the upper and lower tables was evident, with some sclerosis. Well-defined soft tissue opacities were present on each side of the spine and the anterior aspect of the body of T12 showed a hazy, scalloped erosion.

The lesion was explored.

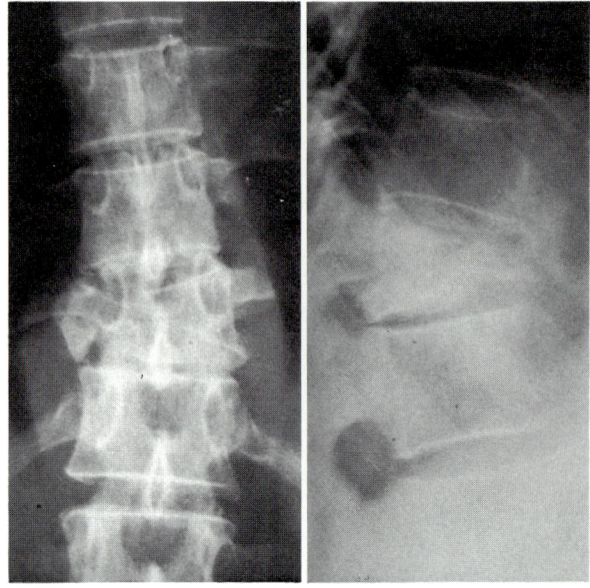

Q1a.

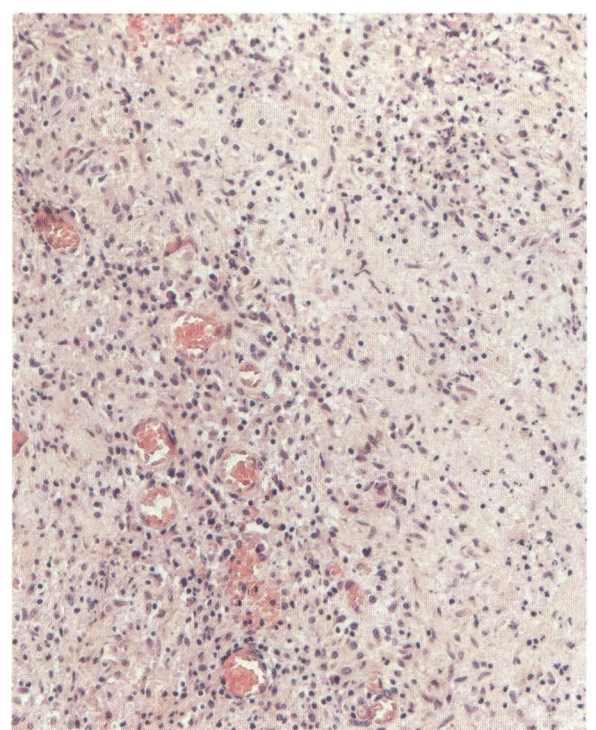

Q1b. (×140)

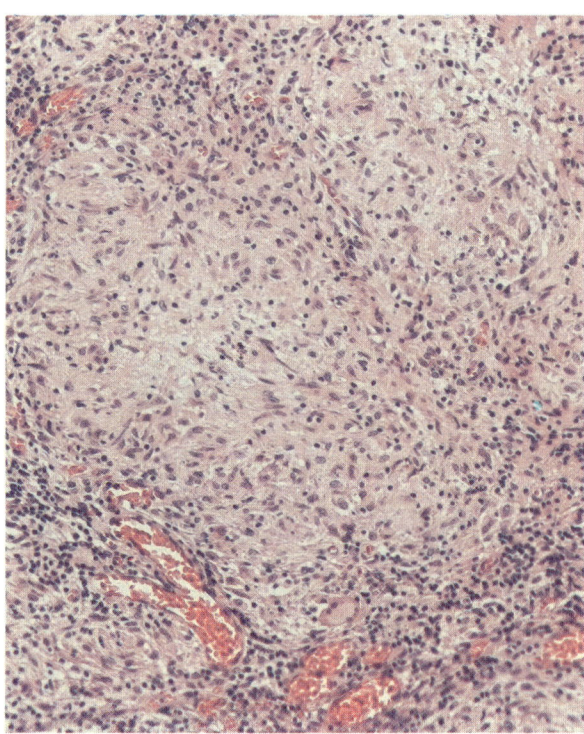

Q1c. (×140)

Q2. This 18-year-old man had complained of mild backache for more than a year.

During recent months the pain had become constant and was aggravated by standing. Clinical examination showed gross limitation of movement and a mildly tender kyphoscoliosis at the thoracolumbar junction.

Radiographs from an examination elsewhere a year earlier were available (Q2a). Narrowing of the T12/L1 intervertebral space had been observed (*arrow*) and a diagnosis of derangement of this intervertebral disc, secondary to Scheuermann's disease, had been suggested. Further examination on this presentation revealed increased narrowing of this intervertebral space, with erosions of the adjacent end-plates. Dense sclerosis had developed in the subchondral portions of these vertebral bodies and organised periosteal reactions were present.

The lesion was explored.

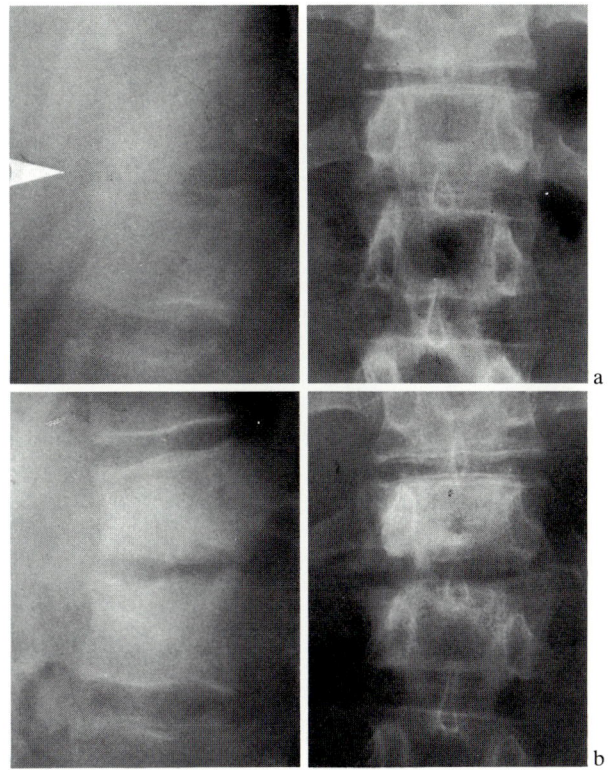

Q2a and b.

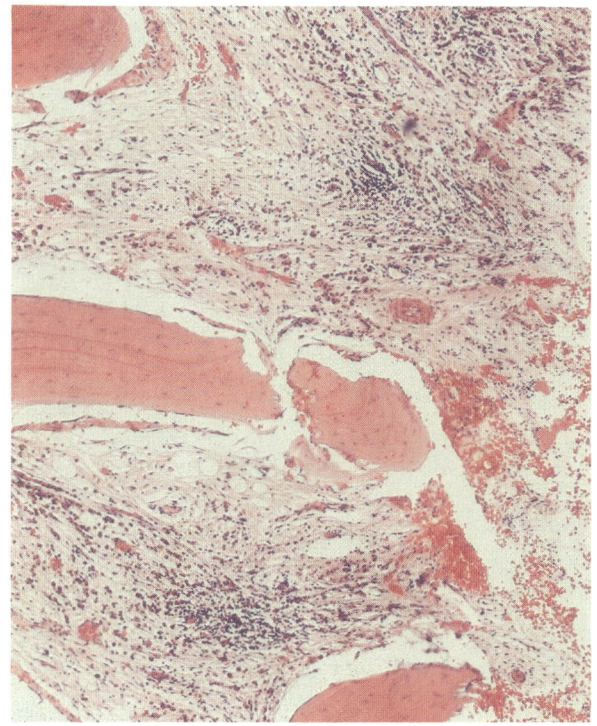

Q2c. (×63)

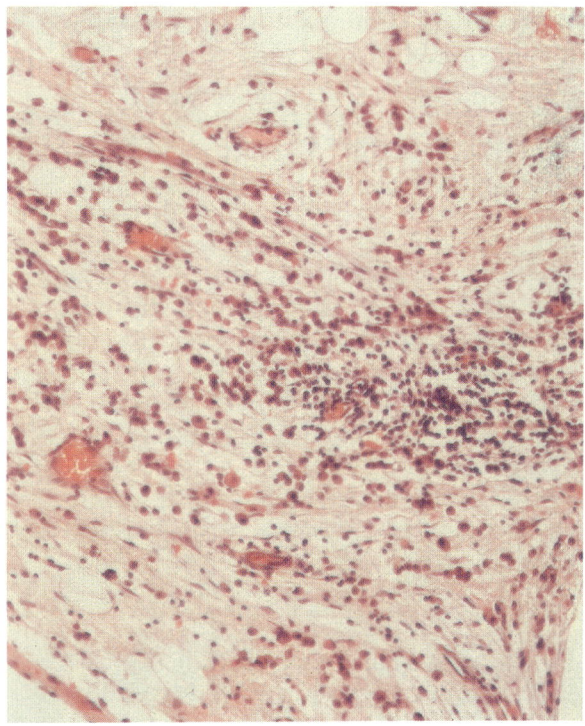

Q2d. (×160)

A1. Tuberculosis of spine (Pott's disease)

The clinical and radiological findings are typical of a chronic inflammatory process. Involvement of more than one vertebral body with erosion of the vertebral plates, coupled with the presence of bilateral paravertebral abscesses, provided a strong indication of tuberculosis being the infective organism, particularly in a patient of this race and origin. In this patient the significant investigations supporting the diagnosis were an elevated ESR (58 mm/h), a reduced haemoglobin level (10.4 g) and a positive tuberculin reaction. In the present case the Mantoux reaction was positive at 1:5000. A negative reaction at 1:1000 or a negative PPD would exclude a diagnosis of tuberculosis.

Despite bed rest and antituberculous therapy, incipient paraparesis developed during the subsequent 6 weeks, demanding active surgical intervention. Anterior decompression and curettage were performed, with the insertion of an anterior graft in the affected spinal segment. The necrotic material from the involved bone and intervertebral disc provided bacteriological confirmation of tuberculosis, subsequent culture demonstrating the organism to be fully sensitive to all the antituberculous drugs. Histological study of this material was undertaken also. Q1b shows the marrow spaces to be occupied by chronic inflammatory tissue. Lymphocytes and plasma cells are present. In addition larger mononuclear cells can be identified, and the tissue has a nodular arrangement which is reminiscent of the 'tubercles' illustrated in the examples of articular tuberculosis described in Exercise 11. Tuberculosis was substantiated even more definitely by the recognition in other areas of tubercles with giant cells (Fig. 1.1) and necrotic—caseous—tissue (Fig. 1.2). This chronic infection had resulted also in clear evidence of bone necrosis, as shown by the dead trabeculae in Fig. 1.3.

Following surgical clearance of the infective focus, the patient recovered rapidly with excellent incorporation of the graft, being well and asymptomatic within 3 months.

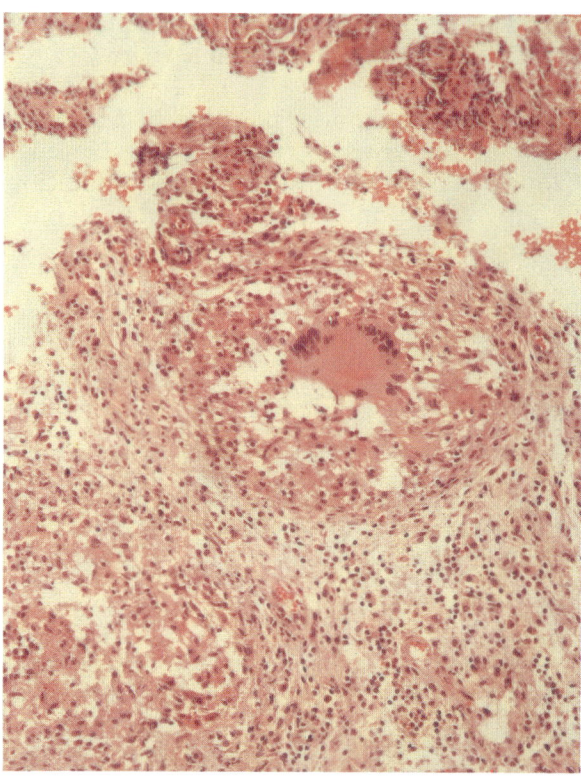

Fig. 1.1. Another field from the same specimen illustrates a classical 'tubercle' with chronic granulation tissue surrounding a giant cell in which many nuclei are arranged with a peripheral orientation. (×140)

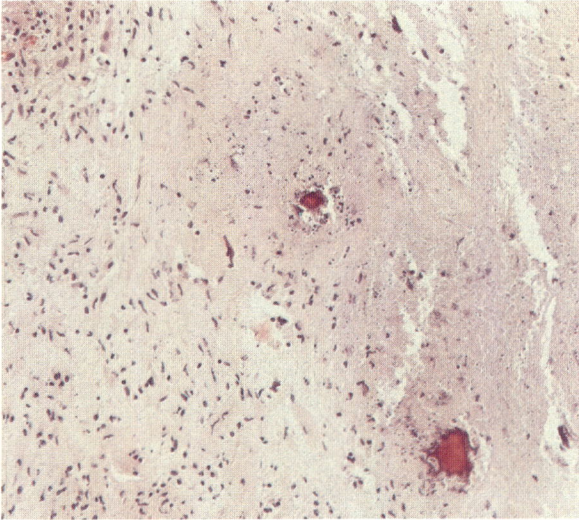

Fig. 1.2. Necrotic caseous tissue with darkly staining foci of calcification. (×125)

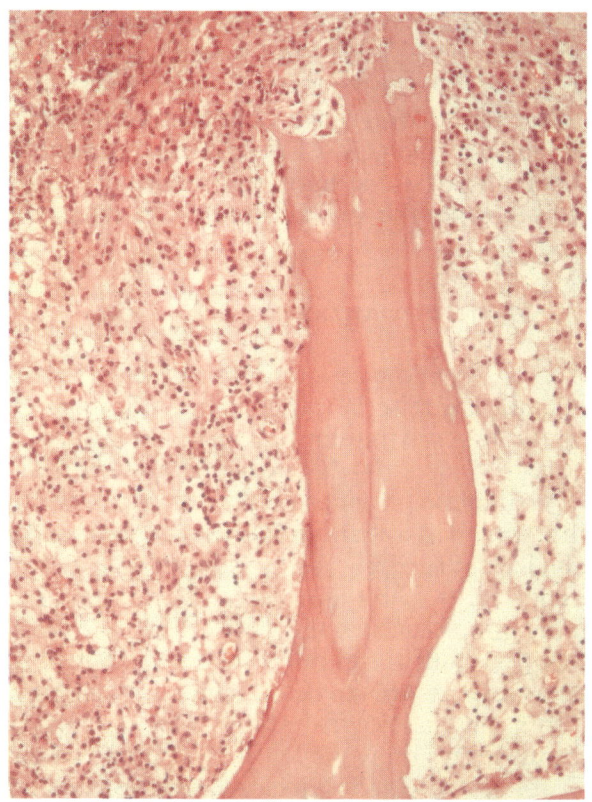

Fig. 1.3. Necrosis of this trabecula is indicated by complete absence of nuclei within the osteocyte lacunae. Some osteoclastic resorption is in progress. Many lymphocytes and plasma cells are present in the adjacent chronic granulomatous tissue. (×140)

Osseous Tuberculosis

This Exercise considers involvement of the skeleton by the tubercle bacillus, excluding the manifestations of articular disease which have been discussed already in Exercise 11. Tuberculosis of the spine, Pott's disease, is much the most common form of skeletal involvement, its incidence exceeding all joint infections and the relatively rare types of osseous lesions encountered elsewhere in the skeleton. Although the incidence of these infections has fallen greatly as a result of improved public health measures and more effective treatment since anti-tuberculous drugs were introduced, the condition is still a scourge in underdeveloped countries. In such areas poverty and inadequate health care may delay diagnosis and, even then, suitable treatment may not be available. In Great Britain, indeed, illness in the immigrant population from such areas as the Indian subcontinent, Africa and the West Indies causes the possibility of tuberculosis to be an early consideration. The disease usually is contracted in childhood, its incidence diminishing, but still continuing, as age advances.

Clinical Features

A. Pott's Disease

The onset of the infection is often insidious, causing at first localised spinal discomfort and progressing only later to mild kyphoscoliosis, which, in severe cases, may become extreme. Generalised symptoms include lassitude, weakness and loss of appetite. Night sweats and intermittent pyrexia may occur. Lymph nodes may be enlarged. Clinical manifestations of pulmonary or renal involvement are surprisingly rare. Cord pressure symptoms leading to paraparesis and culminating occasionally in paraplegia are late and relatively unusual complications. Abscess formation is extremely common and, depending on the site, presents as retropharyngeal, paravertebral or psoas abscesses, which may point virtually anywhere in the vicinity.

B. Other Osseous Lesions

Other osseous lesions are rare. In contrast to pyogenic infections in which bones are more commonly involved than joints, the reverse holds true in the case of tuberculosis. Lesions of this type are heralded usually by mild localised pain and swelling, their recognition depending on radiological examination and their diagnosis on bacteriological culture or histological study.

Radiological Features

A. Pott's Disease

1. Site. Any portion of the spine may be affected, but the lower thoracic and upper lumbar areas are particularly susceptible. The earliest focus of infection is usually in the anterior third of a vertebral body, with subsequent spread to the adjacent intervertebral discs and vertebral bodies. Occasionally a focus may arise in a neural arch, causing destruction of a spinous process or an articular process. Such bizarre lesions are encountered especially in the immigrant population. Although the infection is commonly confined to a single spinal segment, multifocal lesions can occur. Sacro-iliac joint infections, which may be mentioned here as part of the axial skeleton, are almost always unilateral.

2. Appearance. The lesions are primarily destructive, causing irregular areas of osteolysis with hazy and poorly defined margins. When the intervertebral discs are invaded, the normal density of the subchondral bone is lost and erosions of the vertebral plates develop with narrowing of the corresponding intervertebral space. Serial studies show only slow progression of these changes and demonstrate also the gradual development of a kyphoscoliosis. A characteristic feature of Pott's disease is the production of tuberculous pus, sometimes in very large quantities. Consequent abscesses in the thoracic area become evident as sharply defined paravertebral masses, usually bilateral. They may be obscured in an underpenetrated chest radiograph. It is important that their presence behind the heart shadow should not be confused with an unfolded aorta. They may encroach on the spinal canal and contribute to neurological deficits. Abscesses from lumbar lesions distend the outlines of the psoas muscles and those in the neck cause anterior displacement of the trachea. Massive abscess formation may be observed in the rare type of Pott's disease (approximately 2%) known as *subligamentous tuberculosis*. In this entity bony abnormalities at first may be entirely lacking or confined to minimal periosteal reactions on vertebral bodies, but they usually progress ultimately to the classical pattern of bony destruction. In the era before antituberculous medication was introduced, slow healing of the infection was accompanied by contraction of these abscesses and the development of calcification within their walls.

The infective process of Pott's disease is so chronic that, even on presentation, some reactive sclerosis may be evident. Such sclerosis becomes even more prominent if secondary pyogenic infection is introduced through a draining sinus, a complication more common in the pre-antibiotic era than it is today.

B. Other Osseous Lesions

1. Site. As in the case of pyogenic osteomyelitis (see Exercise 10), the hyperaemic areas of metaphyses in immature long bones represent favoured sites. In this instance, however, the growth plate provides no significant barrier to the spread of infection. It must be emphasised again that tuberculous lesions of this type are much rarer than their pyogenic counterparts. Flat bones such as the pelvis, ribs and skull (Pott's 'puffy tumour') may be affected, causing diagnosis to be difficult and to depend often on histological study. Occasionally a bony lesion may develop by direct spread from an infected bursa or tendon sheath. *Tuberculous dactylitis*, with many foci of infection in varying phases of aggression and regression in the small bones of the hands and feet, is now a rarity. Equally rare is the so-called *cystic tuberculosis*, an entity in which multiple foci exhibit a remarkable tendency towards bilateral and symmetrical distribution.

2. Appearance. These osteolytic lesions often resemble pyogenic Brodie's abscesses. They tend to stimulate little or no periosteal reaction. Sequestrum formation is distinctly unusual. In the dactylitic and cystic forms, particularly, the lesions may be expansile.

Pathological Features

Biopsy material, when available, exhibits the same features as those described in articular tuberculosis, namely (a) abundant chronic inflammatory tissue containing numerous lymphocytes and plasma cells, (b) nodular arrangement of 'tubercles', (c) giant cells with peripheral location of nuclei and (d) areas of caseation and necrosis.

Treatment

A. Pott's Disease

During the last decade the great majority of patients have been diagnosed correctly at an early stage. In consequence almost all respond to conservative measures, namely absolute bed rest combined with antituberculous therapy. The routine drugs employed are rifampicin, para-aminosalicylic acid, isoniazid and ethambutol. These medications are administered for a minimum period of 9 months. Provided that medication is continued for this period at least, reactivation does not occur. The patient is mobilised when the erythrocyte sedimentation rate has returned to normal.

In cases of persistent paraplegia, a condition becoming progressively rarer, surgical decompression is performed if 6 weeks of conservative treatment have failed to produce neurological improvement. In tuberculous paraparesis or paraplegia, sphincteric involvement is not an indication for immediate surgical intervention. If adequate facilities are not available, satisfactory decompression can be achieved by a simple costotransversectomy, but a formal anterior decompression, coupled with grafting, is preferable. Anterolateral decompression is indicated only in paraplegia of late onset, when severe deformity precludes an anterior approach. In rare cases of mechanical instability, grafting is clearly required. Laminectomy may be undertaken only when the disease is confined entirely to the posterior vertebral elements, resulting in persistent paraparesis. This procedure, otherwise, is totally contra-indicated.

B. Other Osseous Lesions

Treatment is directed by the site of skeletal involvement. In all cases antituberculous therapy is required. When the bones of the lower limbs are affected, protection from weight-bearing is indicated. Surgical intervention is required only with particularly aggressive lesions for which curettage is usually adequate.

Reference

Seddon HJ (1976) The choice of treatment in Pott's disease. J Bone Jt Surg 58B: 395–397

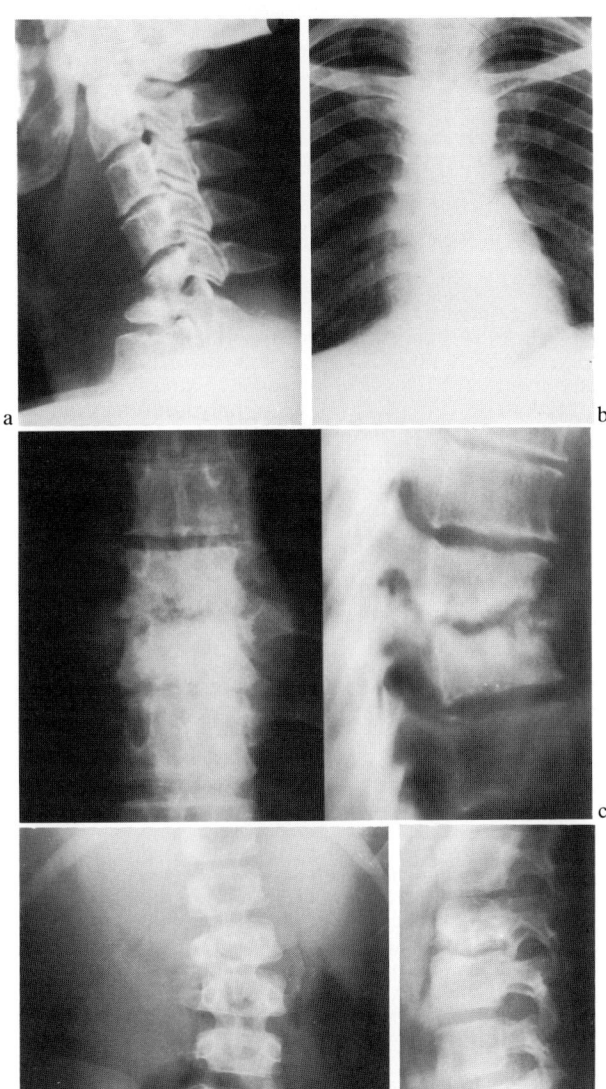

Fig. 1.4. *Spinal tuberculosis—classical examples.* **a** *Cervical.* This 64-year-old man presented with chronic dysphagia and pain in the neck. C5/6 involvement is accompanied by a huge retropharyngeal abscess. **b** *Thoracic.* Routine chest examination of an asymptomatic 32-year-old Nigerian man revealed the shadow of a paravertebral abscess, subsequently confirmed to be tuberculous, lying behind the heart. **c** *Thoracic.* Typical destruction of the adjacent portions of T7 and 8, causing a mild kyphos, in a 44-year-old man with chronic back pain. Smoothly outlined bilateral paravertebral abscesses have formed. At operation more granulation tissue than pus may be found. **d** *Lumbar.* In this 9-year-old boy with intermittent but mild back pain for 18 months, the L3/4 lesion had caused a scoliosis. Observe distension of the right psoas sheath by a large abscess.

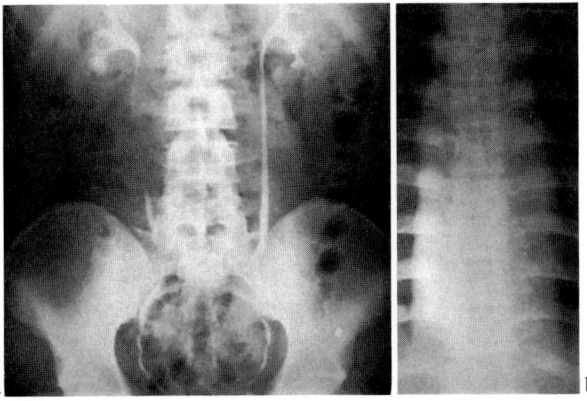

Fig. 1.5. *Subligamentous spinal tuberculosis.* **a** *Lumbar.* Routine investigation of the urinary tract of this 26-year-old Indian man with abdominal discomfort revealed bilateral psoas abscesses with virtually no bone involvement. **b** *Thoracic.* Unusually extensive bilateral paravertebral abscesses, with only minimal bone involvement, were found in this 18-year-old youth, who had complained of pain for several months. Their presence indicated this unusual form of spinal tuberculous infection.

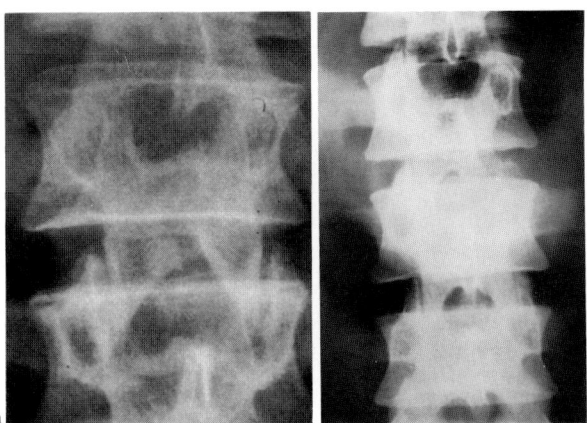

Fig. 1.7. *Spinal tuberculosis—neural arch lesions*—both found in immigrants. **a** Complete destruction of the spinous process of L1. **b** Involvement of left inferior articular process of L3 causing backache of 4 years' duration and recent paraparesis.

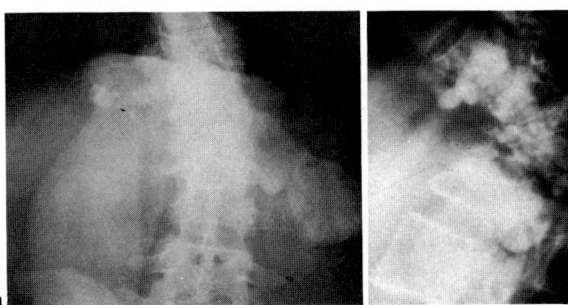

Fig. 1.6. *Spinal tuberculosis—long-standing disease.* Gross destruction of the vertebral bodies and massive calcification of abscesses in this 41-year-old woman had resulted from a childhood infection in the pre-antibiotic era, treated by prolonged decubitus. Calculi were evident in the right kidney—a recognised complication of this treatment. Observe the gross residual kyphosis—today a rarity.

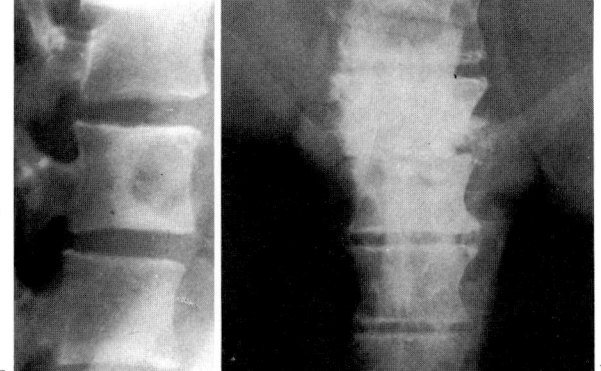

Fig. 1.8. *Spinal tuberculosis.* **a** *Early.* A purely osseous focus in the body of L3. This young male African with back pain for 18 months had been diagnosed initially as having a deranged intervertebral disc. **b** *Late—reactivation due to steroid therapy.* This 60-year-old man had been treated successfully in 1947 for a lesion of the T11/12 level. He was one of the first recipients of streptomycin. In 1981 he developed Addison's disease for which steroid therapy was administered. Within 6 months the old tuberculous focus had reactivated with typical erosions and bilateral paravertebral abscesses, causing paraplegia.

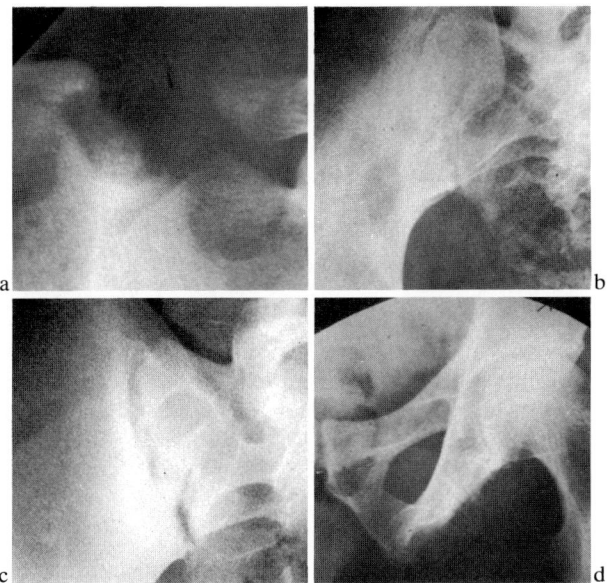

Fig. 1.9. *Osseous tuberculosis—pelvic lesions.* **a** This lytic lesion in the ilium was found in a 23-year-old Indian woman with low back pain, radiating to the ankle for 2 months. The patient's race correctly suggested the diagnosis. **b** A histologically proven tuberculous abscess in the right ilium of a 24-year-old man—another Indian—with a relatively short history of a few weeks' localised pain. In a Caucasian a Brodie's abscess would have been suspected. **c** For comparison a tuberculous infection of the right sacro-iliac joint is illustrated, with extensive articular erosions and reactive sclerosis in a 26-year-old woman who had suffered previously from pulmonary tuberculosis. Such an association is surprisingly unusual. **d** Erosion of the ischium secondary to tuberculous infection of an adjacent adventitious bursa.

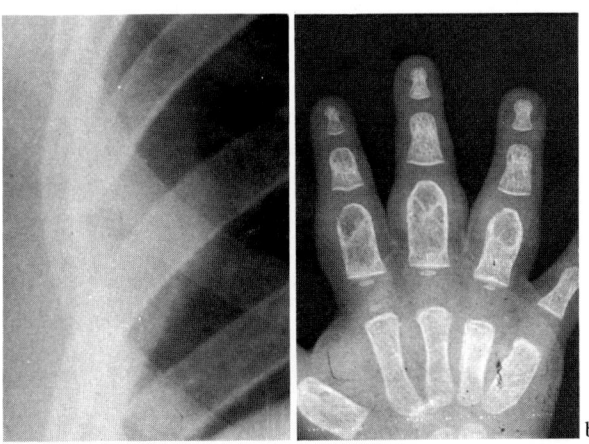

Fig. 1.10. *Osseous tuberculosis—other* manifestations. **a** Destruction of 6th rib with abscess. Lesions of this type are uncommon. **b** *Tuberculous dactylitis.* Many small bones are affected by expansile lytic lesions in differing phases of aggression and repair. The historical term *spina* (a short bone) *ventosa* (inflated with air) was descriptively accurate.

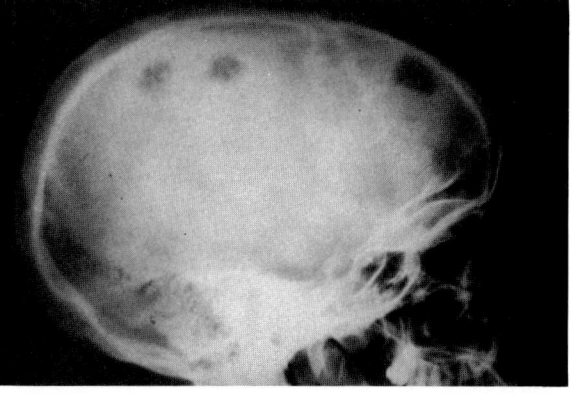

Fig. 1.11. *Osseous tuberculosis—Skull.* Multiple lytic lesions were present in this young man with disseminated skeletal tuberculosis. Individually such foci are known as 'Pott's puffy tumours'.

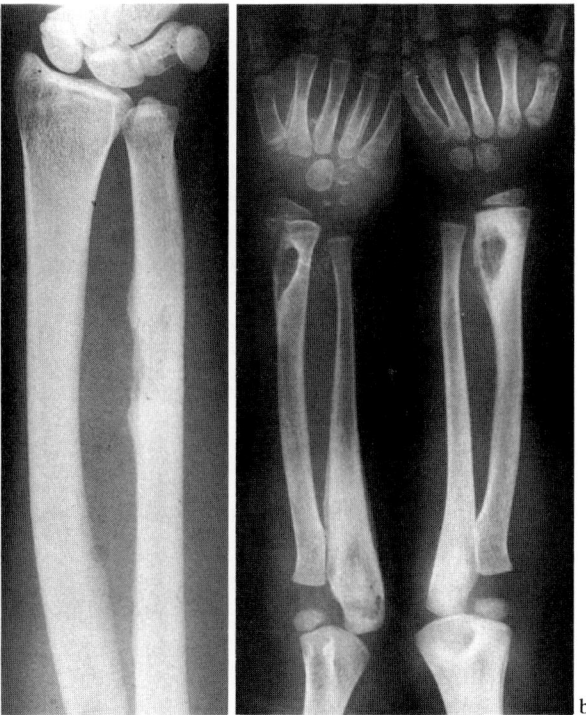

Fig. 1.12. *Osseous tuberculosis—long bones.* **a** *Ulna.* This 49-year-old Indian woman with established renal disease developed in 6 weeks a painful swelling of the right forearm. In other circumstances the destructive lesion might have been regarded as a metastasis. **b** *Disseminated tuberculosis—'cystic' form.* This very rare manifestation of the infection carries a good prognosis and is characterised by remarkably symmetrical and expanding lytic lesions, in the same phase of aggression. Those shown in the forearms of this young English child are typical. The left wrist is affected, but joints often are spared. Observe periosteal reactions on the right metacarpals. The symmetry of the lesions suggests sudden haematogenous dissemination.

A2. Infective discitis

The radiological appearance of this lesion at the time of presentation was typical of a chronic low-grade infection. The erosions of the vertebral plates would probably have been demonstrated more clearly by tomograms, but their presence, together with the organised periosteal reactions and the reactive sclerosis in the vertebral bodies, favoured a pyogenic rather than a tuberculous aetiology. Even in the earlier radiographs, loss of the 'white line' on the inferior table of the body of T12 might well have aroused suspicion of this diagnosis, particularly if a radionuclide scan had been positive. Serological investigations were confirmatory: ESR 59 mm/h, WBC 11 000 per mm^3, Hb 10.2 g, proteins normal, Mantoux test negative at 1:10 000, antistaphylococcal haemolysin 5 units (normal 0.5–2.0).

Culture of material removed from the lesion at operation grew *Staphylococcus aureus* (pyogenes), establishing finally the type of the infective organism, Histological examination showed non-specific inflammatory ('granulation') tissue to have replaced the normal bone marrow. Q2c and d show this tissue to be fibrovascular and to contain numerous lymphocytes and plasma cells. The polymorphonuclear leucocytes which would be expected in an acute staphylococcal osteomyelitis (see Exercise 10) are not present, indicating the indolent nature of this subacute infection. Most examples of acute staphylococcal osteomyelitis develop some histological evidence of bone necrosis. No such necrosis was detected in the present case, even with careful examination of all the available material. Equally, no histological evidence of any specific type of inflammatory process, particularly tuberculosis as in Q1 of this Exercise, was found.

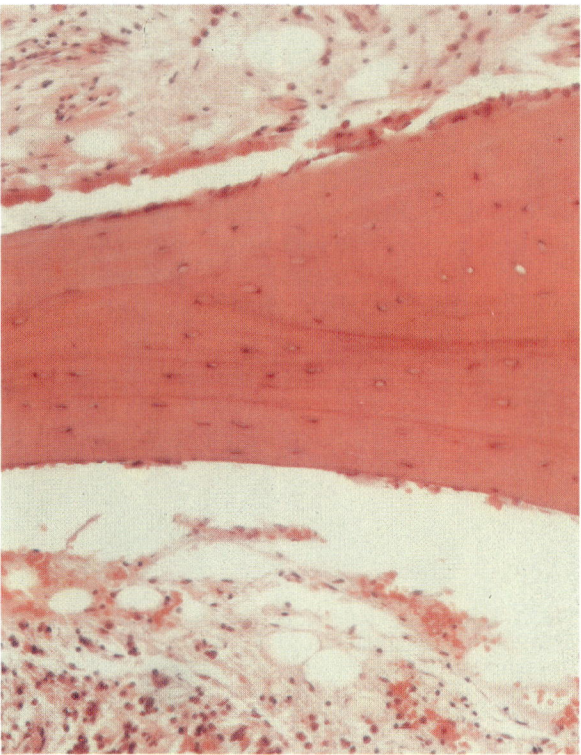

Fig. 2.1. This trabecula from the same specimen consists of viable bone, as indicated by the darkly staining nuclei contained within the osteocyte lacunae. It is surrounded by chronic inflammatory tissue. (×162)

Infective Discitis

Pyogenic spinal infections originate often in intervertebral discs, frequently as a sequel to another focus of infection elsewhere in the body, such as the genito-urinary tract, the skin or the teeth. They are commonest in middle life, but may occur at any age, with a marked predilection for males.

Clinical Features

Chronic and localised back pain is the usual presenting symptom, occurring most frequently in the lumbar area, although any spinal segment may be affected. The disease is rarely fulminating in type and the diagnosis depends largely on radiological findings. The most serious complication is the not infrequent development of partial or complete paraplegia.

Radiological Features

1. Site. As indicated above, the majority of these lesions are unifocal and are recognised most frequently in the lumbar spine.

2. Appearance. The initial abnormality of narrowing of the affected disc space simulates almost exactly derangement of a disc as a result of mechanical stress. Even radionuclide scanning at this stage is equivocal, since both lesions are likely to cause increased uptake of the tracer. The first positive radiological sign is partial or complete loss of the normal and clearly defined density ('white line') of a vertebral end-plate, followed by frank erosions which are evident especially in lateral tomograms. In severe and fulminating infections, these erosions may become so large that the consequent concavities have acquired the descriptive term of 'ballooning'. More commonly the infections are insidious and provoke adjacent reactive sclerosis, even before the erosions can be recognised. An additional and helpful diagnostic feature is the formation of organised periosteal reactions, especially on the anterior aspects of the adjacent vertebral bodies. The presence of both erosions and periosteal reactions, neither features of mechanical disc derangement, permits considerable confidence in the diagnosis of infective discitis. In some cases, however, the infection is so low-grade in type that bacteriological confirmation may never be obtained, although a blood culture occasionally may be positive. Abscess formation is rarely recognisable, but encroachment of granulation tissue on the neural canal, demonstrable by myelography, may induce neurological deficits. As activity subsides, either as a response to conservative antibiotic therapy or following surgical curettage, peripheral bony bridging develops, but bony fusion of the affected bodies is surprisingly uncommon, except in childhood, unlike ordinary osteomyelitis.

Pathological Features

The affected disc is replaced, at least partially, by inflammatory granulation tissue and the cartilaginous elements of the end-plates undergo extensive destruction. In the adjacent and radiographically sclerotic portions of the vertebral bodies the trabeculae are thickened by osteoblastic deposition of new bone, attributed to the localised hyperaemia induced by the infective process. The intervening trabecular spaces are filled by fibroblastic tissue. With the occasional extension of the infection into the vertebral bodies, classical changes of chronic osteomyelitis with areas of necrosis become evident (see Exercise 10).

Isolation of the causative organism from the curetted material is successful in only about two thirds of cases. *Staphylococcus pyogenes* is the most common, followed by *B. proteus* and *E. coli*, although a number of other rarer types of infection may be incriminated.

Treatment

Treatment is essentially conservative. If the causative organism is identified, then the appropriate antibiotic is administered. When it is not, and this is often the case, the condition is treated empirically, preferably using broad spectrum antibiotics. Treatment should be maintained for a minimum of 6 months or until the patient is asymptomatic, with the proviso that the ESR and the antistaphylococcal haemolysin titre have returned to normal. If any suggestion of paraparesis develops, it is essential to explore the lesion. Following curettage, grafting may be required to achieve ultimate stability.

References

Kemp HBS et al. (1973) Pyogenic infections occurring primarily in intervertebral discs. J Bone Jt Surg 55B: 698–714

Menelaus MB (1964) Discitis. J Bone Jt Surg 46B: 16–23

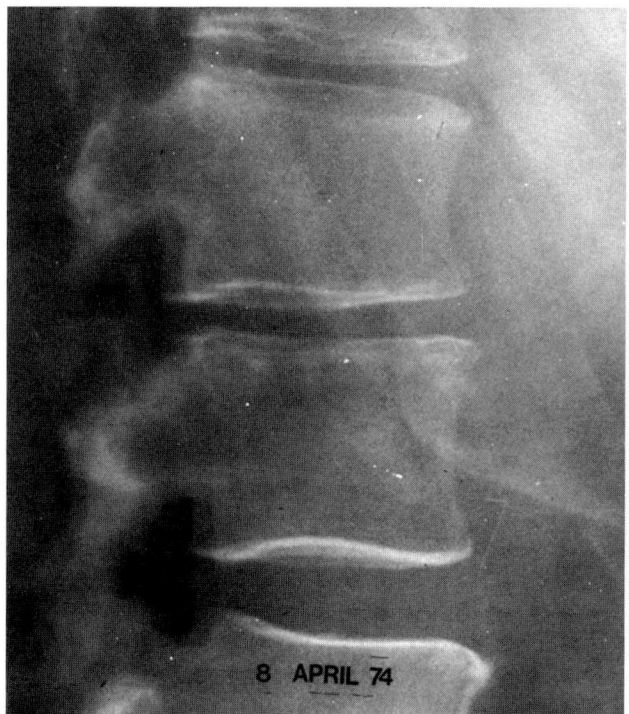 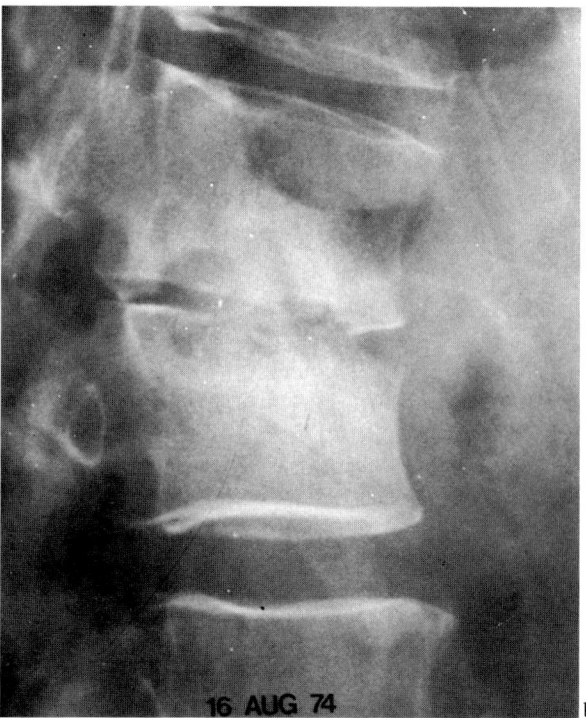

Fig. 2.2. *Infective discitis—early manifestations.* This 67-year-old man had been a poorly controlled diabetic for 14 years and presented with back pain which had been increasing for 5 months. **a** The initial examination, at another hospital, showed narrowing of the L1/2 intervertebral space. Negative agglutination titres at this time were considered to exclude infection and the patient was treated conservatively, but without success, for a prolapsed intervertebral disc. A very important and early radiological sign of infection—namely loss of the 'white line' on the proximal end-plate of the body of L2—was not appreciated. **b** When the patient was referred 4 months later to a special back clinic on account of continued symptoms, typical changes of infective discitis had developed. These consist of increased narrowing of the affected disc space, erosions of the vertebral end-plates and much reactive sclerosis. *Staphylococcus aureus* then was isolated from material obtained by aspiration biopsy.

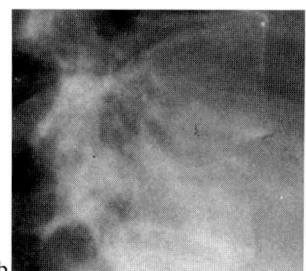 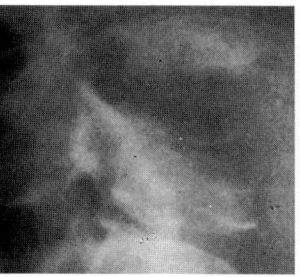 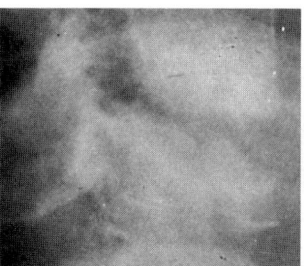 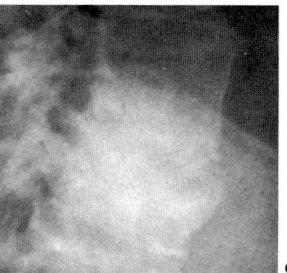

Fig. 2.3. *Infective discitis.* This obese 49-year-old woman had complained of low backache for 2 months. **a** Narrowing of the L4/5 intervertebral space was accompanied by frank erosions of the vertebral end-plates. Blood culture was positive for *Staphylococcus aureus*. **b** Despite appropriate antibiotic therapy and bed rest, the erosions enlarged during the subsequent 7 weeks, illustrating the 'ballooning' which can occur with these infections. Thereafter symptoms subsided and **c** dense sclerosis developed within the next 3 months. Treatment was continued until the titres were normal and **d** the final examination a year after the original presentation showed bony fusions to be almost complete. Direct surgical intervention was not required.

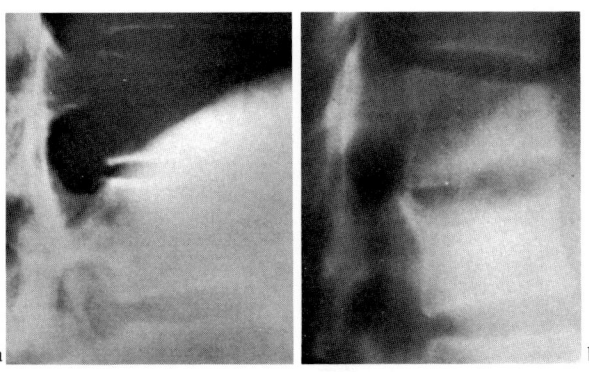

Fig. 2.4. *Infective discitis—source of infection.* **a** The radiographs of this 41-year-old woman with backache of 6 weeks' duration were at first believed to be normal, narrowing of the T11/12 intervertebral space being overlooked. **b** Five months later the diagnosis of infective discitis was obvious and a positive culture for *Staphylococcus aureus* was obtained. This lesion was believed to have originated from infection disseminated from an operation on an infected maxillary antrum 2 months before. Observe the improved detail obtained by tomography.

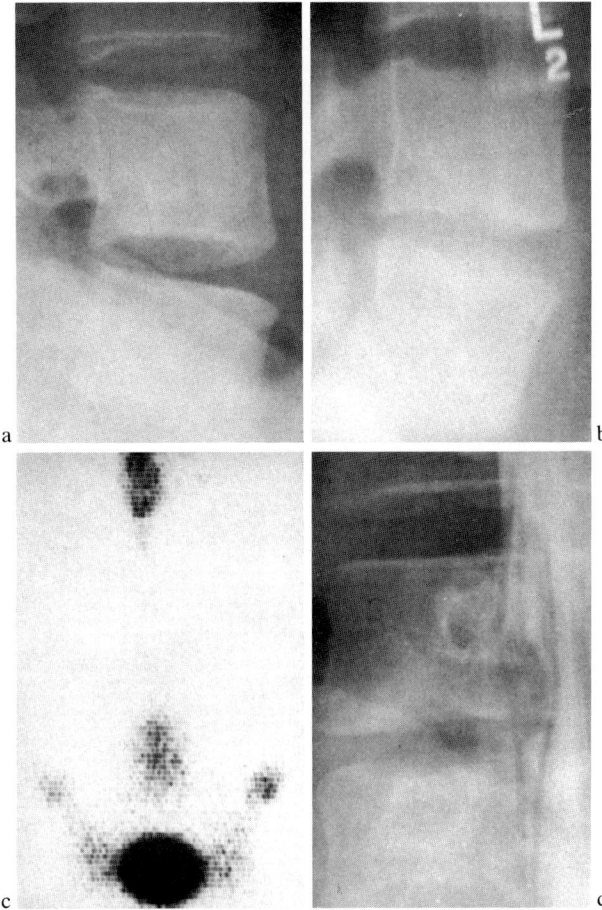

Fig. 2.6. *Infective discitis—abscess encroaching on spinal canal.* This 42-year-old man presented with referred pain and a neurological deficit attributed at first to prolapse of the L4/5 disc. The orthodox lateral film **a** showed slight narrowing of this intervertebral space and reverse slip of the body of L4. **b** Tomography was helpful, suggesting an erosion of the inferior end-plate of L4. **c** As expected, a radionuclide scan was positive, supporting differentiation from a disc lesion. **d** Radiculography demonstrated not only the erosion, but also a filling defect proximal to the L4/5 level. This defect was confirmed at operation to be an abscess. Curettage was performed without grafting, and complete recovery took place in 6 weeks.

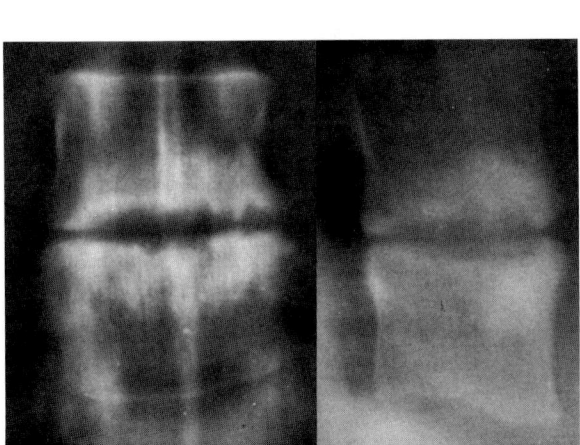

Fig. 2.5. *Infective discitis—periosteal reactions.* In addition to the radiological signs described above, periosteal reactions developing and organising on the adjacent vertebral bodies provide valuable supportive evidence of the diagnosis, permitting definite differentiation from degenerative disc lesions. This 36-year-old woman with typical back pain had a positive staphylococcal titre. The L4/5 lesion was explored, but necrotic material only was found. As not unusually occurs, it proved to be sterile. This infection was believed to have been derived from a dental abscess which had been treated 6 months earlier.

Q1. This 16-year-old boy had complained of pain and swelling of the right thigh for approximately 6 weeks.

On clinical examination a firm and slightly tender swelling was palpable on the postero-lateral aspect of the distal end of the femur. No other abnormality was detected.

Radiological examination showed areas of increased density in the distal portion of the femoral shaft, which was almost surrounded by a clearly defined soft tissue mass. On the lateral and posterior sides of this mass, radiating spicules of bone had formed. At the proximal end of the lesion triangular elevation of the periosteum was evident.

Biopsy was performed.

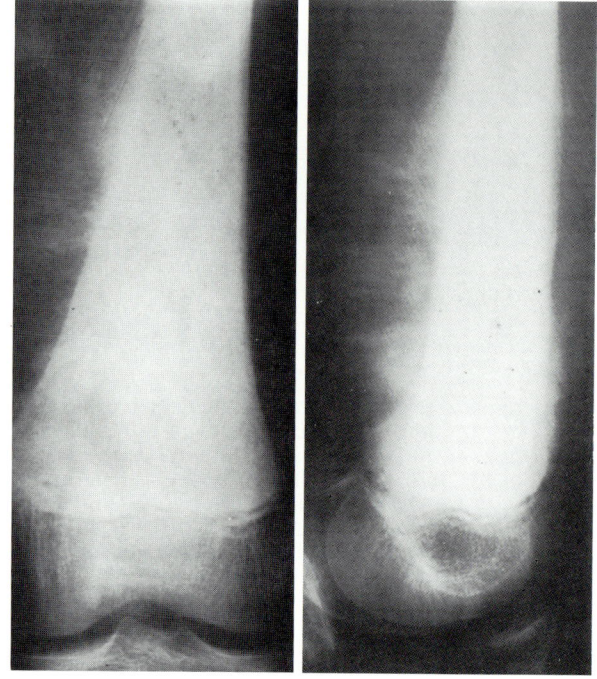

Q1a.

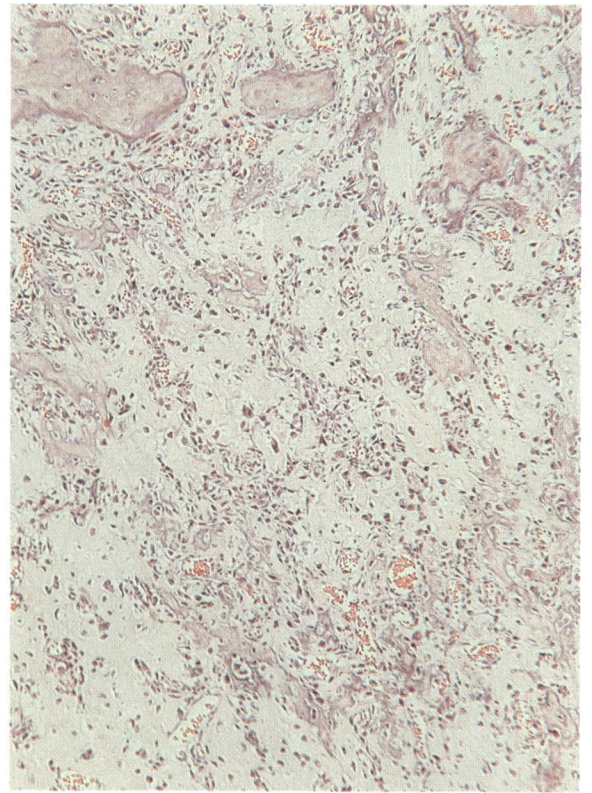

Q1b. (×70)

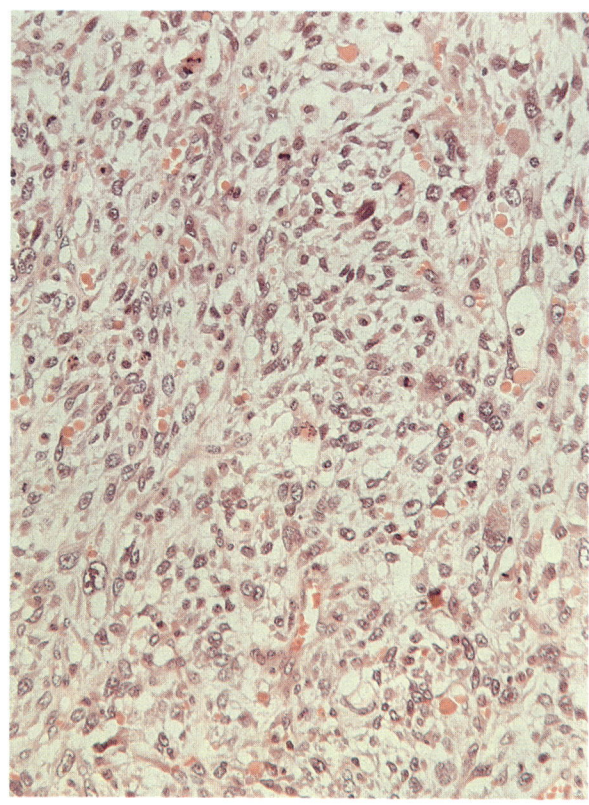

Q1c. (×200)

Exercise 14

Q2. This 60-year-old man had developed pain and swelling of the right knee which had been present for about 9 weeks.

Apart from a mildly tender swelling above the right knee no abnormality was found on clinical examination.

The radiographs showed a large lytic lesion in the distal end of the femur, with poorly defined margins.

A biopsy was performed.

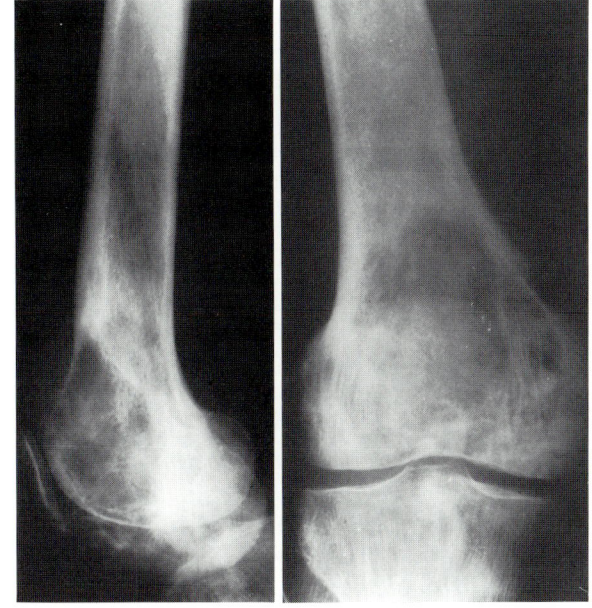

Q2a.

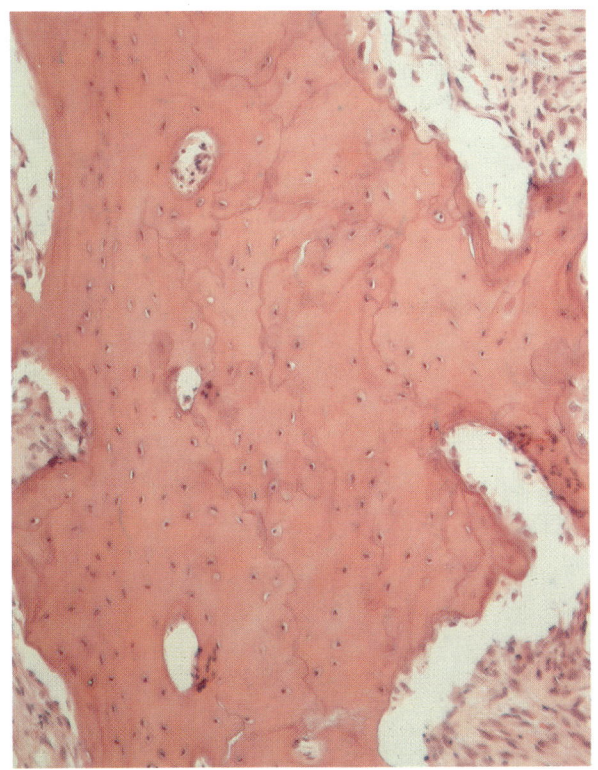

Q2b. (×115)

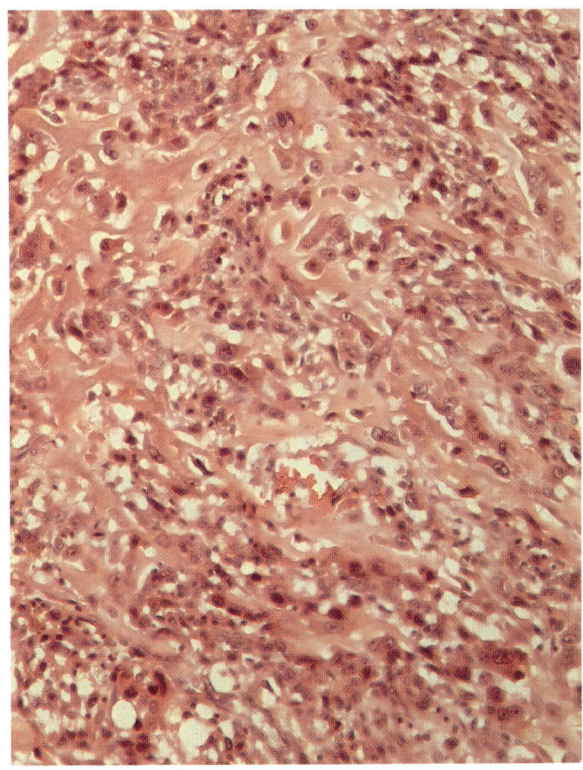

Q2c. (×135)

A1. Osteosarcoma of femur

The radiological appearance of the lesion, with patchy increase in density in the shaft of the femur, the radiating spicules of bone in the extension into the adjacent soft tissues on the lateral and posterior aspects of the bone, and the prominent areas of periosteal reaction (Codman's triangles) at the upper margin, strongly suggested the diagnosis of osteosarcoma. This was confirmed by the biopsy.

Some areas of tumour tissue (Q1b) show conspicuous evidence of bony differentiation, in the form of pale-staining osteoid intercellular matrix and darker calcified bone. Although the general pattern of this tissue strongly suggests a diagnosis of osteosarcoma, cytological evidence of malignancy is more readily found in less differentiated areas (Q1c). Here the variable size and shape of the tumour cells, together with the presence of multinucleated cells and frequent mitoses, all establish that the tumour is malignant.

The rest of the biopsy specimen showed rather different histological appearances, illustrating the variety of structure that can often be found in an osteosarcoma. In some parts of the lesion, particularly in the deeper tissue, the tumour bone has a denser pattern (Fig. 1.1a) and is heavily calcified; this type of tissue explains the increased bone density in the radiograph. As well as tumour bone, areas of tumour cartilage, recognised by its rounded cells and blue staining intercellular matrix (Fig. 1.1b), are present.

Further tissue from the lesion, available from the later amputation specimen, makes it possible to explain the histological basis of the Codman's triangles which were apparent in the radiograph (Q1a). These consist of periosteal new bone, initially deposited in vertical spicules and subsequently remodelled to form horizontal layers on the cortical surface (Fig. 1.1c). Despite immediate amputation this patient died 8 months later with pulmonary metastases.

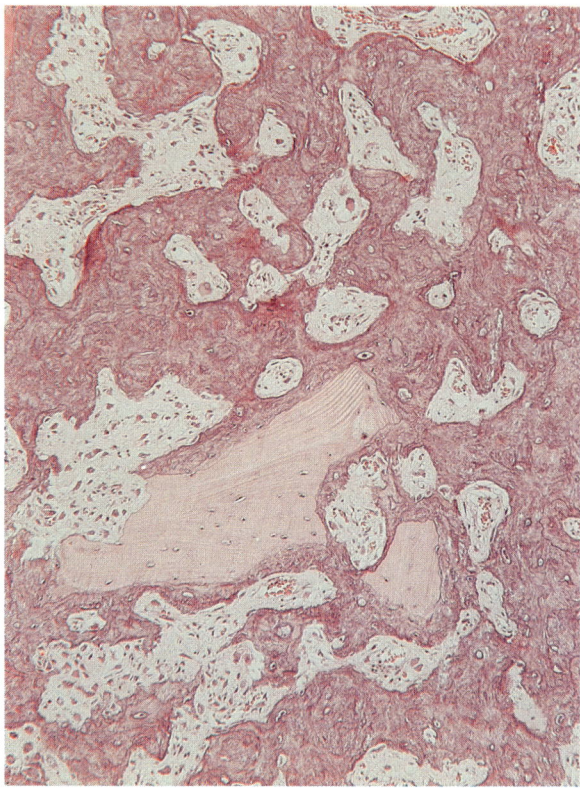

Fig. 1.1a. Part of the biopsy specimen from this case, showing denser, heavily calcified tumour bone from the deeper part of the lesion. (×70)

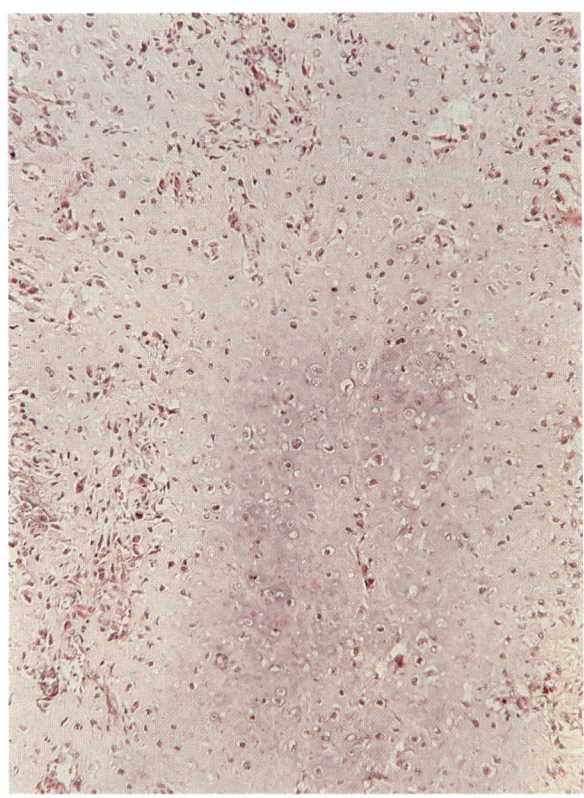

Fig. 1.1b. Another field from the same biopsy, where the tumour tissue shows evidence of cartilaginous differentiation. (×80)

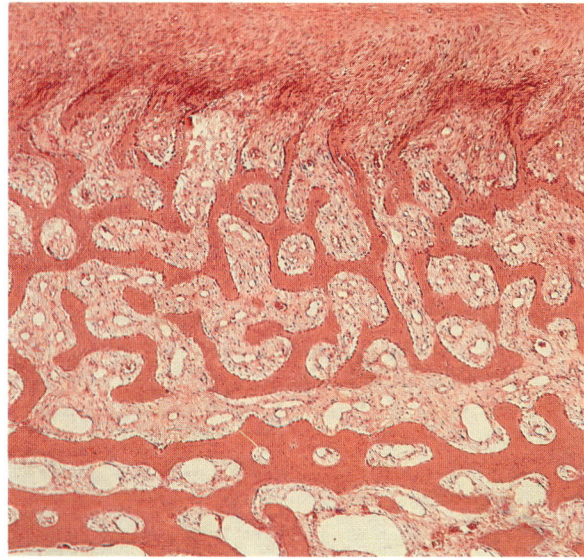

Fig. 1.1c. A section from the amputation specimen, showing the periosteal bone on the surface of the upper part of the shaft of the femur. (×35)

Osteosarcoma

Osteosarcoma is one of the commonest types of primary malignant tumours of bone, accounting for approximately 50% of such cases in published series. Males are more frequently affected than females. Most osteosarcomas occur between the ages of 10 and 20 years, but an increasing incidence in later years, possibly 20%, has been recognised in recent reports. Many of the tumours developing after middle age are associated with Paget's disease. Osteosarcomas sometimes follow radiation damage to bone, usually after a long interval.

Clinical Features

Bone pain is the usual cause of presentation, but this may be so relatively mild that a localised and hard swelling may have already developed without being observed by the patient. Indeed, the tumour may be recognised first on account of a spontaneous pathological fracture in a significant number of cases. Regional lymph nodes may be found to be enlarged though they are not necessarily the site of secondary deposits, but systemic symptoms and signs are not a feature of this disease in the early stages. Such symptoms and signs are only apparent when secondary deposits are widespread, particularly when metastases affect the lungs.

Radiological Features

1. Site. These tumours commonly occur towards the ends of the shafts of long bones, particularly the distal end of the femur and the proximal end of the tibia, although no part of the skeleton is exempt.

2. Appearance. Some appear as aggressive osteolytic lesions, but most of them show some increase in density, diffuse or patchy, because of the neoplastic bone they produce. The zone of transition is usually wide and irregular, a feature always arousing suspicion of malignancy. A clearly defined extension into adjacent soft tissues is often detectable in plain films and tomograms, but is demonstrated in even greater detail by CT scanning. Periosteal reactive bone is commonly present, varying in its degree of organisation. Codman's triangles may be evident, but the classical 'sunray' spicules, projecting horizontally away from the mass, are relatively unusual although a pointer to diagnosis when they are present. Radionuclide scanning is always positive.

3. Differential Diagnosis. The typical radiographic appearance of florid and dense new bone formation rarely presents diagnostic difficulty, but a host of other malignant entities need to be considered in the case of a purely osteolytic lesion. Occasionally an osteosarcoma is mimicked by benign entities. The most important of these is pyogenic osteomyelitis, in which the pattern of *diffuse swelling of the adjacent soft tissues* is an invaluable clue (see Exercise 10). An escape route from the unpleasant task of diagnosing an osteosarcoma may be available when, for example, 'sunray' spiculation is associated with a haemangioma or a fungus infection, when massive periosteal reaction occurs in infantile cortical hyperostosis (although in this instance a malignant diagnosis is made unlikely by the age of the patient) or when an aggressive area of osteolysis has been caused by an eosinophil granuloma. Although osteosarcoma may be encountered in patients beyond the usual age range, osteoblastic metastases, especially from cancer of the prostate and colon, may present an almost identical appearance. Parosteal osteosarcoma, having a much better prognosis than the usual 'central' osteosarcoma, must always be distinguished.

Pathological Features

The usual histological features of osteosarcoma are illustrated well by this case. By definition, osteosarcoma is a 'malignant bone forming tumour', but the histological pattern of the tumour bone is variable, and occasionally can be difficult to distinguish from the reactive bone which may be present in a 'non-osteogenic' tumour, or from the callus tissue of a fracture. The histological distinction from an 'aggressive osteoblastoma' may be difficult, while the presence of large amounts of tumour cartilage in an osteosarcoma may suggest wrongly a diagnosis of chondrosarcoma. Some osteosarcomas contain large numbers of osteoclast giant cells, and this may cause confusion with giant-cell tumour.

The diagnosis in a case of suspected osteosarcoma should be made by planned biopsy. Aspiration biopsy, or drill biopsy, is sometimes advocated, but the advantages of a larger sample of tissue are such that open surgical biopsy is to be preferred. Granted sufficient experience with bone tumours, rapid frozen section diagnosis is possible: many pathologists will, however, prefer to see definitive paraffin sections before making a firm diagnosis. Electron microscopy does not usually provide diagnostic information lacking in ordinary paraffin sections. In addition to sections, imprint preparations always should be prepared. Not only do they provide important cytological information, they can also be used to study enzymes such as acid phosphatase and alkaline phosphatase: the presence of large amounts of alkaline phosphatase reflects increased osteoblastic activity. In a malignant bone tumour, even in the absence of morphological evidence of bone formation, this finding provides presumptive evidence for a diagnosis of osteosarcoma.

Other laboratory investigations are seldom of critical importance in the diagnosis of osteosarcoma. A raised serum alkaline phosphatase is often present, but can be encountered in a variety of other bone lesions. Surgical removal of the primary tumour usually results in the return of serum alkaline phosphatase to normal, but raised values may recur with the development of pulmonary metastases.

Treatment

Treatment of this commonly fatal disease has shown considerable advances during recent years. Formerly the only measures available were either immediate amputation or radiotherapy followed by amputation after an interval of 6 months if no metastases had developed. Both these regimes were relatively ineffective since, on average, a 5-year survival was achieved in only 20% of cases.

Taylor et al. improved the survival rate to 35% by performing a full core biopsy, without an occlusive tourniquet, and proceeding directly to amputation on the basis of frozen sections. *Should a biopsy be performed before referral to the oncological surgeon—and this is unwise—it is essential that the incision should not compromise subsequent amputation flaps.*

In some centres pre-operative radiotherapy was formerly advocated, the dosage being of the order of $5-10 \times 10^3$ rads. This regime was followed by ablation through the most proximal joint or at the site of election for an amputation stump proximal to that joint.

Adjuvant chemotherapy was employed initially only in the presence of metastases. More recently, however, more aggressive regimes of treatment have been introduced for children without CT evidence of metastases. For example, high dosages of methotrexate with citrovorum rescue factor and vincristine are administered prior to any decision regarding surgery. Dependent on the radiological response of the tumour, the options open to the surgeon are either conservative or radical ablation of the limb or endoprosthetic replacement. If the radiological response has been satisfactory, vincristine and citrovorum rescue factor are continued for at least 9 months. If the radiological response has been poor or if pathological examination of the resected section indicates an inadequate response to the initial chemotherapy, then supplementary therapy such as diamino-dichloroplatinum may be used; alternatively, a combination of bleomycin, cyclophosphamide and adriamycin may be added or alternated. The results of these methods of treatment indicate a survival rate of 80% at 4 years in patients without metastases on presentation, but the survival rate when metastases are already present appears to be unaffected.

References

Bleyer WA et al. (1982) Improved three-year disease-free survival in osteogenic sarcoma. J Bone Jt Surg 64B: 233–238

Brostom LA (1979) On the natural history of osteosarcoma. Acta Orthop Scand 183: 9–31

Dahlin DC, Coventry MB (1967) Osteogenic sarcoma: a study of 600 cases. J Bone Jt. Surg 49A 101–110

Jaffe N. Frei E, Traggis D et al. (1974) Adjuvant methotrexate and citrovorum factor treatment of osteogenic sarcoma. N Engl J Med 291: 994–997

Jeffree GM, Price CHG, Sissons HA (1975) The metastatic patterns of osteosarcoma. Br J Cancer 32: 87–107

Mankin H, Lange TA, Spanier SS (1982) The hazards of biopsy in patients with malignant primary bone and soft tissue tumors. J. Bone Jt. Surg. 64A: 1121–1127

Rosenberg SA, Chabner BA, Young RC et al. (1979) Treatment of osteogenic sarcoma. 1. Effect of adjuvant high-dose methotrexate after amputation. Cancer Treat Rep 62: 739–751

Sanerkin NG (1980) Definitions of osteosarcoma, chondrosarcoma and fibrosarcoma of bone. Cancer 46: 178–185

Sutow WW, Gehan EA, Dyment PG et al. (1978) Multi-drug adjuvant chemotherapy for osteosarcoma: interim report of the Southwest Oncology Group studies. Cancer Treat Rep 62: 265–269

Taylor WF, Ivins JC, Dahlin DC et al. (1978) Trends and variability in survival from osteosarcoma. Mayo Clin Proc 53: 695–700

Williams AH, Schwinn CP, Parker JW (1976) The ultrastructure of osteosarcoma: a review of 20 cases. Cancer 37: 1293–1301

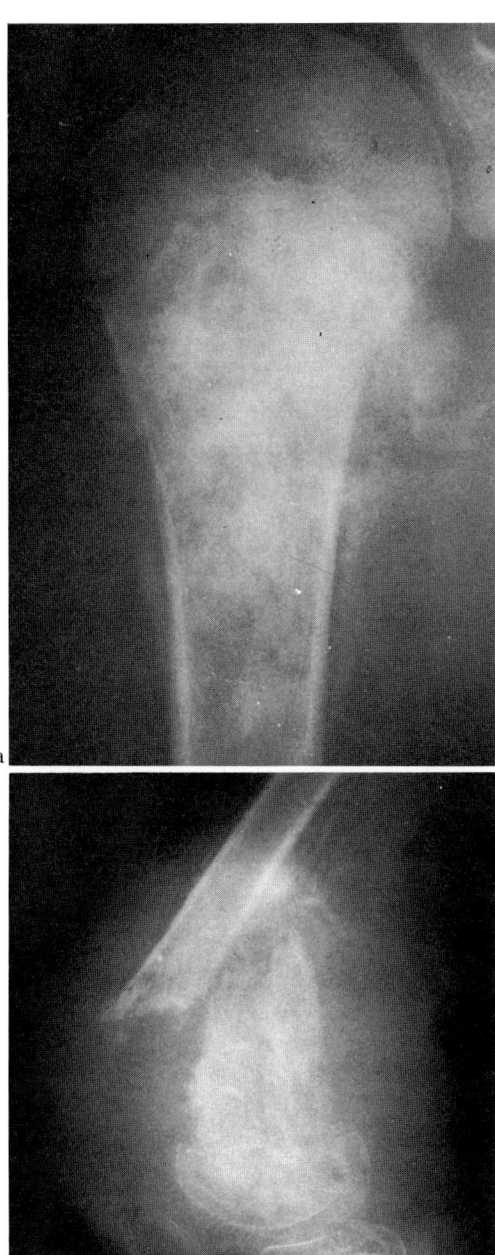

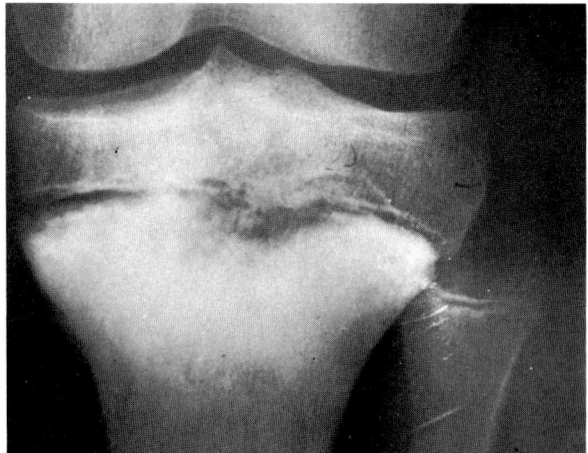

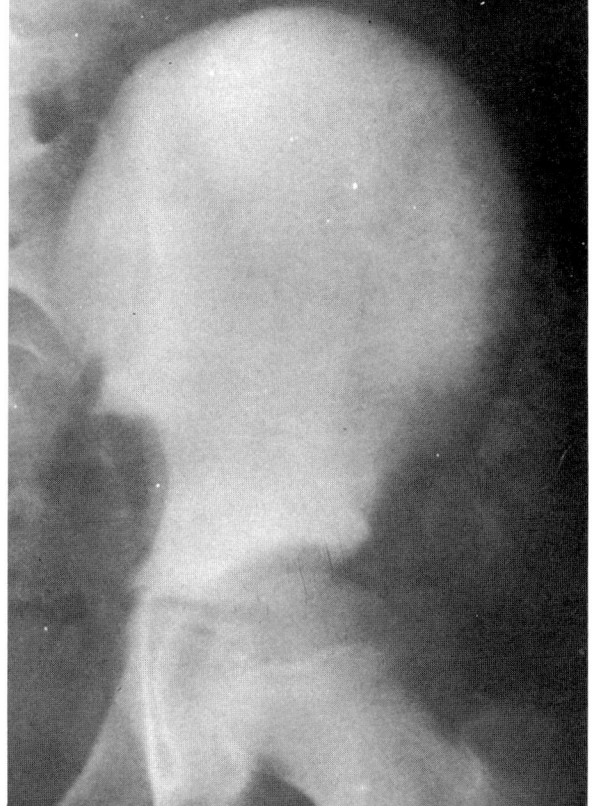

Fig. 1.2. *Osteosarcoma in children—mixed sclerosing and osteolytic lesions.* **a** *Proximal humeral metaphysis* in a 16-year-old boy with pain for 3 months. Tumour bone has formed in the soft tissues and a Codman's triangle is present. **b** *An advanced lesion of the femur*, with a pathological fracture and a huge, well-defined soft tissue extension. The fracture makes the prognosis even worse.

Fig. 1.3. *Osteosarcoma in children—sclerotic lesions.* **a** *Proximal tibial metaphysis* in a 12-year-old girl with no physical signs other than a mild ache for 2 months. This lesion already had traversed the growth plate. **b** *Ilium* in a boy aged 11, who also had complained of pain for only 2 months. Ossification had developed in the soft tissue extension.

Osteosarcoma

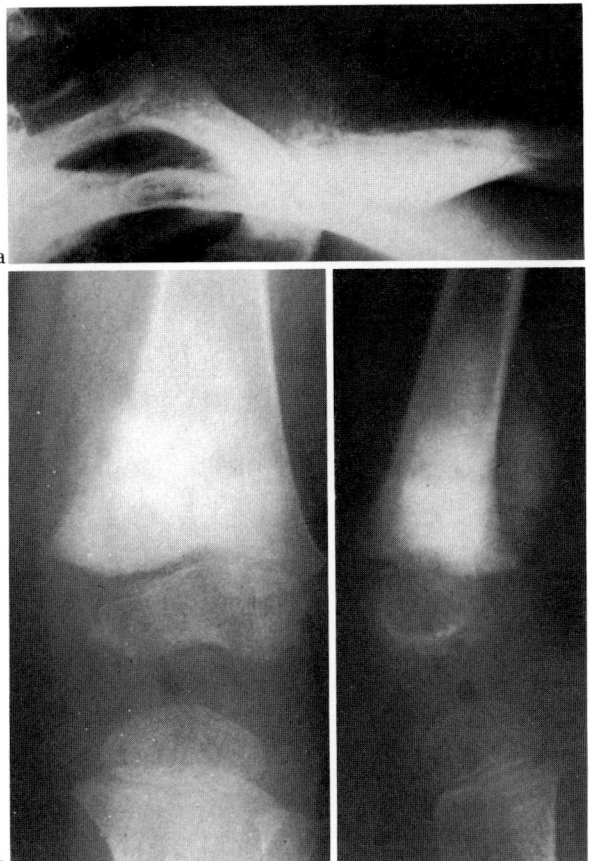

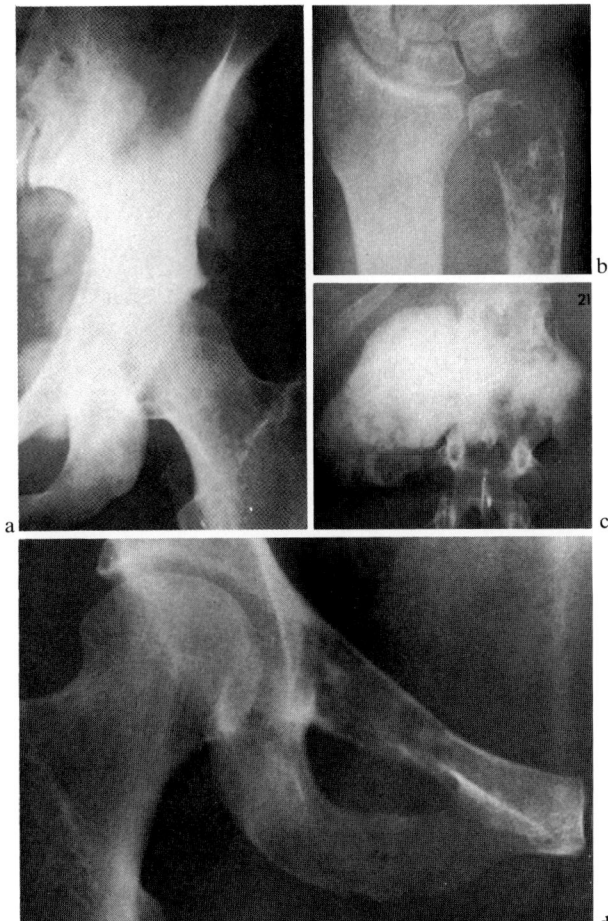

Fig. 1.4. *Osteosarcoma in children—unusual cases.* **a** 'Sunray' spiculation into a well-defined soft mass from an *osteosarcoma of the clavicle* in an adolescent. **b** This typical *osteosarcoma of the distal end of the femur* was confirmed histologically beyond doubt in a female child aged only 18 months. The growth plate so far has provided a barrier to extension of the tumour. The occurrence of this neoplasm under the age of 5 years is *extremely* rare.

Fig. 1.5. *Osteosarcoma in adults* may affect the axial skeleton more commonly than in children. **a** *Pelvic lesion* in a 25-year-old woman with a history of pain for a few months. It is largely sclerotic, with much tumour bone formation in the soft tissues. Pulmonary metastases already were present. **b** *Lytic osteosarcoma of distal end of ulna* in a 29-year-old man. Such lesions can be confused easily with giant-cell tumours. **c** *Osteosarcoma of spine*—a very unusual site of involvement—in a young man with pain in the back. **d** *Lytic osteosarcoma of pubis* in a 50-year-old woman with mild groin pain. The lesion at first was regarded as fibrous dysplasia, but at operation the lymph nodes were involved and histological confirmation was obtained.

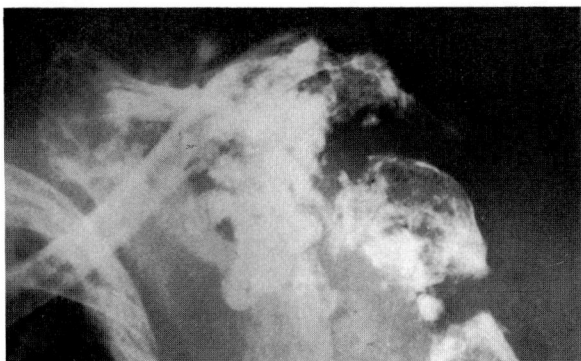

Fig. 1.6. *Post-radiation sarcoma of scapula* in an elderly woman 18 years after treatment for breast cancer. This tumour developed on the superior border of the scapula, causing a painful swelling which contained characteristic bony spicules. Many fractures had occurred in necrotic bones.

A2. Osteosarcoma of femur in Paget's disease

The radiological appearance of the femur, with its pattern of coarse trabeculation and loss of definition of cortical outline, is characteristic of Paget's disease (see Exercise 8). This diagnosis is supported by the presence of similar changes in other parts of the skeleton, including the right tibia and the pelvis (Fig. 2.1). The presence of the osteolytic lesion at the lower end of the femur suggests malignant change, probably an osteosarcoma or a fibrosarcoma.

The biopsy confirmed the diagnosis of Paget's disease, which is established by the presence of bone showing the characteristic mosaic pattern of cement lines (Q2b). In addition, tumour tissue is present, and its structure (Q2c) is that of osteosarcoma, as indicated by the presence of pleomorphic spindle-celled tissue with intercellular bone matrix.

Osteosarcoma in Paget's Disease

Malignant change in Paget's disease has been mentioned above and accounts for a large proportion of the primary malignant bone tumours developing in elderly individuals. The tumours are usually osteosarcomas, but with a predominantly osteolytic radiological appearance. It must be remembered, however, that the skeleton in Paget's disease is by no means immune to metastatic deposits. The development of a pathological fracture carries a particularly grave prognosis, death usually occurring within a few months. Even in the absence of such a fracture survival rarely exceeds 2 years.

References

Price CHG (1962) The incidence of osteogenic sarcoma is south-west England, and its relationship to Paget's disease of bone. J Bone Jt Surg 44B: 366–376

Price CHG, Goldie W (1969) Paget's sarcoma of bone: a study of eighty cases from the Bristol and Leeds Bone Tumour Registries. J Bone Jt Surg 51B: 205–225

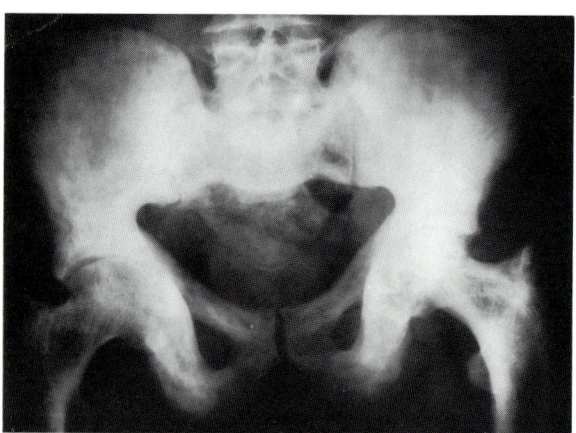

Fig. 2.1. Typical changes of Paget's disease elsewhere in the skeleton of the same patient included widespread involvement of the entire pelvis and the proximal end of each femur.

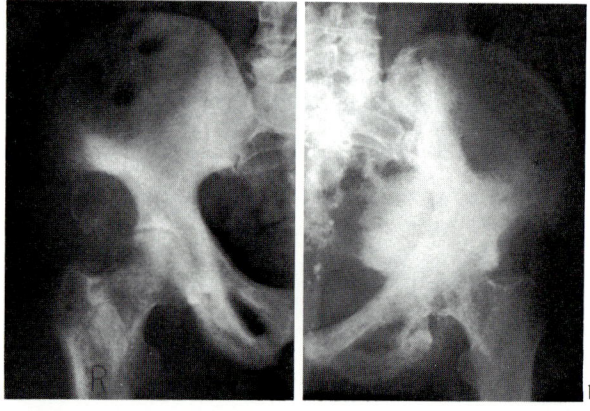

Fig. 2.2. *Osteosarcoma in Paget's disease.* **a** *Lytic lesion in right ilium* in a 60-year-old man who had suffered much pain in the right buttock for 6 months. **b** *Aggressive bone-forming osteosarcoma in left innominate bone* of another elderly man with a similar history. In this patient an osteolytic area had developed also in the left ischial ramus, where an ominous pathological fracture had occurred.

Q1. This 46-year-old woman fell in her garden and injured her right shoulder.

Clinical examination revealed swelling and obvious evidence of a fracture. The fracture was reduced. Despite intensive physiotherapy, normal movement of the gleno-humeral joint was never regained. Sixteen months later, as a sequel to a trivial injury, the shoulder became painful, the patient being aware of a swelling which was increasing rapidly in size. Clinical examination at this time confirmed extreme swelling below the deltoid muscle. Attempts at passive movement of the shoulder evoked acute pain.

The initial radiological examination showed a transverse fracture of the neck of the humerus. Following reduction of the fracture the radiograph confirmed acceptable position of the fragments. At the later presentation, however, it became evident that a large expansile lesion was present, involving the head and neck of the humerus, with extensive cortical destruction. Skeletal survey revealed no other abnormality.

A biopsy was performed.

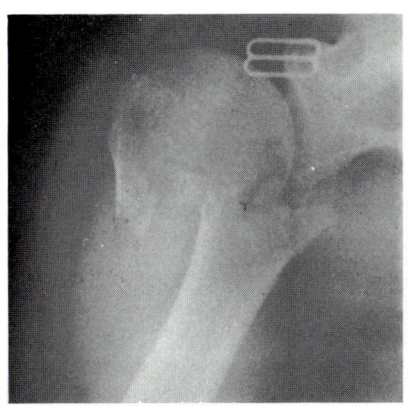
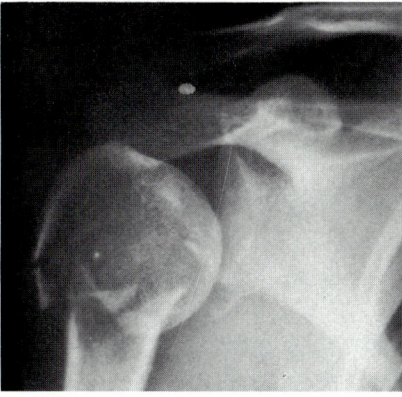
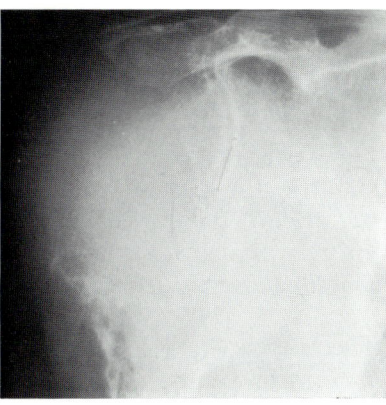

Q1a. Q1b. Q1c.

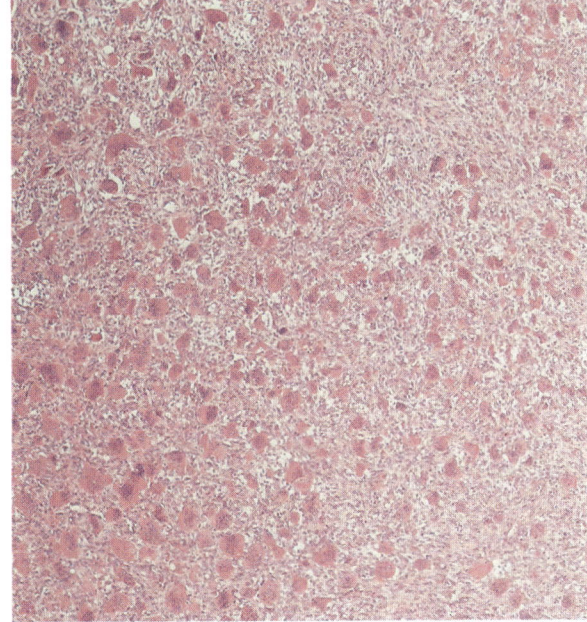

Q1d. (×55)

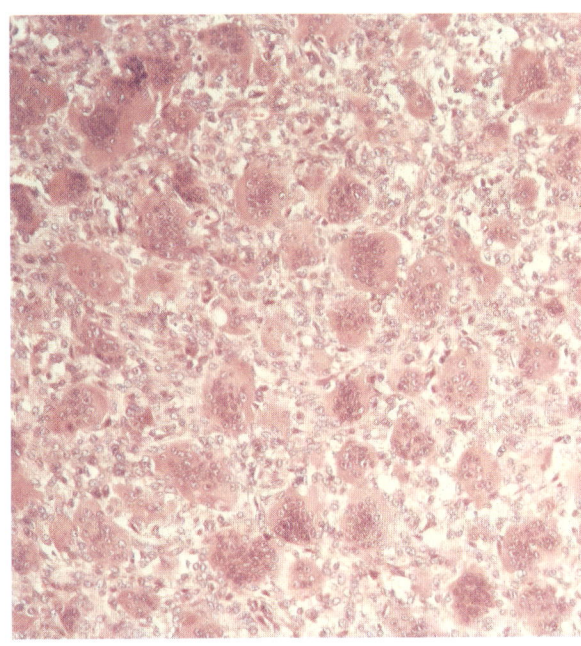

Q1e. (×140)

A1. Giant-cell tumour of humerus

A transverse fracture occurring at this site and at this age is almost invariably pathological. Failure to appreciate this point severely delayed recognition and treatment of this lesion. In the radiograph obtained after reduction of the fracture the extensive area of osteolysis, through which it had occurred, was overlooked. The appearance even at this stage made the diagnosis of an aggressive malignant neoplasm virtually obligatory. By the time of the later study this presumptive diagnosis had become inevitable. Any osteolytic lesion occurring in the latter half of life must arouse primary consideration of a metastasis, in which case the solitary nature of this focus might have suggested a primary tumour of kidney or thyroid (see Exercise 2). The subarticular location and gross expansion of the area of bone destruction, however, were entirely typical of a giant-cell tumour. This diagnosis was offered pre-operatively.

The biopsy established the diagnosis. Q1d and e are representative of the tissue removed at operation and show an appearance which is characteristic of giant-cell tumour. The two basic components of these neoplasms, giant cells and intervening spindle-cell tissue, are evident.

The problem of management of a lesion of the type illustrated is difficult. Local radiotherapy could have been advocated. It would, however, have left the patient with no glenohumeral function and exposed to the subsequent risk of post-radiation malignant change. Excision arthroplasty would have resulted virtually in a flail shoulder. Ideally, massive replacement of the proximal humerus and shoulder joint would have provided the patient with reasonable function.

This procedure was precluded because disuse porosis of the glenoid area of the scapula prevented adequate fixation of a glenoid component. The less satisfactory operation of local excision, with the insertion of a proximal humeral prosthesis, was employed. This replacement allowed the patient a reasonable range of movement and she was able to resume normal activities. Nine years later she continued her work as a schoolmistress and had achieved a reputation in weaving wall tapestries.

Giant-Cell Tumour

Giant-cell tumours represent a significant proportion of all skeletal neoplasms, the incidence varying from 5% to 10% in different series. They cannot be described as being within the groups regarded conventionally as wholly benign or wholly malignant. They occupy a position between these extremes and exhibit a wide spectrum of aggression. Some respond readily and permanently to relatively minor surgical procedures, while a few progress inexorably to metastatic dissemination. As will be seen below, clinical, radiological and histological assessment of the future behaviour of any individual giant-cell tumour is fraught with difficulty and uncertainty.

Giant-cell tumours are encountered most frequently in those between the ages of 20 and 40 years, but a subsidiary peak of incidence occurs later in life between the ages of 55 and 65 years. Fewer than 10% have been observed in the immature skeleton. The sex incidence is equal.

Clinical Features

Most bone tumours are recognised on account of localised pain and swelling. Giant-cell tumour is no exception to this rule. The degree of discomfort engendered by these neoplasms varies considerably, often being unrelated to the size of the tumour at the time of first presentation. Indeed a pathological fracture, involving a large area of bone destruction, may be the initial feature.

Radiological Features

1. Site. These tumours arise characteristically in a subarticular, usually eccentric, location in the end of a long bone; more than half arise around the knee. Occasional exceptions occur in former apophyses such as the greater and lesser trochanter. Much less commonly flat bones, including the pelvis and the scapula, may be affected and a few have been observed in the small bones of the hands and feet. Spinal involvement is rare, except for the sacrum.

2. Appearance. The lesions are always osteolytic and tend to have a wide zone of transition. The overlying cortex frequently is thinned and expanded. Residual ridges of cortical bone may be responsible for linear densities traversing the area of bone destruction.

A number of aggressive osteolytic lesions in the skeleton may simulate the appearance of giant-cell tumour. Of these the most important are aneurysmal bone cyst and the 'brown tumour' of hyperparathyroidism.

Pathological Features

A typical giant-cell tumour is an osteolytic lesion producing some expansion of the terminal portion of a long bone. The tumour tissue is soft and friable, and reddish-brown or grey, with areas of haemorrhage and necrosis. Cystic areas may be present, but are not such a striking feature as in aneurysmal bone cyst. As seen in the present case, the characteristic histological components are the giant cells and the intervening spindle-celled tissue. The giant cells are morphologically similar to osteoclasts. These tumours, therefore, sometimes are referred to as osteoclastomas.

Many other types of bone lesion can contain giant cells, but only giant-cell tumour shows extensive areas of tissue with the even distribution of giant cells illustrated in Q1d and e. In hyperparathyroidism, for example, a 'brown tumour' may contain numerous giant cells, but these are usually arranged in a nodular pattern and are surrounded by areas of reactive bone. The biochemical changes of hyperparathyroidism (hypercalcaemia etc.) will be present. In an aneurysmal bone cyst solid areas of giant-celled tissue are often present, but the cystic appearance of the remainder of the tissue will enable that diagnosis to be established.

Some lesions which regularly contain giant cells were formerly regarded as giant-cell tumour 'variants', but are now considered to be quite separate types of lesion. These include benign chondroblastoma and non-ossifying fibroma, both of which are discussed elsewhere in this work. Occasional osteoclast giant cells can be present in a wide variety of other lesions, including fibrous dysplasia and osteosarcoma. Osteoclast giant cells should not be confused with the entirely different type of cell, the pleomorphic tumour giant cell, which is a feature of most malignant neoplasms, including osteosarcoma, chondrosarcoma and fibrosarcoma.

Histological grading of giant-cell tumours, based on the cellularity and mitotic activity of the spindle-celled component, has been attempted, but is at best uncertain. All giant-cell tumours must be regarded as potentially malignant, but, although many recur locally, few actually metastasise. When metastasis does occur, the lungs are most frequently involved.

Treatment

The majority of these neoplasms are relatively small when first diagnosed. Lesions in the upper limb respond well to curettage, with or without insertion of bone chips. Those in the lower limb require grafting in addition in order to combat the subsequent stress of weight bearing. More aggressive and larger tumours are treated by total excision and prosthetic replacement. The optimal sites for such replacements are the proximal ends of the humerus, femur and tibia and the distal end of the femur. Continued observation for a minimum of 10 years is desirable. Some recurrences have been observed after intervals as long as 20 years. Radiotherapy is employed less commonly than it was in the past, largely on account of the danger of a post-radiation sarcoma developing later in life. When, however, a giant-cell tumour is located in a site inaccessible to adequate surgical treatment, radiotherapy is still of considerable value in controlling its growth and alleviating pain.

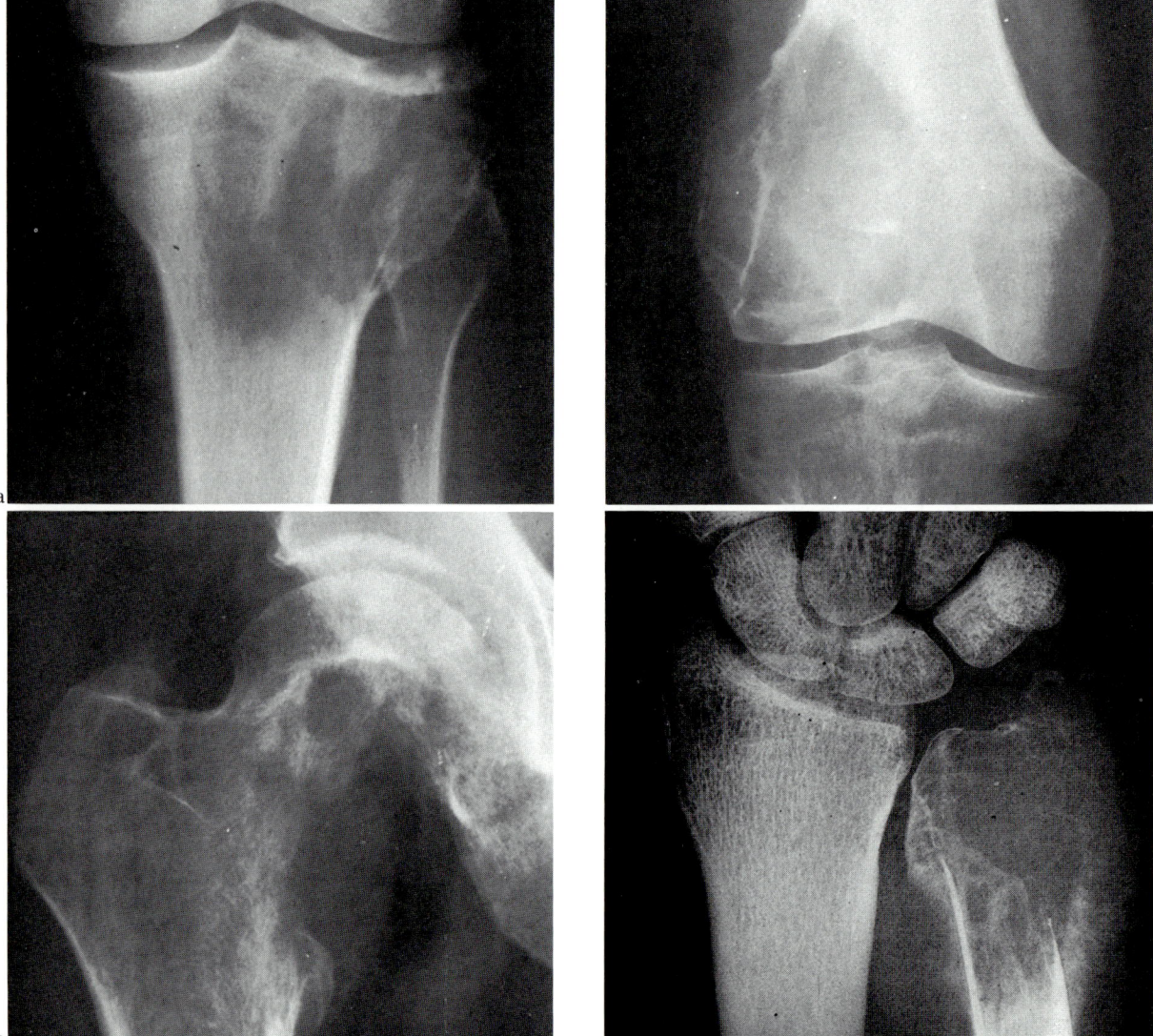

Fig. 1.1. *Giant-cell tumours—typical examples.* **a** *Tibia.* This young man with chronic pain in the knee demonstrates a typical destructive lesion in the lateral condyle. The overlying cortex is thinned and expanded. The endosteal margin has a wide zone of transition. **b** *Lateral femoral condyle.* This destructive lesion was found in a 23-year-old man who had complained of pain and swelling for several months. It exhibits, in a young adult, the characteristic features of a subarticular, eccentric location, expansion and thinning of the overlying cortex and a wide endosteal zone of transition. The tumour is sufficiently large for prosthetic replacement to be considered as a primary method of treatment. **c** *Proximal end of femur.* This 34-year-old man presented with increasing pain in the right hip over a period of 4 months. The same characteristic radiological criteria are present. Prosthetic replacement was undertaken with a very successful result. Although the original prosthesis broke after 5 years, when the patient was moving heavy furniture, requiring insertion of a stronger implant, function was virtually normal 17 years later. **d** *Distal end of ulna.* This typical example shows an even more aggressive pattern with prominent swelling of the soft tissues. The diagnosis was questioned pre-operatively as a possible sarcoma, but was confirmed following excisional biopsy.

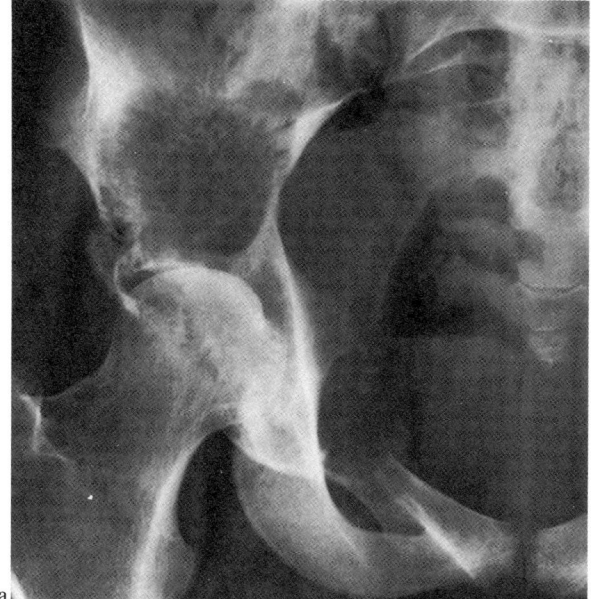
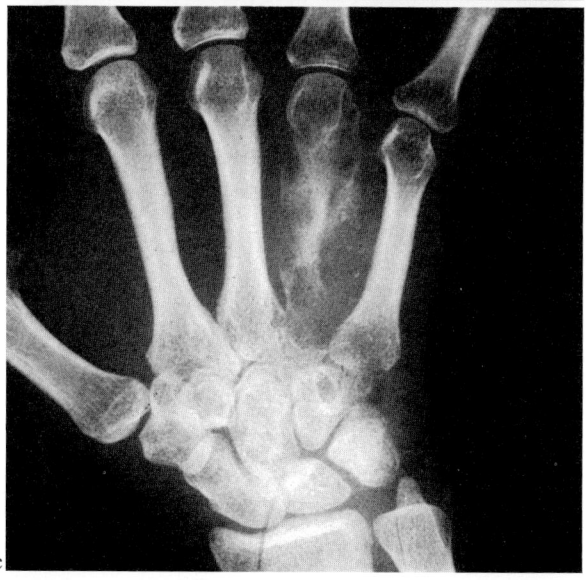
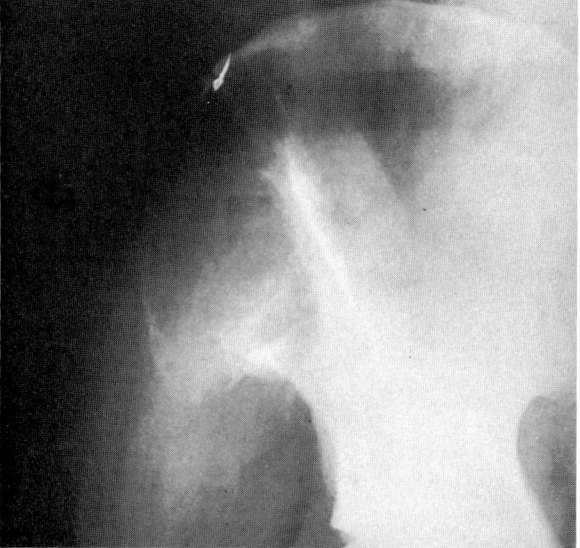
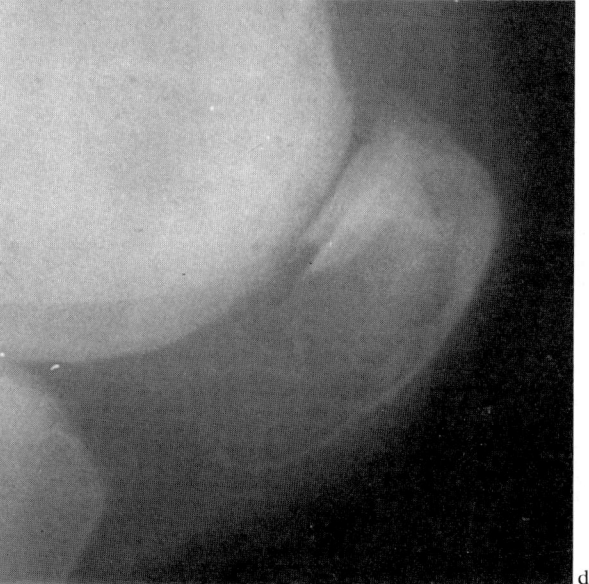

Fig. 1.2. *Giant-cell tumours—unusual sites.* **a** *Acetabulum* in a young woman aged 18. The lesion is subarticular with a wide zone of transition. **b** *Iliac crest* in a 38-year-old man with pelvic pain. This tumour has involved a former apophysis. **c** *4th metacarpal.* Despite the uncommon location in this 26-year-old woman, the lesion exhibits all the classical diagnostic criteria. **d** *Patella*—another subarticular lesion in a young adult with a painful knee. In all these examples the diagnosis was substantiated histologically.

References

Dahlin DC, Cupps RE, Johnson EW (1970) Giant-cell tumor. A study of 195 cases. Cancer 25:1061–1070

Goldenberg RR, Campbell CJ, Bonfiglio M (1970) Giant-cell tumour of bone. J Bone Jt Surg 52A: 619–664

Jacobs P (1972) The diagnosis of osteoclastoma (giant-cell tumour): a radiological and pathological correlation Br J Radiol 45:121–136

Jaffe HL, Lichtenstein L, Portis RB (1950) Giant-cell tumour of bone: its pathological appearance, grading, supposed variant and treatment. Arch Pathol 30: 993–1004

McGrath PJ, (1972) Giant-cell tumour of bone. An analysis of 52 cases. J Bone Jt Surg 54B:216–229

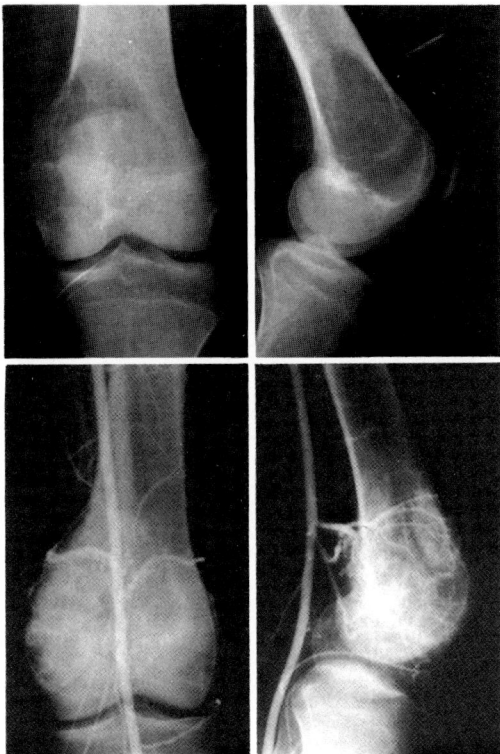

Fig. 1.3. *Giant-cell tumour—early onset.* The diagnosis of this osteolytic lesion in the lateral femoral condyle of a 14-year-old girl was confirmed indubitably on histological grounds. Fewer than 10% of these tumours develop before the skeleton is mature. Typical hypervascularity of the neoplasm was demonstrated by arteriography.

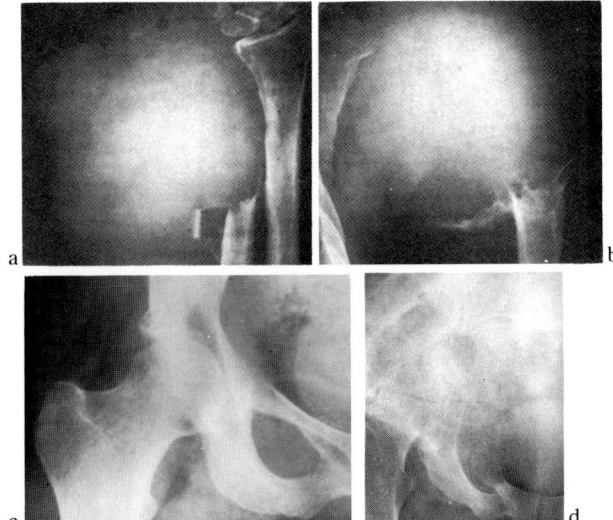

Fig. 1.5. *Giant-cell tumour—advanced lesions.* These enormous expansile tumours in typical locations were found in remote parts of the African continent in **a** the distal end of the ulna in a 23-year-old woman with a painful swelling and **b** the proximal end of the humerus in a 24-year-old woman. **c** and **d** illustrate progression of a giant-cell tumour in a 58-year-old woman. Lack of cooperation between the radiologist, who questioned a destructive lesion in the acetabulum with a soft tissue extension, and the orthopaedic surgeon, originally caused the lesion to be neglected. Persistent pain demanded further examination a year later. At this age the aggressive appearance was suspected to represent a metastasis or a plasmacytoma, the histological diagnosis being unexpected. Following local resection the patient was alive and well, leading a sedentary life, 15 years later.

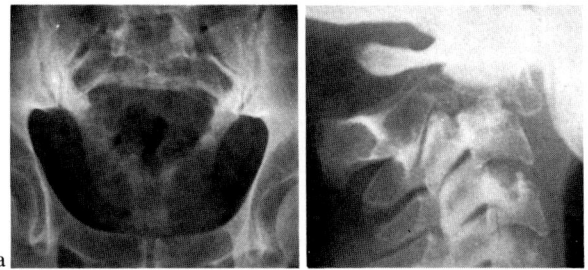

Fig. 1.4. *Giant-cell tumour—spinal lesions* are exceedingly rare. Many of those so diagnosed originally have transpired to be aneurysmal bone cysts on subsequent review of the histological sections. Nevertheless some have been established, most commonly in the sacrum, as in **a** this 27-year-old man with localised pain. Even more surprising was the recognition of **b** this destructive lesion in the body and neural arch of C2 as a giant-cell tumour. It occurred in a 21-year-old woman with pain in the neck for 6 months. No neurological deficit had developed other than mild sensory loss in the C2/3 dermatomes. Partial collapse was associated with a retropharyngeal mass due to extension of the tumour. In both these cases diagnostic preference was given pre-operatively to a chordoma, an entity discussed elsewhere in this volume.

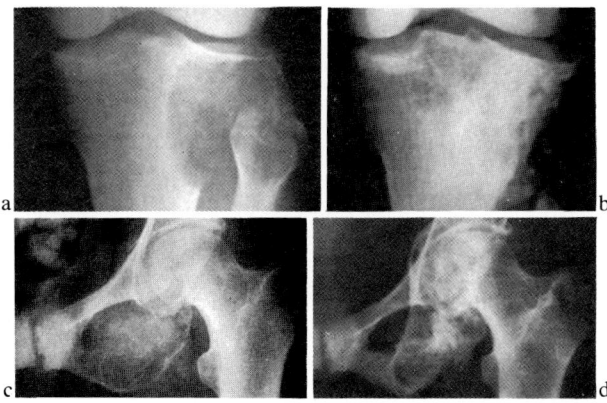

Fig. 1.6. *Giant-cell tumour—response to treatment.* **a** This typical tumour in the lateral tibial condyle of a 45-year-old man was treated by thorough curettage and packing with bone chips derived from the proximal end of the fibula. **b** Ten years later the patient was asymptomatic, the lesion being completely consolidated. **c** A similar tumour in the ischium of a 56-year-old woman responded **d** to similar treatment and adjuvant radiotherapy within a year.

Q1. This 30-year-old man presented on account of a swelling of his left leg. This swelling had developed during the previous 5 years. It had enlarged slowly, but to such a degree that it caused difficulty in putting on and taking off his trousers. Only within the preceding 6 months had the swelling become at all painful.

On clinical examination a large fixed mass was found to arise from the anterior surface of the proximal end of the tibia. It was hard, but not tender. The overlying skin was stretched and shiny. No other abnormality was detected and all routine investigations (including radiological examination of the chest) were normal.

The radiographs showed the mass to be outlined clearly, much of it being lucent, but containing two triangles of greater density extending from an expanded and thinned tibial cortex. The medullary texture of the proximal end of the tibia was itself abnormal, with interspersed areas of lucency and increased density. An organised periosteal reaction was evident on the posterior aspect of the tibial shaft.

A biopsy was performed.

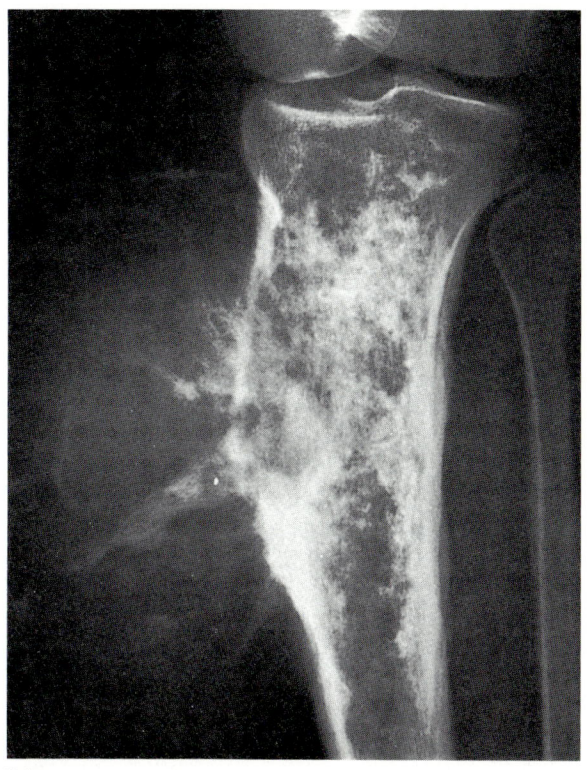

Q1a.

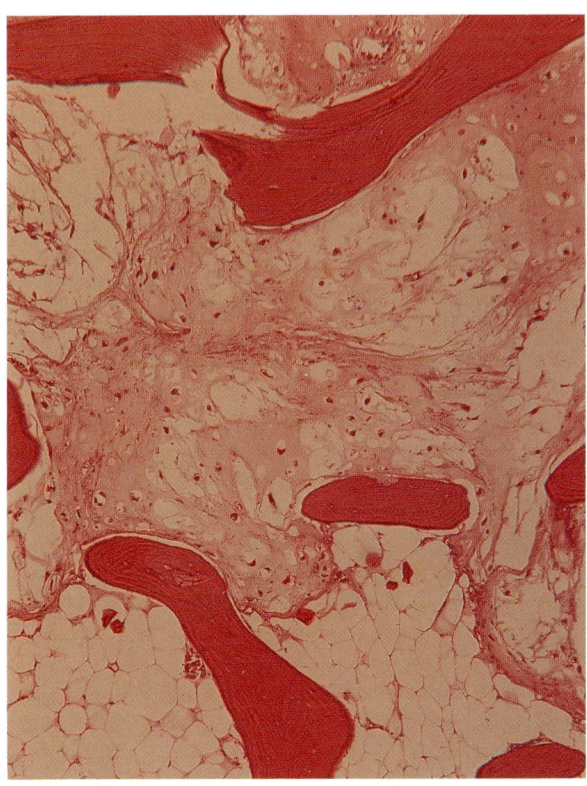

Q1b. (×70)

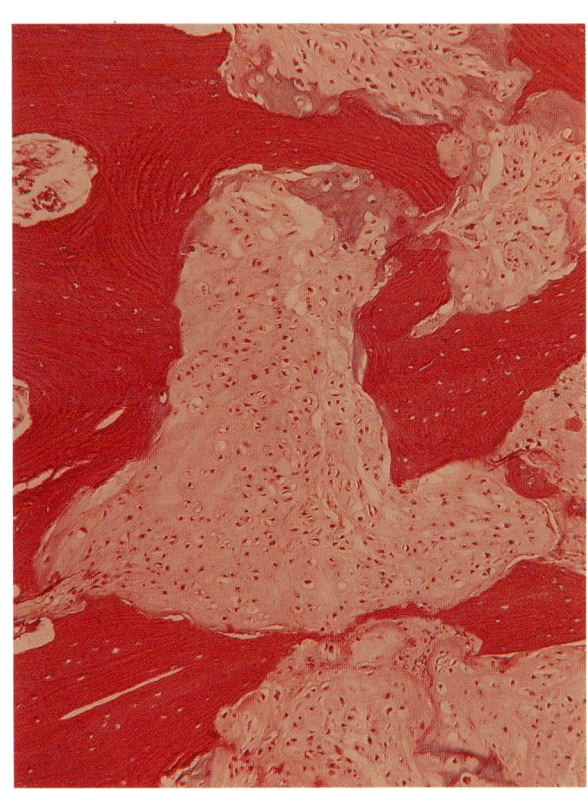

Q1c. (×70)

A1. Chondrosarcoma of tibia

The biopsy established this diagnosis and the limb was amputated above the knee. The histological features of the lesion were demonstrated more satisfactorily in material from the amputation specimen. These features are illustrated in Q1b and c. The former is a section of cancellous bone, with slender trabeculae, and the latter is a section of involved cortical bone. Both are invaded by tumour tissue. In Q1b this tissue is poorly cellular and shows a pink-staining and somewhat fragmented intercellular matrix. The margin of the tumour can be identified clearly where it is extending in the marrow spaces between unresorbed bone trabeculae. In Q1c the same type of tissue is invading cortical bone with extensions into enlarged vascular canals. Tumour cells occupy rounded spaces in the intercellular matrix, a feature characteristic of a cartilaginous neoplasm. The degree of cellularity of the tumour tissue is not great and does not show obvious cytological features of malignancy. The histological evidence of the invasive nature of this lesion is, in the case of tumours of cartilage, an equally important indication of malignancy and establishes the diagnosis of chondrosarcoma.

In Figs. 1.1a and b, derived also from the amputation specimen, the invasive pattern of the tumour is emphasised again. The neoplasm originated centrally within the proximal portion of the tibia and extended through the anterior cortex to form a large lobulated mass. The many minute opacities which are scattered throughout the tumour tissue, as shown in the radiograph of the section, represent focal areas of calcification. The strands of more dense tissue extending outwards from the cortex, which were evident in the clinical radiograph, consist of reactive periosteal bone. The cortex on the posterior side of the tibia is abnormally thick as a result of the organised periosteal reaction.

Histologically, this tumour is to be regarded as a relatively low-grade chondrosarcoma. While many malignant cartilaginous neoplasms are of this type, some are more aggressive and consist of still more cellular tissue, with evidence of pronounced pleomorphism and mitotic activity. Figure 1.2, from another patient, illustrates the histological appearance of such a high-grade chondrosarcoma.

Fig. 1.1. a A photograph of the longitudinally divided tumour in the amputation specimen. Lobular cartilaginous tumour is present in the marrow cavity and extends into the mass on the external surface of the tibia. b Radiograph of a corresponding slice of tissue, illustrating the many minute opacities due to focal areas of calcification and the trabecular pattern of the reactive periosteal bone.

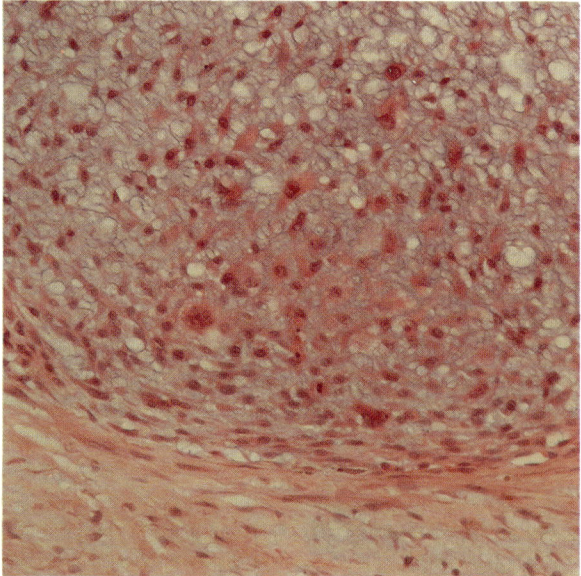

Fig. 1.2. In another high-grade chondrosarcoma, the histological appearance is more malignant in that the tissue is highly cellular and pleomorphic. Tumour giant cells and mitoses are present. ($\times 180$)

Chondrosarcoma

Chondrosarcoma is one of the more common types of primary malignant bone tumour, its incidence being comparable to that of osteosarcoma. Unlike the latter, however, adult patients are most frequently affected, particularly between the ages of 30 and 60 years. Their occurrence earlier in life is comparatively unusual. A distinct male predominance is well recognised. In contrast to the majority of benign cartilaginous tumours (see Exercise 12), which occur mainly in the appendicular skeleton, these malignant cartilaginous neoplasms have a marked predilection for the axial skeleton and the proximal ends of the major limb bones.

In recent years doubt has been cast on the traditional hypothesis that a chondrosarcoma may be secondary to a benign enchondroma, particularly in the shaft of a long bone, although on rare occasions this transition does appear to take place in peripheral bones of the hands and feet. Nevertheless, it is accepted generally that these tumours may arise from the cartilage cap of an osteochondroma, particularly if such excrescences are multiple, as in diaphyseal aclasia. Another secondary form of chondrosarcoma may develop as a complication of enchondromatosis (Ollier's disease). This liability is increased when these cartilaginous lesions in the skeleton are associated with haemangiomas in soft tissues, this combination being known as Maffucci's syndrome.

Clinical Features

As in other types of bone tumour, the presenting signs are those of localised pain and swelling. In general the history of such complaints is long, often extending over many years before medical advice is sought, although in a small number of patients the onset is much more aggressive, pathological fractures occurring occasionally. Recognition of certain subtypes, which are mentioned below, may be aided partially by radiological features of the lesion, but are established more definitely by the histological findings. It is therefore important that an adequate sample is taken at biopsy.

The solitary lesions tend to produce no constitutional disturbance in their early stages. The development of metastatic dissemination usually is delayed for many years, except in particularly aggressive forms and especially when complicated by a pathological fracture.

Radiological Features

1. Site. The vast majority of these neoplasms arise in the central portions of the skeleton, with a special affinity for the pelvis and the proximal ends of the femur and humerus. The ribs, jaw bones, spine and skull may be affected. Despite the frequent occurrence of benign enchondromata in the peripheral small bones of the hands and feet, these tumours only rarely become malignant. Exceptionally a chondrosarcoma may develop in soft tissue with no relation to bone.

2. Appearance. As in other lesions of cartilaginous origin, the offending tissue is radiologically lucent, so that the fundamental abnormality is a zone of osteolysis. Such a tumour arising within a medullary canal may be lobular, causing shallow and well-defined erosions of the endosteal aspect of the cortex. Only with time do the characteristic and pathognomonic foci of calcification appear within the mass of malignant cartilage, therefore reflecting the customary slow growth of the lesion. Simultaneously an organised periosteal reaction on the external surface of the affected bone develops equally slowly. In consequence, the radiological appearance, on presentation, often indicates a lucent, partially calcified, expanding lesion within the medullary cavity. It is surrounded by a fusiform and thickened cortex, comparable in its width to that in the unaffected portion of the bone. Actual penetration of the cortex by the tumour, as in Q1, is followed often by growth of an extra-osseous extension, which may be entirely lucent or contain also the pathognomonic foci of calcification. Such a pattern, indeed, may reveal no obvious involvement of the parent bone and be described as a juxtacortical or parosteal chondrosarcoma. This feature is often evident when the tumour arises, as it does so commonly, in the pelvic bones, especially in relation to the acetabulum. Definition of the margins of an extension of this type may be aided by soft tissue exposures, but are enhanced enormously by CT studies.

When serial radiological examinations confirm the clinical impression of progressive enlargement of the tumour, particularly in the case of a lesion arising from a cartilage-capped osteochondroma, malignancy must be suspected. Spreading of established calcified foci may provide a valuable indication of such growth. As has been mentioned in Exercise 4, however, histological studies after excision of a tumour of this type frequently prove it still to be benign.

Although arteriography usually provides little diagnostic information, demonstration of displaced vessels may assist the surgeon in planning his surgical procedure. Radionuclide scanning, as in the case of most bone tumours, is likely to demonstrate increased uptake of the tracer.

The features described above apply to the low-grade chondrosarcomas, which constitute the majority of these lesions. The much smaller group, which are much more aggressive, may present an appearance almost totally lytic and without the guiding features of calcification and periosteal reaction. In such cases the endosteal zone of transition is wide, the cortex frequently is grossly destroyed and massive extensions into the adjacent soft tissues may be evident.

During recent years certain unusual types of this neoplasm have been reported, their recognition depending largely on histological findings. The entity of 'dedifferentiated' chondrosarcoma is one in which an orthodox low-grade tumour is associated with other, and more malignant, processes. The latter include osteosarcoma, fibrosarcoma and malignant fibrous histiocytoma. Such a diagnosis may be suggested on radiological grounds when the heavily calcified area of an orthodox low-grade lesion is surrounded by an infiltrating area of bone destruction which actually may destroy part of the chondrosarcoma itself. Age, sex and clinical features are all comparable to the orthodox chondrosarcoma. Similar radiological features may be recognised in mesenchymal chondrosarcoma, an entity even rarer. The few cases of this type, however, have occurred in a younger age group. The rarest variant is the clear-cell chondrosarcoma, affecting especially the proximal ends of the femur and humerus and of which the radiological appearance may be deceptively benign, sometimes simulating a chondroblastoma or an osteoblastoma.

Pathological Features

Chondrosarcomas show a marked variation in histological structure. The majority consist of well-differentiated cartilage, with relatively little cytological indication of malignancy. These tumours usually grow slowly and it may be difficult to distinguish them histologically from chondromas. Others are highly cellular and are recognised readily as malignant. The degree of cellularity of the tumour tissue and the presence of large cells and of binucleate or mitotic cells have been cited as useful indications of malignancy in cartilage tumours, but precise histological assessment may be difficult or uncertain, particularly when based on a limited biopsy sample. The same histological criteria, and particularly the numbers of mitotic cells in the tissue, can be used further to grade chondrosarcomas as tumours of low-grade, moderate or high-grade malignancy.

In addition to the usual types of chondrosarcoma, some special varieties are recognised. These are the dedifferentiated chondrosarcoma, the mesenchymal chondrosarcoma and the clear-celled chondrosarcoma. Each of these types has distinctive histological features. They are discussed in more detail elsewhere in this work.

Treatment

Since most of these tumours are of relatively low-grade malignancy and are detected before metastatic dissemination has occurred, wide excision carries an excellent prognosis. It is emphasised that recurrences, when they do take place, may be delayed for many years. While a lesion in a rib, for example, may be removed completely, or one in that common site, the proximal end of the femur, may be replaced successfully by a prosthesis, involvement of the pelvis and spine requires more drastic surgical intervention. Should amputation of a limb prove to be necessary, care should be taken to avoid implantation of tumour cells at the operative site. Pathological fractures inevitably worsen the prognosis, but prosthetic replacement, when feasible, should not be precluded on this account.

All these tumours are notoriously insensitive to radiation therapy, although this technique may be used as a palliative in inoperable cases. Chemotherapy has not proved to be of value.

References

Campanacci M, Guernelli N, Leonessa C, Boni A (1975) Chondrosarcoma. A study of 133 cases, 80 with long term follow up. Ital J Orthop Traumatol 1: 387–414

Evans HL, Atala AG, Romsdahl MM (1977) Prognostic factors in chondrosarcoma of bone. A clinicopathologic analysis with emphasis on histologic grading. Cancer 40: 818–831

Garrison RC, Unni KK, McLeod RA, Pritchard DJ, Dahlin DC (1982) Chondrosarcoma arising in osteochondroma. Cancer 49: 1890–1897

Lichtenstein L, Jaffe HL (1943) Chondrosarcoma of bone. Am J Pathol 19: 553–589

McCarthy EF, Dorfman HD (1982) Chondrosarcoma of bone with dedifferentiation. A study of eighteen cases. Human Pathol 13: 36–40

Salvador AH, Beabout JW, Dahlin DC (1971) Mesenchymal chondrosarcoma. Observation on 30 new cases. Cancer 28: 605–615

Sanerkin NG (1980) The diagnosis and grading of chondrosarcoma of bone. A combined cytologic and histologic approach. Cancer 45: 582–594

Unni KK, Dahlin DC, Beabout JW, Sim FH (1976) Chondrosarcoma: clear cell variant. A report of sixteen cases. J Bone Jt Surg 58A: 676–683

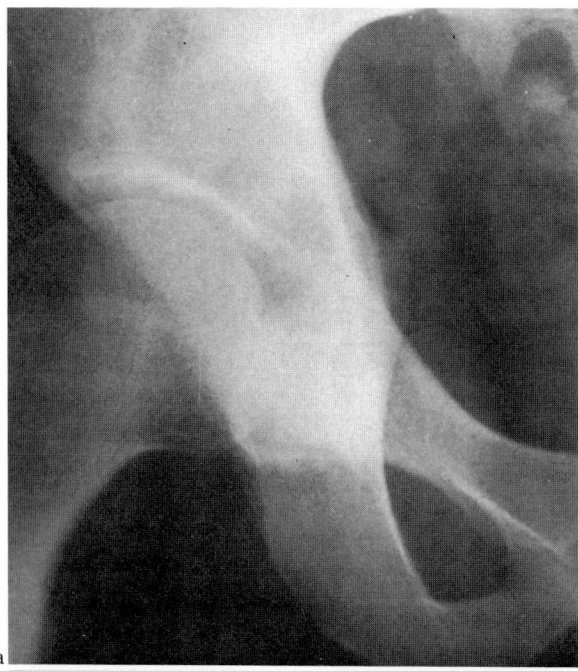

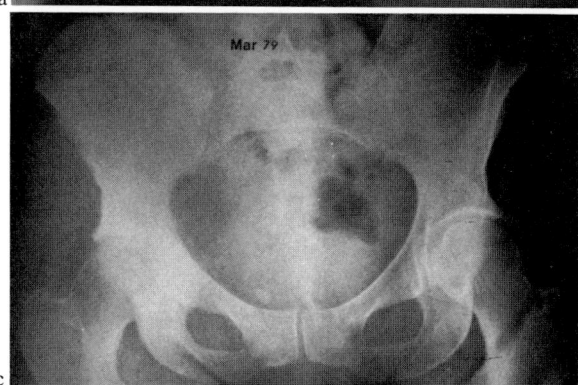

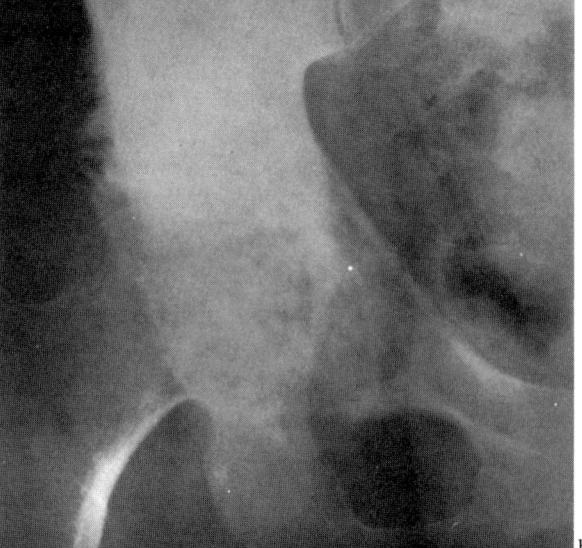

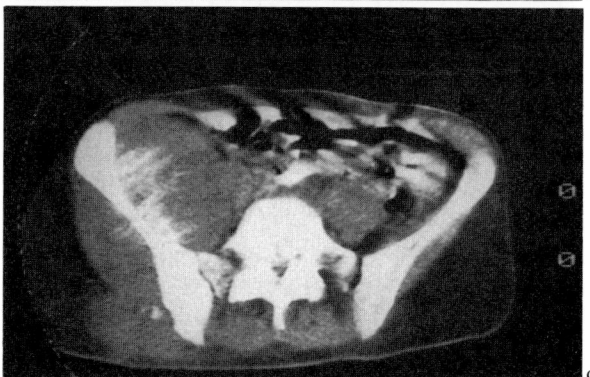

Fig. 1.3. *Chondrosarcoma—pelvis.* The pelvis is the most common site to be affected by these tumours. They tend to progress more rapidly than those arising in long bones and require radical surgical procedures. Hindquarter amputation, however, may prolong life for many years. **a** This 36-year-old man presented with mild pain in the right hip. The significance of the lucent area in the acetabulum and, especially, the well-defined soft tissue mass extending into the pelvic cavity, was not appreciated. **b** Further films obtained 2½ years later, on account of persistent and increasing pain, revealed much more extensive destruction and enlargement of the soft tissue tumour extension. CT had not been invented at the time of these examinations, but would have been invaluable, even on the first occasion. **c** The diagnostic revolution provided by CT is illustrated by the plain film of the pelvis of a 49-year-old woman complaining of constant sciatica, showing a chondrosarcoma in the right ilium with an even larger soft tissue extension, and **d** by the CT study demonstrating the size of this mass on both sides of the affected bone and the strands of calcification radiating into it.

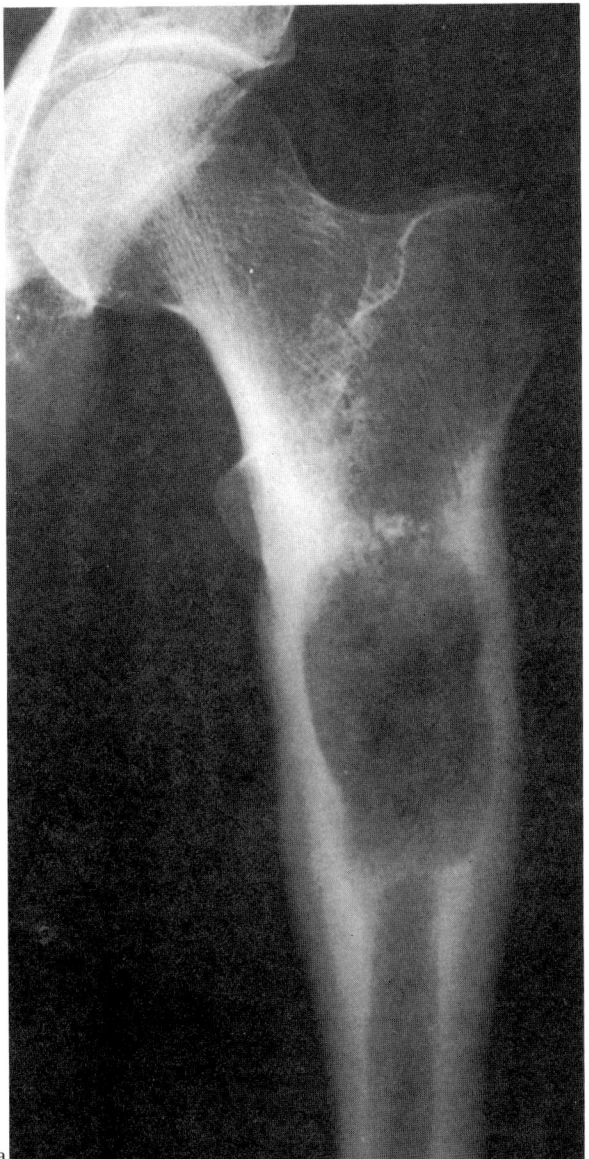
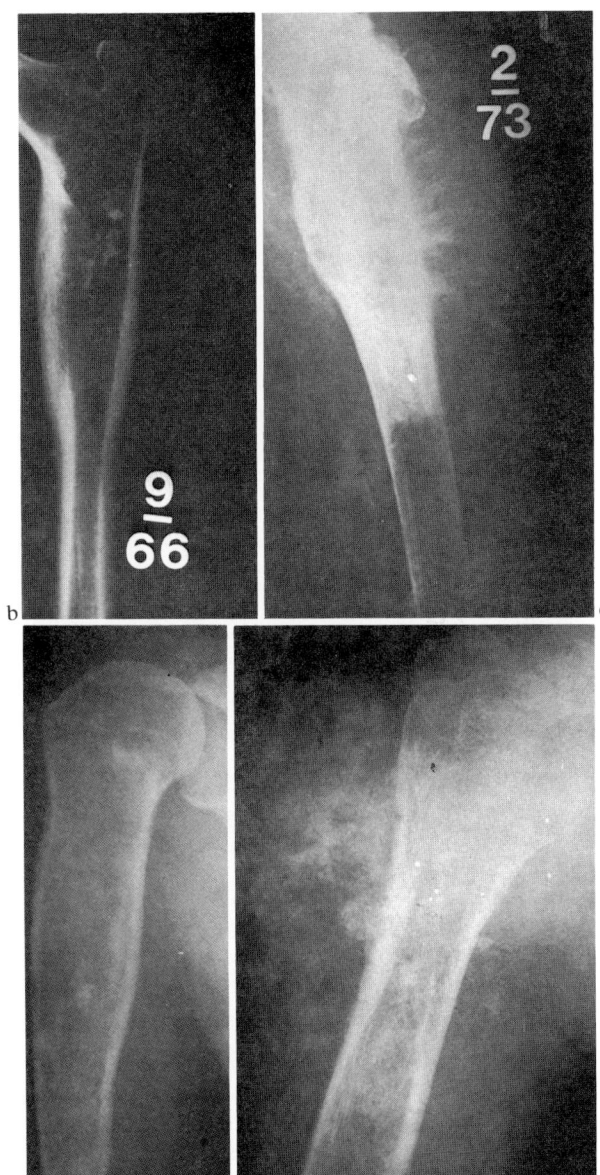

Fig. 1.4. *Chondrosarcoma—proximal ends of femur and humerus* are the next most common sites. **a** This 53-year-old man had complained of mild discomfort in the left thigh for several years. The indolent nature of this tumour is indicated by length of history and radiologically by flecks of calcification within the clearly defined lytic area in the medullary cavity of the femur. Expansion of the tumour has caused scalloped erosions on the internal aspect of the cortex, which itself shows fusiform thickening due to organised periosteal reaction. Lesions of this type are most amenable to prosthetic replacement. **b** This very similar lesion was found incidentally in an elderly woman about to undergo amputation of the leg for vascular insufficiency. It had caused no symptoms and was considered to be benign. **c** Seven years later further examination on account of pain and swelling above the amputation stump showed the tumour to be definitely malignant, with the formation of a large soft tissue mass containing calcification. This case emphasises the malignant potential of these cartilaginous lesions, especially in long bones. **d** Biopsy of this comparable abnormality in the proximal end of the humerus of a 62-year-old man with mild localised pain showed only low-grade malignancy. **e** This 40-year-old man had complained of a painful swelling near the right shoulder. It had developed within a year. The well-circumscribed mass contained much amorphous calcification and was accompanied by irregularity and sclerosis of the adjacent humeral cortex. Such juxtacortical or parosteal chondrosarcomas are uncommon.

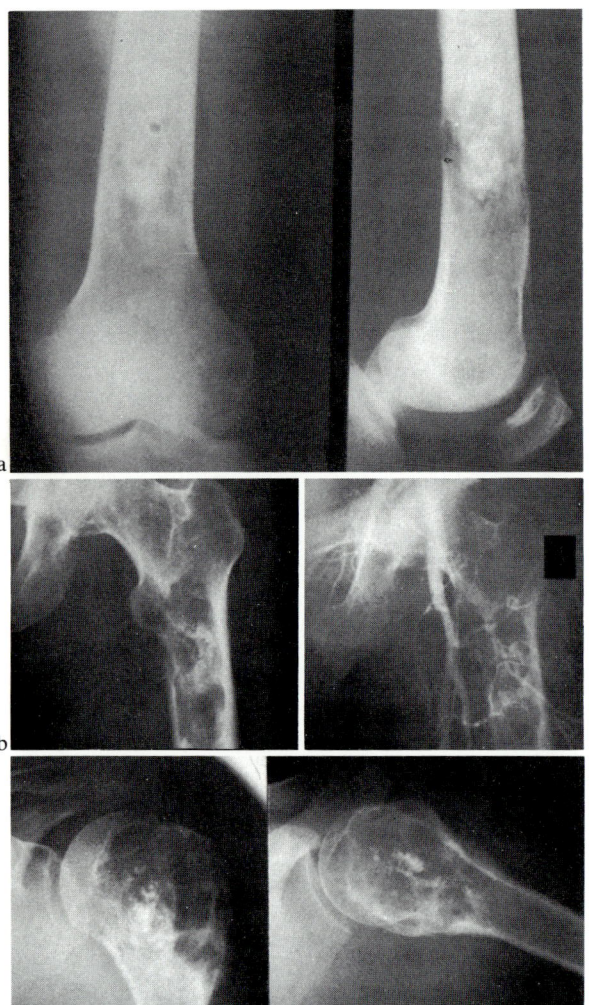

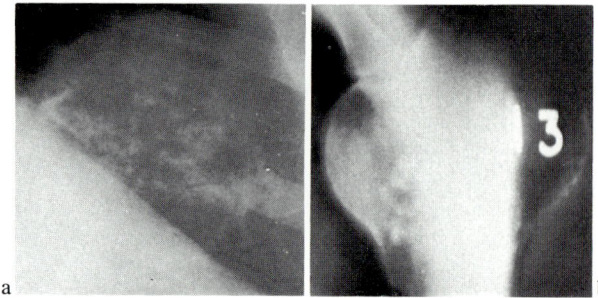

overlying cortex is thinned and expanded. This deceptively benign appearance might suggest a chondroblastoma, but such a pattern has been described with the rare variant of clear-cell chondrosarcoma.

Fig. 1.6. *Chondrosarcoma—other flat bones.* **a** A swelling arising from the posterior segment of the left 7th rib in this middle-aged man had been present for some years and had caused no significant discomfort. It was excised easily, the pre-operative diagnosis having been fibrous dysplasia or a benign enchondroma. Chondrosarcoma can be a great imitator of other entities. **b** Central calcification demonstrated in this tomogram of a sternal swelling in this 48-year-old woman established its cartilaginous nature. In both these cases the histological examinations revealed very low-grade malignancy.

Fig. 1.5. *Chondrosarcoma—aggressive forms.* A minority of these tumours present with a comparatively short and often fulminating history. They carry a more sinister prognosis. The examples shown here were observed before the recent reports of subtypes, but their radiological appearances conform to their descriptions. **a** This elderly man presented with a relatively short history of pain in the thigh. A heavily calcified central opacity in the medullary cavity of the femur is surrounded by a diffuse zone of osteolysis with a wide zone of transition. Destruction of the posterior cortex is evident and no significant periosteal reaction is present. This pattern is comparable to the appearance observed with a dedifferentiated chondrosarcoma. **b** Another highly aggressive lesion in the proximal end of the femur is consistent with the same diagnosis. It occurred in a 64-year-old man with a history of localised pain for months rather than years. Diffuse medullary destruction is associated with endosteal scalloping and a central area of calcification, but no periosteal reaction is evident. Arteriography showed no pathological circulation. Prosthetic replacement in this patient failed completely, death from pulmonary metastases following 3 months later. **c** This chondrosarcoma in the head and neck of the humerus has a sharply defined endosteal margin. The

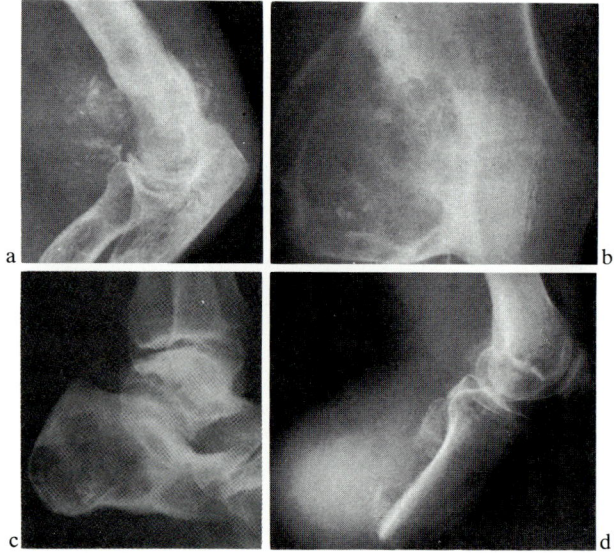

Fig. 1.7. *Chondrosarcoma—peripheral lesions.* Although distinctly less common sites, the occasional occurrence of this tumour in such areas should be appreciated. **a** This very aggressive lesion in the distal end of the humerus was associated with a massive and partially calcified extension into soft tissue. **b** In this 67-year-old man with a painful swelling of the lateral femoral condyle, the lytic, expanding lesion which was detected bore a definite resemblance to a giant-cell tumour, but the patient's age made this diagnosis unlikely (see Exercise 15). Again, this appearance might

have suggested the rare clear-cell variant. **c** This 67-year-old man had complained of pain and swelling of the left heel for only a few weeks, but the radiograph indicated the lesion to be of much longer duration. The irregular area of destruction in the calcaneus contained characteristic foci of calcification. Below-knee amputation was performed, but the tumour **d** recurred in the amputation stump and death from pulmonary metastases followed 6 months later.

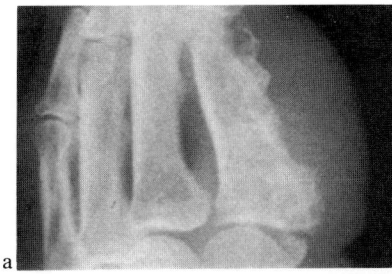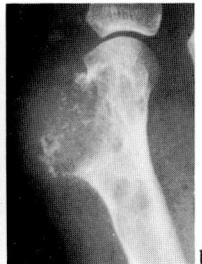

Fig. 1.9. *Chondrosarcoma—digital lesions.* Despite the great frequency of enchondromas in the small tubular bones of the hands and feet, the occurrence of a chondrosarcoma is rare. When they do arise, secondary malignant transformation must be suspected. **a** The swelling in the proximal phalanx of the index finger in this 59-year-old man had been present for many years, but recently had increased in size. This lesion was solitary. The appearance resembles the juxtacortical chondrosarcomas described above, but the mass contains no calcification. **b** A similar swelling of the 5th metacarpal in this 37-year-old man also had enlarged during the previous 2 years. In addition to flecks of calcification within the mass, an obvious enchondroma is present within the proximal portion of the bone. In each of these cases low-grade malignancy was established histologically.

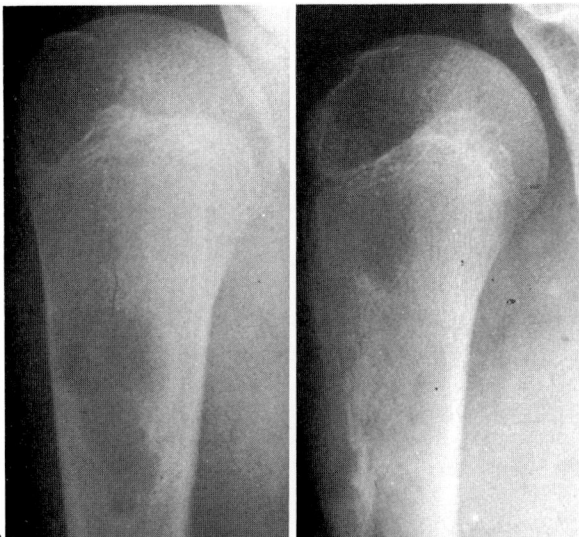

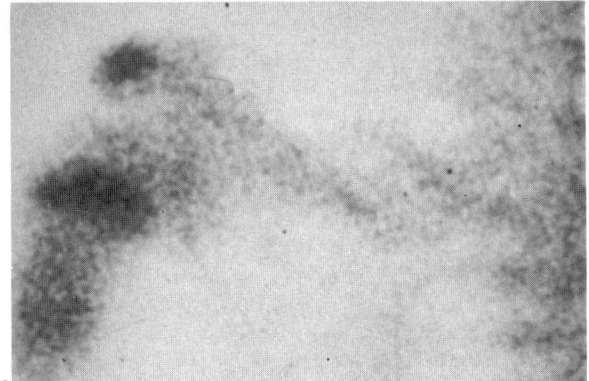

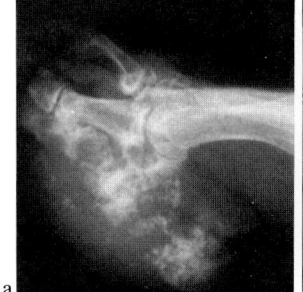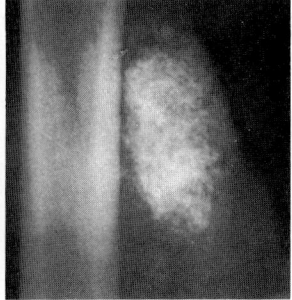

Fig. 1.8. *Chondrosarcoma—onset at early age.* Occasionally this tumour develops in childhood, adolescence or early adult life and is liable to be confused with other malignant tumours. **a** This juxtacortical chondrosarcoma was found in a 16-year-old boy who presented with chronic pain in the right deltoid area, where a swelling was just palpable. Movement of the shoulder was normal. **b** The lytic zone in the lateral cortex of the humerus had provoked some reactive sclerosis and was associated with a small and faintly calcified soft tissue mass. **c** As might be expected, the radionuclide scan was positive.

Fig. 1.10. *Chondrosarcoma—lesions in soft tissue* are rare. **a** The partially calcified mass on the plantar aspect of the forefoot of this 57-year-old woman had been present for 5 years and had enlarged slowly. At operation, surprisingly, no connection with the underlying bone was found. **b** A painful swelling on the medial side of the right thigh had developed in this 56-year-old woman during the preceding 6 months. The mass was mobile and contained much irregular calcification. It proved histologically to be a mesenchymal chondrosarcoma.

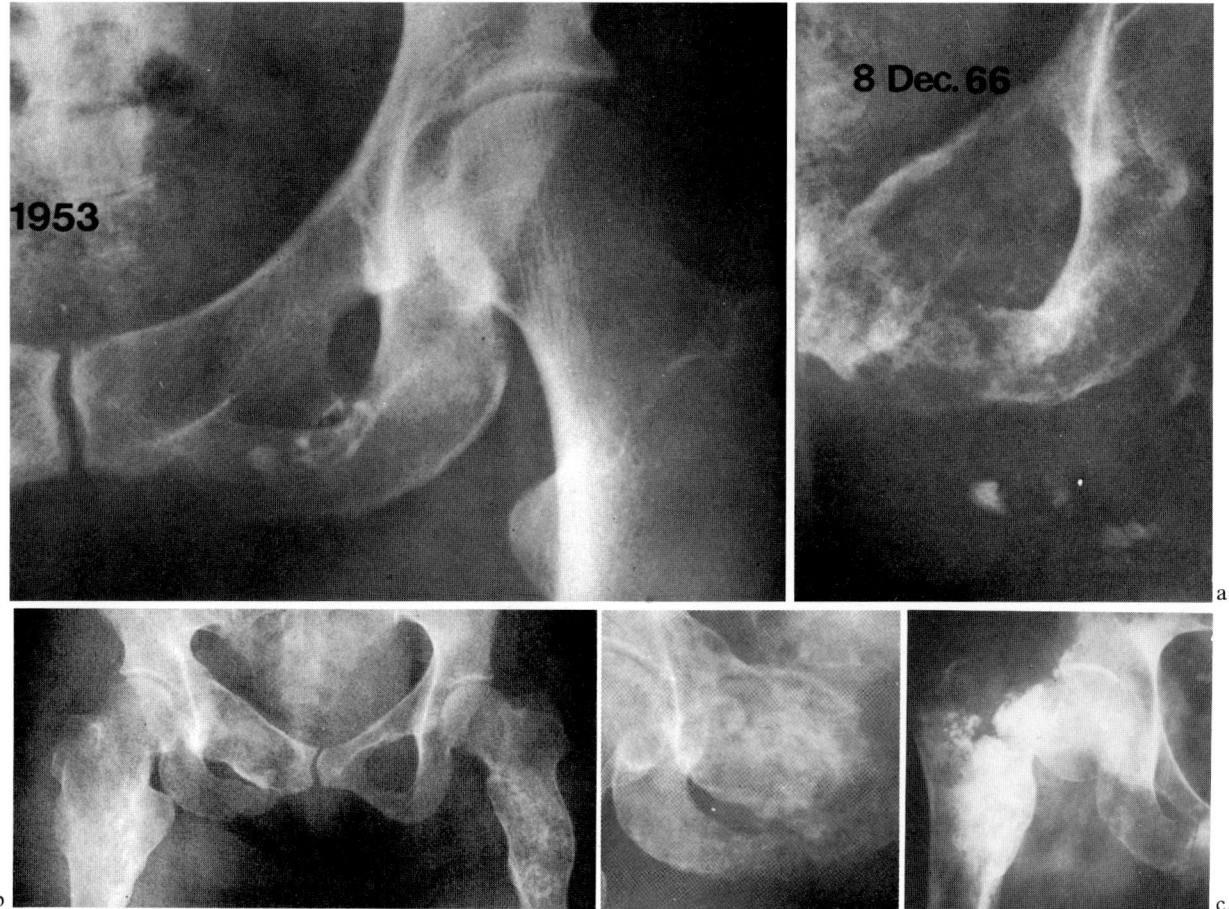

Fig. 1.11. *Secondary chondrosarcoma.* **a** This small osteochondroma arising from the left pubic bone of a 41-year-old woman was an incidental finding in 1953, but when an enlarging painful mass in this region was examined in 1966 all the typical features of a chondrosarcoma had developed. The original focal areas of calcification were spread more diffusely and extensive destruction of bone had become apparent in the superior and inferior pubic rami. **b** This 45-year-old woman with multiple skeletal abnormalities due to enchondromatosis (Ollier's disease, dyschondroplasia) illustrates a typical appearance of this congenital disorder. Lucent expanding areas in the right superior pubic ramus and the proximal ends of the femora contain characteristic foci of calcification, pathognomonic of cartilaginous tissue. The remainder of the skeleton was affected also. **c** Several years later this patient complained of a painful swelling in the right groin and a characteristic appearance of a secondary chondrosarcoma had become evident in the right superior pubic ramus. **d** *Maffucci's syndrome.* This middle-aged woman with enchondromatosis and soft tissue haemangiomas, shown by calcified phleboliths, sustained a pathological fracture of the left femoral neck through an area of bone destruction due to a secondary chondrosarcoma, a common complication of this entity.

Exercise 17

Q1. This 14-year-old boy, with a history of many fractures since infancy, was unable to walk.

On clinical examination multiple deformities were evident, including particularly bowing of the legs and kyphoscoliosis. Dentition was delayed, the muscles were hypoplastic and the sclerae were blue. No family history of bone disease was elicited.

Radiological survey of the skeleton revealed several fractures in varying stages of repair and showed the long bones to be abnormally slender and deformed, with an osteopenic texture and attenuation of the cortices. Muscle wasting was confirmed. Q1a illustrates a typical example, with bowing of long bones and disorganisation of the growth plates, around which circular densities are evident.

A biopsy of the iliac crest was performed.

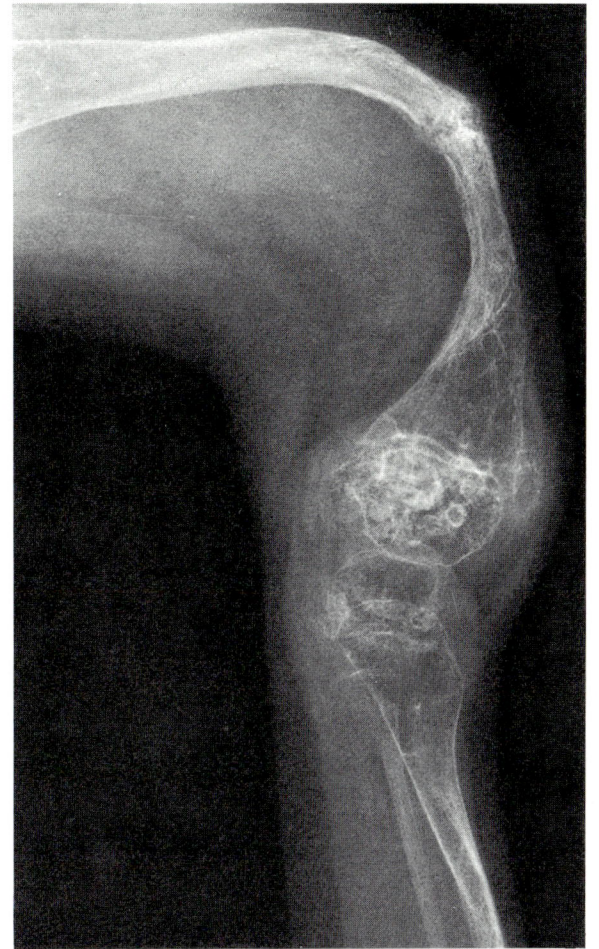

Q1a.

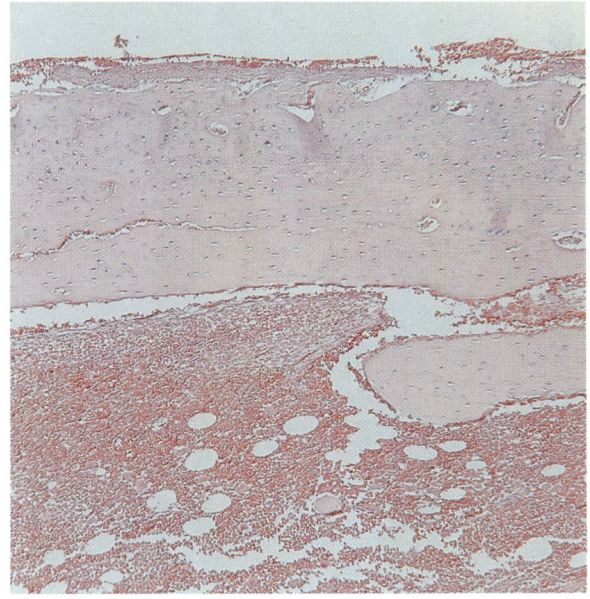

Q1b. (×55)

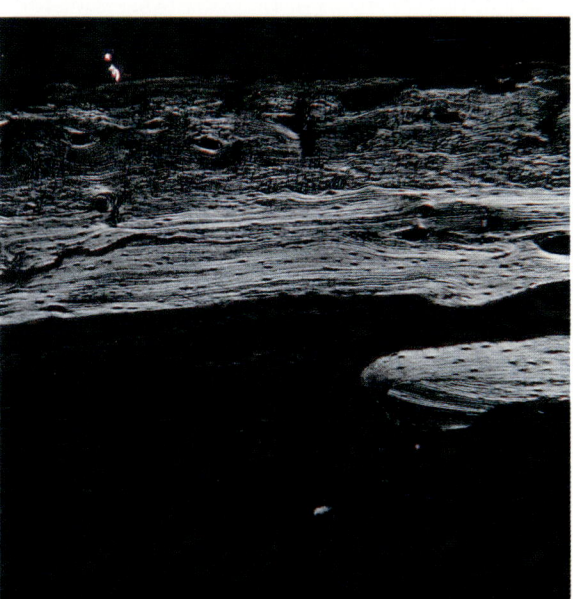

Q1c. (×55) Polarised light

A1. Osteogenesis imperfecta

The clinical and radiological findings in this child established the diagnosis unequivocally. Figure 1.1. illustrates other characteristic radiological features of the disorder in this patient. The biopsy had been undertaken in the course of a general investigation and the material so obtained provides a relatively unusual opportunity to study the histological appearance in this congenital disorder of the skeleton.

The bone of the iliac crest (Q1b and c) is decidedly abnormal, as can be appreciated from comparison with material from the iliac crest of a normal individual of the same age (Figs. 1.2 and 1.3). The cortex is abnormally thin. Although it does consist of lamellar bone, the individual lamellae are thin and indistinct, particularly in the periosteal region shown in the upper part of the field. Osteocyte lacunae are more numerous than in the normal specimen. These changes reflect a general lack of maturity in the bone structure, a feature characteristic of osteogenesis imperfecta.

Figure 1.3 and Q1c show the appearance of normal and abnormal bone when examined in polarised light. This technique, which has many applications in bone pathology, demonstrates any optically active (birefringent; anisotropic) material. The fibrous protein, collagen, is birefringent, and consequently appears either bright or dark according to the orientation of the fibres in relation to the plane of polarisation. Lamellar bone consists of layers of collagen fibres, the orientation of which varies in adjacent lamellae. Because of this, the structural pattern of the tissue is clearly visible when bone sections are examined in polarised light. The same technique enables the distinction between lamellar and non-lamellar bone to be readily made: it also finds use in the identification of certain birefringent crystalline materials such as urates and calcium pyrophosphate.

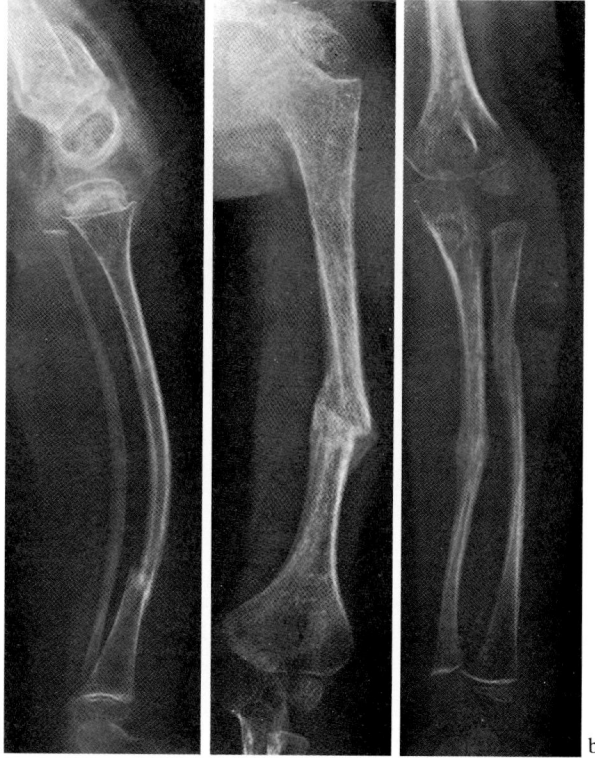

Fig. 1.1. These films of the same patient were obtained at an earlier age. **a, b** and **c** demonstrate the classically slender long bones with early bowing deformities and fractures in varying phases of repair.

Osteogenesis Imperfecta

The term osteogenesis imperfecta is applied to certain genetically determined abnormalities of the skeleton, some of which are inherited as an autosomal dominant, others as a recessive. Osteogenesis imperfecta is the commonest of the genetically determined abnormalities of bone. In some cases the disease is apparent at birth (*osteogenesis imperfecta congenita*), presenting as a severe and fatal form of short-limbed dwarfism, apparently due to a recessive gene. In contrast a later-developing type (*osteogenesis imperfecta tarda*), is recognised usually in childhood or even in adult life and is attributed to a dominant gene. This type, of which Q1 represents a severe example, is characterised also by impaired bony development, with a greater or lesser susceptibility to fracture and secondary deformities.

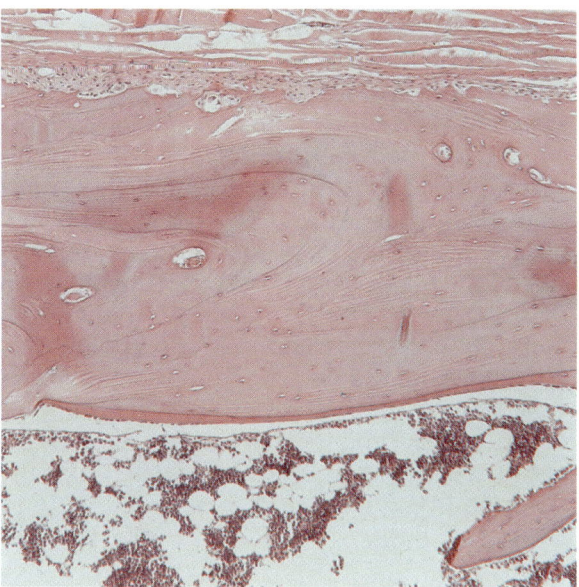

Fig. 1.2. Iliac crest biopsy from normal 14-year-old boy, for comparison with Q1b. The normal cortex is thicker than the cortex in the osteogenesis imperfecta patient. (×55)

Clinical Features

In the *congenital* form failure of ossification is so severe that many cases abort spontaneously or are stillborn. In those who survive for short periods the diagnosis is made obvious by the occurrence of numerous fractures, often causing marked shortening and deformity of the limbs. With the exception of possible elevation of serum alkaline phosphatase, routine biochemical investigations are normal. The radiological appearance, described below, provides confirmation of the diagnosis.

In the *late* form the severity of the disease varies greatly. The factor common to all degrees of the disease is an increased susceptibility to fractures of bones which are, to a greater or lesser extent, osteopenic and poorly formed. Blue sclerae may provide an important diagnostic sign, being due to abnormal collagen formation. Equally, impaired production of dentine results in abnormal and delayed dentition. Softening of the calvarium, with consequent basilar invagination, may cause cranial nerve involvement, often resulting in deafness and visual impairment.

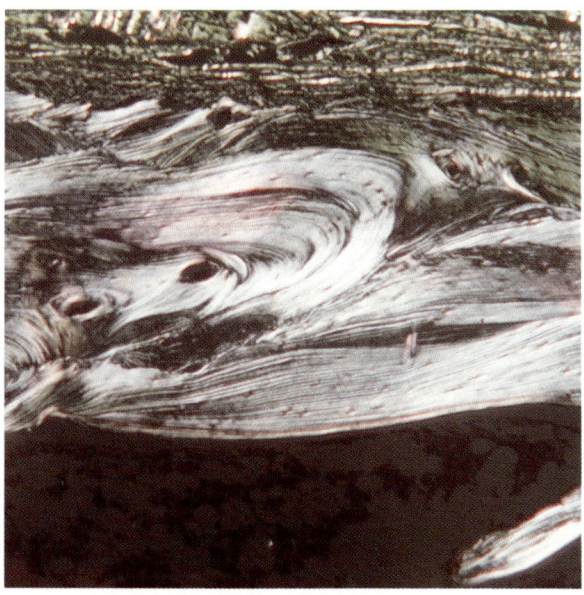

Fig. 1.3. The field shown in Fig. 1.2, seen in polarised light. The bone shows a more mature lamellar structure, with evidence of remodelling. (×55)

Fractures through the thin bones are common, and may lead to severe deformities. The spine commonly shows osteoporosis with biconcave vertebrae. Dislocations of the radial head and acetabular protrusion in association with coxa vara are not uncommon. Characteristic bowing of the femur and tibia is considered to be the result of subclinical fractures. While the fractures usually unite in a reasonably normal fashion, a large mass of hyperplastic callus may develop and even simulate a sarcoma.

Radiological Features

1. Site. The entire skeleton is affected by this generalised congenital disorder.

2. Appearance. The long bones are slender and poorly mineralised, with cortical thinning which may be extremely prominent. Fractures may be discerned in varying phases of repair, occasionally, as mentioned above, with gross hyperplastic callus formation. These fractures, either gross or subclinical, are responsible for the multiple deformities which become evident as age advances. Curvatures of the long bones, of the weight-bearing lower limbs especially, are common. The pelvis may develop a triradiate appearance, the spine a kyphoscoliosis, and defective ossification in the skull is characterised by the presence of numerous wormian bones. In advanced cases basilar invagination may be evident. Supernumerary teeth may reflect delayed dentition.

Pathological Features

The bony abnormalities in osteogenesis imperfecta appear to be due to a defect of bone matrix formation. The amount of bone tissue is reduced. The skeleton fails to show the normal progression from woven bone to lamellar bone, and also fails to undergo the process of maturation and progressive remodelling observed in the normal skeleton. The essential defect appears to be in the osteoblast, and to a lesser extent in other collagen-producing cells such as the fibroblasts of the skin and the sclerae. The precise nature of this defect is unknown. The abnormal bone, as in the present case, shows a poorly formed lamellar structure and contains more osteocytes than mature normal bone. In the severely osteoporotic long bones, secondary changes in the epiphyseal growth plates may occur, as in Q1a. Histologically, the growing cartilage plate (Fig. 1.4) is unsupported because of the failure of development of the metaphyseal spongiosa. Nodules of unsupported cartilage separate from the plate (Fig. 1.5) and are responsible for the 'popcorn calcifications' apparent in the clinical radiographs, as illustrated in the distal end of the femur in Q1a.

Treatment

No specific treatment exists for this generalised disease. Fractures require reduction and immobilisation. Fortunately they usually repair rapidly. Established deformities, particularly of the legs, have responded well to multiple corrective osteotomies to restore normal alignment, stabilisation with intramedullary rods being required.

References

Bullough PG, Davidson DD, Lorenzo JC (1981) The morbid anatomy of the skeleton in osteogenesis imperfecta. Clin Orthop 159: 42–57

Falvo KA, Root L, Bullough PG (1974) Osteogenesis imperfecta: clinical evaluation and management. J Bone Jt Surg 56A: 783–793

Goldman AB, Davidson D, Pavlov H, Bullough PG (1980) "Popcorn calcifications". A prognostic sign in osteogenesis imperfecta. Radiology 136: 351–358

King JD, Bobechko WP (1971) Osteogenesis imperfecta. An orthopaedic description and surgical review. J Bone Jt Surg 53B: 72–89

McKusick VA (1972) Osteogenesis imperfecta. In: Hereditable disorders of connective tissue, 4th edn. C.V. Mosby, St. Louis

Milgram JW, Flick MR, Engh CA (1973) Osteogenesis imperfecta. A histopathological case report. J Bone Jt Surg 55A: 506–515

Sillence DO, Senn A, Danko DM (1979) Genetic heterogeneity in osteogenesis imperfecta. J Med Genet 16: 101–116

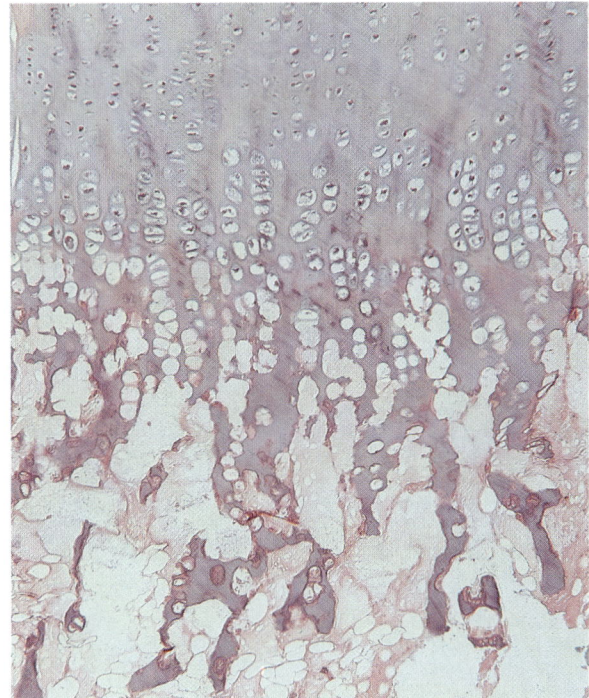

Fig. 1.4. The proximal growth plate of the tibia in another case of osteogenesis imperfecta. Metaphyseal bone trabeculae are absent. (×60)

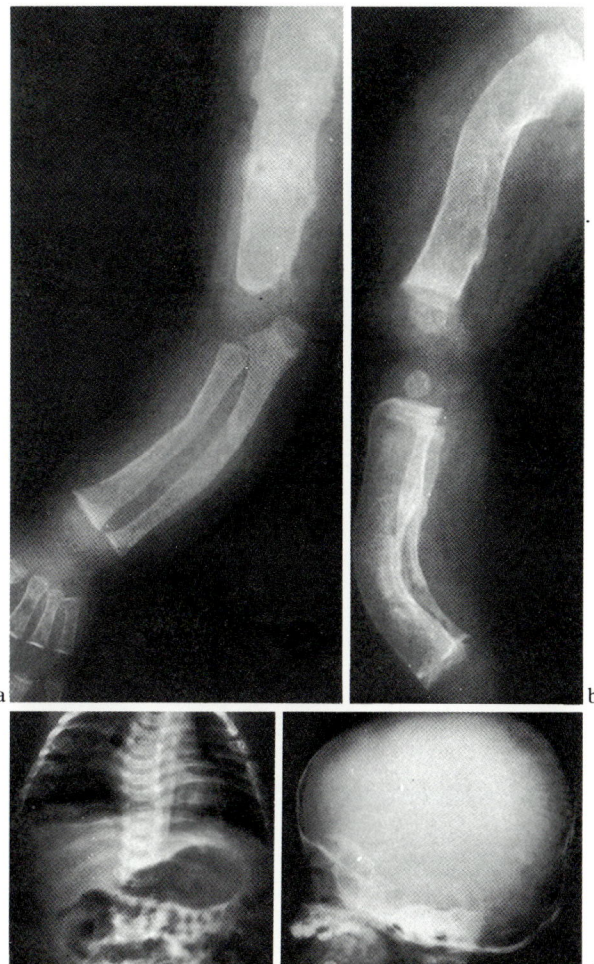

Fig. 1.6. *Osteogenesis imperfecta—congenital form.* The severe manifestations of the disease in infancy are illustrated by numerous fractures in the long bones, in varying stages of repair in **a** the arm and **b** the leg. Gross thinning of the cortex and an osteopenic medullary texture are evident. Widening, shortening and bowing of these long bones reflect intra-uterine infractions which have healed. **c** The ribs have suffered multiple fractures, most of which have united with bulbous expansions. **d** Classical wormian bones are present in the occiput.

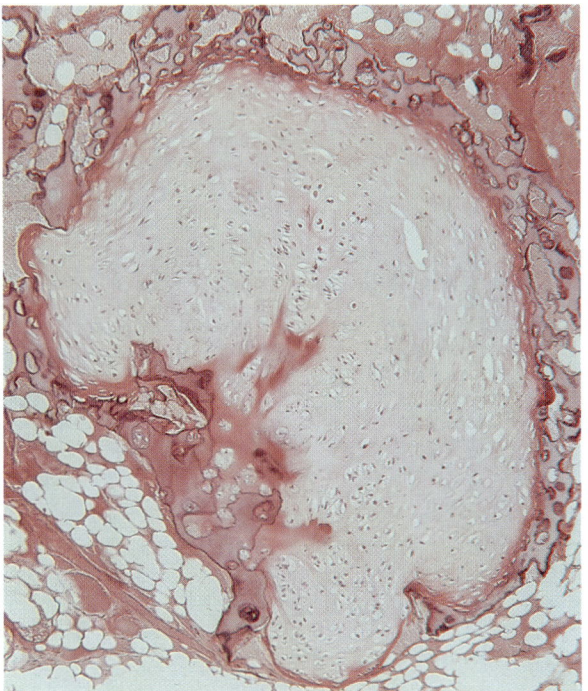

Fig. 1.5. Nodules of displaced growth plate cartilage from distal end of the femur of the case illustrated in Fig. 1.4. (×57)

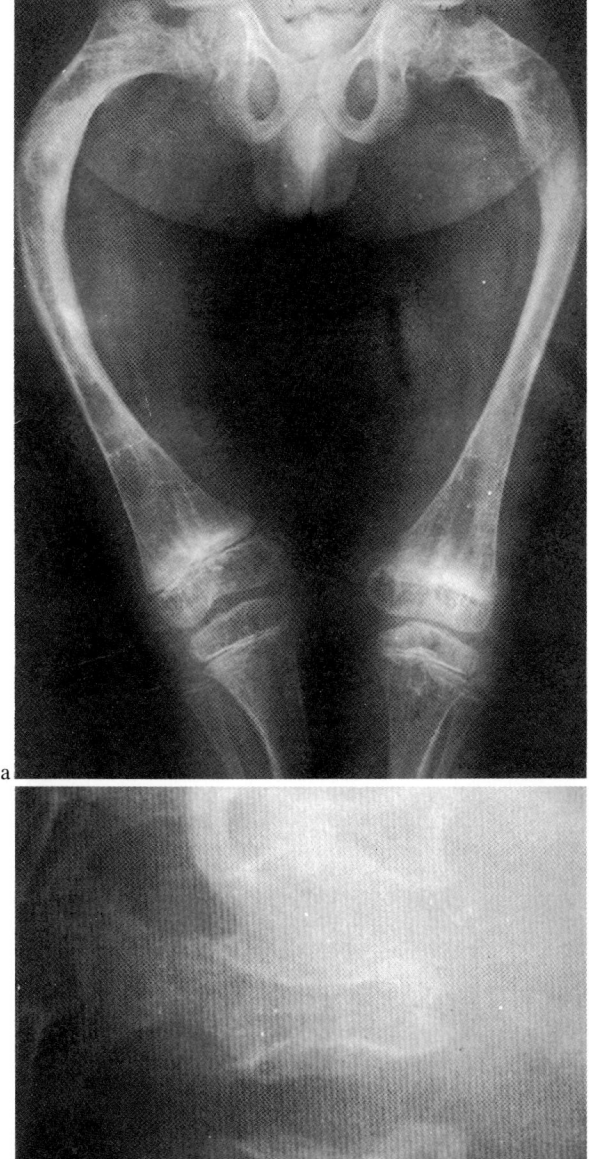

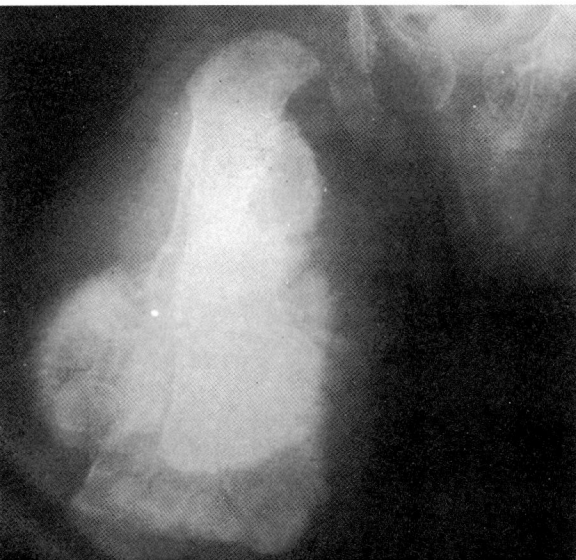

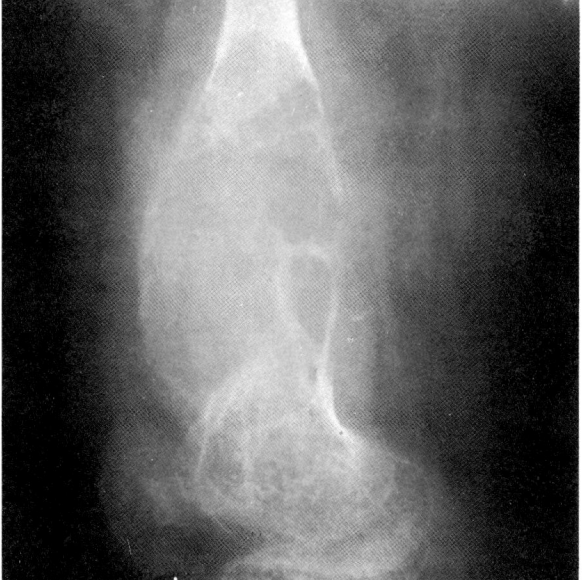

Fig. 1.7. *Osteogenesis imperfecta—late form in older children.* **a** Bowing of femora following repeated infractions. The cortices are thin and the medullae are osteopenic. **b** The fragile vertebral bodies are osteopenic and have undergone partial collapse, the appearance simulating osteoporosis or even leukaemia.

Fig. 1.8. *Osteogenesis imperfecta—pseudotumours.* **a** Hypertrophic callus surrounding a fracture of the femur in a 1-year-old child with the congenital form of the disease might suggest an osteosarcoma, but the rest of the skeleton showed typical changes of the disease. Osteosarcomas, moreover, are excessively rare under the age of 5 years. **b** This 22-year-old woman with long-standing disease developed a painful swelling above the knee. The possibility of a malignant tumour was considered in view of this large cystic lesion.

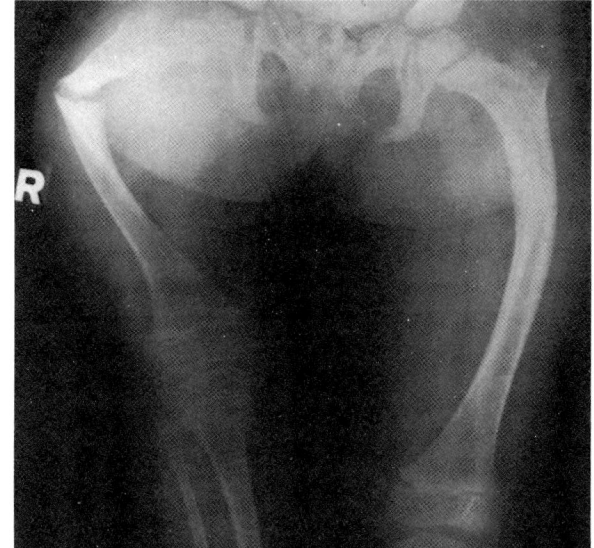
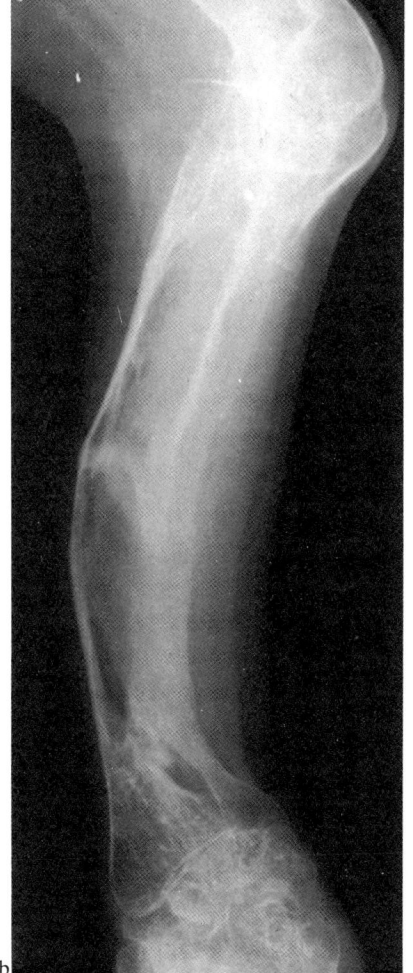
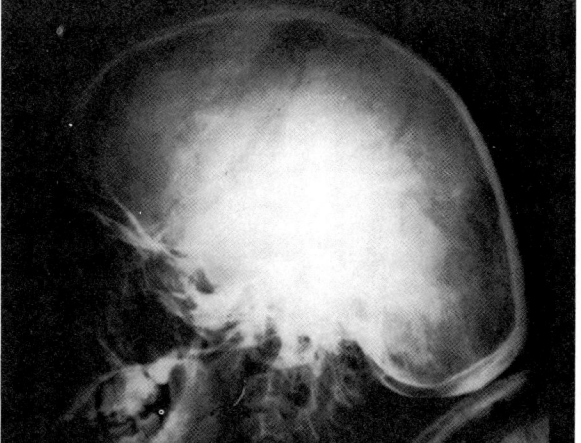
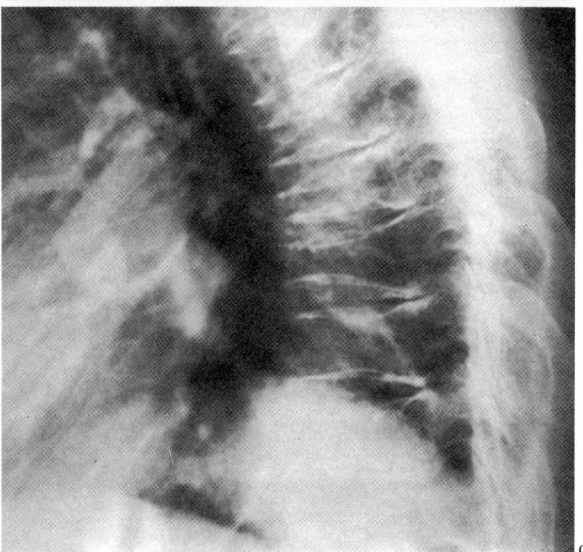

Fig. 1.9. *Osteogenesis imperfecta—less common manifestations.* **a** Occasionally fractures fail to unite and develop a pseudarthosis, as shown in this right femur. Observe typical bowing of the left femur. **b** This disease had been recognised in this woman at the age of 8 years. At the age of 28 severe bowing of the slender bones of the forearms was accompanied by ossification of the interosseous membrane, a feature almost pathognomonic. The radial head was dislocated. **c** Marked basilar invagination of the skull in this 18-year-old man with established disease caused signs of cranial nerve pressure, including deafness. Wormian bones were still present. **d** This 55-year-old woman presented with back pain due to a recent compression fracture of the body of T12. Many other vertebral bodies appeared to have suffered compression fractures, but without causing symptoms. Nevertheless the patient reported an unusual susceptibility to fractures in adolescence and early adult life. Clinical observation of blue sclerae caused the diagnosis of a mild form of osteogenesis imperfecta to be preferred to that of idiopathic osteoporosis (see Exercise 3).

Q1. The patient, a man aged 75 years, had complained of pain and swelling of the knees, ankles and wrists for many years.

On clinical examination the affected joints were found to be swollen and tender, with limitation of movement.

Radiographs of the left knee showed para-articular erosions on the medial and posterior aspects of the tibia and on the lateral femoral condyle, in relation to the attachment of the collateral ligament. Moderate peri-articular osteoporosis was evident. These changes were symmetrical.

A synovial biopsy of the left knee was performed.

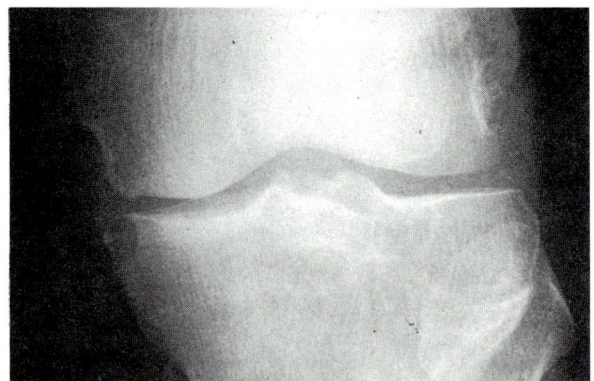

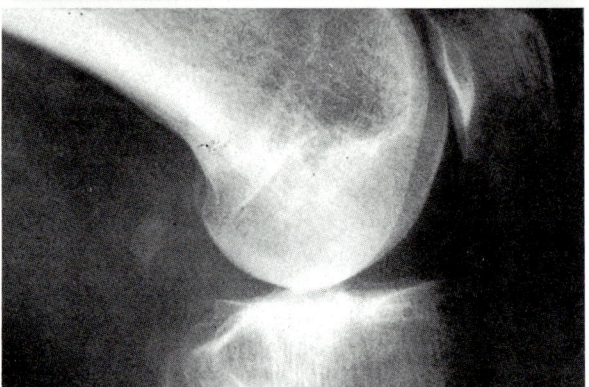

Q1a.

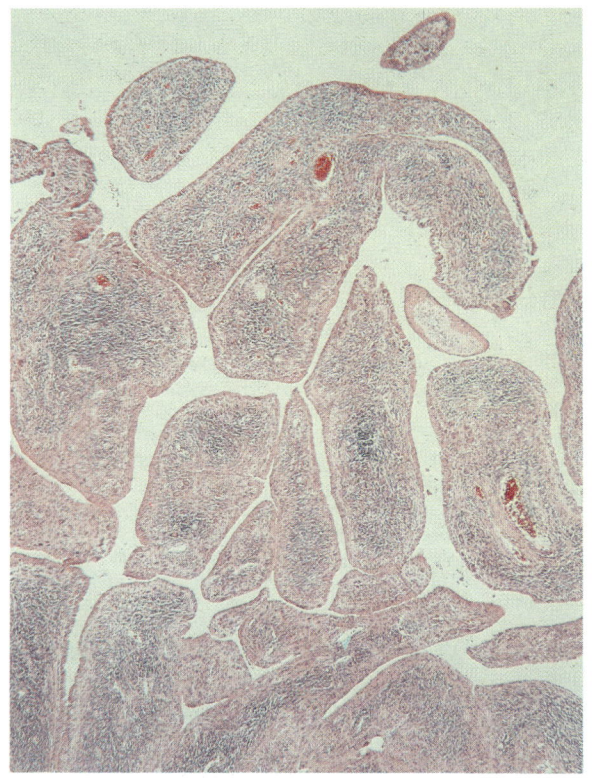

Q1b. (×25)

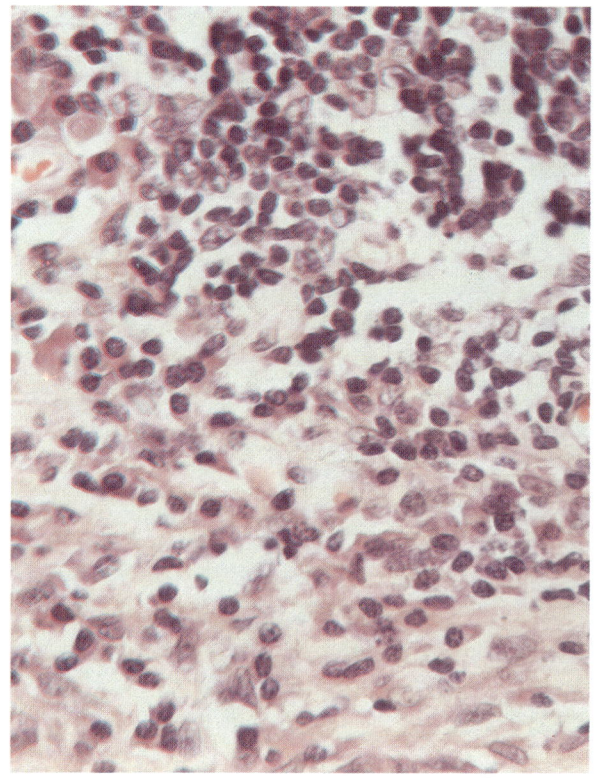

Q1c. (×450)

Q2. This 54-year-old woman had complained of pain and swelling of the right knee for 4 years.

Clinically, she was obese, with a tender swelling of the right knee. The asymptomatic left knee was also swollen, but to a lesser degree. Other joints were not affected.

Radiological examinations showed narrowing of the medial compartment of the joint space, and formation of a small bony excrescence on the inner aspect of the medial condyle of the femur. The proximal end of the tibia is osteopenic. These changes are accompanied by soft tissue thickening consistent with synovial hypertrophy.

A synovial biopsy of the left knee was performed.

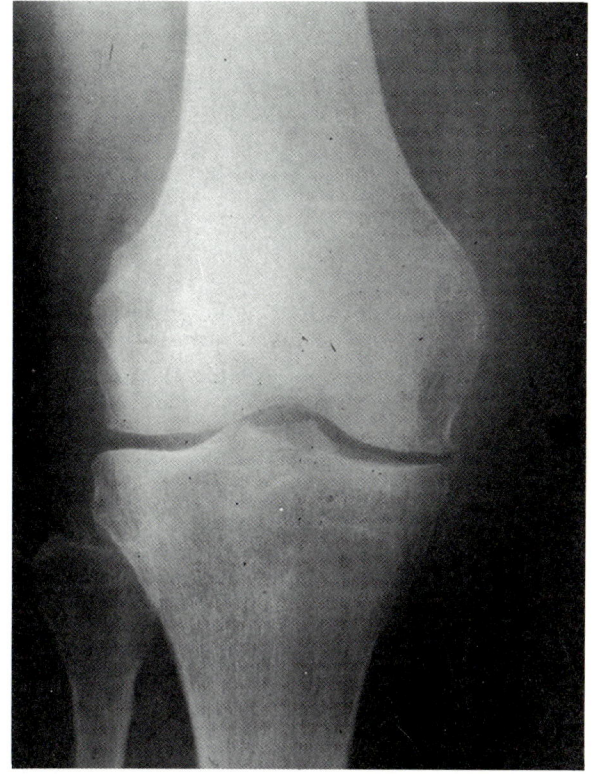

Q2a.

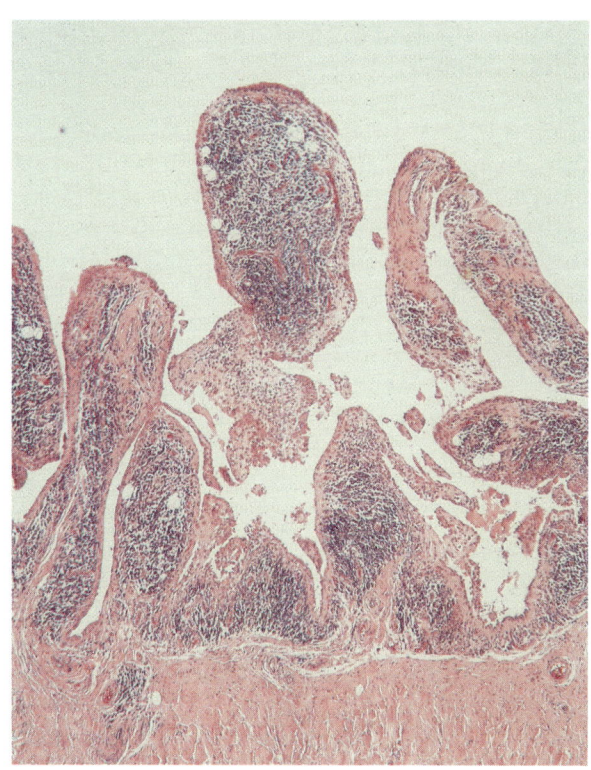

Q2b. (×25)

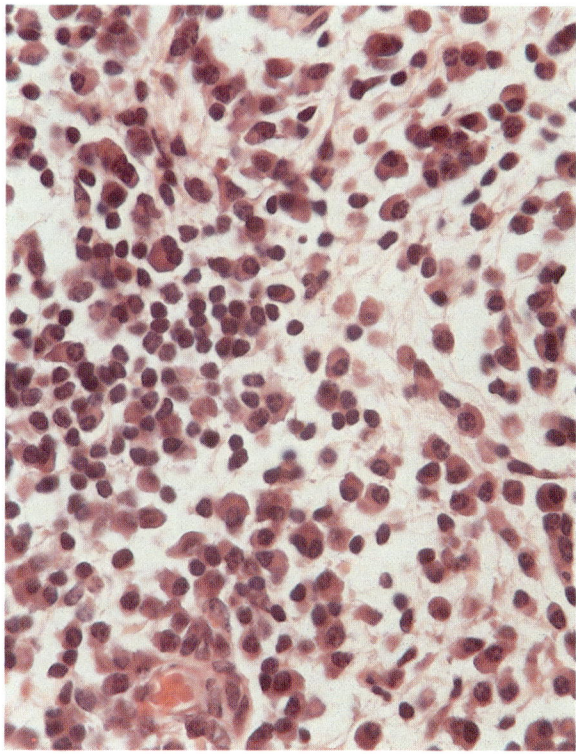

Q2c. (×450)

A1. Rheumatoid arthritis

A clinical diagnosis of rheumatoid arthritis was supported, radiologically, by the classically clear-cut para-articular erosions at the synovial attachments. The osteoporosis in the neighbourhood of the inflamed joint reflected chronic hyperaemia.

At operation, the synovial membrane of the knee joint was thickened, villous and hyperaemic. The articular cartilage appeared normal, except at the margin, where pannus extended a short distance over the cartilaginous surface.

Sections from the synovial biopsy (Q1b and c) show a marked degree of villous synovitis. The villi are crowded with inflammatory cells, including numerous lymphocytes and plasma cells. The lymphocytes appear as small round dark nuclei with little or no surrounding cytoplasm. The plasma cells can be recognised by their more abundant cytoplasm, which stains red, and by the presence, in some of these cells, of a paler zone near the nucleus. These changes are quite characteristic of rheumatoid arthritis, but they are not specific for this condition. In the present case, the diagnosis is supported by other evidence, including the multiplicity of joint involvement, the radiographic changes and other laboratory evidence. In particular, the patient had a high ESR and a positive serological reaction for rheumatoid factor.

Rheumatoid Arthritis

Rheumatoid arthritis is a generalised inflammatory disease affecting many systems of the body, but presenting through involvement of synovial tissues. The aetiology is unknown. A variety of infective agents (diphtheroid organisms, mycoplasmas, viruses) have been considered as causes, but so far without proof. The disease is often regarded as an autoimmune phenomenon because of the frequent presence of circulating antibodies to normal immunoglobulins, referred to as 'rheumatoid factor'. An increased incidence of HLA antigens of the DR4 type in patients with rheumatoid arthritis may possibly indicate an inherited defect in immune regulation.

Rheumatoid arthritis is a common condition, but varies greatly in severity and rate of progress. Some patients are affected so mildly that medical advice is sought, if sought at all, only late in life because of secondary degenerative joint disease. At the other end of the spectrum, the disease may be acute and progressive, particularly in the relatively rare forms recognised in children and adolescents, (Still's disease).

Long regarded as rheumatoid variants, but now to be separated from rheumatoid arthritis, is the group of seronegative spondyloarthropathies (ankylosing spondylitis, psoriatic arthritis, Reiter's syndrome, Behçet's syndrome). These conditions differ from rheumatoid arthritis in that circulating rheumatoid factor is absent, and by a significant association with HLA antigens of the B27 group.

Clinical Features

Middle-aged women are predominantly affected. Early in the course of the disease the involved joints develop pain, swelling and stiffness, frequently symmetrical and often with mild and transient pyrexia. Skin nodules are common, especially over such bony prominences as the olecranon. The erythrocyte sedimentation rate is elevated and serological tests for rheumatoid disease are usually positive when the disease is polyarticular. As a rule the younger the patient, the more aggressive is the disease. Later stages may be marked by joint deformities, such as ulnar deviation of the fingers, or even ankylosis of joints, although secondary degenerative changes in major articulations is a common outcome. Atrophy of bones, muscles and skin may occur.

Radiological Features

1. Site. The metacarpo-phalangeal joints of the hands and the carpus, including particularly the ulnar styloid process, are the commonest sites, together with the metatarso-phalangeal joints of the feet. Major joints may be affected, possibly as solitary lesions, especially the hip, the knee and the shoulder. The cervical spine is involved frequently and, particularly as a pre-operative measure, should be studied always to exclude instability, especially at the atlanto-axial level, in order that inadvertent damage to the spinal cord during anaesthesia may be avoided.

2. Appearance. The earliest abnormality in the acute stage is soft tissue swelling related to the affected synovium. This is followed by subarticular osteoporosis due to the inflammatory hyperaemia and then by the classical erosions at synovial attachments. Diaphyseal periosteal reactions occasionally provide a valuable diagnostic clue, particularly in juvenile rheumatoid arthritis (Still's disease). In the latter condition, accelerated growth of epiphyseal centres and premature fusion of growth plates represent other hyperaemic phenomena. Narrowing of joint spaces reflects destruction of articular cartilage and, in later stages, gross articular disintegration may develop, especially if aggravated by steroid and analgesic therapy. Degenerative joint disease secondary to inflammatory conditions of the rheumatoid type is characterised by minimal or even absent osteophyte formation, owing to the destruction of articular cartilage from which osteophytes originate. For this reason also degenerative subchondral cysts often form. Usually they are small and multiple, but they may be very large and subject to pathological fractures. Space permits illustration of only a few of these features in this Exercise.

Pathological Features

The initial joint abnormality in rheumatoid arthritis is an inflammatory change of the synovial tissues. Inflammatory cells accumulate and the synovial membrane becomes hyperaemic and voluminous, with pronounced villous proliferation. Although neutrophil polymorphs and macrophages may be present, the inflammatory cells are mainly plasma cells and lymphocytes, the latter commonly arranged in focal aggregates (Q1a and b). These features are characteristic of rheumatoid arthritis, but, as shown in Q2, they can occur also in other conditions and must therefore be regarded as non-specific. The synovial lining cells also participate in the inflammatory process and proliferate to form mononuclear phagocytic cells (macrophages) and multinucleate giant cells (Fig. 1.1). The presence of these giant cells in the synovial membrane makes the histological findings more specific, as they are not usually found in osteoarthritis or in other non-specific synovial reactions. They are to be distinguished from the giant cells of tuberculosis (see Exercise 11) and from osteoclasts.

Immunological studies have shown that the rheumatoid synovium contains both B and T lymphocytes. B lymphocytes have as their function the production of antibodies. In rheumatoid arthritis these cells, and the plasma cells—which are derived from them—are the sites of formation of rheumatoid factor and this material can be demonstrated within their cytoplasm. T lymphocytes are involved in cell-mediated immunological reactions. In rheumatoid arthritis they are believed to contribute to the inflammatory process by the secretion of lymphokines and other biologically active substances. Both types of lymphocyte interact with macrophages and influence the phagocytic activities of these cells.

The synovial lining cells, and the phagocytic cells derived from them, frequently contain immunoglobulins and immune complexes which activate the complement system and so accentuate the inflammatory changes present. The same cells contain a variety of lysosomal enzymes which are concerned in the breakdown of proteins in bone, cartilage and other connective tissues.

Changes in the synovial fluid develop as a result of the inflammatory process in the synovial membrane. Their recognition may be useful in diagnosis. Inflammatory cells, particularly neutrophil polymorphs, accumulate. The fluid becomes cloudy and loses its normally high viscosity. The presence of fibrin may lead to clotting, and fibrin deposition is often conspicuous on the surface of the inflamed synovium.

As the synovial changes progress, a pannus of granulation tissue covers and replaces the surfaces of the articular cartilage (Figs. 1.2 and 1.3), extending inward from the margin. The same type of reactive tissue invades the subchondral bone at the joint margin, so producing the bony erosions which are such a characteristic radiological feature of rheumatoid arthritis. Articular cartilage destruction and fibrosis can result ultimately in fibrous or even bony ankylosis of the joint.

Another lesion characteristic of rheumatoid arthritis is the subcutaneous nodule. These nodules are present in about 20% of cases, and are located over bony prominences, particularly along the subcutaneous border of the ulna. Histologically, they consist of fibrous tissue showing conspicuous zones of fibrinoid necrosis, surrounded by radially oriented ('palisaded') connective tissue cells (Fig. 1.4).

Visceral lesions (heart, spleen, kidney, lymph nodes) occur in a minority of cases of rheumatoid arthritis. Amyloidosis, too, may be present in patients with severe disease.

Treatment

The vast majority of cases of rheumatoid arthritis are mild, and respond to simple analgesics, such as aspirin. More severe cases may require such drugs as phenylbutazone or indomethacin, or even gold salts or penicillamine. The value of immunosuppressive or cytotoxic drugs, such as cyclophosphamide and azathioprene, is being assessed currently. Despite their dramatic effects, systemically administered corticosteroid drugs are not ordinarily indicated for the treatment of the articular manifestations of rheumatoid arthritis. This is because of their predictable side effects, which include osteoporosis, often complicated by vertebral fractures. Adjuvant physiotherapy is often of the greatest value. Orthopaedic measures in the acute stage include synovectomy—a surgical answer to a medical problem which is often highly successful—and, in later stages, appropriate treatment of secondary degenerative joint disease. Total replacement of the hip, knee, elbow and finger joints in severe rheumatoid patients now is performed commonly.

The success of reconstructive surgery in this disease, however, is notoriously disappointing, since not only the bones and joints are affected, but also the associated soft tissues and tendons.

References

Gardner DL (1972) The pathology of rheumatoid arthritis. Edward Arnold, London

Glynn LE (1968) The chronicity of inflammation and its significance in rheumatoid arthritis. Ann Rheum Dis 27: 105–121

Harris ED (1981) Pathogenesis of rheumatoid arthritis. In: Kelley WN, Harris ED, Ruddy S, Sledge CB (eds) Textbook of rheumatology. W. B. Saunders, Philadelphia

Ruddy S (1981) The management of rheumatoid arthritis. In: Kelley WN, Harris ED, Ruddy S, Sledge CB (eds) Textbook of Rheumatology. W. B. Saunders, Philadelphia

Sachs JA (1982) HLA systems and rheumatic diseases. In: Berry CL (ed) Bone and joint disease. Springer-Verlag, Berlin Heidelberg New York

Williams RC (1978) Immunopathology of rheumatoid arthritis. Hosp Pract 13: 53–60

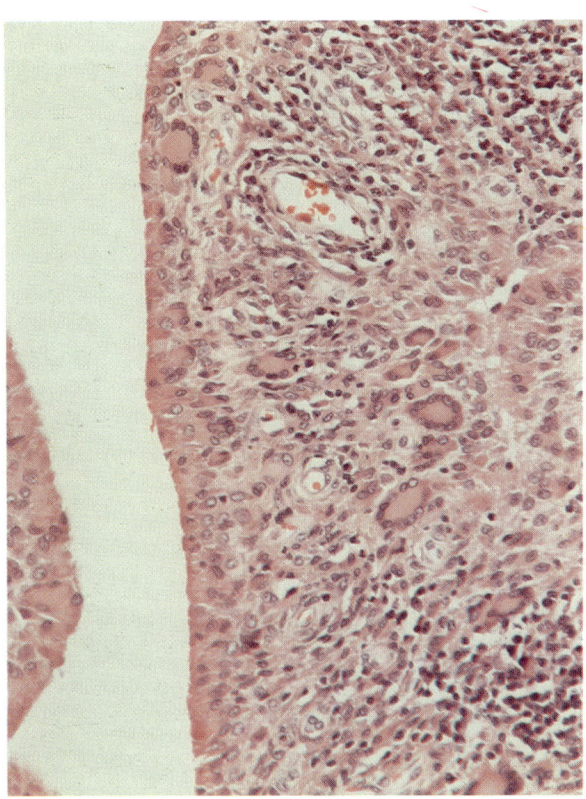

Fig. 1.1. *Rheumatoid arthritis.* Numerous multinucleated giant cells are present in this specimen of rheumatoid synovial membrane. (×450)

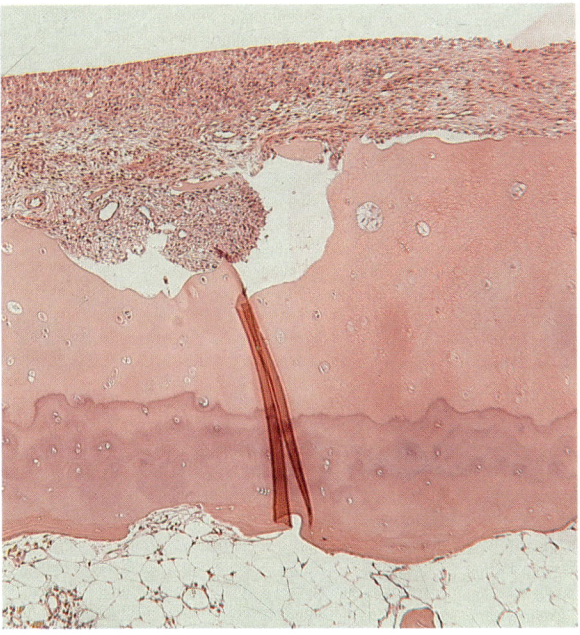

Fig. 1.2. *Rheumatoid arthritis.* The articular cartilage is covered by rheumatoid pannus and already has undergone extensive erosion. (×25)

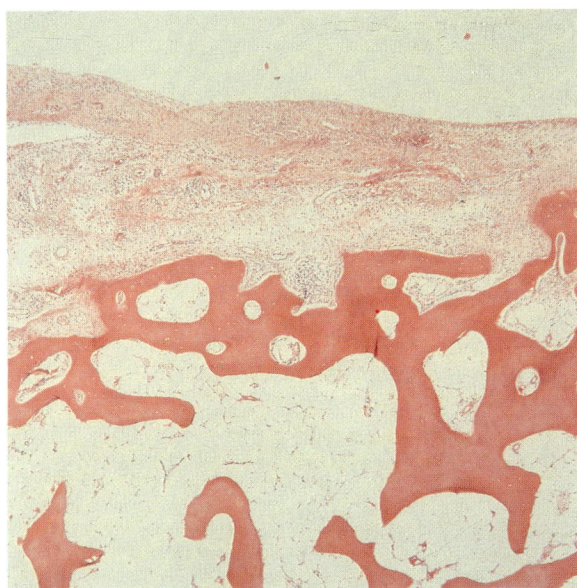

Fig. 1.3 *Rheumatoid arthritis.* This joint surface is shown at a much later stage. The articular cartilage has been destroyed completely and the subchondral bone is covered by pannus. (×25)

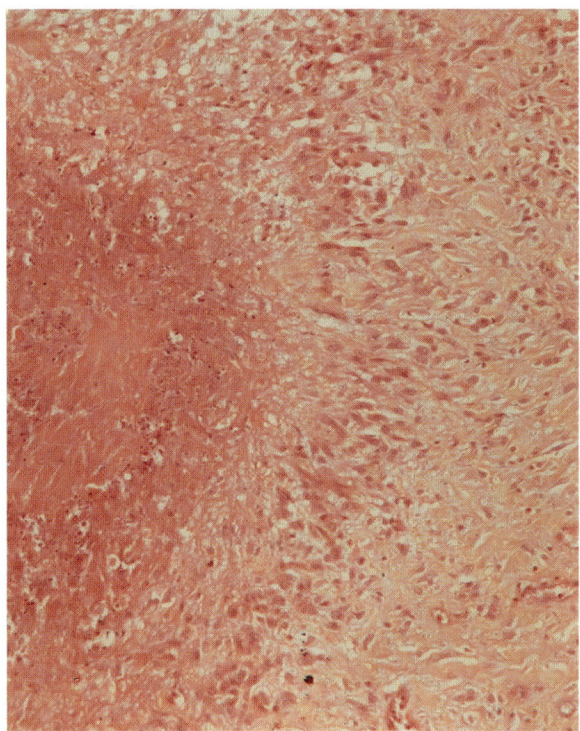

Fig. 1.4. *Rheumatoid arthritis.* Part of a subcutaneous nodule, with palisaded connective tissue cells surrounding a central area of necrosis. (×125)

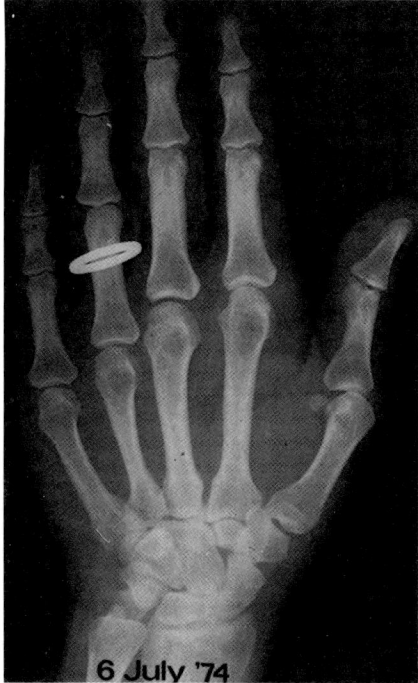
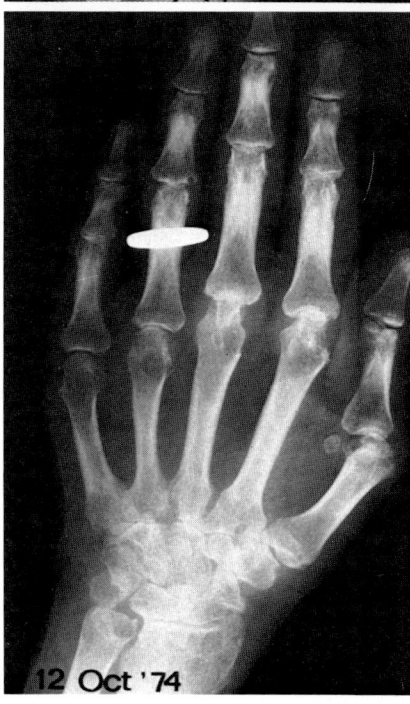

Fig. 1.5. *Rheumatoid arthritis.* This 42-year-old woman, with a history of vague joint pains for 10 years, developed pain and stiffness of the left index finger. Marked soft tissue swelling surrounded the 2nd metacarpo-phalangeal joint. Only 3 months later gross erosions had developed on the 2nd and 3rd metacarpal heads, with generalised subarticular osteoporosis and extensive destruction of the carpus. This progression was unusually rapid. Observe the swelling over the eroded ulnar styloid process.

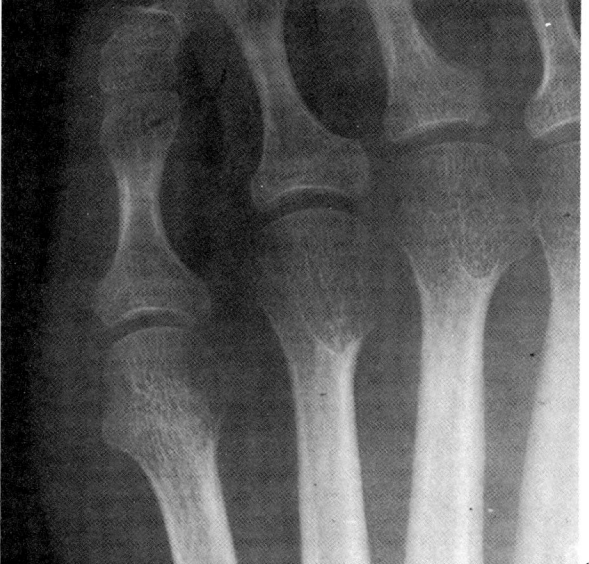
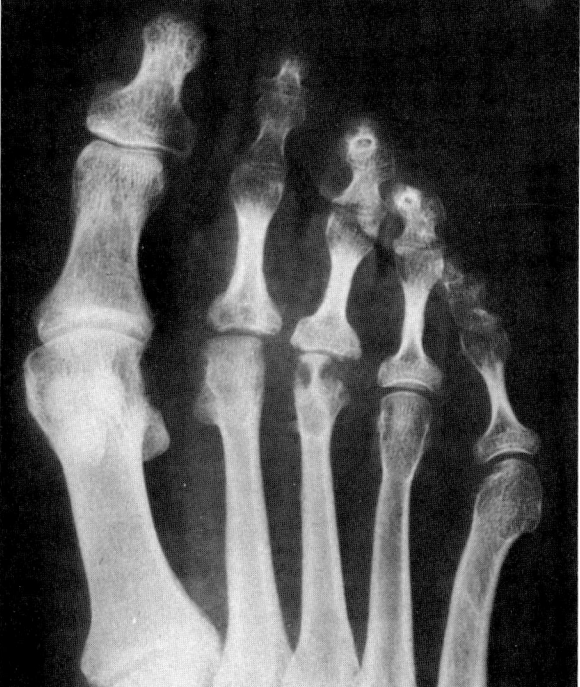

Fig. 1.6. *Rheumatoid arthritis.* **a** Soft tissue swelling had developed around the head of the 5th metatarsal in a 22-year-old woman with painful feet. A typical erosion is evident on the lateral aspect of the bone and generalised subarticular demineralisation is present. The feet are often affected first in this disease. Periosteal reactions were visible on the shafts of the 3rd proximal phalanx. **b** More advanced para-articular erosions are illustrated in a 39-year-old man. Observe narrowing of the 2nd and 3rd metatarso-phalangeal joints.

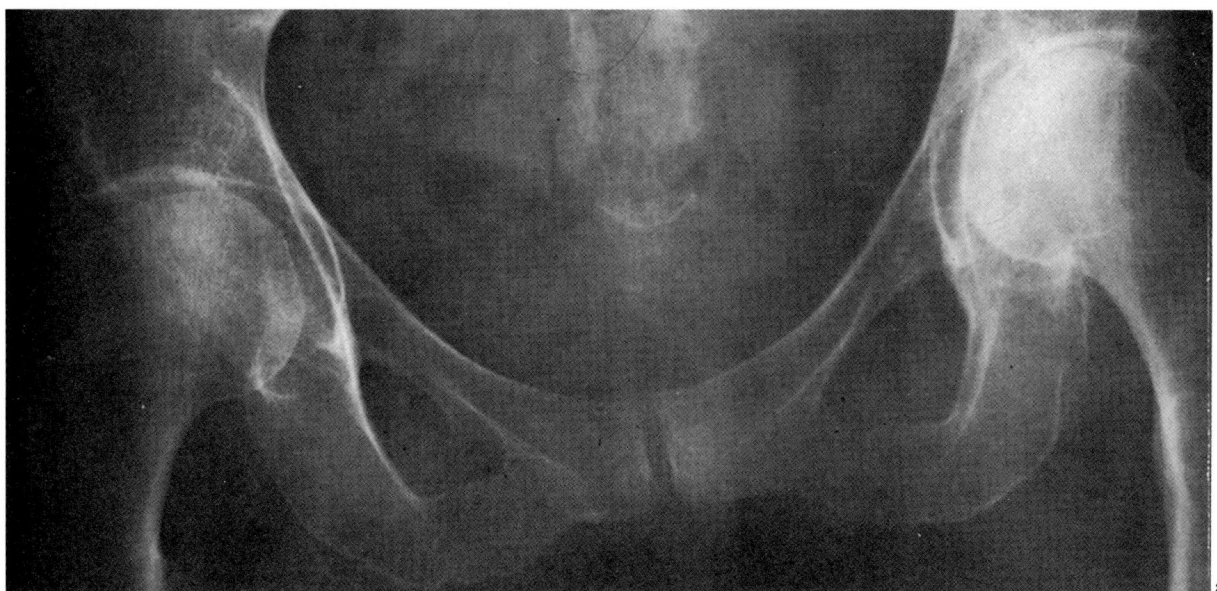

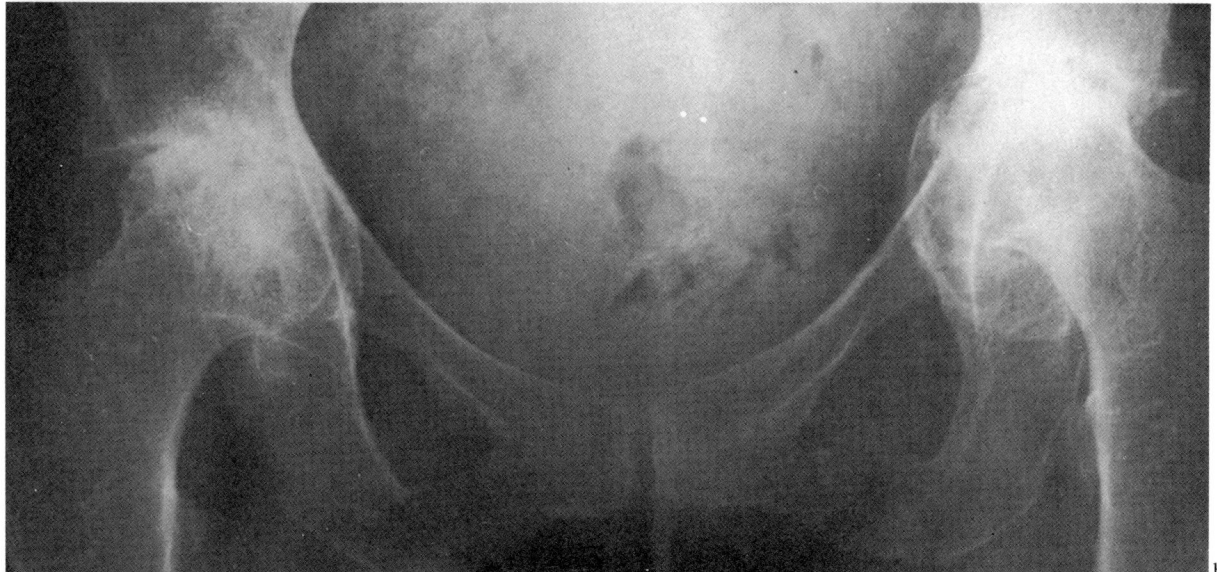

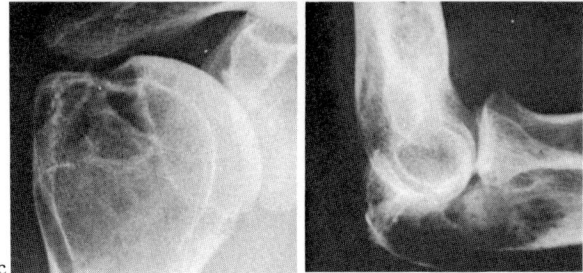

Fig. 1.7. *Rheumatoid arthritis—major joints.* All these patients had longstanding disease. **a** *Hips* with narrowed joint spaces. Reactive sclerosis is present in the left femoral head and acetabulum, but no osteophytes have formed in this 53-year-old woman. **b** Fifteen months later gross deterioration had developed, with medial migration of the left femoral head and a typical protrusio acetabuli deformity. Lesser changes of the same type had affected the right hip. **c** *Shoulder.* The same patient as in Fig. 1.5 had developed, 2 years later, marginal erosions at the capsular attachments of the head of the humerus and a huge subchondral cyst. **d** *Elbow.* This 61-year-old man developed a pathological fracture after a minor injury through another large subchondral cyst in the ulna.

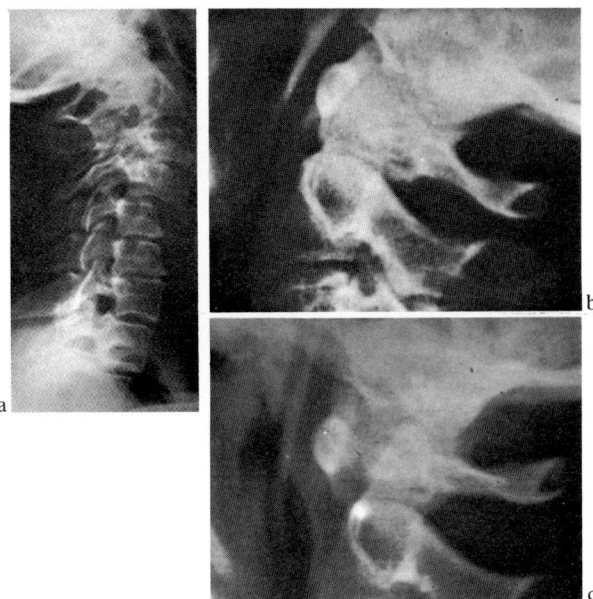
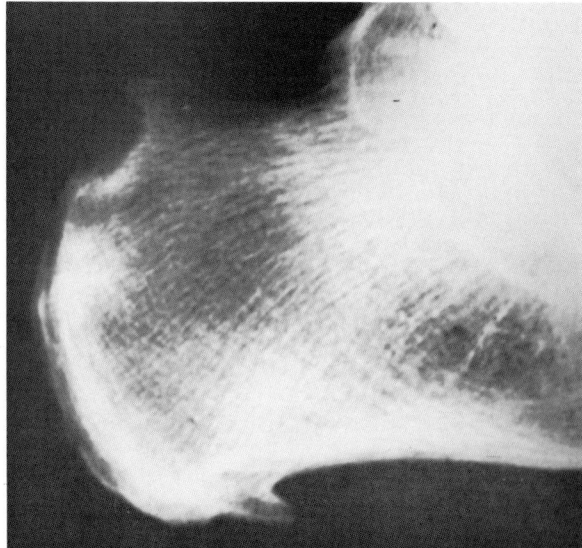

Fig. 1.8 *Rheumatoid arthritis—cervical spine involvement.* The posterior joints, being truly synovial articulations, are especially liable to be affected by the disease, with a particular affinity for the upper cervical area. **a** Gross destruction of the upper posterior joints has caused multiple subluxations, but again no osteophyte formation is visible in this elderly woman with longstanding disease. Of even greater importance is the demonstration of instability, as in this atlanto-axial joint, in a 33-year-old man with early disease, by comparison of lateral films in **b** extension and **c** flexion. Such a finding provides a warning to the anaesthetist.

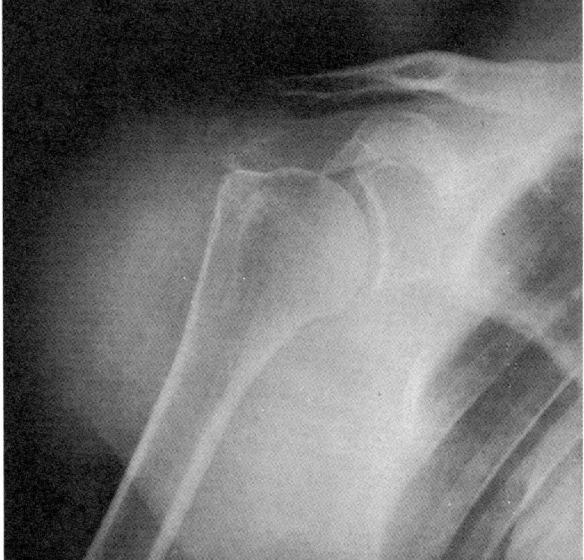
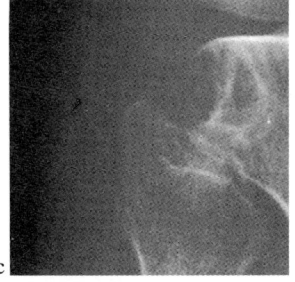
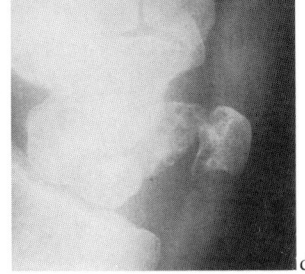

Fig. 1.9 *Rheumatoid arthritis—less common erosions.* **a** *Calcaneus.* This is due to synovitis in the bursa below the Achilles tendon. The plantar spur is common to other arthropathies also, such as psoriasis, ankylosing spondylitis and Reiter's syndrome. This 52-year-old woman had complained of pain in the ankles for 1 year and the lesions were symmetrical. **b** *Lateral end of clavicle.* Such absorption frequently indicates the disease in a chest film. In addition, this 46-year-old woman, with known rheumatoid arthritis for 15 years, had developed a large, virtually painless, rheumatoid cyst in the soft tissues. At operation it contained a multitude of fibrinous bodies resembling grains of rice. **c** *Lateral margin of tibia.* This lesion was shown only with an oblique view in a 56-year-old woman with pain in the knees for 3 years. **d** *Pisiform and triquetrum.* These erosions were the only radiological signs found in a 51-year-old man with painful hands and feet for 2 years. The unorthodox projection in semi-supination was rewarding.

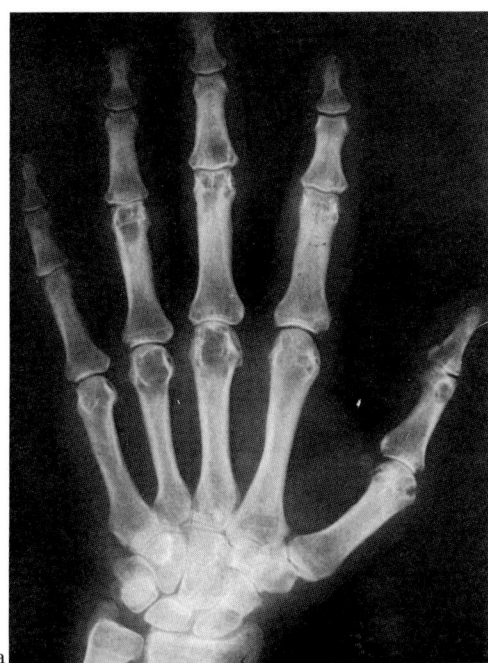

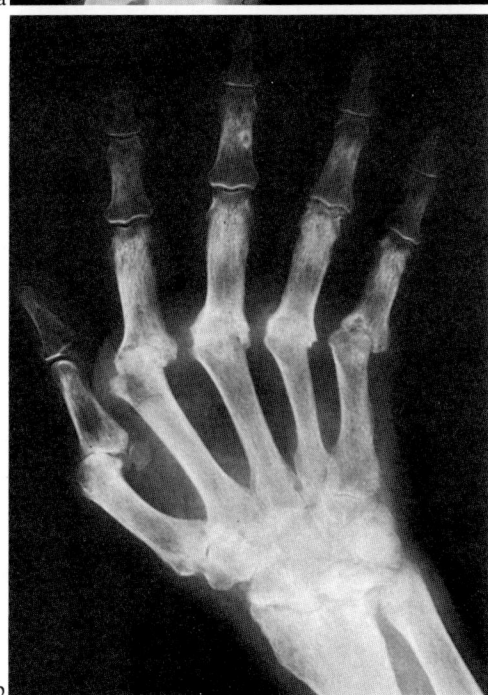

Fig. 1.10 *Rheumatoid arthritis—late effects.* These examples of quiescent lesions in elderly women show **a** narrowed joint spaces, numerous healed erosions and small subarticular cysts and **b** gross destruction of metacarpo-phalangeal joints with characteristic ulnar deviation of the fingers. The radio-carpal joint is eroded with sclerotic margins, and some carpal ankylosis is present. Generalised osteoporosis is due to disuse rather than hyperaemia and is common in the late stages of rheumatoid disease.

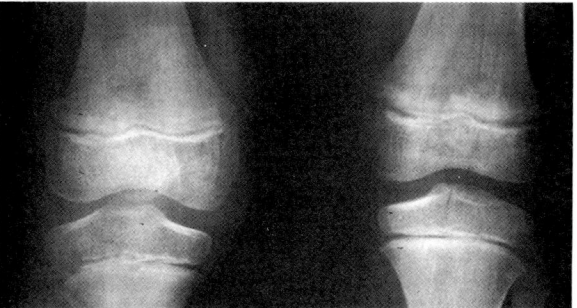

Fig. 1.11. *Juvenile rheumatoid arthritis (Still's disease).* This 6-year-old girl had suffered repeated, but transient, episodes of pain and swelling of the right knee for 3 years. Marked hyperplasia of these major epiphyses was evident, with swelling of the surrounding soft tissues—all attributable to chronic hyperaemia. Histological studies following a synovial biopsy confirmed the diagnosis, but serological tests were negative, as is common in this condition. Synovial tuberculosis and haemophilia can induce identical hyperaemic changes.

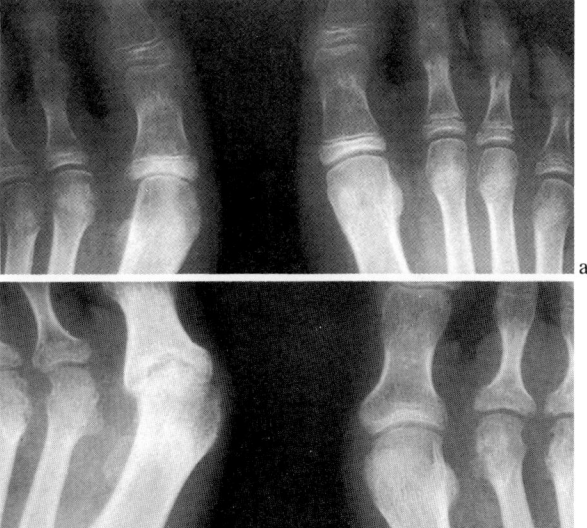

Fig. 1.12. *Juvenile rheumatoid arthritis (Still's disease).* These films of a 14-year-old boy with pain in both feet illustrate several important radiological features of this disease. **a** In 1970 soft tissue swelling due to rheumatoid bursae had separated the 1st and 2nd left metatarsal heads. Hyperaemia had caused generalised subarticular osteoporosis and overgrowth of the epiphysis for the 1st proximal phalanx. It was responsible also for the growth plates of the left proximal phalanges being nearer to fusion than their counterparts. Faint periosteal reactions were evident on the left 3rd and both 1st metatarsal shafts. **b** Marked deterioration had taken place in 1974 with gross destruction of the 1st metatarso-phalangeal joint of the more severely affected left foot, but typical para-articular erosions had developed on the metatarsal heads in both feet.

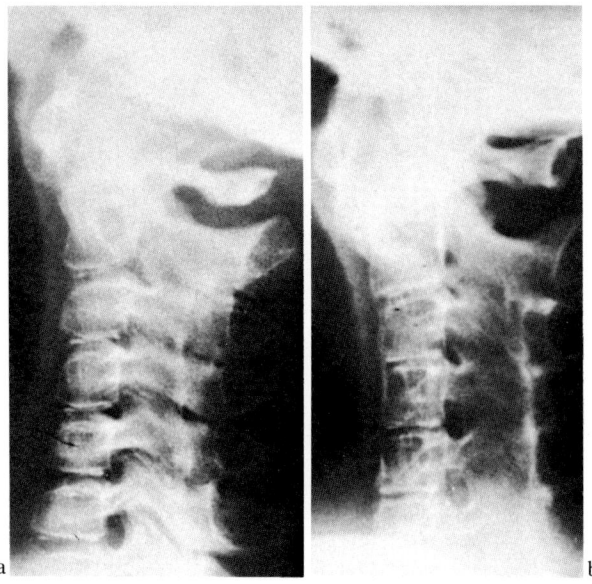

Fig. 1.13. *Juvenile rheumatoid arthritis (Still's disease)— cervical spine.* **a** This 11-year-old girl with multiple lesions had a stiff painful neck. Already the di-arthrodial posterior joints had been eroded. Six years later **b** these joints had ankylosed completely, the appearance simulating a congenital failure of segmentation. Lack of movement of this rigid cervical spine had impaired growth of the vertebral bodies, which remained abnormally small.

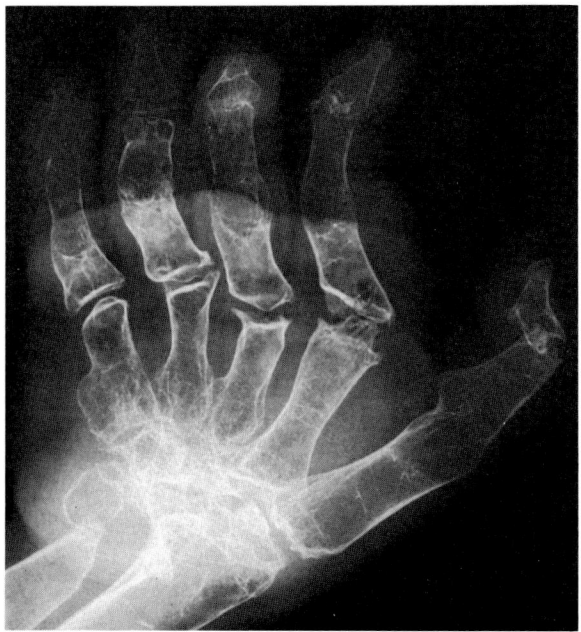

Fig. 1.14 *Juvenile rheumatoid arthritis—late effects.* The metacarpo-phalangeal joints of the fingers and the entire carpus have suffered almost complete attrition in this child with the most severe form of the disease. Many joints are ankylosed. These changes were symmetrical.

A2. Degenerative joint disease (osteoarthritis)

In this case the lack of juxta-articular osteoporosis, as well as the presence of a typical osteophyte on the medial femoral condyle, suggested degenerative joint disease, not uncommon in the knee as a result of former internal derangement or the increased stresses induced by obesity.

At operation, the synovial membrane of the knee joint in this case, as in the previous one, was thickened, villous and hyperaemic. The articular cartilage on each of the joint surfaces was soft and fibrillated, but no involvement of the marginal tissue by pannus had taken place.

Sections from the synovial membrane show histological changes which are very similar to those in the previous case. There is a marked degree of villous synovitis, and here too, the inflammatory cells include many lymphocytes and plasma cells. Serological tests for rheumatoid factor were negative. The histological changes in this case are to be regarded as a non-specific synovial reaction, a pattern not uncommon in degenerative joint disease (see Exercise 3).

Seronegative Spondyloarthropathies

Brief reference may be made to some of the entities regarded formerly as variants of rheumatoid arthritis, but presently accepted as a group of separate disorders. In these conditions rheumatoid factor is absent. HLA antigens of the B27 group are present in a high proportion of these patients, indicating a genetically determined predisposition to disorders of this type. In contrast, HLA B27 antigens are found in only 4% of patients with rheumatoid arthritis, this incidence being comparable to that in normal individuals.

Ankylosing Spondylitis

Young adult males are particularly affected by this disease, women being relatively immune. The HLA B27 incidence is 96%. The severity of the disorder varies greatly. In many instances spontaneous arrest may occur at an early stage, while, less commonly, inexorable progression may culminate in gross and crippling disability.

Clinical Features

Low back pain of insidious onset is the common presenting complaint and in many instances may be the only symptom. In more severe cases manifestations frequently may be systemic, the patient exhibiting mild pyrexia, loss of weight and an elevated ESR. Progressive spinal stiffness develops, ascending from the lumbar spine, usually accompanied by thoraco-lumbar kyphosis. As the thoracic spine becomes involved, expansion of the thoracic cage diminishes progressively, so that the patient is forced to resort to diaphragmatic breathing. The manubrio-sternal joint and the attachments of major muscles often become painful. In severe cases the cervical spine may be involved, ultimately causing a kyphosis of the entire spine. The final complication in a minority of these unfortunate individuals is the development of erosive changes in peripheral joints, culminating frequently in complete ankylosis.

Radiological Features

1. Site. The disease becomes evident first by symmetrical involvement of the sacro-iliac joints. Other sites to be affected early, but virtually always after the sacro-iliac joints, include the manubrio-sternal joint and the 12th costo-vertebral joints. Spinal changes begin in the lumbar area and extend proximally to the dorsal and cervical regions. In later stages accentuation of major muscle and ligamentous attachments is common, often reflecting the rigidity of the axial skeleton.

2. Appearance. The characteristic and earliest abnormalities are symmetrical erosions of the articular sufaces of the sacro-iliac joints with development of reactive subchondral sclerosis. When the disease begins in late adolescence, recognition of abnormalities of this type may be difficult, since, at this age, the sacro-iliac articular margins are normally hazy and poorly defined. Similar destructive lesions may be observed around the manubrio-sternal joint, the 12th costo-vertebral joints and the posterior joints of the spine. As the disease progresses, these posterior joints ankylose and the vertebral bodies lose their anterior concavities to become square in appearance. Syndesmophytes then form around the intervertebral spaces and, in advanced disease, fuse to contribute to spinal rigidity. Thereafter the intervertebral discs may calcify. Erosions of the cortex of vertebral bodies are known as Andersson lesions. Occasionally they become so extensive at a single level, usually in the lower dorsal area, that destruction at a solitary residual site of mobility, the Romanus lesion, may simulate infective discitis (see Exercise 13). Prominences of muscular attachments, especially on the ischial tuberosities and lesser trochanter, may develop as a result of chronic stress. The formation of a plantar calcaneal spur at the insertion of the long plantar ligament is a feature common to all these arthropathies and is often a sequel to previous plantar fasciitis.

Pathological Features

In ankylosing spondylitis the principal sites of histological change are the bony insertions of ligaments and joint capsules ('entheses'). In the spine, the earliest changes take the form of erosive inflammatory lesions, characterised by collections of lymphocytes and plasma cells, in the peripheral part of the annulus fibrosus of the intervertebral disc and the adjacent bone. These early changes are followed by fibroblastic proliferation and reactive bone formation which leads to the formation of syndesmophytes, the bridges of bone which ultimately may unite the vertebral bodies. Similar lesions occur at other sites of ligamentous attachment. In peripheral joints, particularly the hip, knee and shoulder, ankylosis may follow.

Treatment

It is fortunate that in many patients with this disorder the symptoms and signs are relatively minor and spontaneous cessation of activity of the process is common. Relief of pain may be provided by various analgesics. Remedial physiotherapy is usually of value in maintaining an acceptable degree of mobility and preventing deformity until the condition becomes quiescent. In the past radiation therapy was favoured, since such treatment undoubtedly relieved pain, but did not restore mobility. Radiation therapy, however, has been modified or even abandoned since recognition of its subsequent association with blood dyscrasias, notably leukaemia.

For advanced cases, orthopaedic surgery has a place in the provision of prosthetic replacements of major joints and even in the hazardous operation of spinal osteotomy. The great relief offered by the last procedure in correcting gross kyphosis is appreciated by the patient when he no longer is obliged to have his eyes fixed on his feet. All patients with advanced disease should be warned to keep the arms free when walking to offer protection in case of a fall. Failure to observe this rule, when the hands are kept in pockets, has resulted in spinal fractures, sometimes fatal.

References

Ball J (1971) Enthesopathy of rheumatoid and ankylosing spondylitis. Ann Rheum Dis 30: 213–223
Brewerton DA, Cathrey M, Hart FD, James DCO, Nicholls A, Sturrock RD (1973) Ankylosing spondylitis and HL-A27. Lancet I: 904–907
Dihlmann W (1979) Current concepts of ankylosing spondylitis. Skeletal Radiol 4: 179–188
Schlosstein L, Terasaki PI, Bluestone R, Pearson CM (1973) High association of an HL-A antigen, W27, with ankylosing spondylitis. N Engl J Med 288: 704–706

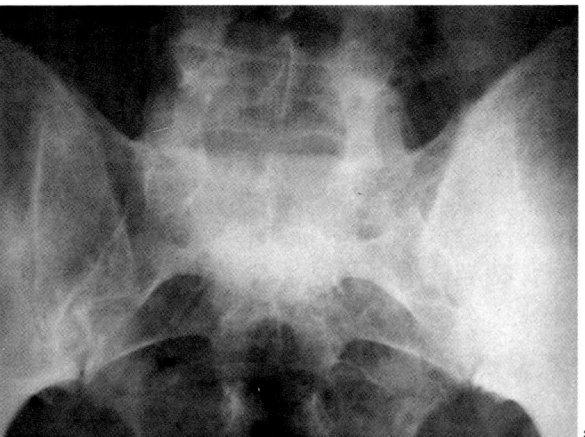
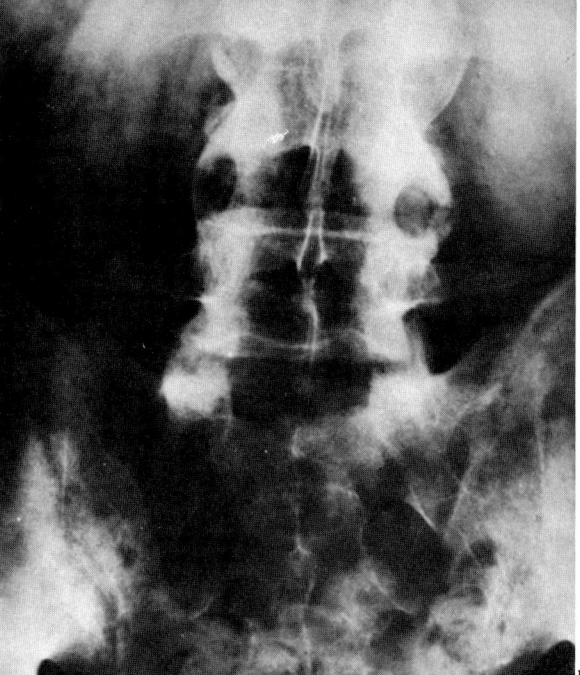

Fig. 2.1. *Ankylosing spondylitis—sacro-iliitis* is the commonest early radiological sign of the disease. **a** This 44-year-old man had complained of mild back pain for 1 year. The very early erosions of the sacro-iliac joints were not appreciated. Symptoms were intermittent and not severe. On occasion relief was sought with analgesics. **b** Three years later, however, significant, but not very painful, spinal stiffness had developed. By this time the erosions were much more extensive and presented a classical appearance. Typical changes were present also in the lumbar spine, as shown by the presence of syndesmophytes with ossification of the intervertebral ligaments (the 'bamboo' spine).

Ankylosing Spondylitis

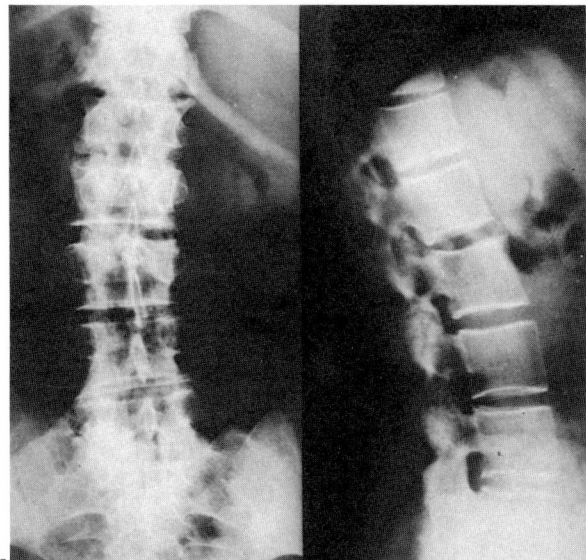

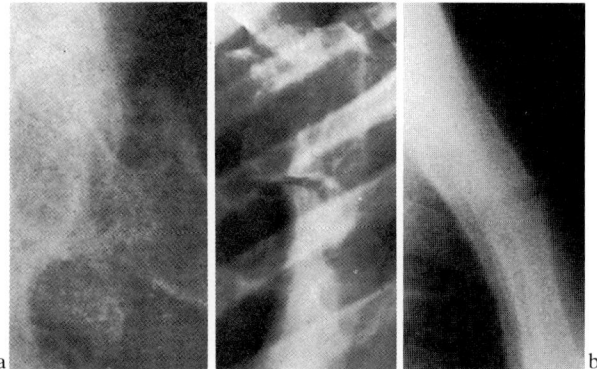

Fig. 2.3. *Ankylosing spondylitis—other early sites of skeletal involvement.* Recognition of such lesions may support the diagnosis when involvement of the sacro-iliac joints is dubious. **a** The *12th costo-vertebral joint* shows typical erosions in a patient with established disease. **b** Similar changes are present in the *manubriosternal joint* of this 47-year-old man, in whom sacro-iliac erosions already had been detected.

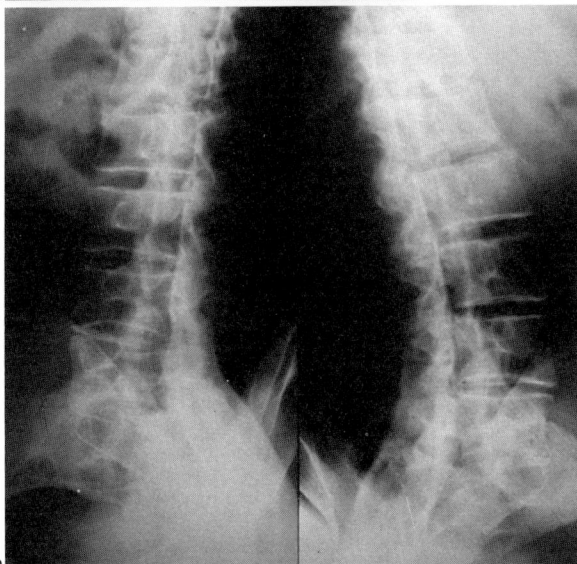

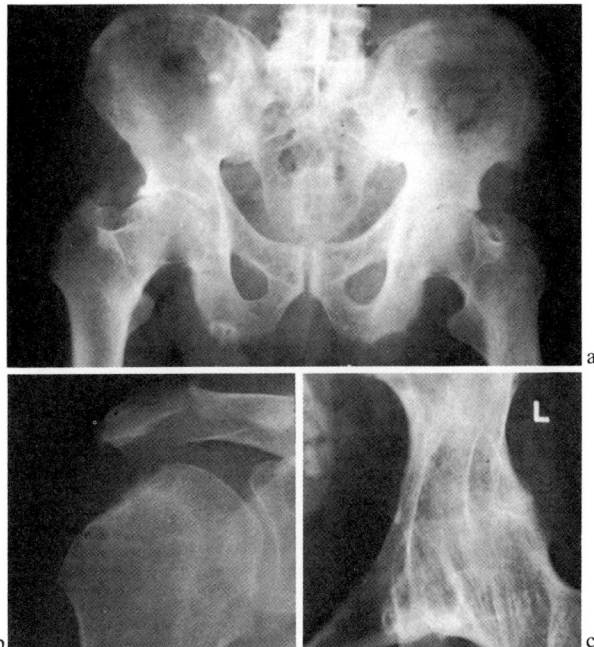

Fig. 2.2. *Ankylosing spondylitis—spinal involvement.* This 33-year-old woman had been aware of increasing and slightly painful stiffness of her lumbar spine for 2 years. In addition to obvious symmetrical erosions of the sacro-iliac joints, similar changes had affected the posterior intervertebral joints, as shown in the oblique projections. Several of these joints already were near to ankylosis. The lateral view shows the typically square shape of the vertebral bodies, due to bone absorption of their superior and inferior corners, with loss of their normal anterior concavities. This case emphasises the relatively advanced stage of the disease which may be present on first presentation. The sex of the patient was unusual, for only one woman is affected for every ten men.

Fig. 2.4. *Ankylosing spondylitis—advanced disease.* **a** This pelvis shows complete ankylosis of the sacro-iliac joints. Massive accentuation of the muscular attachments on the iliac bones, greater trochanters and ischial tuberosities is the result of chronic stress at these sites. **b** Similar avulsion of the origin of the long head of the triceps is evident in relation to this affected shoulder, with erosion of the lateral side of the humeral head. **c** This hip has been ankylosed totally by the disease.

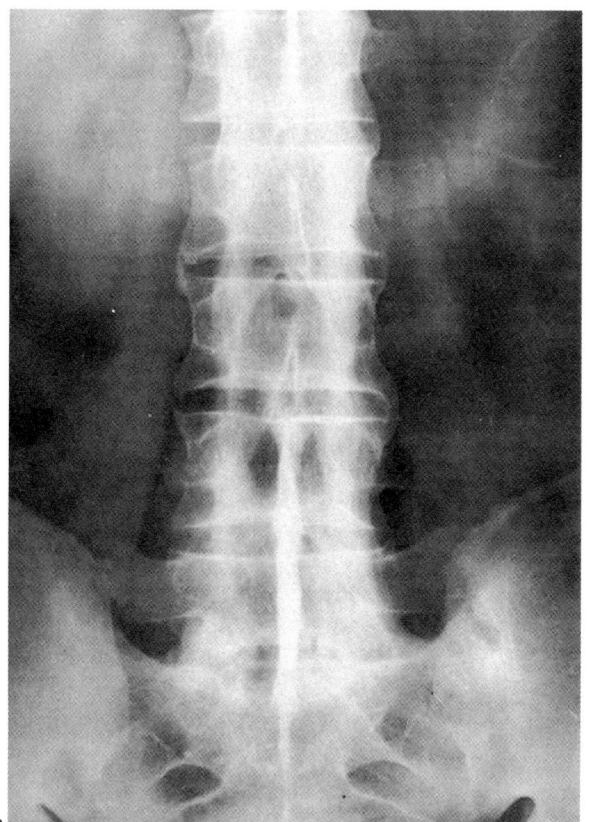
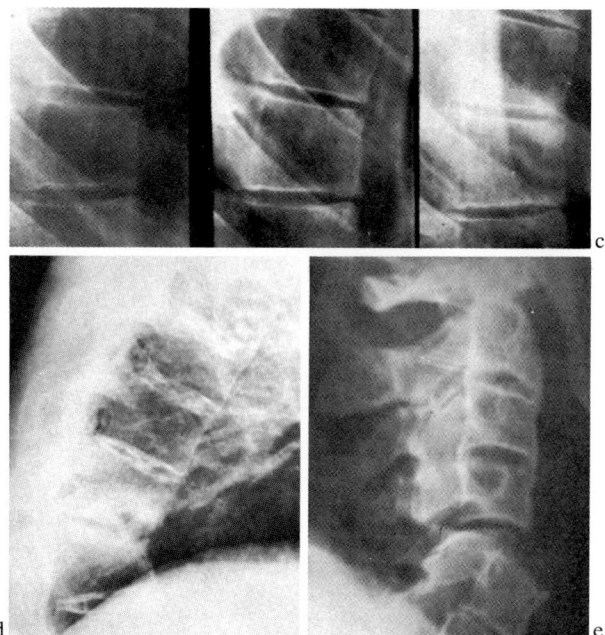
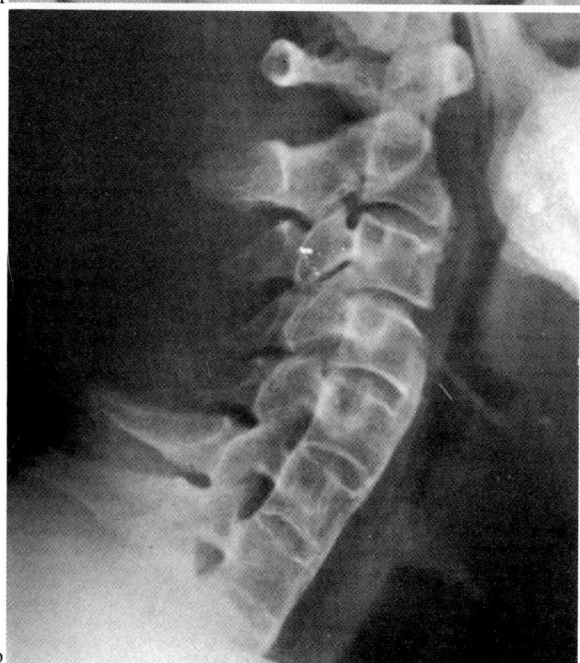

Fig. 2.5. *Ankylosing spondylitis—further spinal manifestations.* **a** Ligamentous ossification with fusion of syndesmophytes produces the classical 'bamboo' appearance as shown in this lumbar spine. **b** Typical ligamentous ossification in the cervical spine in advanced disease. **c** This 47-year-old man with established disease developed pain and tenderness in the upper thoracic spine. These serial studies, obtained over a period of 20 months, show an erosion typical of the Andersson lesion, developing on the antero-superior corner of T5, subsequently followed by reactive sclerosis. Observe the square vertebral bodies. **d** Another man of the same age presented with more severe pain in the lower thoracic area. In addition to classical vertebral squaring, extensive destruction is evident in the adjacent portions of the bodies of T11 and 12, with much reactive sclerosis. This appearance is known as the Romanus lesion and reflects chronic stress at a site of residual mobility in a spine otherwise rigid. It should not be confused with infection. Paradoxically, anterior spinal fusion is required. Posterior fusion is doomed to failure. Observe, incidentally, calcification of intervertebral discs, a finding not uncommon in later stages of the disease. **e** This C4/5 fracture dislocation followed an unguarded fall by an elderly man with known disease. It caused tetraplegia and subsequent death.

Psoriatic Arthritis

Dermatological manifestations of psoriasis may be encountered in as many as 4% in population studies, this incidence being comparable to rheumatoid arthritis, with which condition a significant coincidental association exists. Articular manifestations of the disease, however, are relatively uncommon. HLA B27 is present in half these patients. Clinically these manifestations are responsible for the same pain and stiffness of joints as in other arthropathies. Articular erosions are similar in type to those of rheumatoid arthritis. These erosions, however, have a different distribution, exhibiting a marked predilection for the terminal interphalangeal joints of digits. Another differentiating feature is the formation of incomplete ('floating') syndesmophytes in the lumbar spine. As in all these arthropathies, sacro-iliitis may be evident. The histological appearance of these 'enthesopathic' (insertional tendinitis) lesions is similar to those occurring in ankylosing spondylitis. The changes affecting the synovial membrane of joints are comparable to those observed in rheumatoid arthritis.

References

Avila R, Pugh DG, Slocumb CH, Winkelmann RK (1960) Psoriatic arthritis: a roentgenologic study. Radiology 75: 691–702

Bywaters ECL, Dixon AS (1965) Paravertebral ossification in psoriatic arthritis. Ann Rheum Dis 24: 313–331

Romanus R, Yden S (1952) Destructive and ossifying spondylitic changes in rheumatoid ankylosing spondylitis (pelvi-spondylitis ossificans). Acta Orthop Scand 22: 89–98

Sherman M (1952) Psoriatic arthritis. Observations on the clinical, roentgenographic and pathologic changes. J Bone Jt Surg 34A: 831–852

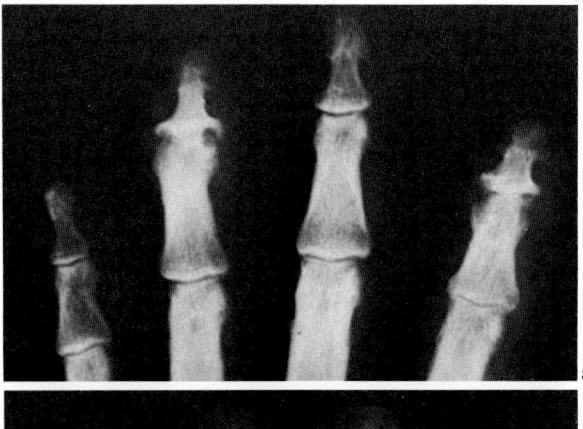
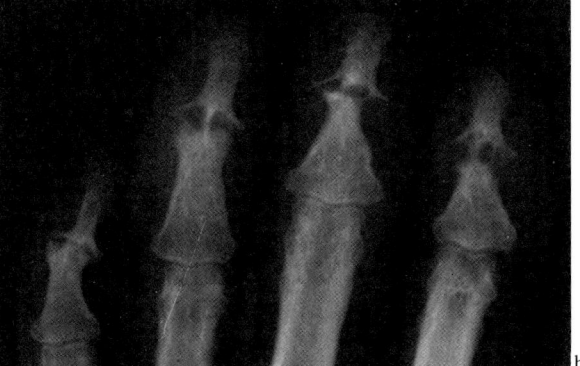
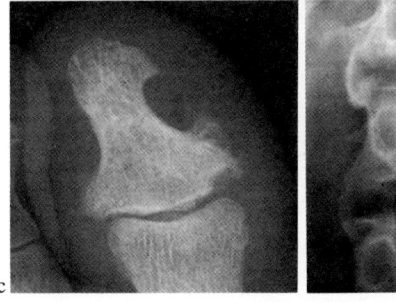
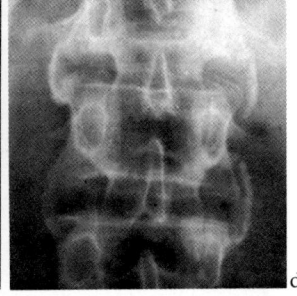

Fig. 3.1. *Psoriatic arthritis.* **a** The arthritic changes in the distal interphalangeal joints include erosions of the articular surfaces and bony spur formation on both sides of the bases of the distal phalanges. Such an appearance is suggestive immediately of psoriasis. **b** More advanced changes of the same type demonstrate classical pointing of the distal ends of the middle phalanges and progressive enlargement of the peripheral bony spurs around the bases of the distal phalanges. This 'cup and pencil' appearance is typical of the later stages of the disease. **c** This 42-year-old man presented with mild pain and swelling of the right big toe. The erosion on the medial side of the base of the distal phalanx and the formation of a medial bony spur constitute abnormalities characteristic of a psoriatic arthropathy and represent classical radiological features of the disease. **d** In this patient with established psoriasis, examination of the lumbar spine revealed massive syndesmophyte formation. Some of these syndesmophytes lie loose in the soft tissues ('floating syndesmophytes'), a helpful diagnostic appearance.

Reiter's Sydrome

This syndrome consists of a classical triad of arthritis, non-specific urethritis and conjunctivitis and has long been regarded as having a venereal origin in young adult men. Eye involvement, however, often is lacking and the urethritis may be replaced by inflammatory conditions of the bowel, such as ulcerative colitis or Crohn's disease. Acute episodes of arthritic pain develop in the feet, often associated with plantar fasciitis, with a predilection for the 1st interphalangeal joint and the metatarso-phalangeal joints. Articular erosions with subarticular demineralisation occur and often are accompanied by exuberant periosteal reactions, which are much more florid than those observed occasionally in rheumatoid arthritis. Irregular bony spurs on the calcaneus tend to be larger and more prominent than in other arthropathies. Later stages are likely to be marked by extensive destruction of the affected joints, syndesmophyte formation and sacro-iliitis. In contrast to ankylosing spondylitis, the last-mentioned is frequently unilateral. Histological study of affected synovium again reveals an appearance similar to that of rheumatoid arthritis. HLA B27 is found in three quarters of patients with this rare disease.

References

Brewerton DA et al. (1973) Reiter's disease and HL-A27. Lancet II: 996–998

Weinberger HW, Ropes MW, Kulka JP, Bauer W (1962) Reiter's syndrome: clinical and pathologic observations. Medicine (Balt) 41: 35–91

Wright V (1965) Diagnosis of Reiter's syndrome. Rheumatism 21: 30–34

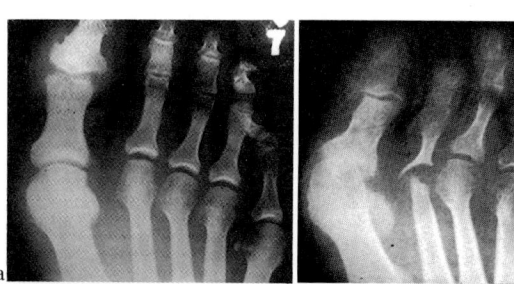
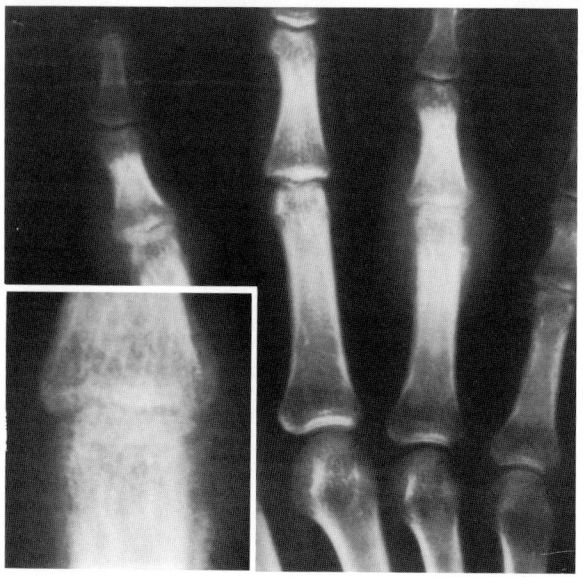
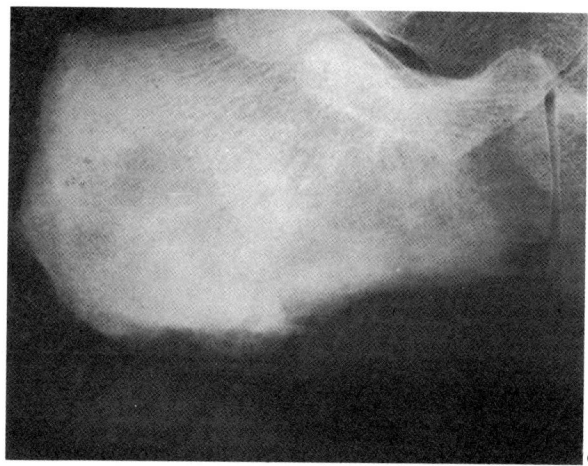

Fig. 4.1. *Reiter's syndrome.* **a** This 32-year-old man developed acute pain and swelling of the right big toe. Extensive erosions were evident around the interphalangeal joint. An associated non-specific urethritis had been present for 2 years. This patient had no ocular symptoms or signs, but involvement of the other foot followed in a few weeks. **b** Eight years later the residual effects of the disease were apparent. In addition to destruction of the 1st interphalangeal joint, gross disintegration of the 2nd metatarso-phalangeal joint had taken place. An erosion was present on the head of the 3rd metatarsal and a diaphyseal periosteal reaction was evident on the 3rd proximal phalanx. The left foot showed similar appearances. **c** Exceptionally the hand may be involved. Painful swellings around the 2nd and 4th proximal interphalangeal joints in this 25-year-old man were associated with acute conjunctivitis and a long-established non-specific urethritis. Observe, in addition to articular erosions, the exuberant diaphyseal periosteal reactions. **d** Similar florid new bone formation was present on the calcaneus of this young man with Reiter's syndrome.

Inflammatory (Erosive) Osteoarthritis

Middle-aged women are affected particularly by this unusual condition, in which the lesions are confined almost entirely to the interphalangeal joints of the hands, causing a resemblance to psoriatic arthritis. It is marked clinically by intermittent episodes of sudden onset of pain and swelling. Peripheral osteophytes form and erosions develop, unlike rheumatoid arthritis, on central portions of the articular surfaces. These erosions are clearly defined by sclerotic margins and usually progress slowly. The rheumatoid factor is invariably negative. Histological studies demonstrate non-specific inflammatory changes with villous hypertrophy of synovium.

References

Martel W, Stuck KJ, Dworin AM, Hylland RG (1980) Erosive osteoarthritis and psoriatic arthritis. A radiologic comparison in the hand, wrist and foot. Am J Roentgenol 134: 125–135

Peter JB, Pearson CM, Marmor L (1966) Erosive osteoarthritis of the hands. Arthritis Rheum 9: 365–388

Resnick D, Niwayama G (1981) In: Diagnosis of bone and joint disorders. W. B. Saunders, Philadelphia, pp. 1356–1358

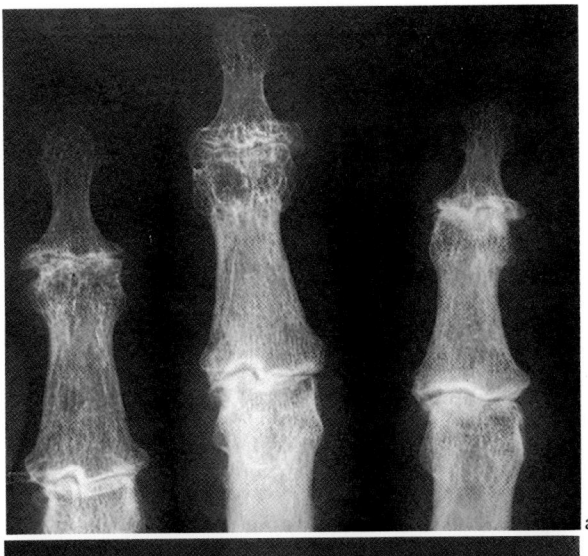
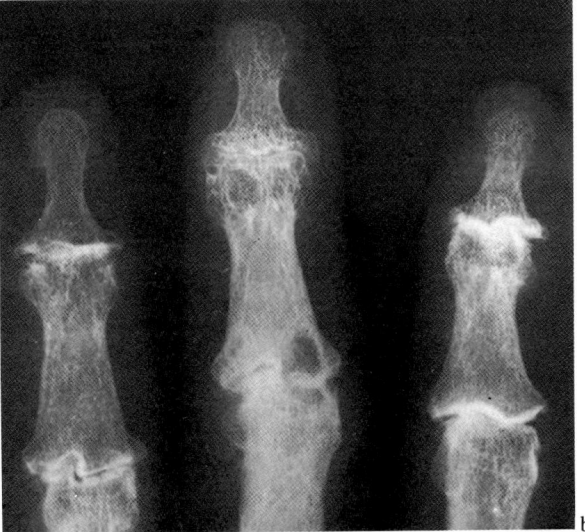

Fig. 5.1. *Inflammatory (erosive) osteoarthritis.* This 46-year-old woman reported successive episodes of sudden pain and swelling of the small joints of the fingers. No clinical evidence of psoriasis was detected and the rheumatoid factor was absent. **a** Observe narrowing of the joint spaces, peripheral osteophytes around the distal interphalangeal joints and central erosions on the bases of the 3rd and 4th middle phalanges. The other hand was affected similarly. **b** Two years later these abnormalities had progressed, with some subarticular cyst formation. The possible outcome of spontaneous ankylosis, however, had not developed.

Behçet's Syndrome

This even rarer syndrome, of unknown aetiology, does not show an association with HLA B27. The condition is characterised by ulceration of the mouth and genitalia, iritis and polyarthritis. Major joints, particularly the knee, tend to be affected, synovial biopsy showing non-specific inflammatory changes, but often without significant radiological abnormality. Of importance is the development of sacro-iliitis in approximately one third of patients, so that confusion with ankylosing spondylitis may arise.

Reference

Caporn N, Higgs ER, Dieppe PA, Watt I (1983) Arthritis in Behçet's syndrome. Br J Radiol 56: 87–91

Diffuse Idiopathic Skeletal Hyperostosis (DISH) (Forestier's Disease)

This rare and peculiar ossifying diathesis of uncertain aetiology affects males more than females. Unlike ankylosing spondylitis it occurs late in life and is recognised usually on account of spinal pain and stiffness. Limitation of movement becomes apparent first in the cervical and lower thoracic areas, but symptoms of pain and stiffness of peripheral joints may precede such symptoms and signs. The radiological appearance is unique. Flowing hyperostosis is due to ossification of the anterior longitudinal ligament and the adjacent connective tissues. These paravertebral bony masses grow slowly and become much more pronounced and robust than the ossified syndesmophytes observed in ankylosing spondylitis (compare Fig. 2.5b). Moreover, the intervertebral disc spaces tend to be of normal width, the anterior concavities of the lumbar vertebral bodies persist and, most importantly, the integrity of the posterior joints and the sacro-iliac articulations is maintained. In recent years Resnick has drawn attention to the extraspinal manifestations of this condition. Calcified and ossified prominences at the attachments of muscles and ligaments, in the presence of normal sacro-iliac joints, may suggest the diagnosis even before the pathognomonic spinal abnormalities are demonstrated. Pathological studies have shown the abnormal bone to develop by a process of extending calcification and ossification in the ligamentous tissue adjacent to vertebral bodies. In contrast to ankylosing spondylitis, obliteration of the disc itself does not occur.

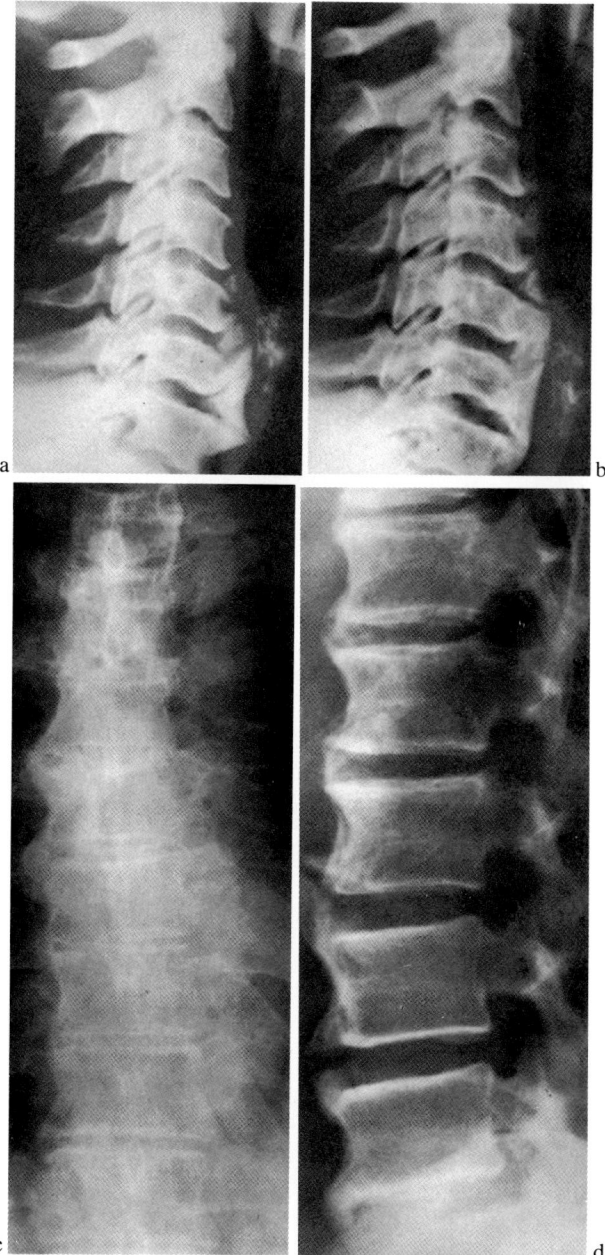

Fig. 6.1. *DISH*. These films of a 65-year-old man who presented with mild pain and stiffness of the neck illustrate **a** prevertebral ossification from C4 to T1 inclusive, which **b** had become even more massive 5 years later. At this time involvement of the thoracic spine **c** had developed, typically on its right side. **d** Similar changes were then evident in the lumbar spine, with preservation of the disc spaces and posterior intervertebral joints. Observe the normal contour of the vertebral bodies. The sacro-iliac joints were normal.

References

Forestier J, Lagier R (1971) Ankylosing hyperostosis of the spine. Clin Orthop 74: 65–83

Resnick D, Shaul SR, Robins JM (1975) Diffuse idiopathic skeletal hyperostosis (DISH); Forestier's disease with extraspinal manifestations. Radiology 115: 513–524

Resnick D, Niwayama G (1976) Radiographic and pathologic features of spinal involvement in diffuse idiopathic skeletal hyperostosis (DISH). Radiology 119: 559–568

Q1. This 12-year-old boy, previously asymptomatic, suddenly experienced sharp pain in the region of the left hip.

Clinical examination revealed tenderness in the upper thigh but a full range of painful movement of the left hip.

The radiographs revealed a large osteolytic lesion in the intertrochanteric portion of the femur. In the lateral projection a minute infraction through the thinned cortex was considered to have been responsible for the acute onset of pain.

The lesion was explored.

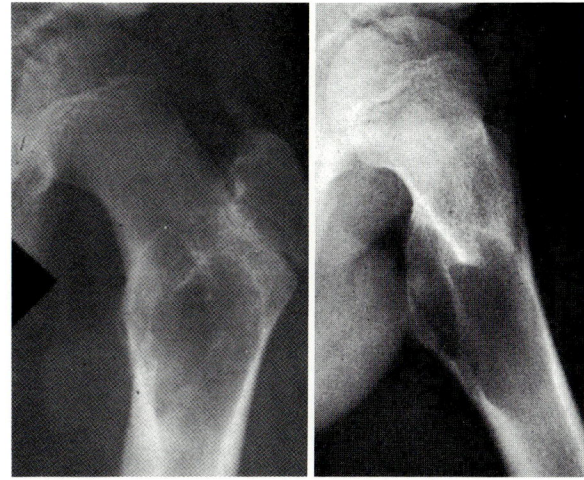

Q1a.

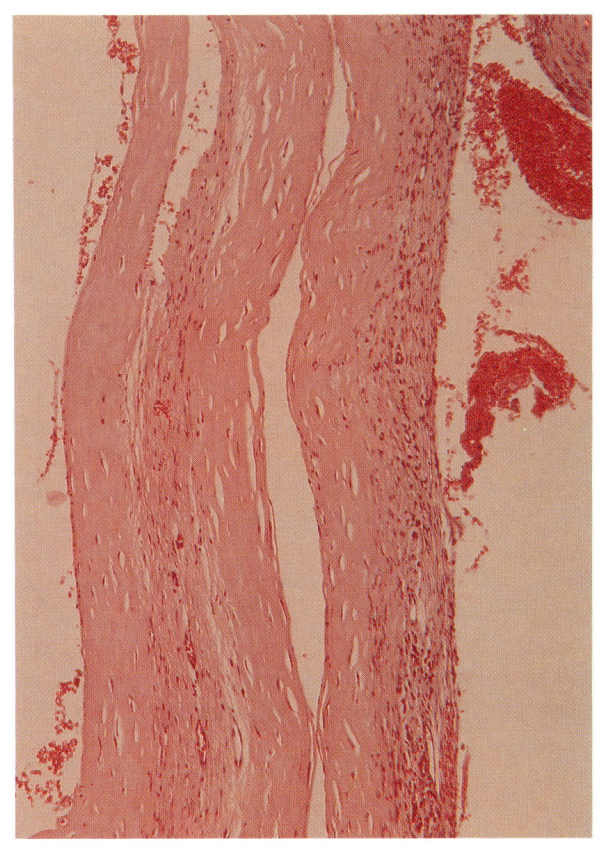

Q1b. (×84)

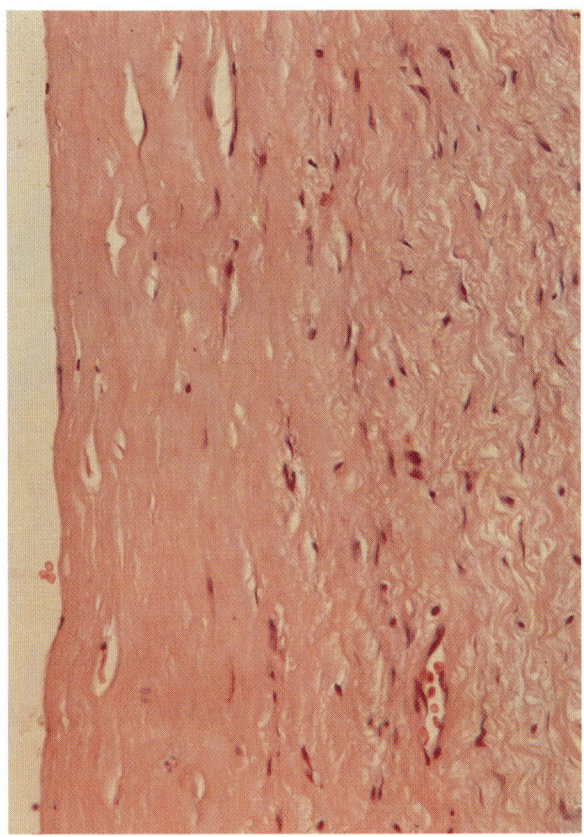

Q1c. (×120)

A1. Simple (unicameral) bone cyst

The radiological appearance in this case was not specific. While it was undoubtedly consistent with a bone cyst, a similar pattern may be observed with other entities, particularly benign fibrous lesions, such as an aneurysmal bone cyst, a non-ossifying fibroma (see Exercise 6) or even fibrous dysplasia (see Exercise 1).

At operation the lesion was found to be a cyst filled with clear fluid. Q1b and c are from the small amount of tissue that was curetted from its wall. They show a thin layer of fibrous tissue which has become folded during processing, and which now appears doubled on itself. It is not possible to say which is the inner, and which the outer, surface of the cyst wall. This case illustrates the essentially 'negative' features of the tissue that is usually obtained from curettage of a simple bone cyst. The diagnosis is established, as it were, by exclusion. The histological appearance of the tissue, in addition to its small amount, is not consistent with any alternative diagnosis, such as aneurysmal bone cyst or any type of solid lesion.

Simple (Unicameral) Bone Cyst

The lesion referred to as a simple bone cyst (sometimes as 'solitary bone cyst' or 'unicameral bone cyst') occurs commonly in young children, usually in the metaphysis of a long bone. A very few cases of multiple cysts of this type have been reported.

Clinical Features

Simple bone cysts are sometimes discovered as an incidental radiological finding, but commonly they come to clinical attention because of a pathological fracture.

Radiological Features

1. Site. The vast majority occur in the proximal end of the humerus, initially involving the metaphysis but frequently being carried by growth into the shaft. Other long bones to be affected include the femur and, less often, the tibia. Rather exceptionally lytic lesions in such flat bones as the calcaneus and cuboid prove to be simple cysts.

2. Appearance. The lesion is essentially osteolytic with a narrow sclerotic border and thinning of the cortex. Expansion of the affected bone is rarely a feature, unlike the aneurysmal bone cyst with which it may be confused so easily. Ridges of residual cortical bone may give the lesion an apparently multilocular appearance.

Pathological Features

At operation, an uncomplicated cyst appears as a rounded cavity, containing clear fluid and lined by a thin layer of fibrous tissue. Haemorrhage occurs following fracture, and the development of reactive tissue and fracture callus (often with areas of xanthomatous tissue or amorphous calcification) can produce a more bulky lining membrane or cyst wall.

Treatment

Curettage and packing of the cavity with bone chips is advisable in the case of the young child with a pathological fracture, but even then a significant recurrence rate exists and the procedure often requires repetition on one or more occasions. It may be performed prophylactically when the cyst is of incidental discovery in order to avoid an almost inevitable fracture. Occasionally these cysts fill in spontaneously, usually as a sequel to a fracture, particularly if the patient already has reached adolescence.

The method of treatment by injection of steroids, a recent innovation, is still under trial.

References

Boseker EH, Bickel WH, Dahlin DC (1968) A clinicopathologic study of simple unicameral bone cysts. Surg Gynecol Obstet 126: 550–560

Capanna R, Dalmonte A, Gitelis S, Campanacci M (1982) The natural history of unicameral bone cyst after steroid injection. Clin Orthop 166: 204–211

Cohen J (1977) Unicameral bone cysts. A current synthesis of reported cases. Orthop Clin North Am 8: 715–736

Sadler A, Rosenheim F (1964) Occurrence of two unicameral bone cysts in the same patient. J Bone Jt Surg 56A: 1557–1560

Scaglietti O, Marchetti PG, Bartolozzi P (1982) Final results obtained in the treatment of bone cysts with methyl-prednisilone acetate (Depo-Mechol) and a discussion of results achieved in other bone lesions. Clin Orthop 165: 33–42

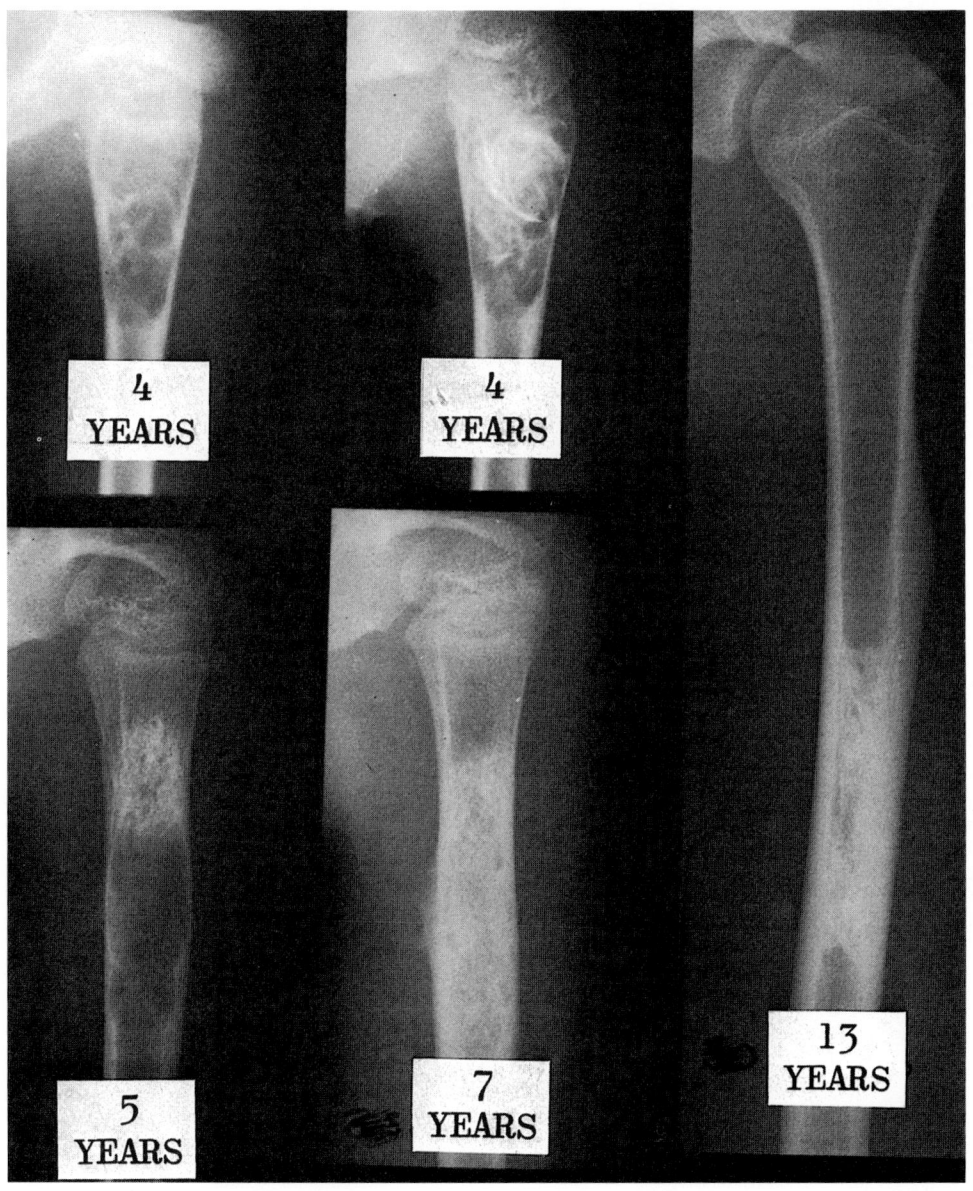

Fig. 1.1. *Simple cyst of humerus—life history*. Serial studies of a lesion arising at the site most frequently affected—the proximal humeral metaphysis—with a characteristic pathological fracture in a 4-year-old child. Observe the recurrence after initial curettage and packing with bone chips, requiring further surgery. At the age of 13 the area of residual sclerosis illustrates the effect of major growth of the humerus at its proximal end.

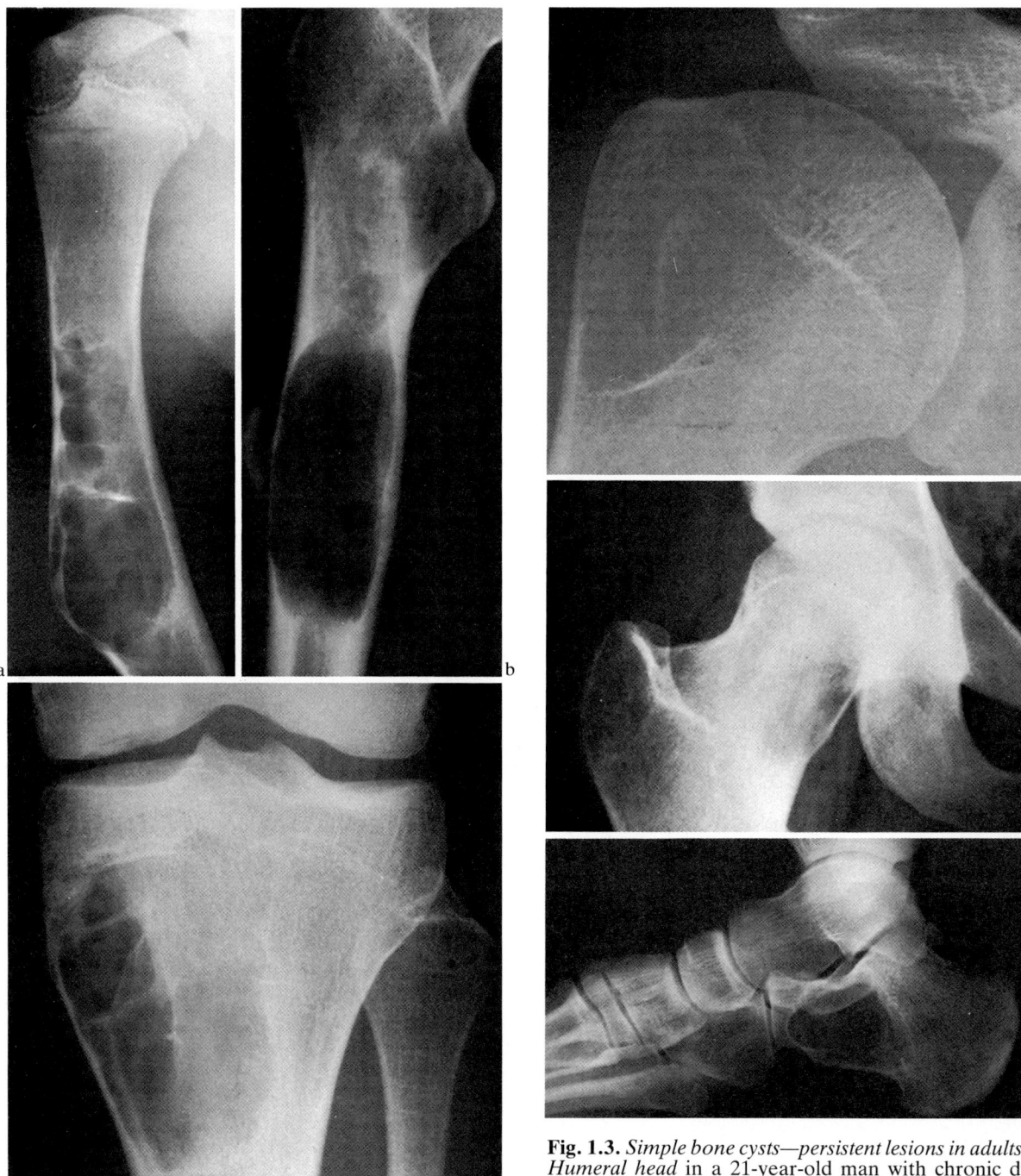

Fig. 1.2. *Simple bone cysts—less common manifestations.* **a** *Recurrence in humerus* with satellite lesions in a 10-year-old boy. **b** *Pathological fracture of femur* in a 14-year-old girl. **c** *Tibial lesion* in a 17-year-old female presenting with symptoms due to osteochondritis dissecans of medial femoral condyle.

Fig. 1.3. *Simple bone cysts—persistent lesions in adults.* **a** *Humeral head* in a 21-year-old man with chronic dull pain in the upper arm. Pre-operatively a chondroblastoma had been suspected. **b** *Neck of femur* in a 20-year-old woman complaining of groin pain. This rather unusual lesion had been regarded as fibrous dysplasia. **c** *Calcaneal cyst* in a 20-year-old woman with pain in the heel, attributed to a minor infraction.

Exercise 20

Q1. This 10-year-old boy complained of persistent pain in the neck following a twisting injury incurred by a fall 10 days before.

No abnormality other than localised muscle spasm was detected on clinical examination. In particular no abnormal neurological signs were elicited to suggest long tract involvement. All routine laboratory investigations were negative.

The radiographs revealed marked flattening of the body of C3 with swelling of the adjacent retropharyngeal soft tissues.

This lesion was biopsied and material submitted for culture.

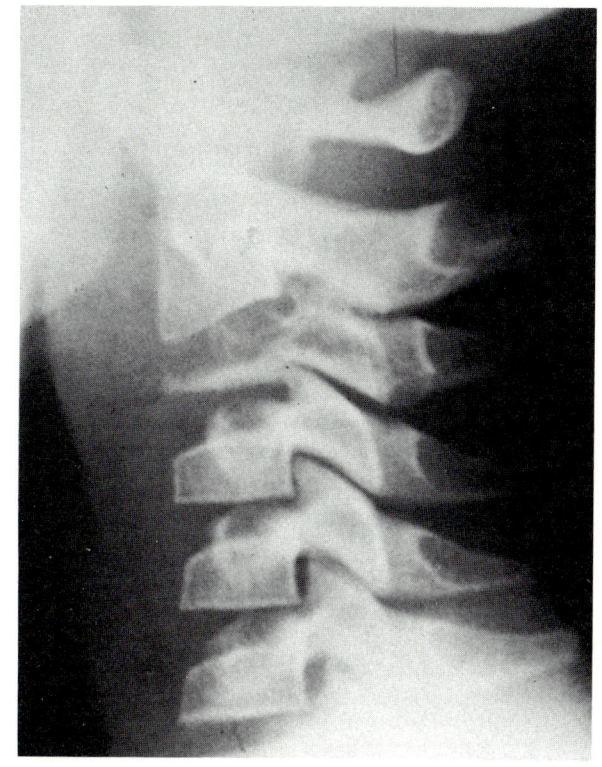

Q1a.

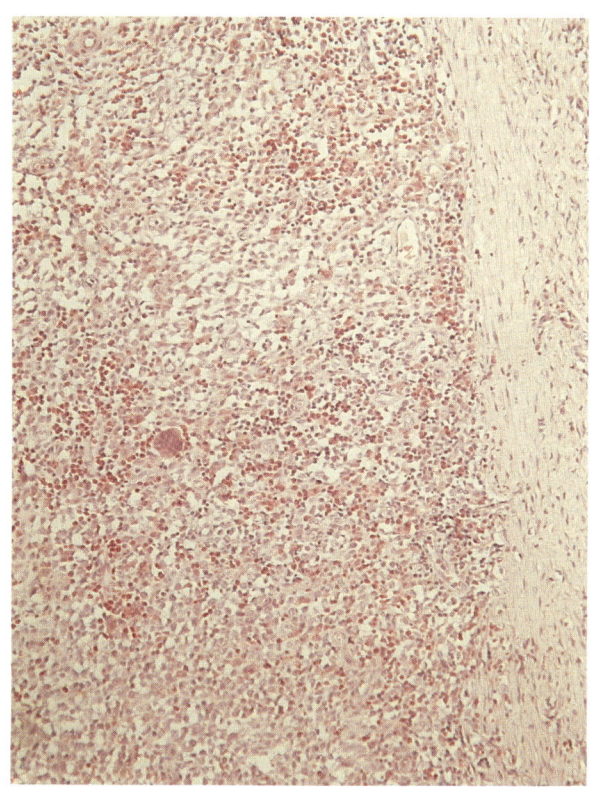

Q1b. (×96)

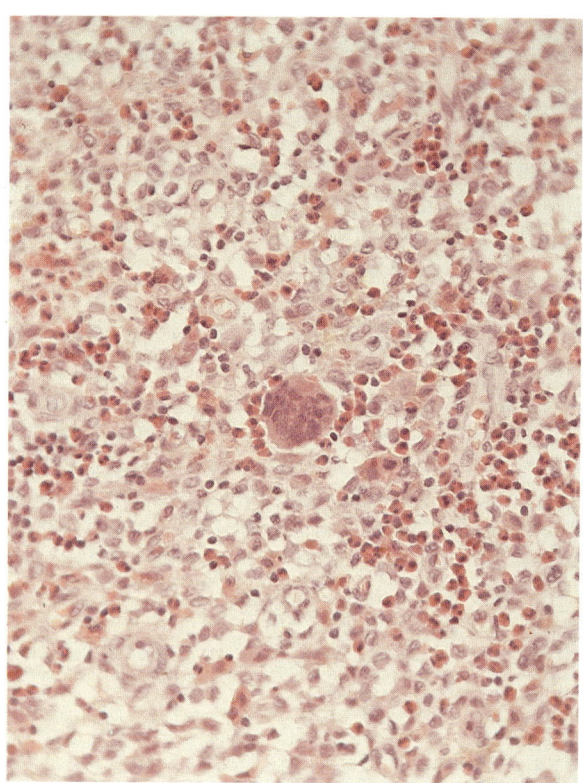

Q1c. (×240)

A1. Eosinophil granuloma of C3

The extensive destruction of the upper portion of the affected body excluded the possibility, suggested by the clinical history, of a compression fracture. No growth was obtained on culture, excluding infection. The most common cause of a vertebra plana deformity of this type in a young patient is eosinophil granuloma, which was the diagnosis offered pre-operatively. The soft tissue swelling was attributed to a recent haemorrhage, a common complication of these lesions when vertebral bodies are involved.

The biopsy specimen (Q1b and c) showed cellular tissue made up of palely staining mononuclear cells, smaller darker polymorphonuclear leucocytes and scattered multinucleate giant cells. At first sight, the cellularity of the tissue might suggest a malignant tumour, but the lesion is, in fact, an eosinophil granuloma.

The eosinophil granules of the polymorphonuclear leucocytes can be identified in an ordinary haematoxylin and eosin section, where they appear larger and brighter than the granules of ordinary neutrophil polymorphs. The distinction can be made more easily in sections stained with Chromotrope R (Fig. 1.1a), in which the eosinophil granules appear bright red. If the polymorphs are not identified as eosinophils, these lesions can sometimes be mistaken, histologically, as being due to a bacterial infection.

Occasionally the distinctive eosinophil cells are infrequent (Fig. 1.1b). The mononuclear cells then can simulate the appearance of a malignant tumour. The histological distinction between eosinophil granuloma and Hodgkin's disease of bone, in which eosinophil cells also may be present, can be difficult.

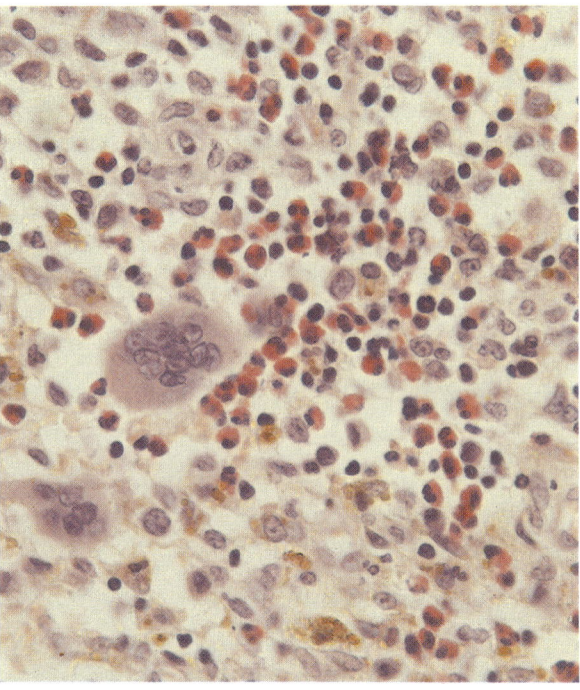

Fig. 1.1a. In this section specially stained with Chromotrope R, the eosinophil cells stand out clearly because of the bright red appearance of their cytoplasmic granules. (×440)

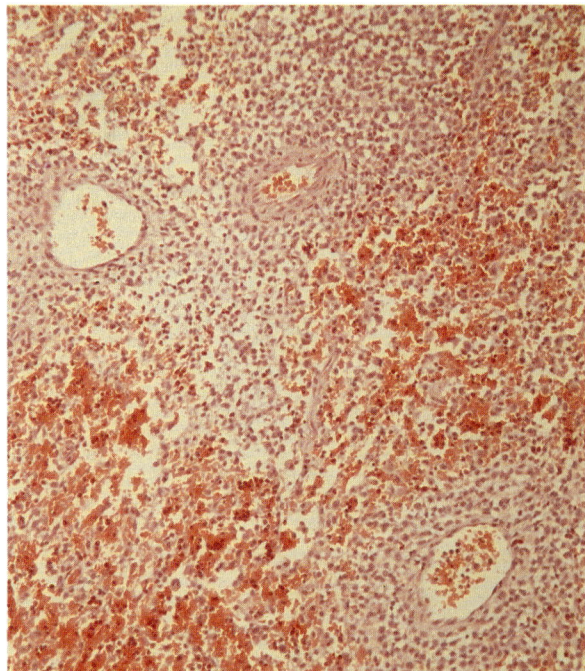

Fig. 1.1b. Another area of tissue from the same lesion, where eosinophil cells are few or absent and where the appearance of the mononuclear cells might suggest the possibility of a malignant tumour. (×96)

Histiocytosis

The majority of cases of eosinophil granuloma of bone have been solitary lesions, although occasional cases, perhaps 10%, either present with multiple lesions or subsequently develop them. Rarely, lesions in other tissues, usually the lungs or the skin and mucous membranes, may be present. For many years a histological similarity has been noted between eosinophil granuloma and certain disseminated lesions of bone marrow and visceral organs (Hand-Schüller-Christian disease; Letterer-Siwe disease). Both of these are characterised by the presence of histiocytes and by the accumulation of lipid material, although eosinophil cells are not always a feature of these forms of disseminated histiocytosis. The term 'histiocytosis X' is sometimes used to refer to the whole group of cases and it has been established that cases initially presenting with atypical eosinophil granuloma of bone can develop subsequently the pituitary involvement and diabetes insipidus of Hand-Schüller-Christian disease.

Clinical Features

The clinical spectrum presented by these disorders varies widely, but it is generally accepted that they have a common origin and that improvement or deterioration in the physical status of these patients may alter the nomenclature of the diagnosis. The older the patient the better the prognosis. It is fortunate that the mildest manifestation of the disease, the solitary eosinophil granuloma, is also the commonest. Occasionally such lesions are so lacking in symptoms and signs that they are detected only by chance during an incidental radiographic examination. More often, however, they cause low-grade pain and possibly localised swelling at the affected site. In cases of this type skeletal survey, in this instance more reliable than radionuclide scanning, may disclose additional and asymptomatic areas of involvement elsewhere in the skeleton, a valuable aid to diagnosis. An important feature to appreciate is that these patients are rarely systemically ill, unless, rather unusually, pulmonary infiltration develops. Routine laboratory investigations are essentially normal. The great majority of these lesions are encountered in childhood and adolescence, but, somewhat exceptionally, solitary eosinophil granulomas have been observed in middle age, when they tend to be confused with foci of chronic infection. Males are affected more frequently than females.

The more severe entity of disseminated histiocytosis, often described as Hand-Schüller-Christian disease, occurs only in about 5% of the whole group. In contrast to the more benign lesions, it affects young children, who are usually systemically ill. Multiple skeletal lesions, in the same phase of aggression or repair, are accompanied by anaemia, thrombocytopenia, visceral involvement, including hepatomegaly and splenomegaly, and pulmonary infiltration. The formation of bullae and fibrosis may precipitate cor pulmonale. Chronic infections of the mouth and otitis media may be present. The classical triad of defects in the calvarium, diabetes insipidus and exophthalmos is, in fact, rare, the last two features being attributable to the fortuitous development of destructive lesions in relation to the pituitary fossa or the posterior wall of an orbit.

The worst form of disseminated histiocytosis, Letterer-Siwe disease, is very unusual, occurring in probably fewer than 1% of the entire group. Infants under 2 years are affected, again with visceral and pulmonary involvement and high fever suggesting generalised sepsis. The outcome is usually fatal, often before widespread skeletal involvement becomes manifest.

Radiological Features

1. Site. Seventy-five per cent of eosinophil granulomas occur in the axial skeleton, with a predilection for the spine, pelvis and skull. The remainder are located in major long bones. We have encountered none in the bones of the hands and feet, even with disseminated disease.

2. Appearance. Characteristically the lesions are osteolytic with clearly defined margins and a narrow zone of transition. In the healing phase the peripheral edges become sclerotic and bone repair eventually restores a normal bone structure. The relatively common involvement of vertebral bodies causes typical vertebra plana, especially in children. Remarkably, complete restoration of these structures may be demonstrated by serial examinations during the remaining years of growth. Differential destruction of the inner and outer tables of the skull may cause the typical pattern of bevelled edges. Lesions in long bones lie within the spongiosa. If the cortex is eroded, overlying periosteal reactions develop. When multiple eosinophil granulomas are detected, rarely more than four or five, some may be in an active phase of destruction while others are undergoing repair. It is wise to remember that a solitary eosinophil granuloma may simulate a malignant primary neoplasm, particularly a Ewing's tumour. The clinical well-being of the individual, however, is of value in excluding that more sinister diagnosis. Routine chest films are desirable to exclude pulmonary infiltration.

In disseminated histiocytosis a very large number of similar osteolytic lesions are likely to be present, all in the same phase of aggression. They are situated not only in the axial skeleton, but also in the major long bones with a special affinity for metaphyseal areas.

Pathological Features

Histologically, as already noted, lesions of eosinophil granuloma consist of mononuclear cells which can be identified as histiocytes, and eosinophil polymorphonuclear leucocytes. The histiocytes frequently contain lipid material, particularly in long-established lesions. Ultrastructurally, the histiocytes of eosinophil granuloma, and of disseminated histiocytosis, have been reported to show the characteristically outlined inclusion bodies of Langerhans' cells.

Treatment

In those instances when an eosinophil granuloma is solitary, it is essential to biopsy the lesion to obtain categorical pathological confirmation of the diagnosis. However, as mentioned above, many solitary eosinophil granulomas regress spontaneously without treatment, so that the child's parents may be reassured with some confidence. More painful lesions appear to respond well to low dose radiotherapy though this has not been clearly demonstrated. In the more severe forms of disseminated histiocytosis improvement has been obtained with administration of steroids and of broad spectrum antibiotics. The latter have been directed particularly to combat the relatively common complications of pulmonary involvement and sepsis of the mouth and ear.

References

Green WT, Farber S (1942) 'Eosinophilic or solitary granuloma' of bone. J Bone Jt Surg 24: 499–526

Jaffe HL, Lichtenstein L (1944) Eosinophilic granuloma of bone. Arch Pathol 37: 99–118

Lichtenstein L (1953) Histiocytosis X. Integration of eosinophilic granuloma of bone, "Letterer-Siwe disease", and "Schüller-Christian disease" as related manifestations of a single nosologic entity. Arch Pathol 56: 84–102

McCullough CJ (1980) Eosinophilic granuloma of bone. Acta Orthop Scand 51: 389–398

Nezelof C, Frileux-Herbert F, Cronier F, Sachot J (1979) Disseminated histiocytosis X. Analysis of prognostic factors based on a retrospective study of 50 cases. Cancer 44: 1824–1838

Otani S (1957) A discussion on eosinophilic granuloma of bone, Letterer-Siwe disease and Schüller-Christian disease. J Mount Sinai Hosp 24: 1079–1092

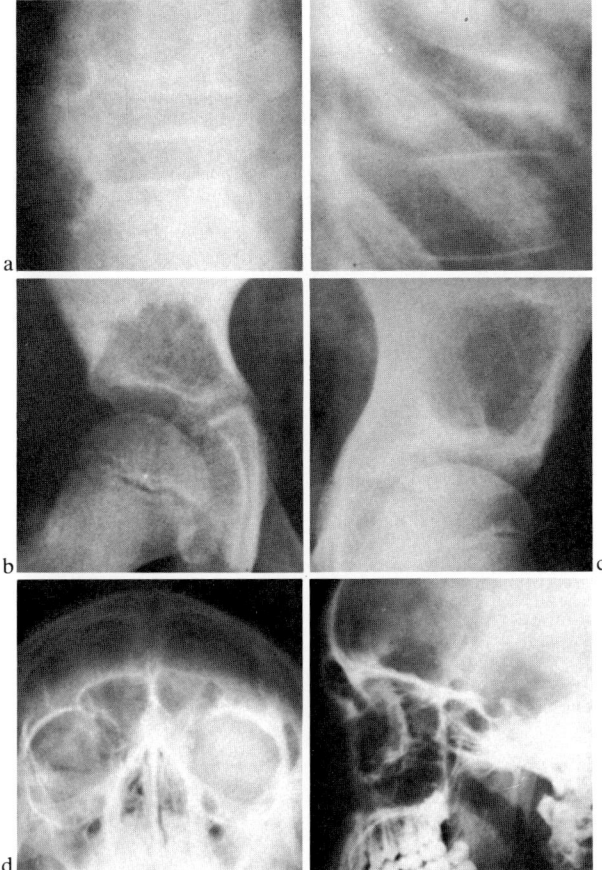

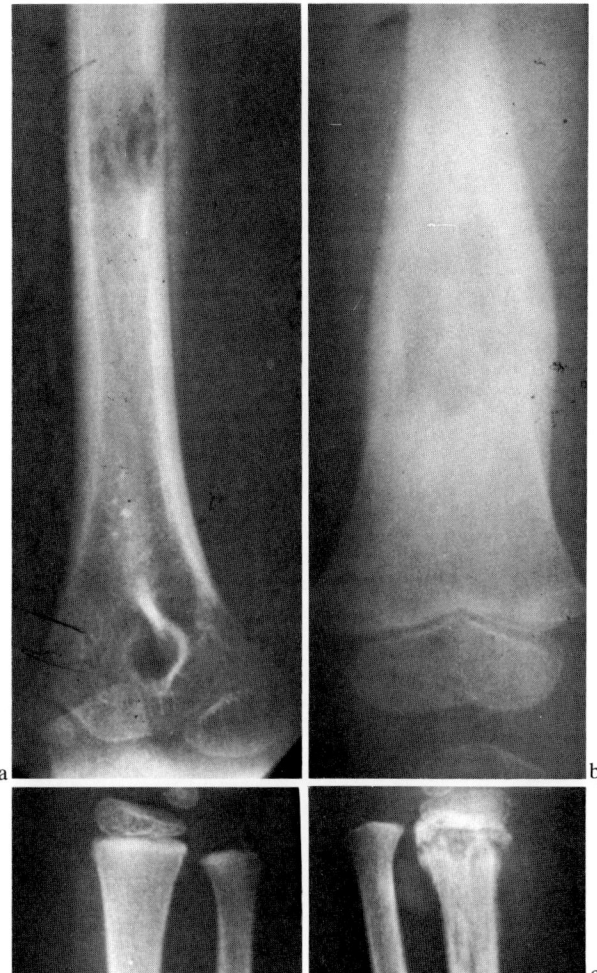

Fig. 1.2. *Solitary eosinophil granuloma—axial skeleton.* **a** *Body of T8.* This 8-year-old girl who had complained of mild thoracic pain for several weeks presented with a sudden onset of a minimal paraparesis, a most unusual complication. Decompression was successful and histological confirmation was obtained. The extreme compression of the body of T8 represents the classical 'silver dollar' sign. Bilateral paravertebral shadows represented recent haemorrhages which were responsible for the sudden onset of neurological signs. **b** *Right acetabulum.* This destructive lesion has clearly defined margins without reactive sclerosis and was the cause of moderate pain in the hip of a 6-year-old boy. **c** *Left ilium.* A similar lesion in this 9-year-old girl was detected only after she had reported mild pain above the left hip for 1 week. The sclerotic margin of the lytic area indicated healing already to be progressing, so that this abnormality had been virtually asymptomatic. **d** *Left frontal bone.* This 10-year-old boy developed exophthalmos due to a retro-orbital eosinophil granuloma. The margins of the lesion are slightly irregular, but are not sclerotic, indicating activity. Although initially solitary, another typical focus developed a few weeks later in a parietal bone.

Fig. 1.3. *Solitary eosinophil granuloma—long bones.* **a** *Humerus.* This destructive lesion, causing pain and swelling of the left arm in a 7-year-old girl, was regarded at first as a focus of pyogenic osteomyelitis. At operation no pus was found and the diagnosis was established histologically. The lesion is located mainly within the humeral shaft, but the cortex has been breached and an extensive periosteal reaction has developed. Observe the radiological similarity, not only to acute osteomyelitis, but also to a Ewing's tumour. **b** *Femur.* Another eosinophil granuloma in a young boy with only mild pain is clearly in a healing phase and is surrounded by organised periosteal new bone. The diagnosis was confirmed by biopsy. **c** *Radius.* This remarkable case involved a 7-year-old boy who presented with a painful swollen wrist. The radiographs at that time revealed no bony abnormality, but in the space of a month destructive changes in the distal end of the bone caused a confident diagnosis of acute osteomyelitis to be offered. No evidence of such infection was found at operation or on culture and this surprising diagnosis was established histologically.

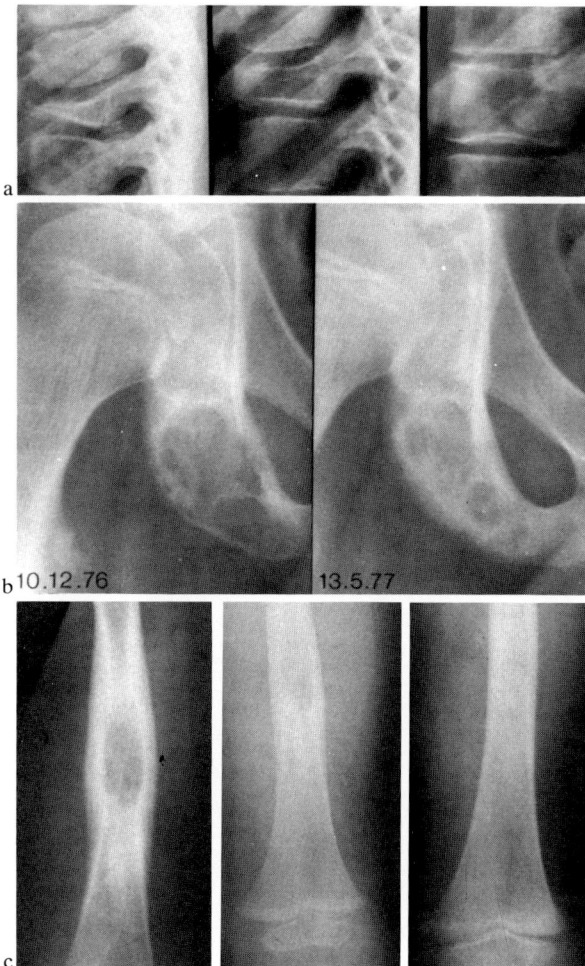

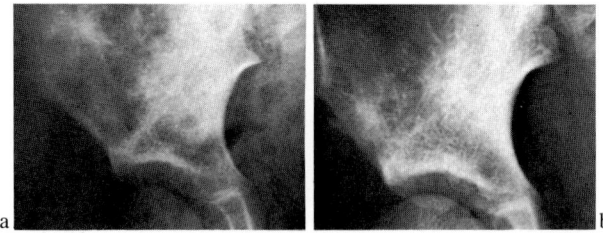

Fig. 1.5. *Eosinophil granuloma—response to treatment.* **a** This lesion in the ilium of a 3-year-old girl responded well to curettage and low dose radiation therapy as shown **b** 2 years later. Radiation therapy is of questionable value.

Fig. 1.4. *Eosinophil granuloma—evolution.* **a** *Spine.* Gross vertebra plana in a 6-year-old boy followed at 5- and 21-year intervals, illustrating the remarkable degree of reconstitution which may take place. Although no histological confirmation was obtained in this case, eosinophil granuloma is the most common cause of this abnormality, so that an expectant attitude may be adopted. **b** *Ischium.* This was one of several lesions in a boy aged 11. It was found after a minor injury causing localised pain, presumably due to a minor and unrecognisable infraction. Symptoms regressed rapidly and 6 months later the lesion was healing. **c** *Femur.* Similar spontaneous repair is illustrated in a 4-year-old boy by serial examinations at intervals of 3 and 14 months. A biopsy had been performed to exclude the possibility of a Ewing's tumour. Eosinophil granuloma always deserves consideration as a helpful alternative to malignant disease.

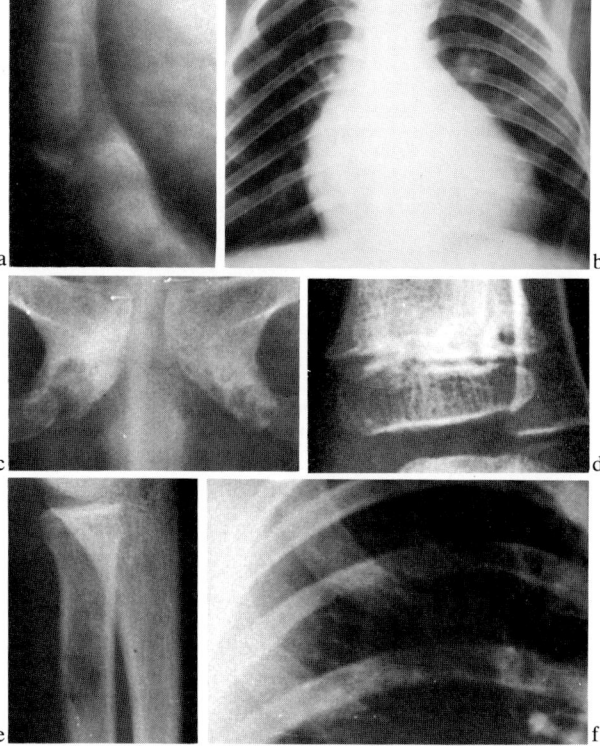

Fig. 1.6. *Eosinophil granuloma—multiple lesions.* **a** A tender swelling of the sternum in this 3-year-old child prompted a skeletal survey, which disclosed other lesions in varying stages of activity. **b** Healed lesions were evident in the anterior ends of the right fifth and the left fourth and sixth ribs, with residual fusiform swelling. **c** More active areas of bone destruction were present in the ischio-pubic junctions and, interestingly, **d** the distal tibial metaphyses (see Fig. 2.1a). Biopsy of the sternum confirmed the diagnosis. **e** In another patient, a 13-year-old girl, examination for pain below the elbow revealed this osteolytic focus in the radius. On skeletal survey, more accurate than radionuclide scanning, although in this instance positive, a further lesion was found **f** in a rib. Biopsy of the radial lesion again was confirmatory.

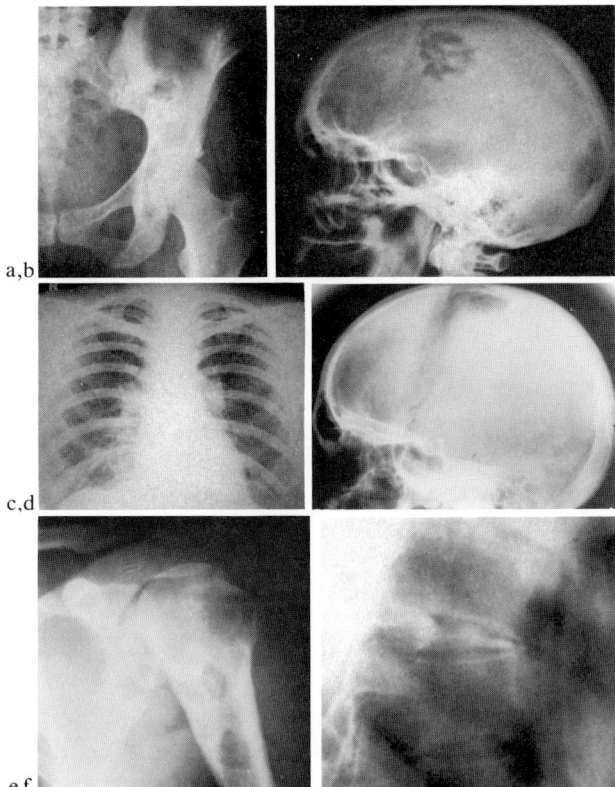

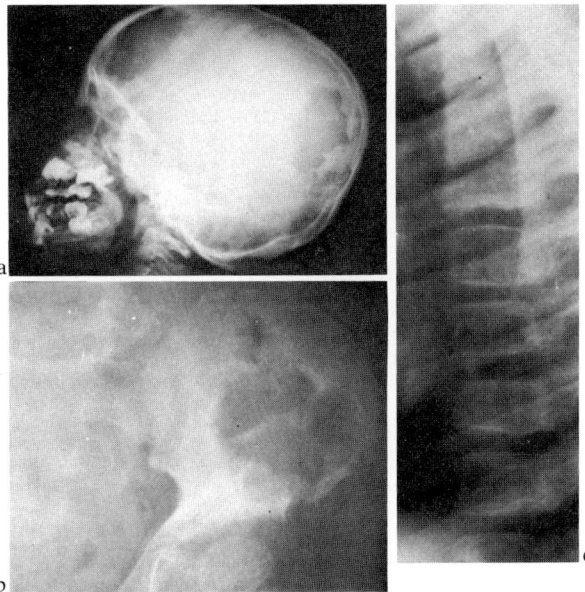

Fig. 1.7. *Eosinophil granuloma—lesions in adults* are relatively unusual, being found in about 10% of cases. They are often multiple, cause only low-grade symptoms and rarely occur after the age of 35. In most cases they resemble chronic pyogenic infections. **a** *Ilium*. These typical healing lesions were found in a 22-year-old woman with mild pain in the groin. Other more aggressive, but asymptomatic lesions **b** were present in the calvarium, and diffuse and typical reticulo-nodular infiltration **c** was evident in the lungs. As is not unusual, no pulmonary symptoms were reported. **d** *Calvarium*. This unusual osteolytic area in the vault of the skull of a 35-year-old woman, with a localised tender swelling, was proved histologically to be an eosinophil granuloma presenting at a late age. Differential destruction of the tables of the skull has caused the margins of the lesion to have a typically duplicated, or 'bevelled edge' appearance. **e** *Humerus*. Healing lesions resembling Brodie's abscesses in a 23-year-old man in whom further foci were present in the pelvis and both femora. **f** *Spine*. Classical vertebra plana of T8 was found in a 29-year-old Indian with back pain for 1 year. Because of his race a bizarre manifestation of tuberculosis was diagnosed preoperatively. All these cases emphasise the confusion with chronic infections which can be caused by this disease.

Fig. 1.8. *Hand-Schüller-Christian disease*. Widely disseminated lesions were present in this young child with this severe systemic disease. **a** The cranial vault shows several sharply defined lucent areas, this pattern being described classically as 'geographic'. **b** Other foci of osteolysis involved the pelvis. **c** In the spine similar lesions were present in many vertebral bodies, some of which had undergone partial collapse. Note that all these areas of bone destruction are in the same phase of aggression.

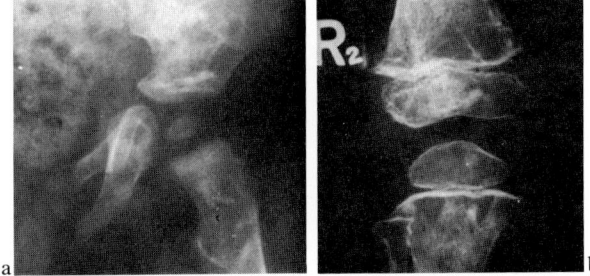

Fig. 1.9. *Letterer-Siwe disease*. Examples of disseminated lesions of this entity are illustrated in **a** the pelvis and left femur of an infant and **b** around the knee of an older child. The latter destructive areas exhibit a predilection for the metaphyses. The remainder of the skeleton was widely affected. In both cases pulmonary infiltration was prominent. Children with this disease often die before bone involvement develops.

Chronic Granulomatous Disease

Chronic granulomatous disease together with its causation in infancy is well documented. It is recognised as a triad consisting of infection of the gastro-intestinal tract, the respiratory system and the skeleton. The last particularly affects the small bones of the hands and feet. The outcome is invariably fatal. The disorder described below may represent a milder manifestation of this condition.

The 'Lazy Leucocyte' Syndrome

More recently a number of patients have presented in late childhood and adolescence with mildly painful skeletal lesions. Their destructive nature, combined with relatively unimpressive clinical findings, has caused the diagnosis of multiple eosinophil granulomas to be considered. Re-assessment, however, has indicated this disease to be a sequel to disorders of leucocyte function. From studies of this function in vitro, it appears that the entity is attributable to an abnormal response to infection by bacteria, which usually are non-pathogenic. These lesions have occurred only in patients whose immunological response is compromised by the inability of the leucocyte to destroy the causative organism— the 'lazy leucocyte' syndrome.

Clinically and radiologically the condition is characterised by a multifocal, chronic (hypertrophic) granulomatous process. Initially the lesions became apparent as juxta-metaphyseal areas of bone destruction adjacent to a growth plate or as slowly progressive zones of sclerosis in flat bones. The metaphyseal lesions, if unrecognised and untreated, frequently progress to become hypertrophic and sclerotic. Florid bony overgrowth, indeed, may cause mechanical restriction of movement of an adjacent joint. In late adolescence, following premature fusion of a growth plate, a joint may become involved and subsequently ankylose.

When treated empirically with perfusions of normal serum, coupled with broad spectrum antibiotics, the early metaphyseal lesions may resolve. Healing of established metaphyseal lesions and of the sclerosing lesions in flat bones does not exhibit such a favourable response.

Histologically, the changes in the bone marrow are those of a non-specific inflammatory process, with a preponderance of neutrophils as opposed to eosinophils.

The condition is apparently benign. A few of these patients have developed a normal immunological response when they reach adult life.

Reference

Wolfson JJ et al. (1969) Bone findings in chronic granulomatous disease of childhood. J Bone Jt Surg 51A: 1573–1583

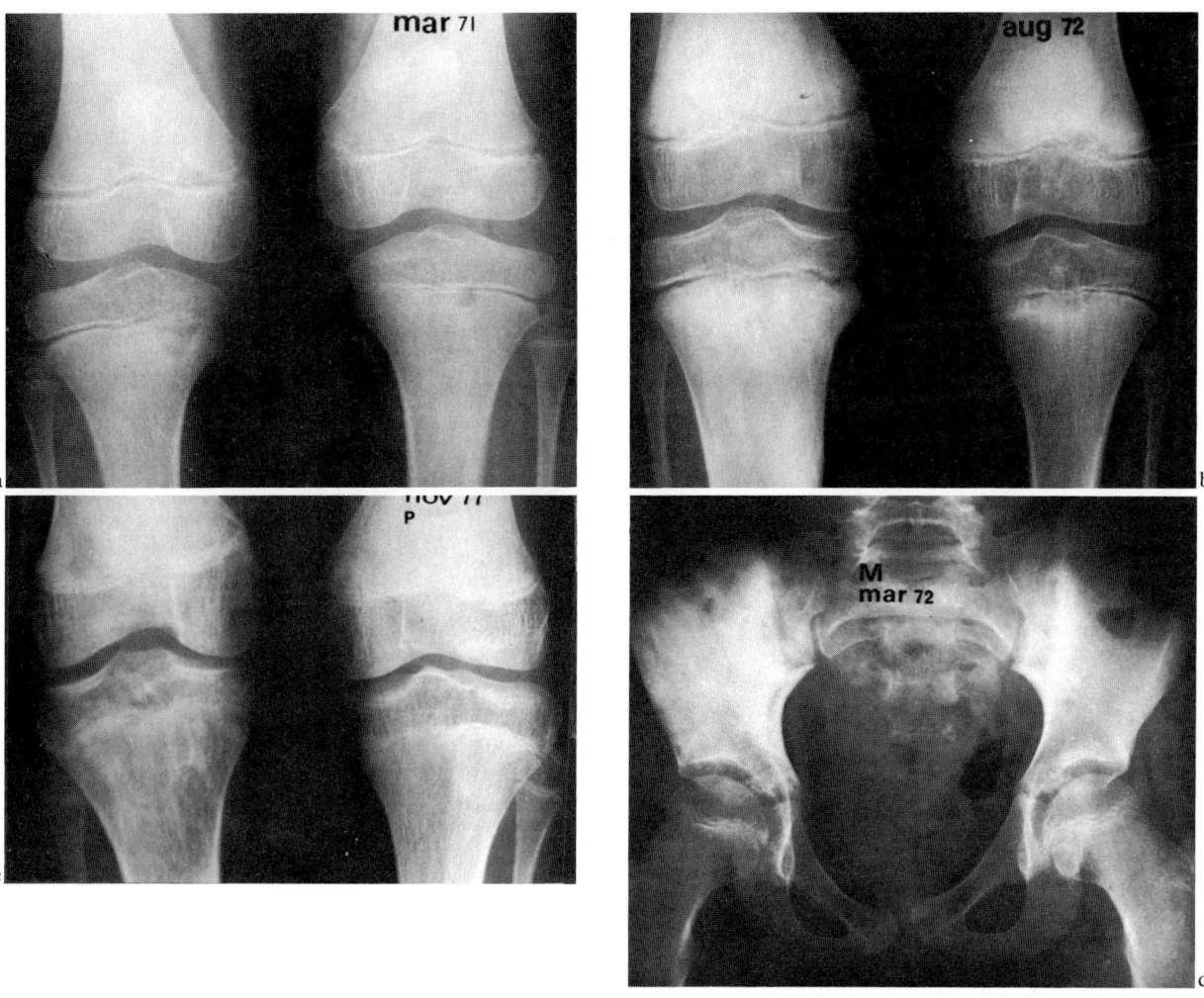

Fig. 2.1. *The 'lazy leucocyte' syndrome.* This 8-year-old girl presented with mild discomfort around both knees and the left elbow. Typical lytic lesions were present in the metaphyses around these joints. **a** Lucent areas in the distal femoral and proximal tibial metaphyses of the right knee were surrounded by a thin zone of reactive sclerosis. **b** Eighteen months later diffuse sclerosis had developed in both these metaphyses, together with more extensive involvement of the left knee. The child eventually responded to broad spectrum antibiotics. **c** Six years after the first presentation the sclerosis had regressed, but the growth plates were fusing prematurely. **d** Another child with a similar history developed this sclerotic area in the right ilium in addition to metaphyseal lesions.

Q1. This 13-year-old girl had complained of intermittent aching below the right ankle for approximately 2 years. In recent months the pain had become more severe, and was worse during the night than in the day; it was found to be relieved by aspirin.

Clinically, apart from tenderness elicited over the neck of the talus, no abnormality was detected.

Radiological examination revealed an osteolytic lesion, with a sclerotic margin, deep to the superior cortex of the neck of the talus. Suspicion of a central density, round in shape and contained within the lytic area, was confirmed by tomography.

The lesion was explored.

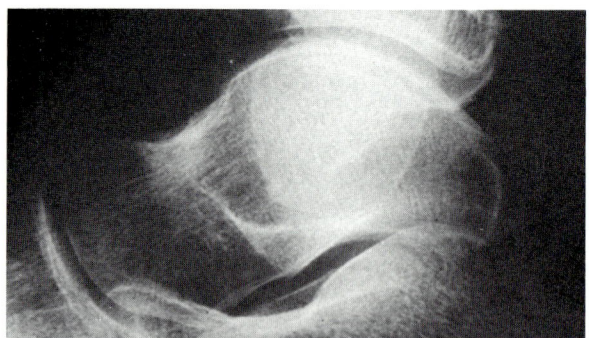
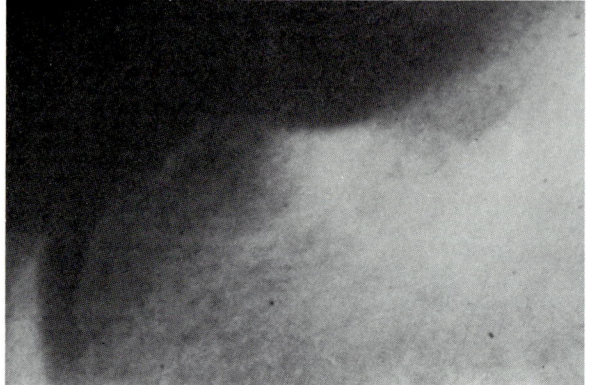

Q1a.

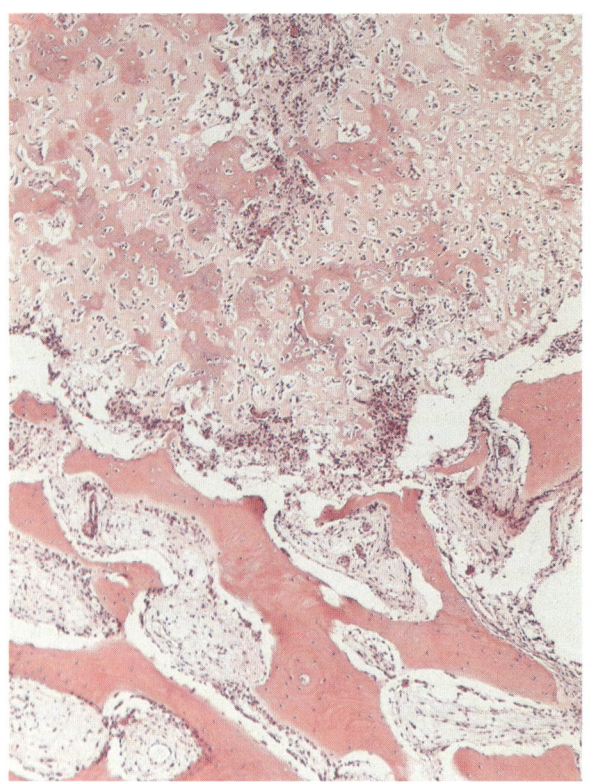

Q1b. (×46)

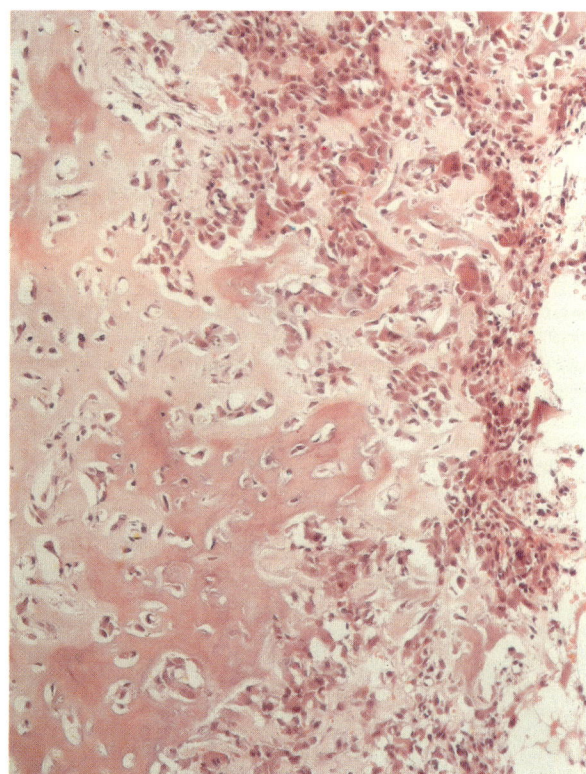

Q1c. (×120)

Q2. This 14-year-old girl had complained of pain and stiffness of the neck for 1 year. She attributed her symptoms to an earlier injury to her neck.

Clinical examination revealed generalised restriction of movement and a painful torticollis. Localised tenderness was elicited over the mid-cervical area.

On radiological examination an expanding lytic area was observed in the neural arch of C5.

This lesion was explored.

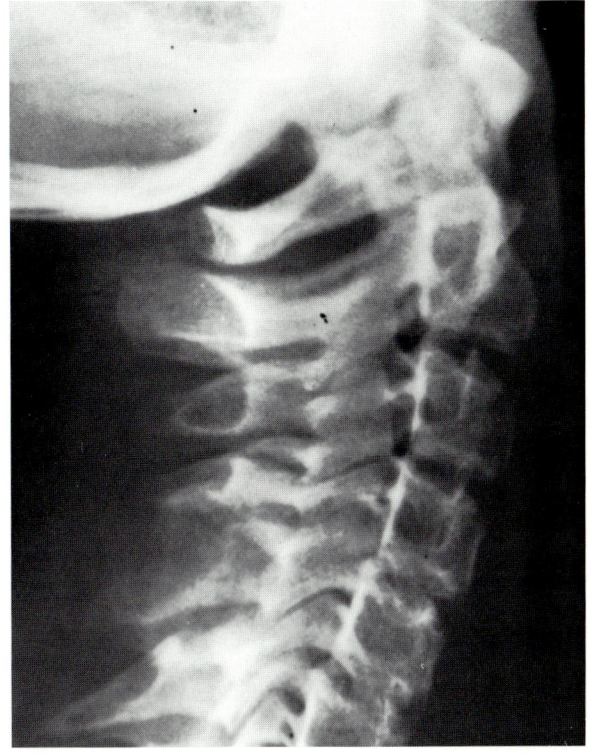

Q2a.

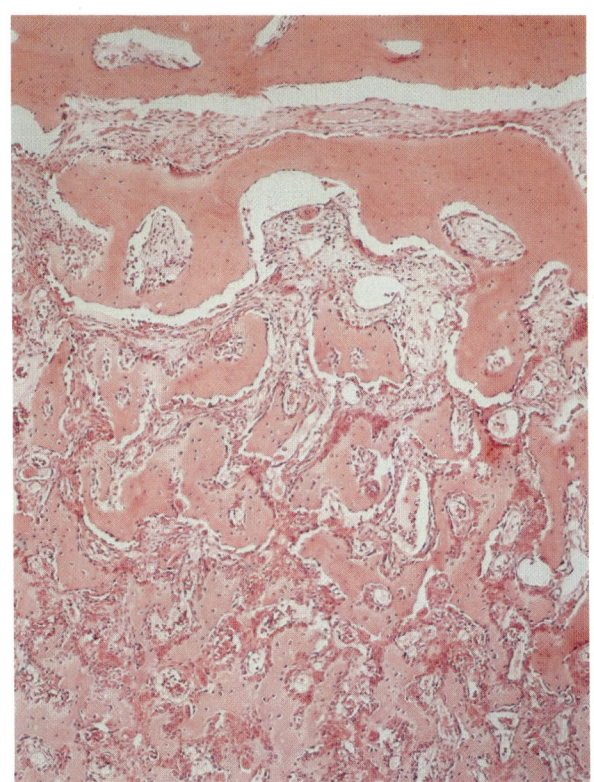

Q2b. (×68)

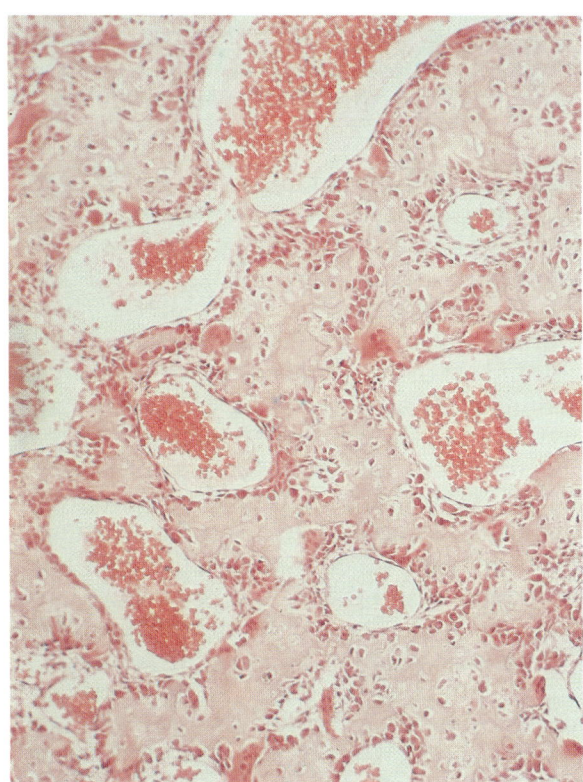

Q2c. (×160)

A1. Osteoid osteoma of talus

The radiological appearance of a small circumscribed osteolytic area containing a central rounded area of increased density strongly suggested the diagnosis of an osteoid osteoma, although the possibility of a Brodie's abscess with a central sequestrum also had been considered. It should be noted, however, that a sequestrum in a Brodie's abscess is almost always linear, and not round, in shape. Retrospective examination of a radiograph obtained at first presentation, 2 years earlier (Fig. 1.1), did indicate that the abnormality had begun to develop at that time, when radionuclide scanning undoubtedly would have been positive. Routine blood investigations, including the antistaphylococcal titre, were normal, and no history of a recent infection could be obtained. Another important clue to the diagnosis of osteoid osteoma was the relief of pain by aspirin.

At operation, the lesion could be identified by a local increase in vascularity of the involved area of the neck of the talus. It was locally resected and the specimen showed, on naked eye examination, a central area of gritty tissue surrounded by cortical and cancellous bone.

Histologically, the findings are typical of an osteoid osteoma. Q1b shows, above, part of the central 'nidus' of osteoblastic tissue, with, below, some thickened bone trabeculae from the surrounding zone of reactive bony sclerosis. Q1c illustrates a more magnified view of part of the periphery of the nidus. The staining reaction of the tissue permits distinction, even in the decalcified section, of areas of darker calcified bone and paler osteoid tissue (uncalcified bone). This tissue contains numerous osteoblasts and some scattered osteoclasts, but it does not have the cellularity or pleomorphism that would be expected in a malignant tumour, such as an osteosarcoma. The small size of the nidus (approximately 1 cm in diameter) is characteristic of osteoid osteoma and aids distinction from a benign osteoblastoma. Excision of the tumour was followed by immediate and permanent relief of pain.

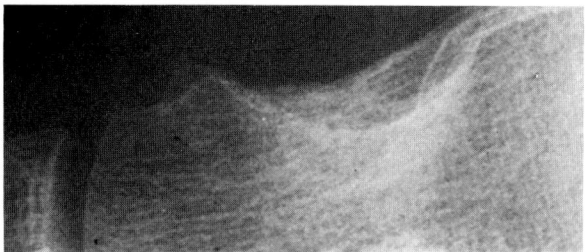

Fig. 1.1. This is the film of the patient in Q1, which had been regarded as normal 2 years earlier. Even then an opaque 'nidus' could be discerned.

Osteoid Osteoma

This lesion, long regarded as being inflammatory, now is accepted generally as a benign osteoblastic neoplasm. Histologically, it is related closely to benign osteoblastoma, from which it is distinguished mainly by size, skeletal distribution and its characteristic clinical symptomatology.

Clinical Features

Males are affected twice as commonly as females. Almost all cases are recognised before the age of 30, with the majority occurring in childhood and adolescence. Localised bone pain, usually worse at night, is the presenting complaint. The pain often is relieved dramatically by aspirin. When the lesion is subcutaneous, the associated hyperaemia may cause localised swelling and erythema.

Radiological Features

1. Site. Any bone may be affected, but the diaphyses of the long bones are most frequently involved. Lesions of the proximal end of the femur account for more than half the cases. Spinal lesions almost invariably involve a neural arch and, if adjacent to an articular facet, usually cause a painful scoliosis. In such cases the lesion is located at the apex of the concavity. These tumours may occur also in the small bones of the hands and feet, but involvement of such bones as the pelvis and skull is rare.

2. Appearance. A circular area of lucency, less than 1.5 cm in diameter, is typical. It usually contains a central round density described as the 'nidus'. Surrounding reactive sclerosis is usually evident, its quantity depending on (a) duration of lesion, (b) location in bone—least in medulla and most in relation to cortex and periosteum and (c) age—the younger the patient, the greater the response. Intra-articular lesions, as in Q1, produce less reactive bone because of the absence of periosteum. Periosteal reactions may occur remote from the tumour and even in an adjacent bone, reflecting surrounding hyperaemia. A similar hyperaemic response is slight overgrowth of an affected long bone in childhood.

Arteriography, by showing a blush in the nidus in the venous phase, may be of value in distinguishing an osteoid osteoma from an osteomyelitic sequestrum (see Exercise 10).

Radionuclide scanning will show increased uptake of the tracer even *before* frank radiological changes develop. It can be of use in identifying and locating a small nidus as a preliminary to, or during, surgical removal.

Pathological Features

The gross appearance of a typical osteoid osteoma is illustrated in Figs. 1.2a and b. The nidus is the neoplastic part of the lesion. It consists of osteoblastic tissue, usually with prominent capillary blood vessels and scattered osteoclasts. This osteoblastic tissue contains variable amounts of osteoid and calcified bone, the latter being responsible for the central radiological density. Histological distinction must be made from other osteoblastic lesions, such as fibrous dysplasia and osteosarcoma. The tissue of the nidus contrasts (Q1c) with the thickened trabeculae of the surrounding sclerotic bone and any periosteal new bone. These tissues, as well as the nidus, can show a marked increase in vascularity.

Treatment

Excision, provided it removes the nidus completely, is curative and relieves the pain immediately. It appears probable that untreated lesions eventually undergo spontaneous involution after an interval of 5–10 years.

References

Colton CL, Hardy JG (1980) Experience with a sterilisable radiation probe for detecting bone seeking isotope. J Bone Jt Surg 62B: 259

Freiberger RH (1960) Osteoid osteoma of the spine: a cause of backache and scoliosis in children and young adults. Radiology 75: 232–236

Jaffe HL (1935) 'Osteoid osteoma'. A benign osteoblastic tumor composed of osteoid and atypical bone. Arch Surg 31: 709–728

Jaffe HL, Lichtenstein L (1940) Osteoid osteoma. J Bone Jt Surg 22: 645–682

Lindbom A, Lindvall N, Soderberg G, Spjut H (1960) Angiography in osteoid osteoma. Acta Radiol 54: 327–333

Lisbona R, Rosenthall L (1979) Role of radionuclide imaging in osteoid osteoma. Am J Radiol 132: 77–80

Swee RG, McLeod RA, Beabout JW (1979) Osteoid osteoma. Detection, diagnosis and localization. Radiology 130: 117–123

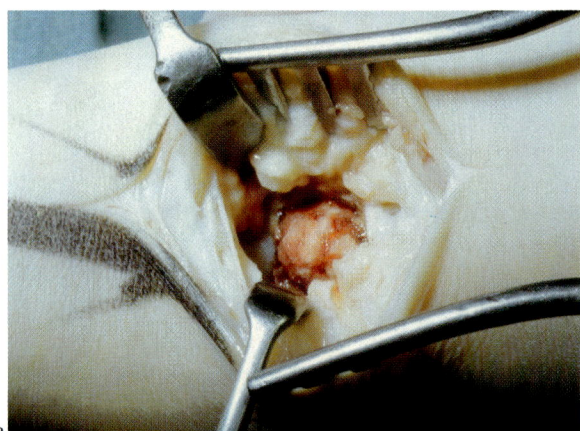

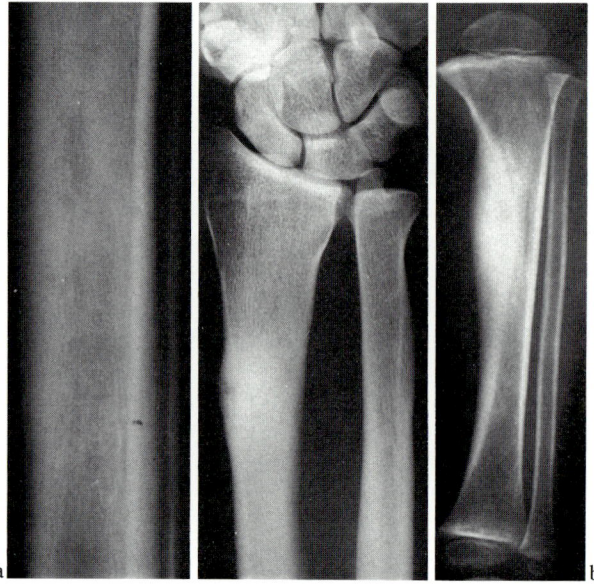

Fig. 1.2. Another osteoid osteoma in the neck of the talus shown at operation **a** before and **b** after excision of the small, rounded, well-demarcated nidus. The vascular nature of the tumour and its surrounding bone can be appreciated. This 22-year-old woman had complained of persistent pain. The ankle was swollen and local vasodilation and point tenderness over the lesion were observed. This circumscribed tumour (1 cm in diameter) was shelled out easily from the parent bone.

Fig. 1.4. *Osteoid osteoma—degrees of reactive sclerosis.* **a** *Intramedullary*, in tibia of a 12-year-old girl with localised pain for 5 months. Only an oval lucency is visible. **b** *Cortical* in radius of a 24-year-old man with long-standing pain. **c** *Parosteal* in tibia of a 4-year-old boy, exhibiting particularly florid reactive bone formation.

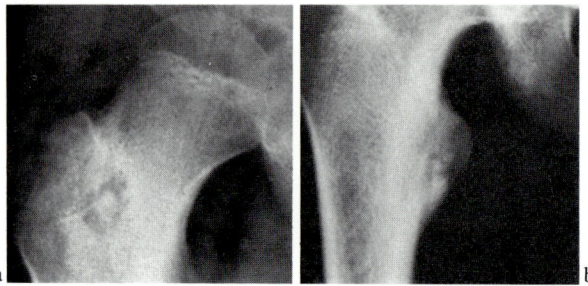

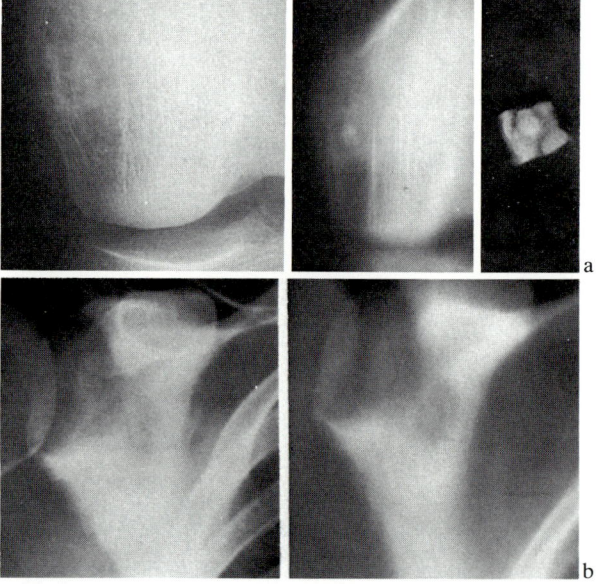

Fig. 1.3. *Osteoid osteoma—most common site is proximal end of femur.* These examples show **a** a 10-year-old girl with pain for 3 months, wakening her at night, and **b** an intramedullary lesion in the lesser trochanter of a 22-year-old woman. It contains two central densities.

Fig. 1.5. *Osteoid osteoma—value of tomography.* **a** Plain film diagnosis was speculative in this lesion of the medial femoral condyle of a 24-year-old man, but the tomographic appearance was typical. The radiograph of the excised specimen (*right*), importantly, confirmed that the entire tumour had been removed. **b** This scapular osteoid osteoma had caused prolonged pain at the unusually late age of 40 in this female nurse. Observe periosteal reaction remote from the lesion.

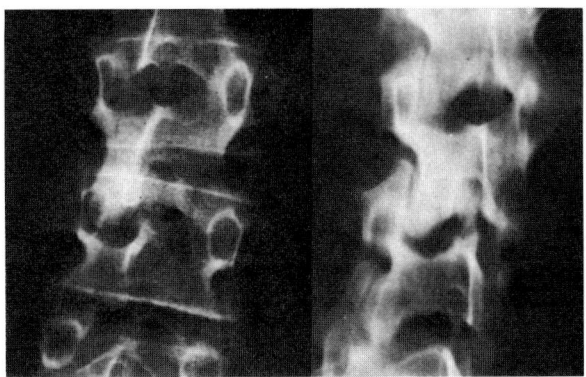

Fig. 1.6. *Osteoid osteoma of neural arch of L2.* This 13-year-old girl developed a painful scoliosis which persisted for many months before the sclerosing lesion in the right inferior articular process was observed. Tomography then demonstrated the nidus conclusively. It was situated, characteristically, in the apex of the concavity of the scoliosis.

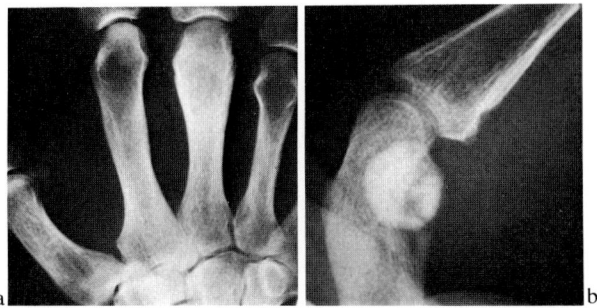

Fig. 1.8. *Osteoid osteoma—involvement of small bones.* **a** 3rd metacarpal in a 28-year-old man. **b** Neck of proximal phalanx of middle finger of a 21-year-old man, with increasing pain and swelling for 9 months. This lesion is intracapsular, hence no overlying periosteal reaction, but remote reactions attributable to hyperaemia are visible on the dorsal aspect of the affected bone *and* on the middle phalanx.

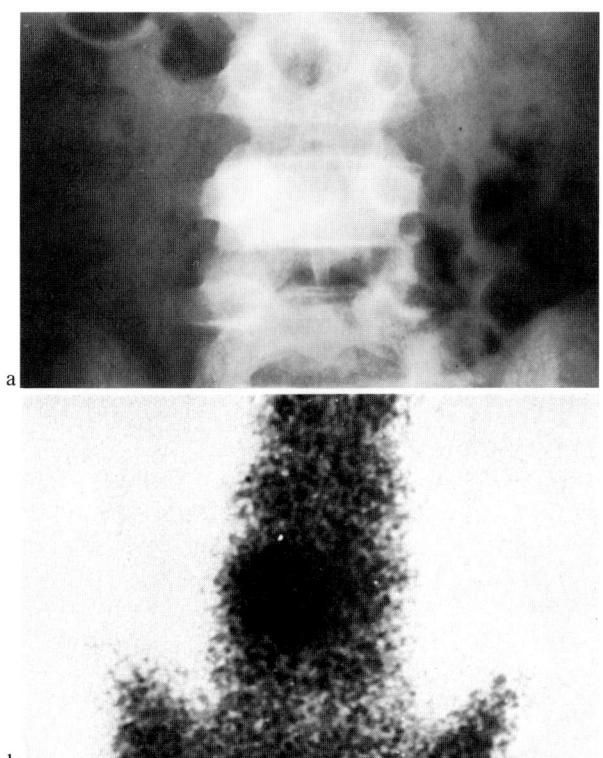

Fig. 1.7. *Osteoid osteoma of neural arch of L4.* Back pain in this 6-year-old boy was of much shorter duration. The sclerosing lesion in the base of the right pedicle of L4 was investigated at once by a radionuclide scan which proved positive. The lesion was excised, with immediate relief of pain. Histological confirmation of the diagnosis was obtained.

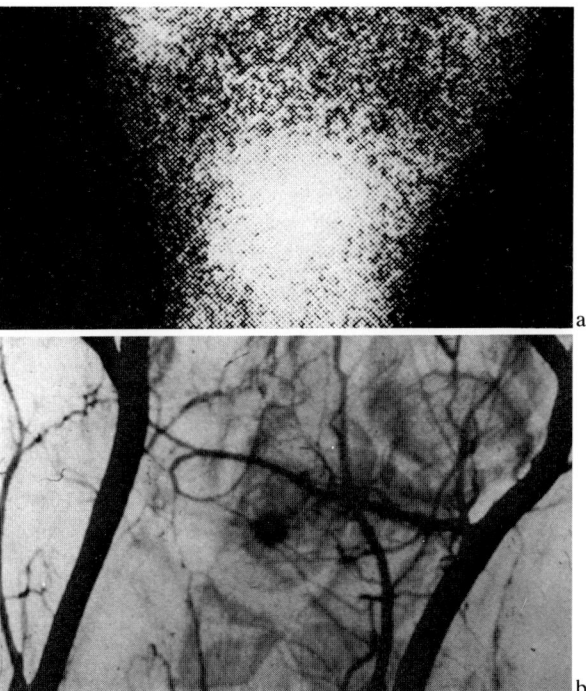

Fig. 1.9. *Osteoid osteoma of capitate.* This unique case, included by courtesy of Dr. L. Lateur and Prof. A. L. Baert, emphasises the value of other methods of diagnostic imaging in this disorder. Pain in the wrist of several months' duration in this 24-year-old man had responded to aspirin, but plain films and fine-section tomograms were inconclusive. **a** A radionuclide scan showed diffuse increase of uptake of the tracer in the carpus, but the actual localisation of the nidus depended finally **b** on the demonstration of a vascular blush in the subtraction film obtained during the venous phase of an arteriogram. Lateur L, Baert AL (1977) Localisation and diagnosis of osteoid osteoma in the carpal area by angiography. Skeletal Radiol 2: 75–79

A2. Benign osteoblastoma of spinous process of C5

The clinical findings, in a patient of this age, coupled with an expanding osteolytic lesion in the spinous process and laminae of C5 pre-operatively suggested the diagnosis of benign osteoblastoma.

At operation, a mass of solid and highly vascular tissue, 2×3 cm in size, was found, expanding the bone of the neural arch (Fig. 2.2). Histologically (Q2b and c) the lesion consists of vascular osteoblastic tissue. The expanding cortical bone is evident in the upper part of Q2b. The tissue contains a network of trabecular structures, many of which are covered by a layer of osteoblasts (Q2c). Scattered osteoclasts are also present. These histological components are similar to those present in the osteoid osteoma illustrated in Q1 and, as in that case, they indicate that the lesion is a benign osteoblastic tumour. Less osteoid tissue is seen in the present case and the bone tissue has a more pronounced trabecular pattern. Combined with the size of the lesion, which is more than 1.5 cm in diameter, these features establish a diagnosis of benign osteoblastoma.

The patient's symptoms were permanently alleviated by the removal of the tumour.

Benign Osteoblastoma

These tumours are related closely to osteoid osteomas, but differ from them in size, clinical presentation and skeletal distribution and also by being distinctly rarer. They occur particularly in children and young adults, males being affected more commonly than females. In contrast to osteoid osteoma, osteoblastomas usually show progressive, although slow, growth. Some behave in a locally invasive fashion and the term 'aggressive osteoblastoma' has been applied to them. They often recur locally, but have not been reported to metastasise. The transformation of an osteoblastoma to an osteosarcoma has been recorded, but is exceedingly rare. Such an apparent change in the nature of the lesion is to be explained usually by the erroneous diagnosis of an osteosarcoma as an osteoblastoma.

Clinical Features

The clinical features are not distinctive. Although pain is sometimes present, it is not as intense as in an osteoid osteoma and is not relieved by aspirin. Since these tumours develop so slowly, the history of localised discomfort and pain frequently is measured in years rather than months. Unilateral spinal lesions, particularly if situated on one side of a vertebra, represent another cause of painful scoliosis. If the neoplasm encroaches on the spinal canal, long tract pressure signs ensue.

Radiological Features

1. Site. Approximately half these tumours affect the spine, although other parts of the skeleton may be affected, including tubular and short bones. As in the case of osteoid osteoma, involvement of the skull, facial bones and ribs is very rare.

2. Appearance. Osteoblastomas present a remarkably varied radiological pattern, varying from large zones of extreme density, which may simulate a malignant bone-forming tumour such as an osteosarcoma, to extremely expansile areas which closely resemble such entities as aneurysmal bone cyst, giant-cell tumour or benign fibrous lesions. In an appropriate age group this diagnosis deserves consideration when any bizarre solitary lesion is encountered, especially if a prolonged history indicates its nature to be benign.

Pathological Features

The typical osteoblastoma is larger than 1 cm in diameter. Indeed, some attain a diameter of 10 cm. or more. Usually they lack the surrounding sclerosis which is such a characteristic feature of many osteoid osteomas.

Histologically, like osteoid osteoma, osteoblastoma is a benign osteoblastic tumour and consists of bone and osteoid tissue, with a vascular stromal tissue. Osteoblasts usually cover the bony surfaces. Scattered osteoclasts may be present and are sometimes conspicuous. In osteoblastomas, the bone and osteoid tissue is often arranged in a trabecular pattern (Q2b), while in osteoid osteoma it has a more diffuse arrangement (Q1b). The histological similarity between these entities has led to their description together as the 'osteoid osteoma–osteoblastoma complex'.

Histological distinction from osteosarcoma (see Exercise 14) is made by the absence of cellular and nuclear pleomorphism and by the more regular trabecular pattern in osteoblastoma.

Treatment

When the lesion is potentially removable by an appropriate surgical procedure, it is essential that an adequate margin of normal bone is also removed to prevent recurrence. Where the lesion is too extensive for such a procedure, osteoblastomas have responded successfully to radiotherapy, despite the established belief that they are insensitive to this treatment.

References

Byers PD (1968) Solitary benign osteoblastic lesions of bone. Osteoid osteoma and benign osteoblastoma. Cancer 22: 43–57

Dorfman HD (1973) Malignant transformation of benign bone lesions. In: Proceedings of Seventh National Cancer Conference. American Cancer Society, pp. 901–913

Jaffe HL (1956) Benign osteoblastoma. Bull Hosp Joint Dis 17: 141–151

Lichtenstein L (1956) Benign osteoblastoma. Cancer 9: 1044–1052

Mayer L (1907) Malignant degeneration of so-called benign osteoblastoma. Bull Hosp Joint Dis 28: 4–13

Schajowicz F, Lemos C (1976) Malignant osteoblastoma. J Bone Jt Surg 58B: 202–211

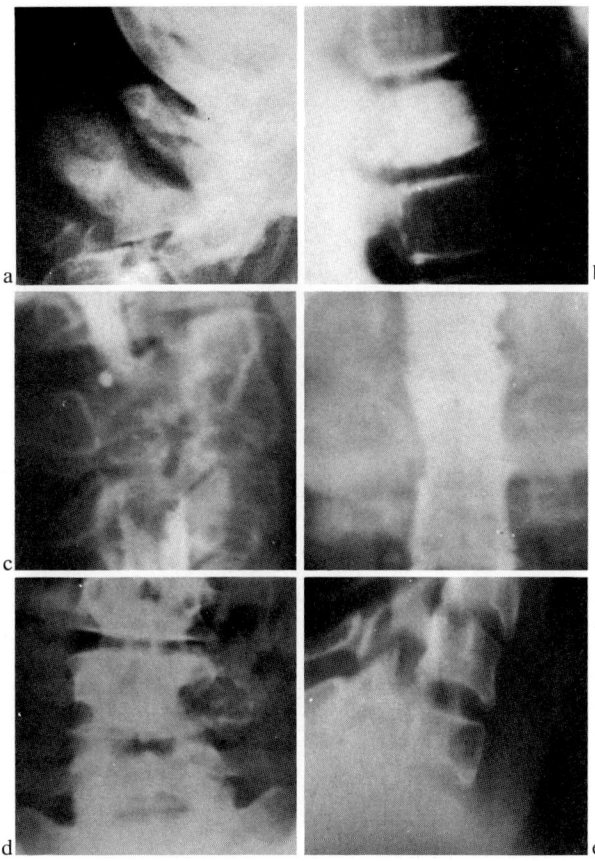

Fig. 2.1. *Benign osteoblastoma—spinal lesions*, mainly arising in neural arches and all productive of prolonged low-grade pain. **a** *Spinous process of C2* in a young adult. The central nidus, surrounded by an expansile zone of lucency, is sufficiently large to permit differentiation from an osteoid osteoma. **b** *Neural arch of T9*. Expansion of the tumour has caused pressure erosion on the vertebral body and has stimulated much reactive and unusually dense sclerosis. **c** *Pedicle of C2*. This 34-year-old butcher complained of chronic pain aggravated by chopping meat. This lesion is lytic and expansile, encroaching on the neural canal, as shown in the myelogram. **d** *Body of L3*. This grossly expanding tumour had caused a painful scoliosis for 2 years in an 18-year-old youth. It lies typically within the apex of the concavity of the scoliosis. Observe the resemblance to an aneurysmal bone cyst. **e** *Body of C6*. This 28-year-old woman presented with the relatively short history of 6 months' neck pain. The lytic area in the slightly expanded vertebral body, shown best in this tomogram, also was suspected to be an aneurysmal bone cyst. At operation solid tissue was found and the diagnosis was established histologically. Vertebral bodies are affected much less frequently than neural arches, but in both types encroachment on the neural canal may cause neurological symptoms and signs.

Fig. 2.2. *Benign osteoblastoma—lesions of long bones.* **a** *Tibia.* A classical osteoblastoma had caused this 12-year-old boy to complain of chronic pain below the knee for over a year. The nidus is large and is more poorly defined than is usual with its smaller counterpart, the osteoid osteoma. The surrounding zone of lucency consists of uncalcified osteoid tissue. The tumour has expanded the bone and localised hyperaemia has induced dense reactive sclerosis. **b** *Fibula.* In this instance the central lucency contains no central density, but has stimulated peripheral bone formation. It had caused chronic pain above the ankle of this young man for many months. **c** *Neck of femur.* This expansile and partially ossified osteoblastoma resembles a blister, one of the bizarre patterns not uncommonly encountered in this entity. This 24-year-old woman gave a history of groin pain for nearly 3 years.

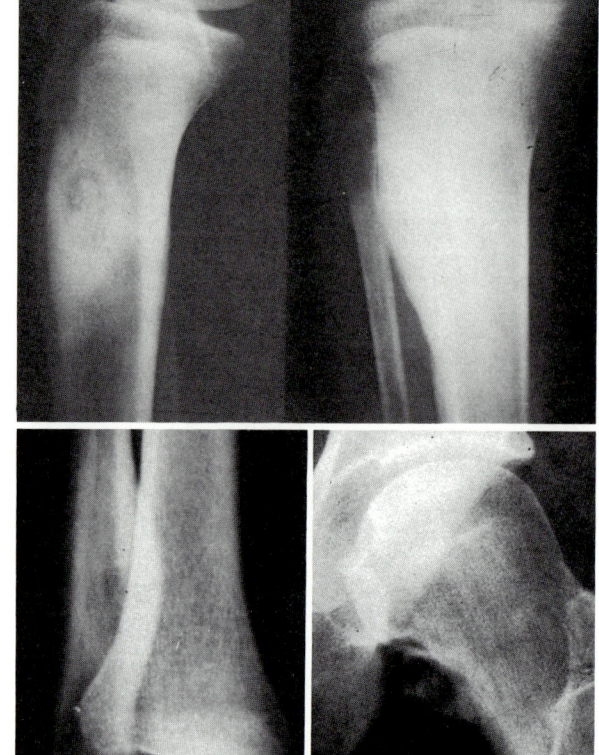

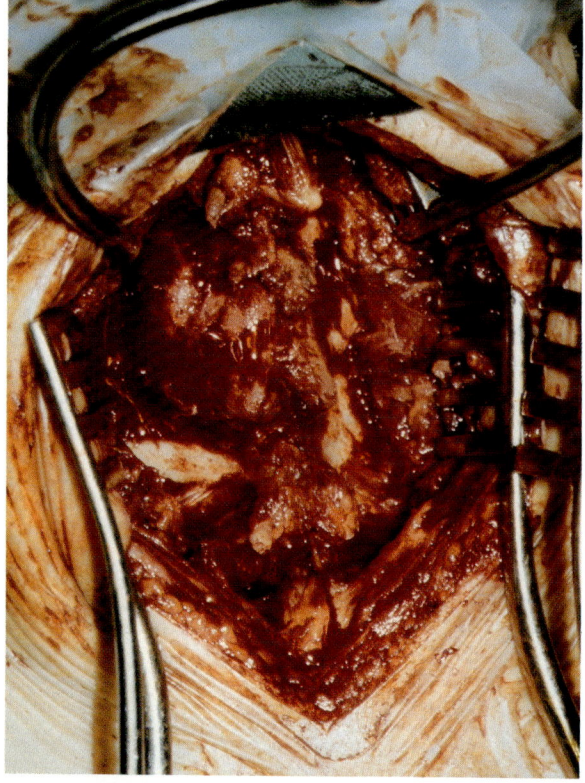

Fig. 2.3. Photograph of the benign osteoblastoma of the patient in Q2 at operation. It is larger than the osteoid osteoma illustrated in Fig. 1.2a and b, but is equally vascular. Excision of the lesion was immediately curative.

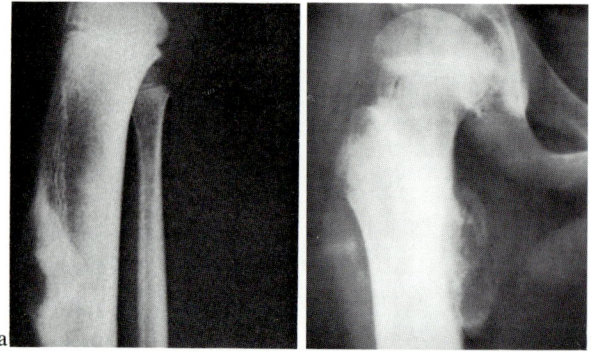

Fig. 2.4. *Benign osteoblastoma—periosteal lesions.* Further examples of the 'blister' appearance. **a** *Tibia* in an 8-year-old child. This tumour bears some resemblance to a non-ossifying fibroma (see Exercise 6). **b** *Femur* in an adolescent. Such bizarre patterns should arouse suspicion of the correct diagnosis.

Benign Osteoblastoma

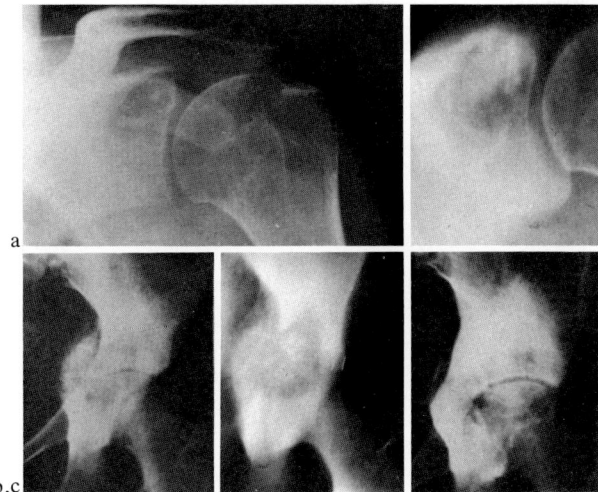

Fig. 2.5. *Benign osteoblastoma—lesions of flat bones* are uncommon and also present misleading appearances. **a** *Scapula*. This 29-year-old man had complained for over a year of increasing pain in the right shoulder which failed to respond to analgesics. Irregular areas of ossification within the lucent defect were demonstrated more satisfactorily in the tomogram. **b** *Acetabulum*. Similar central and poorly defined ossification was evident in the tomogram **c** of this expanding osteolytic lesion in a 16-year-old girl who had complained of a painful limp for many months. Consolidation **d** followed 18 months later after successful curettage, with complete relief of symptoms.

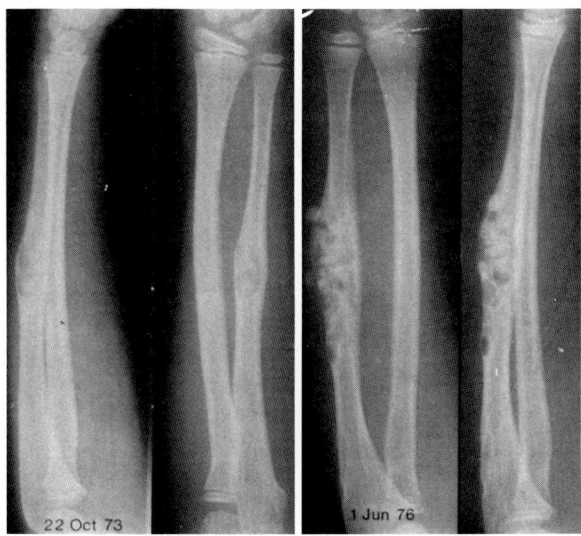

Fig. 2.7. *Benign osteoblastoma—recurrent lesion*. This series illustrates a typical benign osteoblastoma of the ulnar shaft, which caused a painful swelling of the forearm in a 9-year-old girl. The earlier studies showed an expansile lytic lesion containing irregular central densities. The diagnosis was confirmed histologically. Curettage at that time presumably was incomplete, since symptoms recurred and the appearance was much more florid 3 years later. The histological report then described the lesion as an aggressive osteoblastoma.

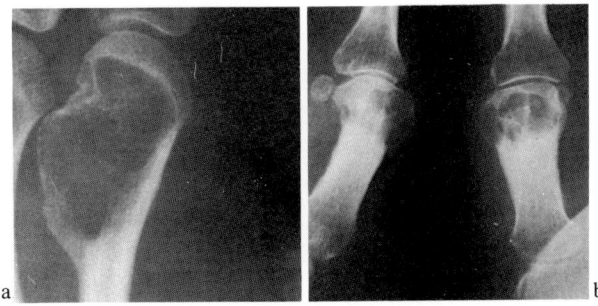

Fig. 2.6. *Benign osteoblastoma—peripheral lesions*. **a** This expanding lucent defect in the neck of the 2nd metacarpal of a 17-year-old girl was associated with a mildly painful swelling which had developed over many months. The similarity to an aneurysmal bone cyst is obvious. **b** Another benign osteoblastoma which had caused pain and swelling at the base of the thumb for many months in a 34-year-old man. Although a central and irregular density can be identified, a giant-cell tumour (see Exercise 15) was suggested pre-operatively.

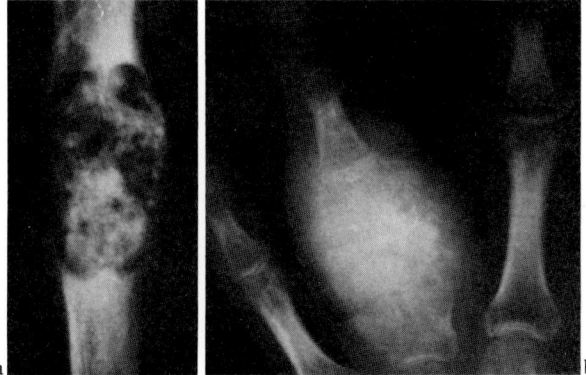

Fig. 2.8. *Benign osteoblastoma—aggressive forms*. Although relatively rare, these tumours occasionally present radiological patterns which inevitably arouse suspicion of malignancy. **a** *Humerus*. The destructive lesion has expanded and thinned the cortex. It caused chronic pain and was detected only at the unusually late age of 56 in this man. Abundant and irregular new bone has formed within the defect. Perhaps the clearly defined endosteal margin with a narrow zone of transition permits differentiation from an aggressive malignant tumour. **b** *4th proximal phalanx*. This tumour has destroyed completely the overlying cortex and has produced a huge soft tissue swelling with central areas of ossification.

Exercise 22

Q1. This 14-year-old girl had complained of intermittent discomfort in the lumbosacral region for 2 years.

This area had become painful during the previous 3 months, with the development of a localised swelling on the left side of the lumbosacral junction.

Clinical examination confirmed the presence of a hard and palpable swelling, but revealed no other abnormality. In particular, no neurological deficit was detected.

Radiological studies showed a large and clearly defined soft tissue mass on the left side of the lower lumbar spine, with extensive destruction of the left side of the body and neural arch of L5. The superior articular surface was preserved, but had undergone a minor degree of collapse. A myelogram performed at another hospital 2 months previously had been reported to be normal.

The lesion was explored and biopsied.

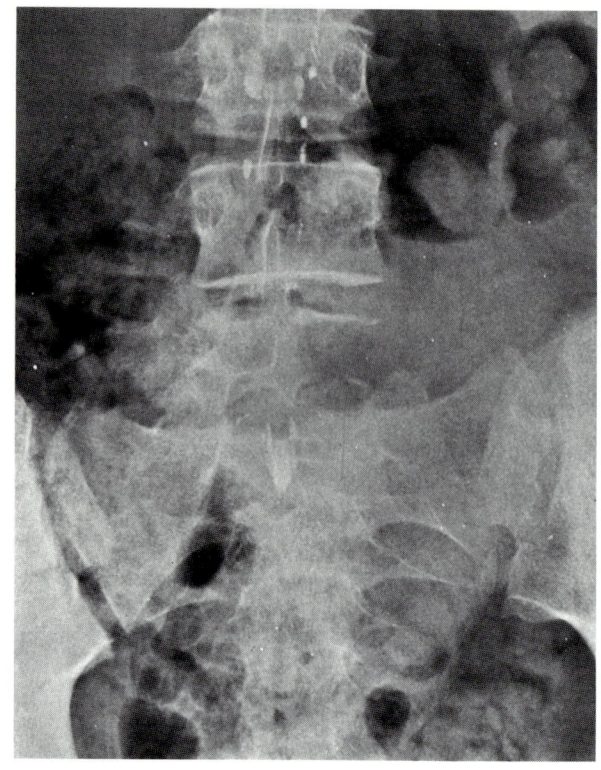

Q1a.

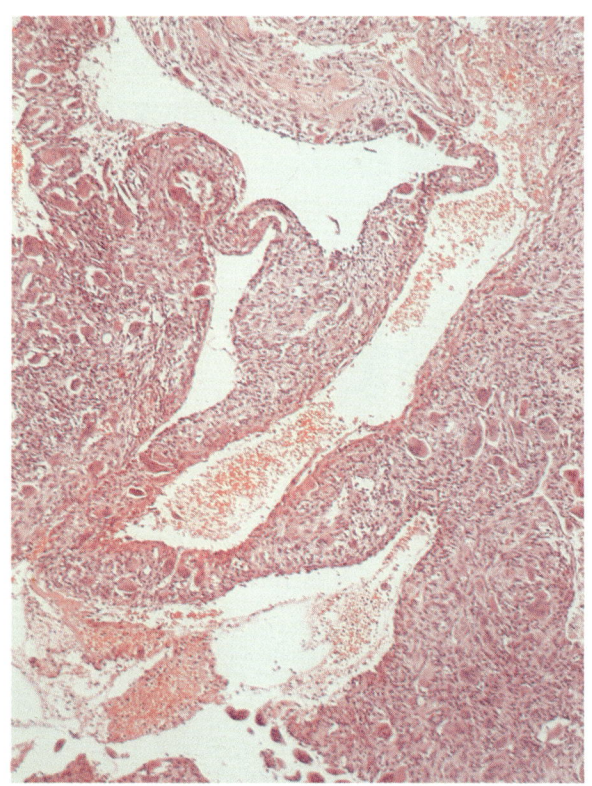

Q1b. (×50)

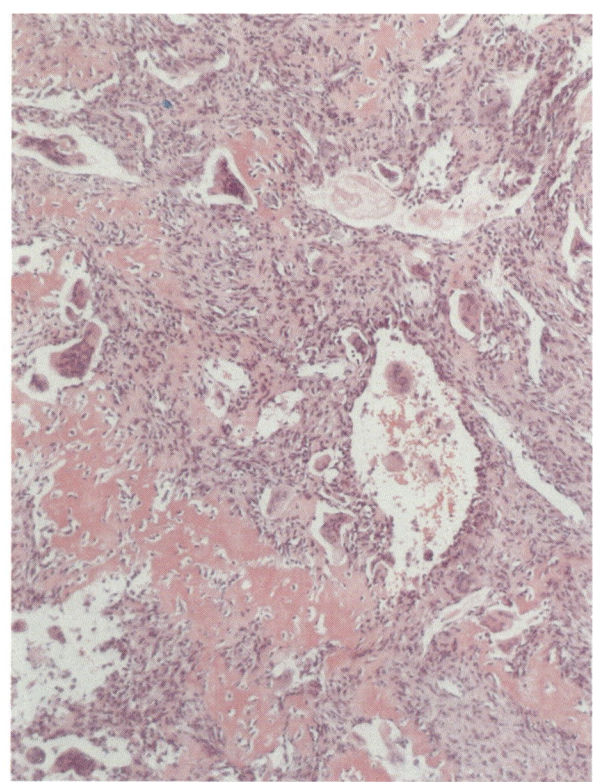

Q1c. (×88)

Q2. A 17-year-old boy complained of a mildly tender and painful swelling on the flexor aspect of the arm, just above the elbow.

He declared that this swelling had developed during the course of weeks rather than months. The swelling was obvious clinically. Palpation confirmed localised tenderness and slight increase in warmth. The overlying skin appeared normal. Flexion of the elbow was limited.

Radiologically, a large expanding lesion was demonstrated on the anterior aspect of the distal end of the humerus, with reduction of the thickness of the cortex to that of an egg-shell. The endosteal margin was clearly defined, but an irregular area of medullary osteolysis extended towards the distal end of the bone.

The lesion was explored and biopsied.

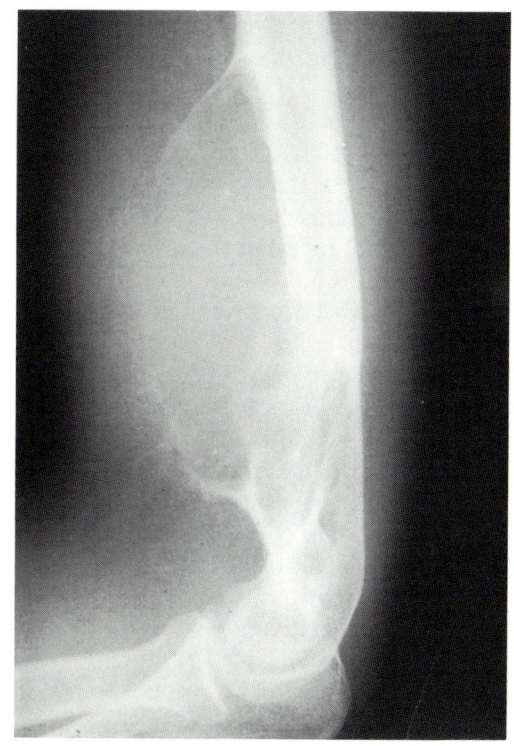

Q2a.

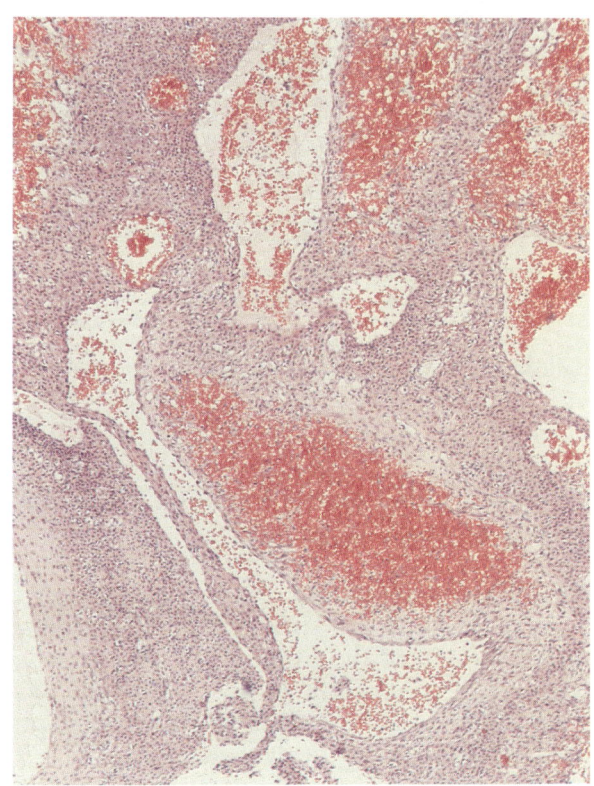

Q2b. (×45)

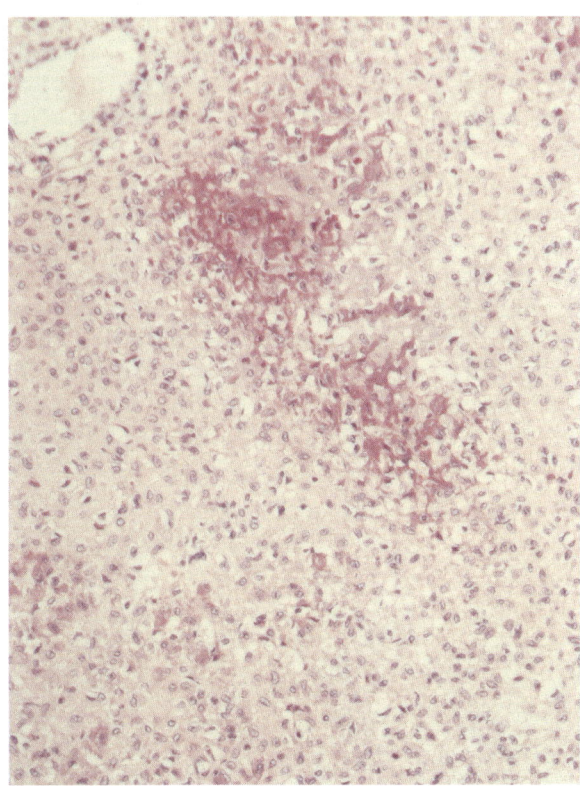

Q2c. (×150)

A1. Aneurysmal bone cyst of L5

The presence of such a large osteolytic lesion in the body and neural arch of L5, with its adjacent soft tissue mass, raised a number of diagnostic possibilities. If the abnormality was due to malignant disease a metastasis at this age was considered to be unlikely, but the possibilities of a malignant round-cell tumour or an osteolytic sarcoma lay within the differential diagnosis. Another, more benign, entity—an aneurysmal bone cyst—was suggested and this diagnosis was established histologically. A CT scan had been performed at the time of the myelogram 2 months previously (Fig. 1.1a) and when this procedure was repeated (Fig. 1.1b) remarkable enlargement of the lesion was evident. The rapidity of growth provided considerable support for the correct diagnosis.

At operation, using a posterior approach, the lesion was found to consist of a mass of vascular tissue, destroying the neural arch of the vertebra and extending towards the adjacent spinal muscles. Tissue removed from this site shows the appearance illustrated in Q1b and c. The combination of vascular spaces, giant cells and reactive bone (Q1c) is characteristic of aneurysmal bone cyst. No malignant tissue could be identified. After the removal of the posterior part of the mass, and the arrest of very considerable haemorrhage from the vascular lesion, a posterior fusion was performed. At a subsequent operation, the anterior part of the mass was removed and an anterior stabilising procedure carried out. All the tissue that was removed showed the histological features of aneurysmal bone cyst, with no indication of another underlying lesion.

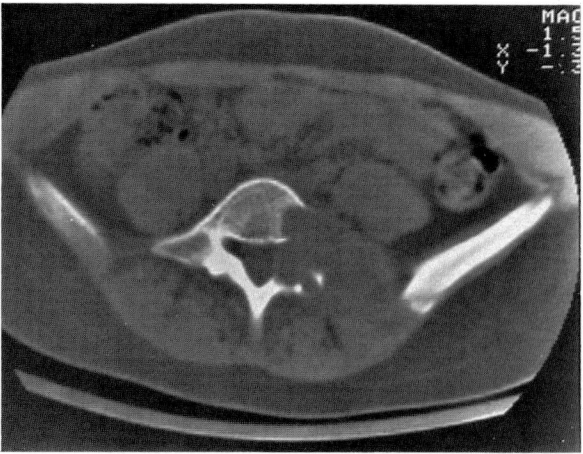

Fig. 1.1a. *CT scan of the lesion at the time of presentation.* Much of the left side of the neural arch and part of the body of L5 had been destroyed, with a considerable extension into the soft tissues.

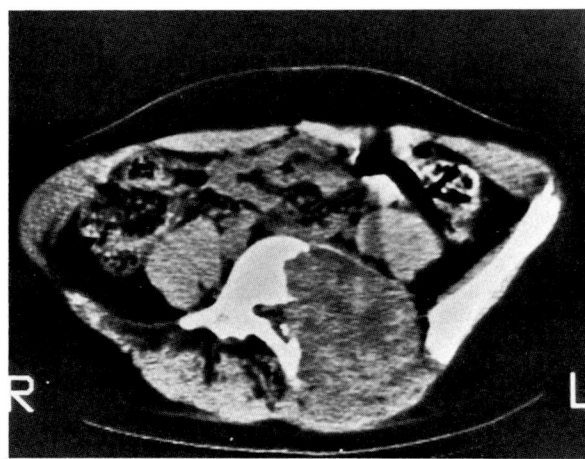

Fig. 1.1b. *CT scan 2 months later.* Observe the rapid growth of this aneurysmal bone cyst, with enlargement of the soft tissue mass and much more osseous destruction and encroachment on the neural canal, indicating the necessity for adjuvant radiotherapy.

A2. Aneurysmal bone cyst of humerus, secondary to a chondroblastoma

The extreme expansion of bone with marked cortical thinning and the well-defined endosteal margin of the lesion are characteristic features of aneurysmal bone cyst, which was the radiological pre-operative diagnosis. The area of medullary destruction represented chondroblastoma tissue persisting in the region of the growth plate.

At operation, the lesion was cystic and haemorrhagic. A thorough curettage was carried out. The features shown in Q2b and c are representative of the material so obtained. The vascular spaces and strands of haemorrhagic spindle-celled tissue (Q2b) are consistent with aneurysmal bone cyst, but large areas of solid tissue also are present and their structure, with rounded cells and patchy calcification of the intercellular material (Q2c), establishes a diagnosis of chondroblastoma, an entity discussed elsewhere in this work. The lesion is, in fact, a chondroblastoma with the formation of a *secondary* aneurysmal bone cyst. The term 'cystic chondroblastoma' has been used to describe this type of lesion (Schajowicz and Gallardo 1970).

Aneurysmal Bone Cyst

This unusual vascular lesion, whose nature is still obscure, is accepted generally as a benign bone tumour. Prior to its recognition as a distinct entity by Jaffe and Lichtenstein in 1950, cases were often regarded as cystic variants of giant-cell tumours. In many instances a history of previous trauma can be elicited, a fact which may be significant. Recently, the occasional development of an aneurysmal bone cyst as a lesion secondary to some other, pre-existing, abnormality has been recognised, as in Q2.

Clinical Features

Aneurysmal bone cysts usually occur in older children and young adults and have no sexual predilection. They tend to have a relatively rapid onset, developing in a few weeks or months with increasing pain and swelling. Gross pathological fractures are uncommon, but attention to these tumours is drawn frequently by minor infractions of an attenuated cortex. Encroachment on the neural canal by spinal lesions may precipitate neurological deficits and even paraplegia.

Radiological Features

1. Site. Any bone may be affected. Approximately half occur in major long bones, especially towards their ends, and a quarter in the spine. Less common locations include the small bones of the hands and feet, the ribs, the clavicle and even, exceptionally, the skull.

2. Appearance. The lesions are entirely osteolytic, expanding and thinning extremely the overlying cortex and disrupting its continuity. Discrete extensions into adjacent soft tissues often develop, which may, in turn, cause pressure erosions on neighbouring bones. The endosteal margin tends to be serpiginous and usually develops a narrow zone of transition with a thin sclerotic reaction. Serial studies show these tumours to enlarge rapidly, some doubling their size within a few weeks, a feature matched by virtually no other skeletal abnormality. Occasionally, however, some aneurysmal bone cysts are so aggressive in their appearance and behaviour that malignancy, justifiably, may be suspected.

Angiography of these lesions usually shows hypervascularity in the peripheral vessels, but no central accumulation of the medium. Radionuclide scanning demonstrates increased uptake of the tracer. CT scanning is of value in assessing the exact size of the tumour and establishing its cystic nature.

Pathological Features

On surgical exploration, an aneurysmal bone cyst appears typically as a honeycomb of cystic spaces, separated by septae of solid and often haemorrhagic tissue. Histologically, numerous vascular channels can be identified; the intervening solid tissue usually contains large numbers of giant cells and areas of reactive bone formation. Histological distinction from a giant-cell tumour sometimes can be difficult. To make a diagnosis of giant-cell tumour, large areas of solid giant-celled tissue must be identified (see Exercise 15).

'Secondary' aneurysmal bone cyst has been reported in a variety of bone lesions, including non-ossifying fibroma, chondroblastoma, giant-cell tumour and fibrous dysplasia. Careful histological examination of all the tissue from an aneurysmal bone cyst is necessary in order to exclude the presence of an underlying lesion.

Treatment

Curettage and packing with bone chips is usually curative. Recurrences are less common than with the so-called 'simple' or unicameral bone cyst (see Exercise 19). Some lesions, indeed, respond excellently to no more than the surgical insult of a biopsy. Adjuvant radiotherapy with a dosage of 2000—3000 rads is of value in more aggressive aneurysmal bone cysts, especially those to which surgical access may be difficult, as in some spinal and sacral locations. On rare occasions amputation of a limb may be required in the case of unusually aggressive and recurrent lesions.

References

Biesecker JL, Marcove RC, Huvos AG, Mike V (1970) Aneurysmal bone cysts. A clinicopathological study of 66 cases. Cancer 26: 615–625

Bonakdarpour A, Levy WM, Aegerter E (1978) Primary and secondary aneurysmal bone cyst. A radiological study of 75 cases. Radiology 126: 75–83

Buraczewski J, Dabska M (1971) Pathogenesis of aneurysmal bone cyst. Cancer 28: 597–604

Dabska M, Buraczewski J (1969) Aneurysmal bone cyst. Pathology, clinical course and radiologic appearance. Cancer 23: 371–389

Hay MC, Paterson D, Taylor TK (1978) Aneurysmal bone cysts of the spine. J Bone Jt Surg 60B: 406–411

Jaffe HL (1950) Aneurysmal bone cyst. Bull Hosp Joint Dis 11: 3–13

Levy WM, Miller AS, Bonakdarpour A, Aegerter E (1975) Aneurysmal bone cyst secondary to other osseous lesions. Am J Clin Pathol 63: 1–8

Lichtenstein L (1950) Aneurysmal bone cyst. Cancer 3: 279–289

Schajowicz F, Gallardo H (1970) Epiphyseal chondroblastoma of bone. A clinico-pathological study of 69 cases. J Bone Jt Surg 52B: 205–226

Tillman BP, Dahlin DC, Lipscomb PR (1968) Aneurysmal bone cyst. An analysis of 95 cases. Mayo Clin Proc 43:478–495

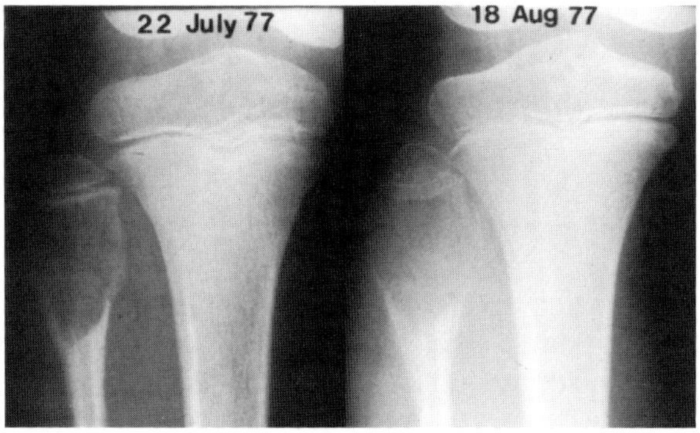

Fig. 1.2. *Aneurysmal bone cyst—rate of growth.* **a** This 10-year-old boy developed sudden pain below the knee in relation to a slightly tender swelling which had developed during the previous few weeks. A pathological infraction had occurred through the slender cortex of the typically expansile lesion in the proximal metaphysis of the fibula. **b** Only 4 weeks later the cyst had doubled in size. Curettage and packing with bone chips was followed by reconstitution of bone and only a residual zone of sclerosis.

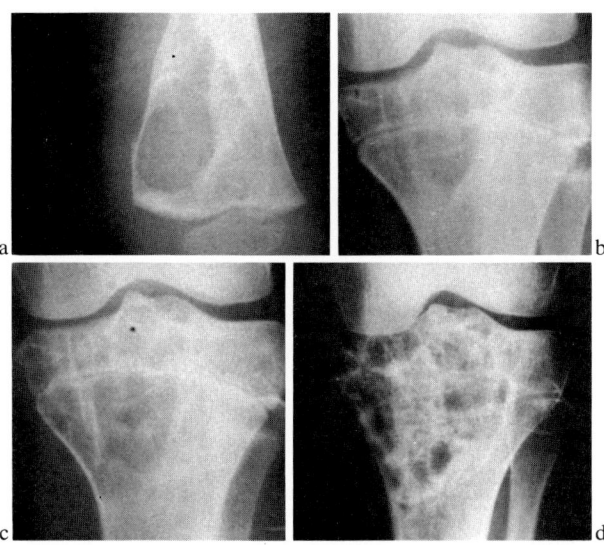

Fig. 1.3. *Aneurysmal bone cyst—long bones in children.* **a** This 2-year-old boy developed a painful swelling above the left knee. The metaphyseal location in the femur of this clearly defined and expansile cyst is typical. **b** An exceptional example of a similar metaphyseal lesion, in the proximal end of the left tibia of a 10-year-old boy with localised pain, which actually traversed the growth plate and which **c** enlarged greatly during the subsequent 3 months. After radical curettage and packing with bone chips considerable sclerosis **d** had developed a year later, but at the expense of premature epiphyseal fusion.

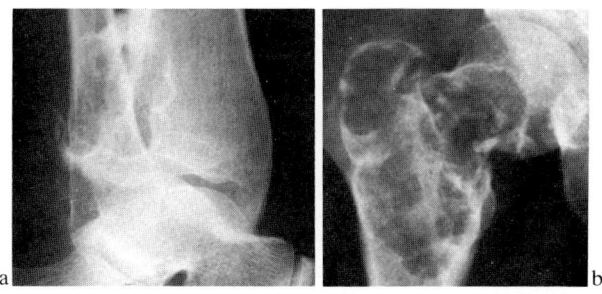

Fig. 1.4 *Aneurysmal bone cyst—long bones in adults.* **a** The appearance of this lytic expanding lesion in the distal end of the tibia of a young man with ankle pain is characteristic. Part of the attenuated cortex has been destroyed and a typical serpiginous endosteal margin is sclerotic with a narrow zone of transition. **b** Attention to this classical aneurysmal bone cyst was called by a pathological fracture of the femoral neck. The tumour shows the same radiological features. The patient was a 36-year-old woman who admitted to transient episodes of discomfort during the preceding 3 years.

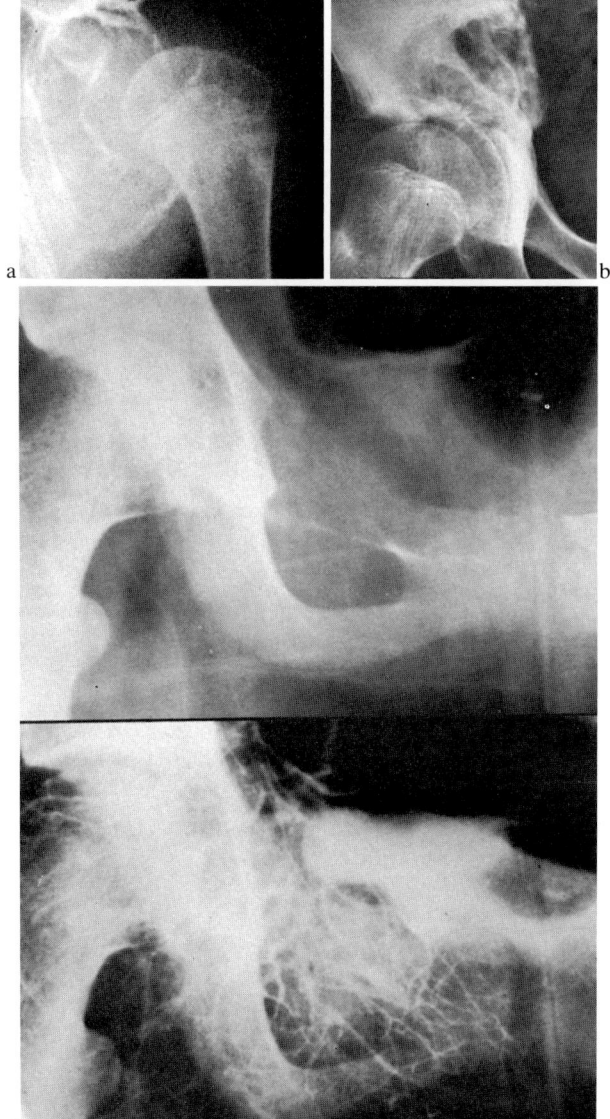

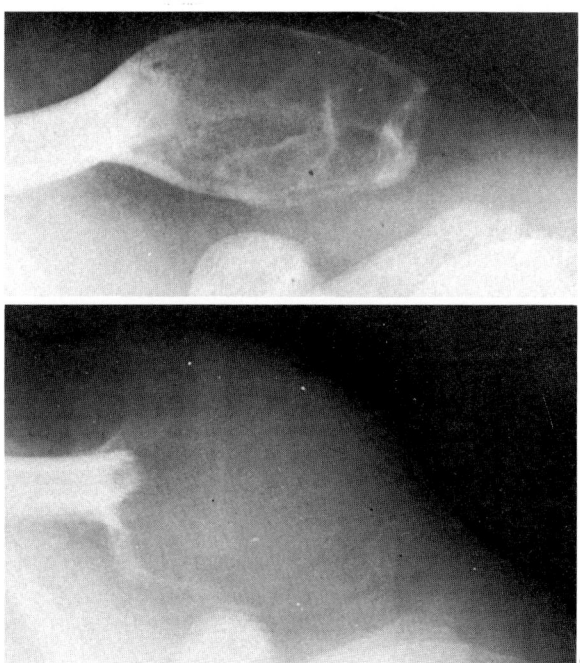

Fig. 1.5. *Aneurysmal bone cyst—flat bones.* **a** This typical lesion in the scapula of a 6-year-old girl was discovered incidentally following a minor injury. Clinically the expansile mass was palpable, but painless. Despite curettage, two recurrences subsequently required operative clearance before satisfactory healing occurred. **b** On the other hand, this similar lesion in the ilium of a 10-year-old boy with low-grade pelvic pain responded promptly to a single surgical curettage. **c** This lesion of the public ramus in a 16-year-old girl with pain in the groin was suspected pre-operatively to be a Ewing's tumour. Arteriography showed characteristic *peripheral* hypervascularity, with no obvious accumulation of the contrast within the tumour itself. **d** Another flat bone lesion in the outer end of the clavicle of a 12-year-old boy who had sustained a minor injury. Observe the extremely rapid growth of the tumour which took place during the following 2 months, emphasising a characteristic sequence of events with these neoplasms.

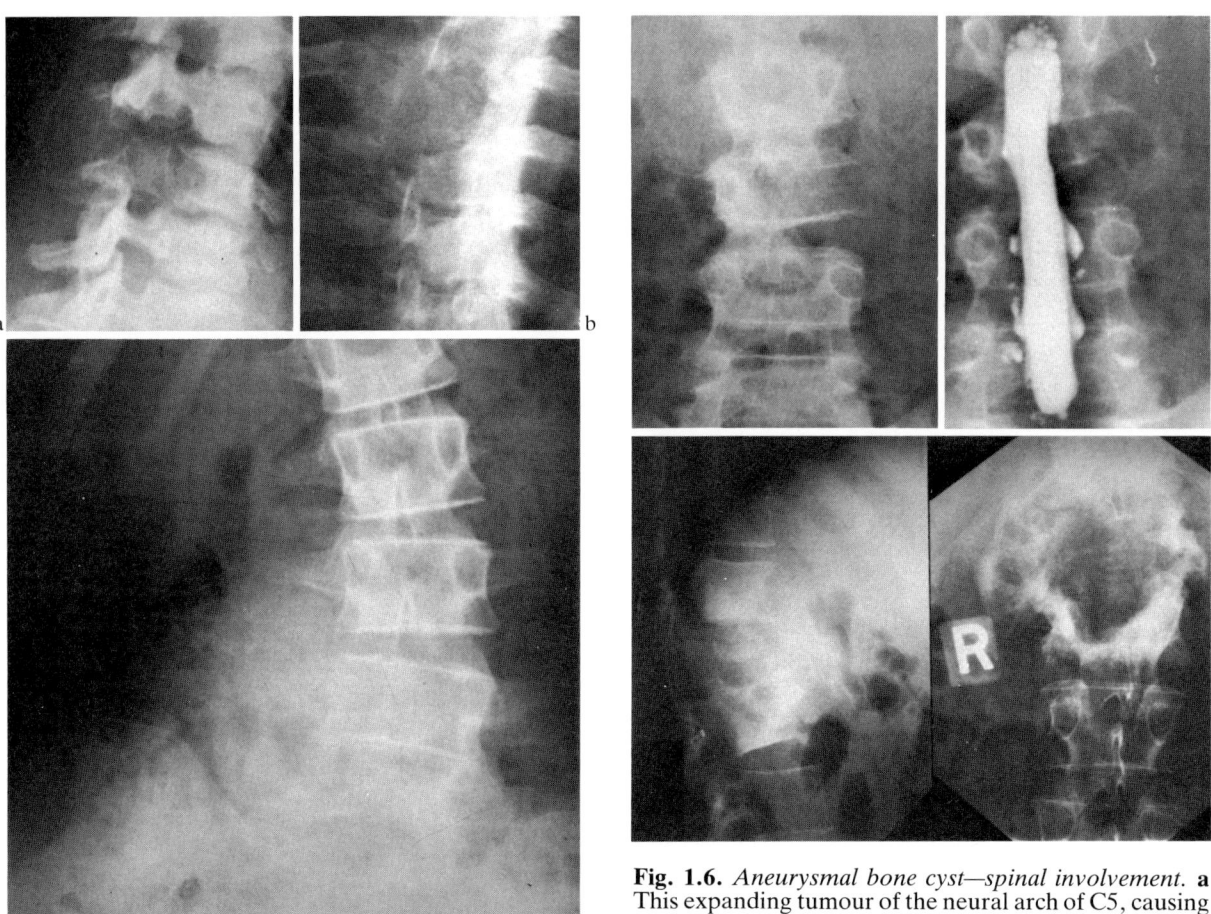

Fig. 1.6. *Aneurysmal bone cyst—spinal involvement.* **a** This expanding tumour of the neural arch of C5, causing neck pain in a young adult, is outlined by a peripheral density of egg-shell thickness and has caused pressure erosion on the adjacent lamina of C4. **b** A similar lesion of the body and neural arch of T5 found in a young man with girdle pain. **c** This tumour of L5 in a 12-year-old girl was situated typically within the apex of the concavity of the secondary scoliosis which it had caused. The child had complained of intermittent low back pain for 2 years. Myelography revealed a spinal block associated with extensive destruction of the right side of the body and neural arch. An excellent response to radiotherapy healed the lesion within a year. **d** This similar lesion involving the left side of L3 in a 10-year-old girl caused symptoms at first attributed to a prolapsed intervertebral disc. The tumour was detected only after removal of an ineffective plaster cast. Myelography showed encroachment of the expanding mass onto the left L4 nerve root. Curettage was curative. **e** This unusually severe lesion occurred in the body and neural arch of L2 in a 22-year-old man complaining of back pain for several months. Secondary pressure erosion had affected the adjacent vertebral bodies. Not surprisingly, a more sinister diagnosis was suspected pre-operatively and the nature of the lesion was established finally on histological grounds.

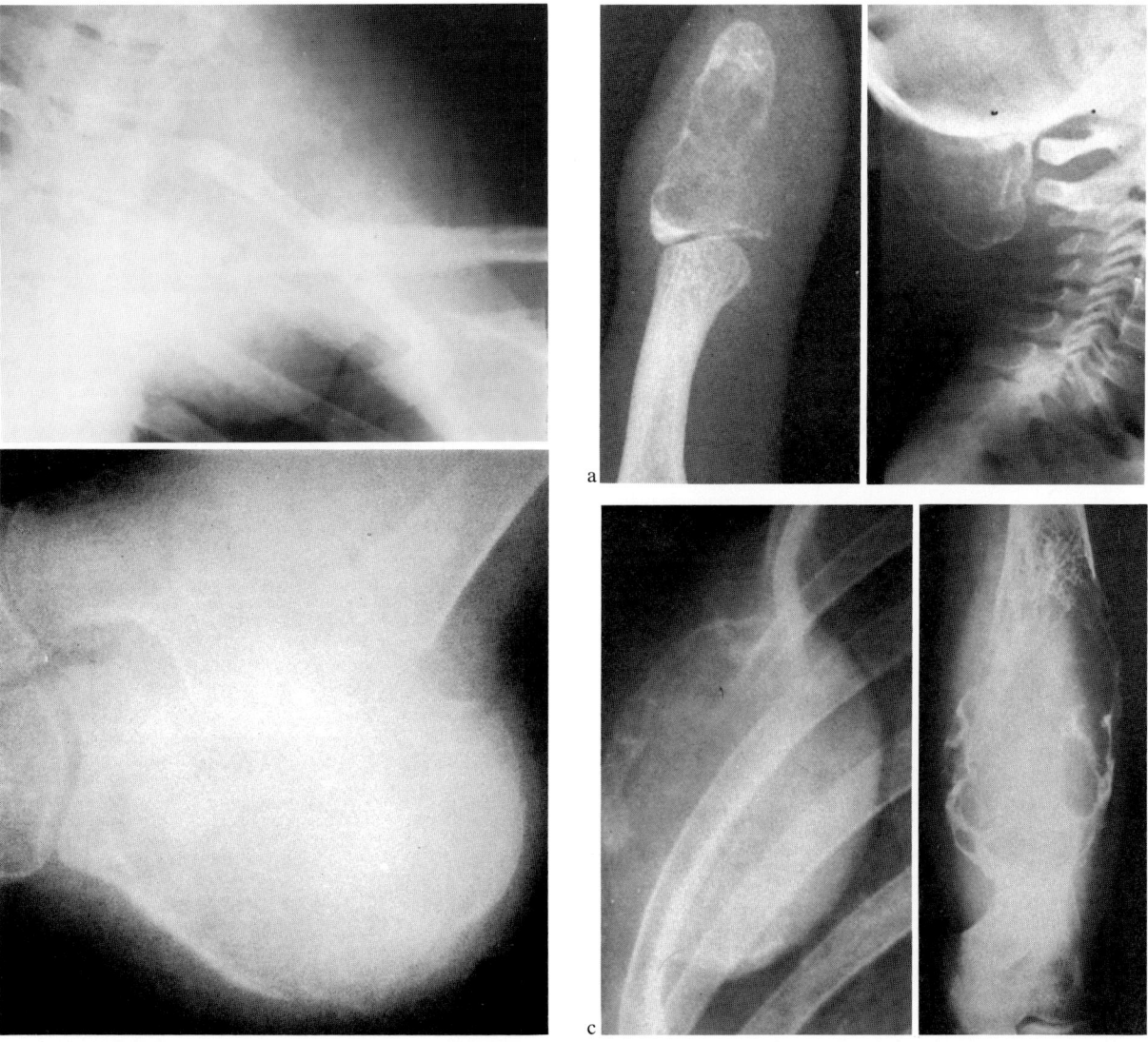

Fig. 1.7. *Aneurysmal bone cyst—aggressive lesions.* In a small number of cases these tumours grow so rapidly and cause such extensive and irregular destruction of the affected bone that the radiological appearance must provoke suspicion of malignancy. **a** *1st left rib.* This huge lesion caused a large painful swelling which developed within 6 months in an 18-year-old girl. Pre-operatively a haemangiosarcoma was suggested. An excellent response to radiotherapy was obtained, with contraction and sclerosis of the tumour. The patient was alive and well 12 years later. **b** *Calcaneus.* This painful and destructive aneurysmal bone cyst in a 10-year-old girl not only failed to respond to radiotherapy, but also to curettage on several occasions. Treatment in this instance was so unsuccessful that ultimately amputation was accepted.

Fig. 1.8. *Aneurysmal bone cyst—unusual locations and manifestations.* **a** *Terminal phalanx* of middle finger in a young adult with a painful swelling. **b** *Occiput* in a 2-year-old child. The tender mass developed within a few weeks. **c** *Rib*, causing a tender and rapidly enlarging swelling of the chest wall of this 32-year-old woman. **d** *Humerus.* This 15-year-old boy had developed a painful and tender swelling in the left arm during the previous year. Six months before that he had sustained a pathological fracture through a lytic medullary lesion, regarded pre-operatively as a unicameral bone cyst. At operation, however, the abnormal tissue was solid and proved histologically to be fibrous dysplasia. This case therefore is an example of a *secondary* aneurysmal bone cyst.

Q1. This 61-year-old woman was admitted to hospital because of a painful swelling over the shaft of the 3rd metacarpal bone, present for 6 months.

She also complained of 'rheumatism', particularly affecting her right hip and knee.

Clinical examination showed a tender swelling of the knuckle, with hypo-aesthesia of the pulp of the middle finger.

The radiographs demonstrated the presence of an expanding lytic lesion involving the head and neck of the third metacarpal, through which a healing pathological infraction was evident. Generalised osteopenia had affected all the bones of the hand.

A biopsy was performed.

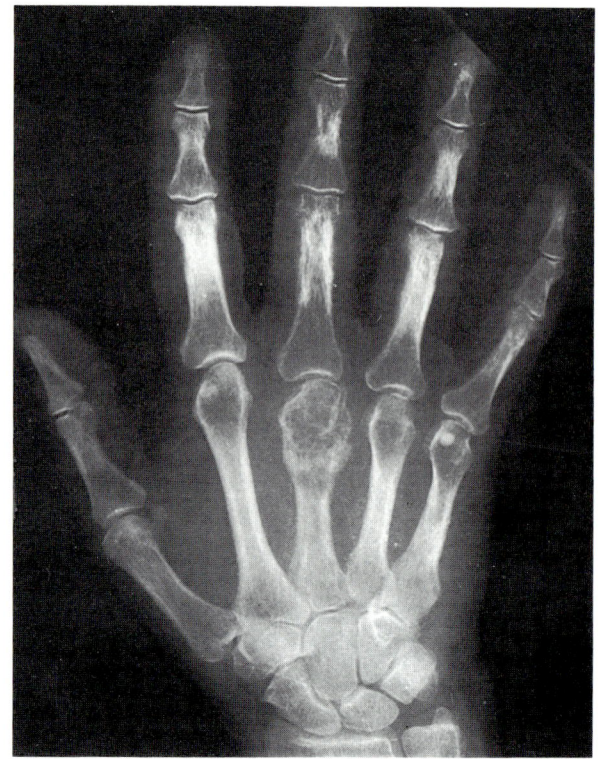

Q1a.

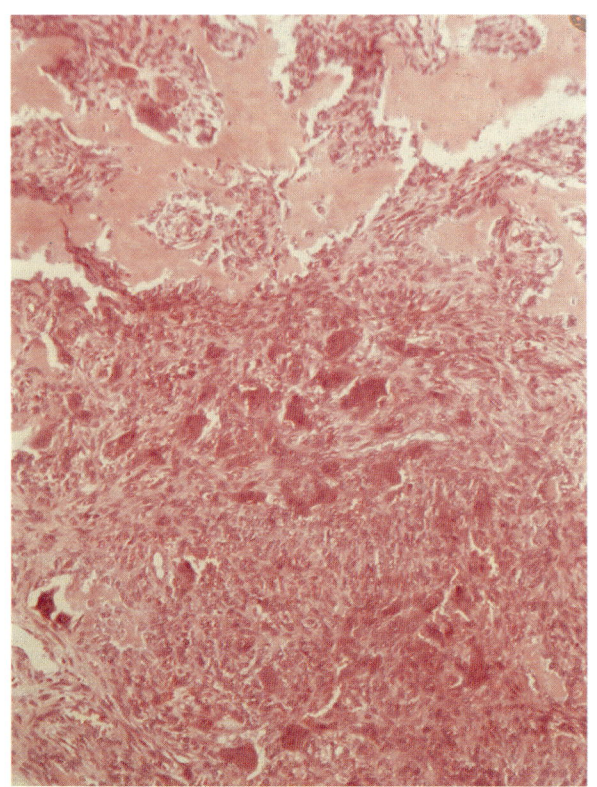

Q1b. (×105)

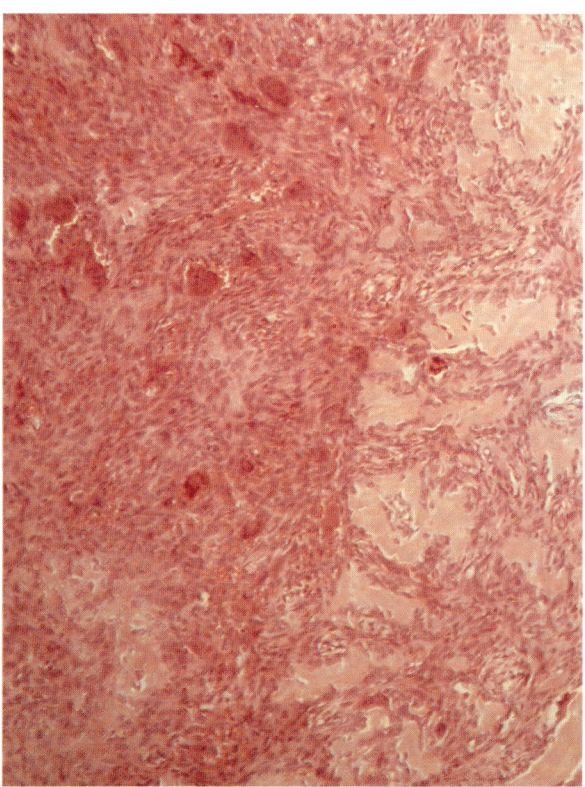

Q1c. (×105)

Q2. This 56-year-old female was admitted to hospital because of pain in the shoulder which had been present for some months.

This patient also complained of 'rheumatism', particularly affecting her hips, buttocks, thighs and feet.

On clinical examination, a tender swelling of the scapula was palpated, with limitation of all movements of the shoulder.

Radiological examination confirmed the presence of a large, expanding osteolytic lesion of the scapula, extending from the subarticular portion of the glenoid fossa and having a clearly defined endosteal margin with a narrow zone of transition.

A biopsy was performed.

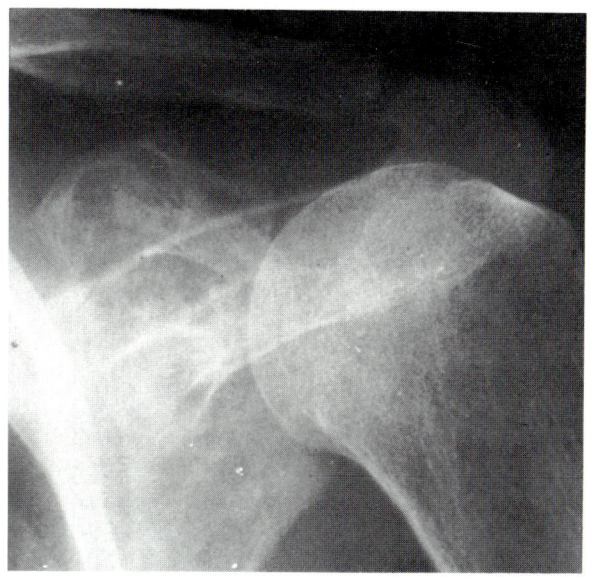

Q2a.

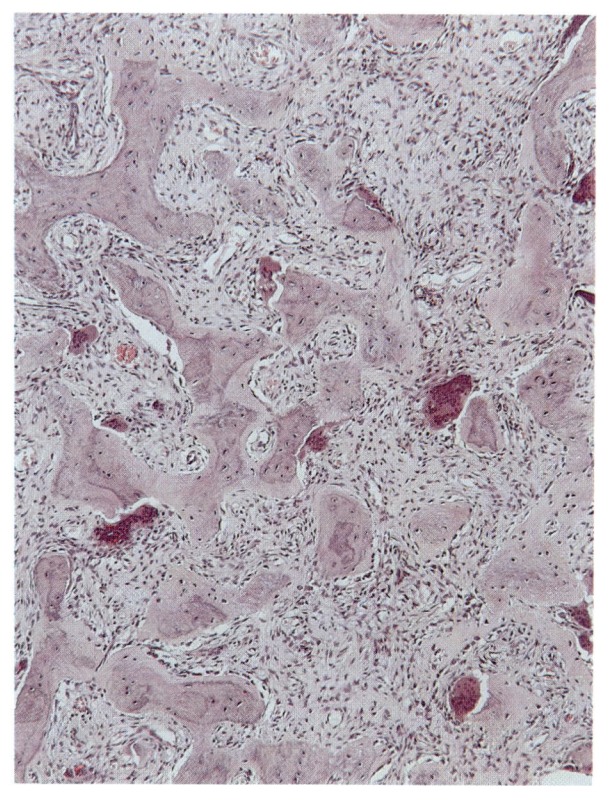

Q2b. (×67)

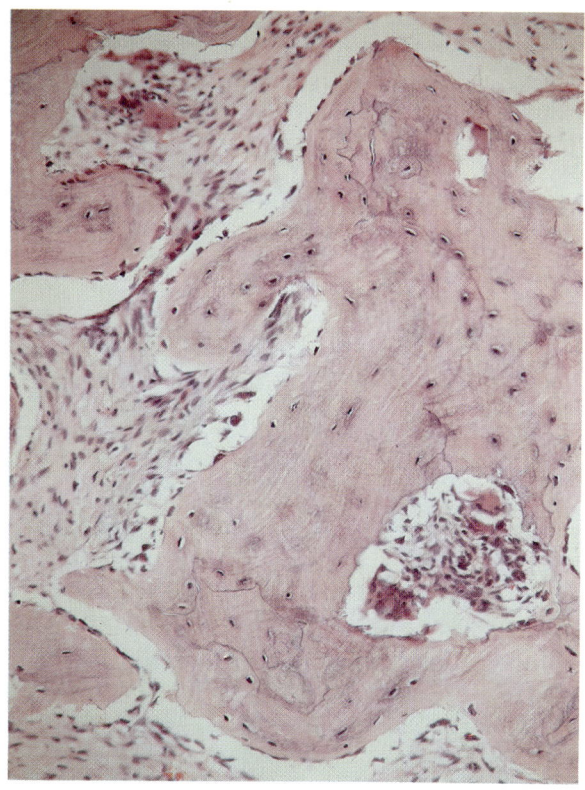

Q2c. (×110)

A1. Primary hyperparathyroidism

In hyperparathyroidism, biochemical and radiological evidence normally alerts the clinician to the diagnosis. In this case, however, the pertinent information was overlooked, and the surgeon explored the lesion under the erroneous impression that it was a bone tumour. The subarticular location of this destructive and enlarging bone lesion would, at an earlier age, certainly have been consistent with a giant-cell tumour, the presumptive pre-operative diagnosis. The correct diagnosis of hyperparathyroidism, however, should have been suggested by the association of this osteolytic area, particularly in an elderly patient, with the diffuse osteopenia. The latter had been ascribed to disuse osteoporosis (see Exercise 3), but, in addition, the radial aspects of the shafts of middle phalanges of the middle and ring fingers had lost their normal cortical outline and had become excessively concave. This feature, indeed, represents a classical radiological sign of this disorder and is illustrated in greater detail in Fig. 1.2a. As might have been expected, skeletal survey revealed further manifestations of hyperparathyroidism elsewhere in the skeleton. The diagnosis was established finally by the biochemical findings, and specifically by the greatly elevated serum calcium, the low serum inorganic phosporus, the raised serum alkaline phosphatase and the increased urinary calcium:

Serum calcium	13.4 mg% (3.3 mmol/litre)
Serum inorganic phosphorus	2.4 mg% (0.8 mmol/litre)
Serum alkaline phosphatase	26.2 KA units (185 IU/litre)
Urinary calcium	455 mg in 24 h (11.4 mmol in 24 h)
Blood urea nitrogen	24.4 mg% (4.0 mmol/litre)

As may be appreciated, opportunities for histological study in this entity are infrequent. The biopsy (Q1b and c) shows a combination of spindle-celled tissue containing osteoclast giant cells and trabeculae of newly formed reactive bone. These changes are completely consistent with a diagnosis of hyperparathyroidism, but they illustrate the close histological resemblance to giant-cell tumour which can occur in this condition (see Exercise 15).

Following operation, discussion of the clinical, radiological, biochemical and histological data made it clear that not only did the patient have primary hyperparathyroidism, but that the metacarpal lesion was part of this condition, representing a classical 'brown' tumour.

The patient's neck was explored and a parathyroid adenoma was removed from the lower pole of the right lobe of the thyroid. Following operation the raised serum calcium returned rapidly to normal, and a few weeks later the serum alkaline phosphatase, too, was normal. The radiological abnormalities regressed also, a normal bone texture being restored within a few months and dense sclerosis developing within the 'brown' tumour (Fig. 1.1).

This case illustrates the importance of co-ordinated discussion of clinical, radiological and laboratory data in cases of bone disease.

A2. Secondary hyperparathyroidism in osteomalacia

As in the previous case (Q1), biochemical abnormalities should have alerted the clinician to a diagnosis of metabolic bone disease. Once again this pertinent information was overlooked, and the surgeon explored the lesion on the assumption that it was a localised—and presumably solitary—lesion of the scapula.

In this instance the expanding lytic lesion in the scapula caused a wide differential diagnosis to be offered radiologically. An osteolytic metastasis, especially from a renal or thyroid primary tumour, was preferred initially to a giant-cell tumour arising relatively late in life. The possibility of a plasmacytoma was considered. Although mentioned pre-operatively, a 'brown tumour' of hyperpara-

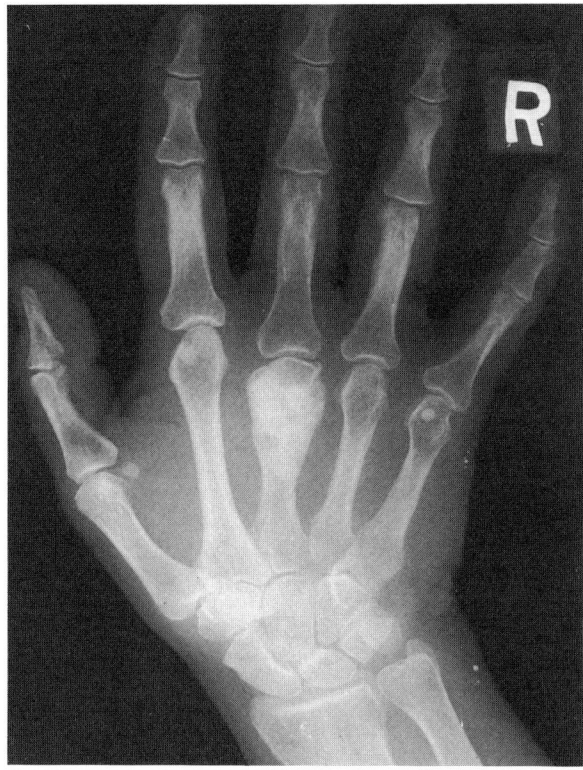

Fig. 1.1. Five months after excision of the parathyroid adenoma the 'brown tumour' had been replaced by dense sclerotic bone and the osteopenia and subperiosteal erosions had regressed completely.

thyroidism—the correct diagnosis—was not supported by frank evidence of such a disorder in other radiological studies, including particularly the hands.

The biopsy (Q2b and c) showed replacement of the normal bone by fibrous tissue containing many newly formed trabeculae and prominent osteoclast giant cells. These histological changes are not specific. In Q2b the appearances perhaps could result from fibrous dysplasia or even atypical Paget's disease. The numerous irregular cement lines in Q2c might be thought to support the latter diagnosis. The cement lines, however, do not show the typical 'mosaic' pattern of Paget's disease, and merely represent the accelerated bone turnover caused by excess circulating parathyroid hormone. The underlying osteomalacia might be suspected from the pale-staining tissue on the surfaces of many of the bone trabeculae in Q2b. Its presence was confirmed subsequently by the demonstration of large amounts of osteoid tissue in appropriately stained undecalcified sections from an iliac crest biopsy (see Q2b in Exercise 3).

The all-important biochemical findings, performed after the biopsy, indicating a major error in diagnostic approach, were as follows:

Serum calcium	8.8 mg% (2.2 mmol/litre)
Serum inorganic phosphorus	2.5 mg% (0.8 mmol/litre)
Serum alkaline phosphatase	80 KA units (610 IU/litre)
Blood urea nitrogen	22 mg% (3.5 mmol/litre)

The greatly elevated serum alkaline phosphatase was a non-specific indication of bone disease, while the low serum calcium was consistent with osteomalacia. At this time a hitherto unappreciated factor in the patient's history was reconsidered. At the age of 28 years a gastrojejunostomy for a duodenal ulcer had been performed. The diagnosis is one of osteomalacia due to intestinal malabsorption following the gastric surgery. The lesion of the scapula is a manifestation of the secondary hyperparathyroidism induced by the low serum calcium. It is a reminder that secondary hyperparathyroidism need not be accompanied by the high serum calcium which is characteristic of primary hyperparathyroidism.

As expected in malabsorption osteomalacia, the patient responded well to treatment with vitamin D and calcium, with resolution of the radiological abnormalities in the skeleton, improvement of the 'rheumatic' pains, and the return of the serum calcium and alkaline phosphatase to normal.

Hyperparathyroidism

The hormone elaborated by the parathyroid glands controls osteoclastic activity and regulates renal excretion of phosphorus. Excessive parathyroid activity is accompanied by elevation of the serum calcium level and increased loss of calcium and phosphorus in the urine. The increased bone turnover is indicated by increased urinary hydroxyproline excretion. In *primary* hyperparathyroidism the excessive activity is due usually to a parathyroid adenoma or, less often, to parathyroid hyperplasia. In only 1% of cases is a carcinoma responsible. Primary hyperparathyroidism is more common in women than men. It was originally regarded as a rare disease but more recently the incidence had been estimated at 1 per 2000 in the population. Although biochemical findings of a raised serum calcium and a low serum phosphorus strongly suggest the diagnosis, confirmation by demonstrating a high circulating level of parathyroid hormone (by immunoassay) is appropriate. Parathyroid antisera differ in their sensitivity and specificity, and conflicting results are sometimes obtained.

A low serum calcium, whatever the cause, will stimulate parathyroid function and hyperplasia of the parathyroid glands, causing *secondary* hyperparathyroidism. The most important of these causes is renal failure resulting in phosphate retention, but others include osteomalacia and rickets of almost any origin.

The hormone calcitonin, produced by the thyroid, is essentially antagonistic to parathyroid hormone.

Clinical Features

Most cases of primary hyperparathyroidism present because of urinary calculi. Symptomatic or radiological bone disease is present in only about 20% of cases. These patients, in whom skeletal involvement is the presenting feature, are subject to urolithiasis and occasionally develop nephrolithiasis. In a smaller group neither nephrolithiasis nor overt bone disease occurs, the disease presenting only with evidence of hypercalcaemia. It has been postulated that these variants are due to different degrees of activity within parathyroid adenomas. One type grows slowly, is of low activity and is associated with nephrolithiasis. In these patients elevation of the serum calcium is not excessive and the tumour itself is relatively small. Symptoms are prolonged (mean duration 6.8 years). In contrast, patients with overt bone disease have much larger tumours, a higher serum calcium level and a shorter (mean 3.6 years) symptomatic period (Lloyd et al.).

The clinical manifestations of this disorder, therefore, can be divided into those attributable to hypercalcaemia, to bone disease and to renal disease.

Hypercalcaemia may cause a variety of misleading symptoms which may delay diagnosis, such as anorexia, indigestion and constipation. Rapidly rising levels of serum calcium lead to nausea and vomiting, frequently accompanied by generalised lassitude and severe muscle weakness. Exceptionally, a palpable swelling may be present in the neck, but occasionally the primary tumour arises in an ectopic focus in the mediastinum.

Overt skeletal abnormalities develop in approximately a quarter of patients with primary hyperparathyroidism, so that they do not necessarily accompany hypercalcaemia, although bone pain and tenderness are commonly present. In such cases, mobilisation of calcium results in characteristic radiological features described below. Their clinical effects include deformities and pathological fractures. The latter, indeed, may occur spontaneously and draw attention to the disease. The most common injury of this type is a compression fracture of a vertebral body.

Urinary tract symptoms due to hypercalcaemia usually present early as polydipsia and polyuria, as a result of the diuresis associated with the increased excretion of calcium. The formation of renal calculi is common. Especially when such calculi are bilateral this diagnosis always should be considered. Population studies have shown that at least 5% of patients presenting with recurrent renal calculi have a parathyroid adenoma. A later complication in patients with bone disease is the development of nephrocalcinosis due to the deposition of calcium phosphate in renal papillae; this contributes to hypertension and ultimate renal failure.

As mentioned above, secondary hyperparathyroidism is a sequel to diseases which produce a persistently low serum calcium, particularly rickets, osteomalacia and chronic renal failure. In an attempt to restore a normal calcium–phosphorus balance the parathyroid glands respond by reactive hyperplasia. These patients have low or normal values of serum calcium, but radiological and histological studies demonstrate changes in bone comparable to those encountered in the primary form.

Secondary hyperparathyroidism may lead on to a tertiary form in which an autonomous parathyroid adenoma develops and then causes hypercalcaemia. It is a particular problem in patients with renal failure treated by regular dialysis.

Radiological Features

1. Site. A parathyroid tumour itself may be detected, sometimes with the aid of a barium swallow or by more sophisticated investigations, including ultrasound and CT scanning. Since the primary effect of the disease in the skeleton is to mobilise calcium phosphate, all bones may be affected, causing diffuse and non-specific osteopenia. Localised radiological abnormalities are not detectable in earlier stages. The initial and specific sign is subperiosteal resorption of bone. This feature almost invariably develops first on the radial aspects of the middle phalanges of the index and middle fingers. Other typical skeletal sites to be affected in the same way, but nearly always occurring after the phalangeal lesions, include the outer ends of the clavicles (sometimes permitting the entity to be recognised on routine examination of the chest), the medial aspects of the proximal ends of the tibia and femur, the ischial tuberosities and the margins of the symphysis pubis. Loss of the specialised cortex, the lamina dura, around the roots of the teeth may be a helpful sign, but is less specific than was regarded formerly. In advanced stages excessive resorption of terminal phalanges may be apparent. Cystic lesions ('brown tumours') may be detectable in later stages, but exceptionally, as in Q2, may be the only diagnostic feature. They are said to have a predilection for facial bones, but may be encountered anywhere in the skeleton. They are subject to pathological fractures, which may result in residual deformities even after successful treatment.

2. Appearance. Widespread and generalised osteopenia is characteristic. This osteopenia becomes even more prominent in the bones of a limb following a pathological fracture. In the skull it causes a rather granular appearance. The subperiosteal erosions have poorly defined margins and may be detected more easily in their earliest stage with magnification techniques. The 'brown tumours' which develop relatively late in the disease usually are evident as well defined and often expansile osteolytic areas. The solitary lesion, as in Q1, may simulate a giant-cell tumour or other benign cystic forms of bone disease, such as aneurysmal bone cysts or fibrous dysplasia. Indeed, the resemblance to the latter may be very striking after successful excision of the primary tumour. Exceptionally dense sclerosis develops during the process of repair. Multiple 'brown tumours' may arouse consideration in differential diagnosis of osteolytic metastases, myelomatosis or histiocytosis. The appearance created by such multiple lesions was described in the past as 'osteitis fibrosa cystica', a term somewhat unsatisfactory as it was used also in connection with fibrous dysplasia.

As indicated above, renal calculi or nephrocalcinosis may suggest the diagnosis. Calcification in soft tissues may occur in the primary form of the disease in the menisci of the knee, articular cartilage (being one cause of chondrocalcinosis) or even synovial membranes. It is, however, less striking than the diffuse and generalised deposition of calcium phosphate which occurs in the terminal stages of renal failure with secondary hyperparathyroidism, when mobilisation from bone continues while urinary excretion is impaired.

In secondary hyperparathyroidism most of the changes described above are superimposed on those of the primary disorder, such as rickets, with lucent metaphyses, or osteomalacia, with Looser zones. These entities themselves may cause complicating deformities, such as bowing of the long bones of the legs from childhood rickets or compression of the pelvis from osteomalacia. 'Brown tumours', however, are distinctly less common, possibly because the patient is either treated successfully for the underlying disorder or, in the case of renal failure, does not survive long enough for them to develop. A feature which still lacks a valid explanation is the dense sclerosis which often occurs in the vertebral end-plates, producing the so-called 'sandwich vertebra' or 'rugger jersey' spine. This appearance is observed only rarely in the primary form of the disease.

Pathological Features

The primary effect of parathyroid hormone on bone is the stimulation of osteoclastic resorption, although not all cases of primary hyperparathyroidism show histological evidence of this, even when quantitative morphometric studies of biopsy material are carried out. When sufficiently active, osteoclastic resorption is followed by fibrous replacement of bone, resulting in the 'osteitis fibrosa' of older terminology. Changes may be diffuse or focal, resulting in generalised rarefaction of bone or in localised lesions where haemorrhage, reactive bone formation and cystic change may also be found. These localised lesions are often referred to as 'brown tumours'.

While the osteoclast is clearly the main agent of bone resorption in hyperparathyroidism, the idea of osteocytic resorption has also been discussed, but still remains controversial.

Treatment

In primary hyperparathyroidism, the treatment consists of the identification and the removal of the primary adenoma. Such operations may be technically difficult and may require exploration of the mediastinum. Multiple adenomata may be encountered. When generalised hyperplasia is present, only 200 mg of parathyroid tissue should be left. When correctly performed, the clinical results from these procedures are excellent. An iatrogenic complication has occurred infrequently after inadvertent total excision of the parathyroids, resulting after an interval of a few weeks in post-operative tetany. This entity, due to a drastic reduction in the serum calcium level, causes hyperexcitability of nerve and muscle, demonstrated clinically by a positive Chvostek sign. Muscular spasms occasionally have been sufficiently severe to cause bilateral and spontaneous fractures of the femoral necks. Tetany may occur also in the rare congenital and idiopathic disorders of hypoparathyroidism, pseudohypoparathyroidism and pseudopseudohypoparathyroidism.

In secondary hyperparathyroidism, treatment is directed to the control of the underlying disorder.

In tertiary hyperparathyroidism the condition should be treated by parathyroidectomy.

References

Genant HK et al. (1973) Primary hyperparathyroidism. Radiology 109: 513–524
Habener JH, Potts JT (1978) Parathyroid physiology and primary hyperparathyroidism. In: Avioli LS, Krane SM (eds) Metabolic bone disease, vol 2. Academic Press, New York
Lloyd HM (1968) Primary hyperparathyroidism. An analysis of the role of the parathyroid tumour. Medicine (Balt) 47: 53–71
Wells SA, Leight GS, Ross AJ (1980) Primary hyperparathyroidism. Current problems in surgery. Year Book Medical Publishers, Chicago London. 17, 18 398–463

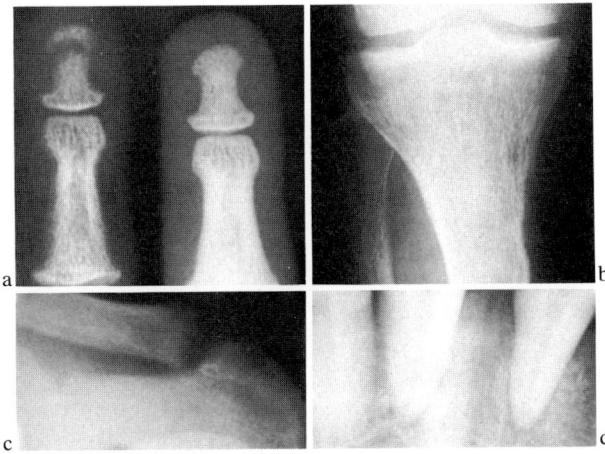

Fig. 1.2. *Hyperparathyroidism—classical erosions.* **a** *Phalanx.* Typical cortical resorption is illustrated on the radial aspect of the middle phalanx of an index finger. Observe also the generalised osteopenia and the lucency below the tuft of the terminal phalanx, Compare these changes with the normal control. **b** *Proximal end of tibia.* The erosion on the medial aspect of the tibial shaft has occurred at a common site. The generalised osteopenia in this 62-year-old woman was found on examination for pain in both knees. Observe incidentally meniscal calcification. Typical erosions then were demonstrated in the hands. **c** *Outer end of clavicle.* Such an erosion can provide a diagnostic clue in a chest film. Its margin, typically, is poorly defined. **d** *Teeth.* Absorption of the specialised cortex surrounding the roots of the teeth— the lamina dura—provides a valuable, but not infallible, diagnostic sign.

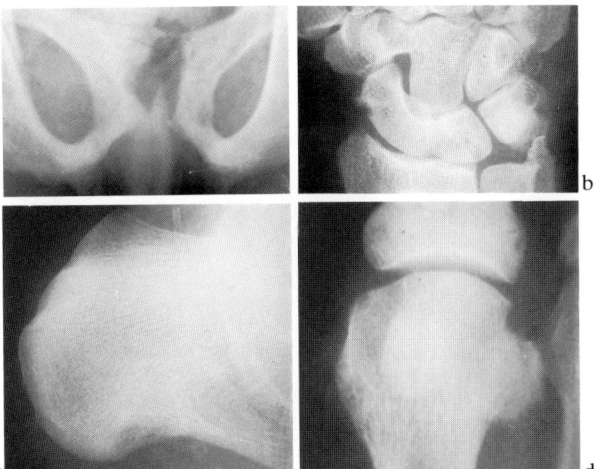

Fig. 1.3. *Hyperparathyroidism—erosions at less common sites.* In each of these cases the hands also were affected. **a** *Ischial tuberosities and symphysis pubis.* **b** *Styloid processes of radius and ulna and scaphoid.* **c** *Calcaneus* at attachment of plantar fascia. Note vascular calcification. **d** *Sesamoid of hallux.* Resorption on the phalanges of the feet is very rare, possibly because they are subjected to less stress than the phalanges of the hands.

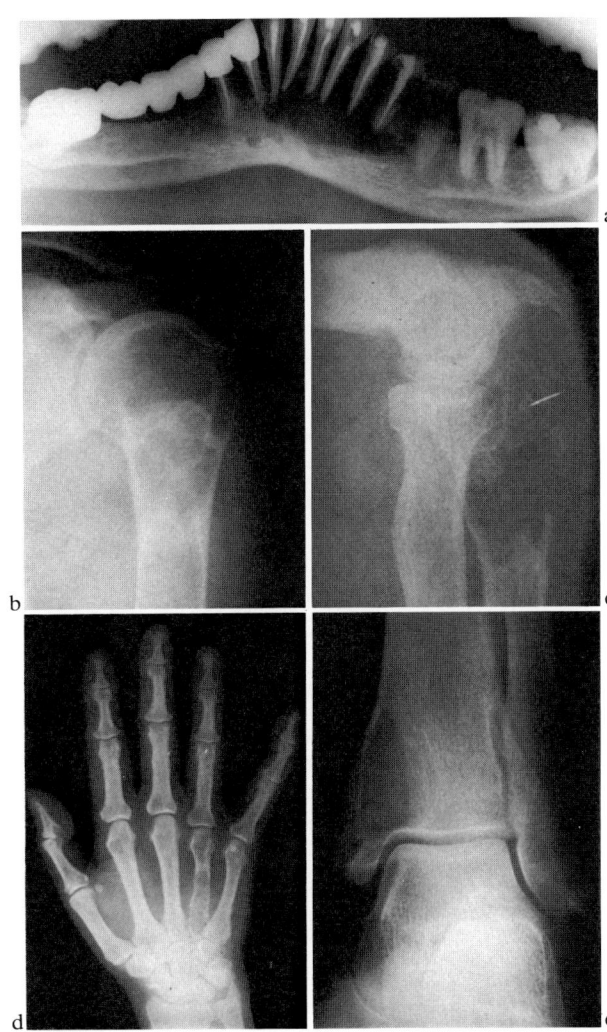

Fig. 1.4. *Hyperparathyroidism—'brown tumours'.* Some examples of these expanding lytic lesions, which are found usually in post-menopausal women presenting with localised bone pain. In each case phalangeal erosions confirmed the diagnosis. **a** *Mandible.* Involvement of the facial bones is common. Observe resorption of the lamina dura. **b** *Head of humerus.* Erosion of the outer end of the clavicle provides a diagnostic clue. **c** *Ulna* with a pathological fracture and generalised osteopenia. **d** *2nd and 4th metacarpals* with numerous phalangeal erosions. **e** *Medial malleolus of tibia*, with characteristic osteopenia.

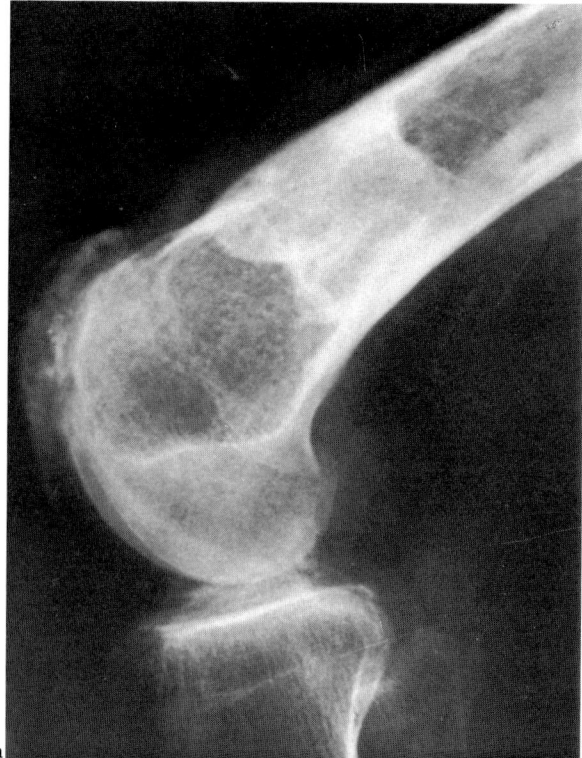

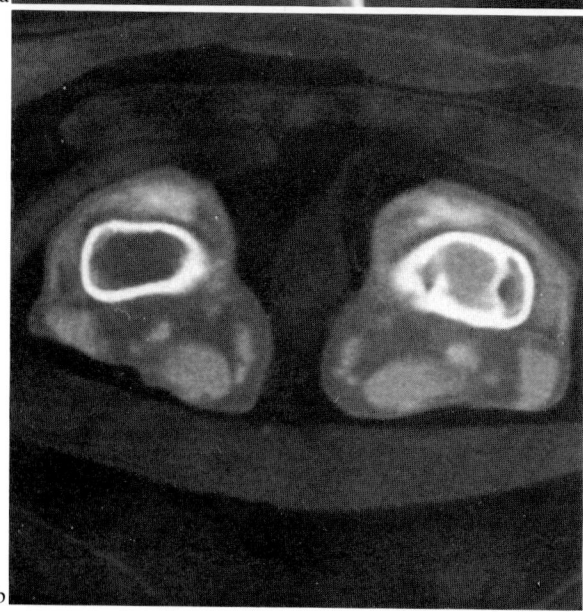

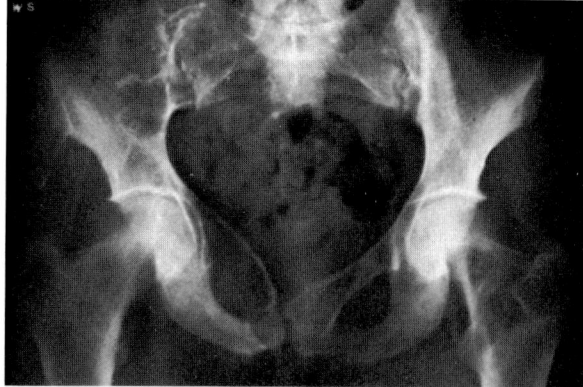

Fig. 1.5. *Hyperparathyroidism—value of CT.* **a** Another example of 'brown tumours' in the distal end of the femur in a patient with established disease. **b** The CT scan demonstrates excellently the size of this lesion.

Fig. 1.6. *Hyperparathyroidism—sequel of surgical treatment.* **a** This 24-year-old woman presented with classical symptoms of polydipsia, polyuria and pelvic pain. Numerous 'brown tumours' were present in the pelvis and femoral necks. Observe incidentally subperiosteal resorption of the femoral necks and the margins of the symphysis pubis. Symptoms were relieved promptly by excision of a large parathyroid adenoma. **b** Two years later the patient was asymptomatic. All the lesions had consolidated with some residual deformity, the appearance then resembling fibrous dysplasia.

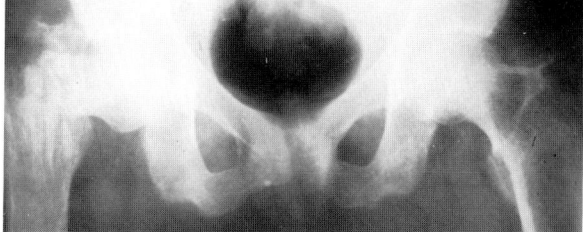

Fig. 1.7. *Hyperparathyroidism—post-operative tetany.* This 43-year-old woman presented with renal colic. Rather unusually, a urinary calculus was associated with overt bone disease, including generalised osteopenia and erosions on the ischial tuberosities and symphysis pubis. Multiple parathyroid adenomas were excised, but inadvertently total parathyroidectomy was performed at the same time. The serum calcium fell to 3.3 mg% (0.8 mmol/litre) and tetany ensued. Muscular spasms were sufficiently severe to cause this spontaneous fracture of the left femoral neck.

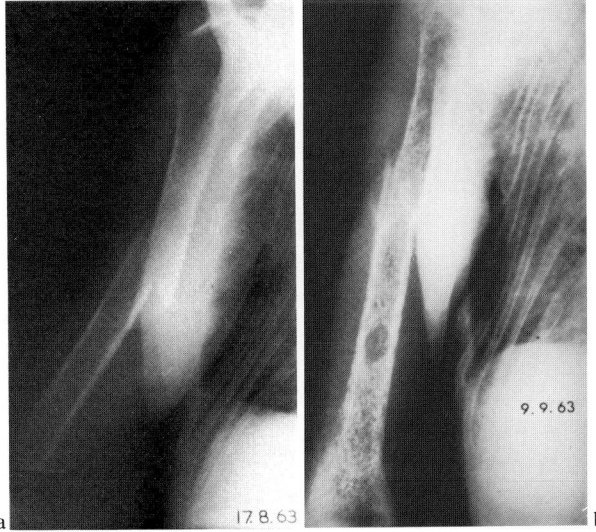

Fig. 1.8. *Primary hyperparathyroidism.* A spontaneous and pathological fracture of the right humerus drew attention to this disorder in a 51-year-old man. This series illustrates nearly all the classical features of overt bone disease in primary hyperparathyroidism. **a** The oblique fracture had occurred through a demineralised humerus in which the rounded lucency of a 'brown tumour' was evident. **b** Only 24 days later the osteopenia and the 'brown tumour' became much more pronounced, presumably as a result of the hyperaemia caused by the fracture. In both studies deformities of the ribs were evident. **c** The slender deformed ribs, many of which were fractured, were clearly evident in a film of the chest. Other stigmata included erosion of the right clavicle and scoliosis due to vertebral collapse, as shown **d** in the lumbar spine. Classical nephrocalcinosis was present. **e** Typical changes were present in the hands, particularly the right, in this film obtained 24 days after the injury. **f** The granular pattern of osteopenia in the skull was typical of the disorder. Following excision of three parathyroid adenomas, the patient made an excellent recovery.

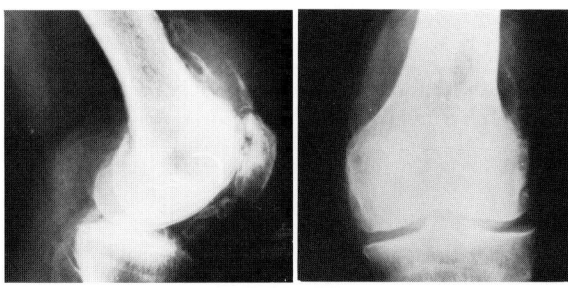

Fig. 1.9. *Primary hyperparathyroidism—ectopic calcification.* This 72-year-old woman, who complained of increasing pain in the knees for 7 months, also gave a history of constipation, thirst and polyuria for the previous year. In addition to the usual features of osteopenia and erosions, especially on the patella, less common calcification of the menisci and articular cartilage was evident. The condition is one important cause of chondrocalcinosis or hydroxyapatite deposition disease. These changes were symmetrical. Even more unusual was extensive calcification of the synovial membrane. Typical changes in the hands confirmed the diagnosis and immediate improvement was achieved by excision of a parathyroid adenoma.

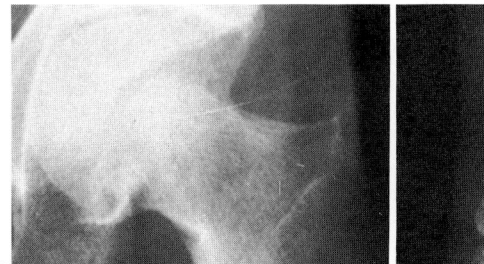

Fig. 2.1. *Secondary hyperparathyroidism in osteomalacia.* Radiological examination following the positive biochemical findings in the patient in Q2 revealed **a** a typical Looser zone on the medial side of the left femoral neck. Retrospective study of films of the hands did reveal **b** a concavity suspicious of an erosion on the radial side of the middle phalanx of the right middle finger. As indicated above, very exceptionally a 'brown tumour' may develop before the usual earliest sign of subperiosteal phalangeal resorption develops.

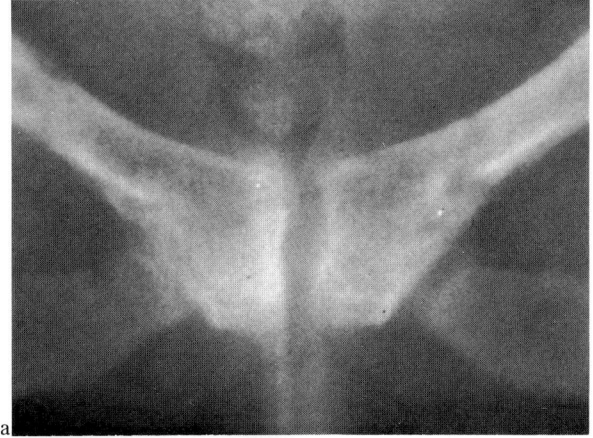
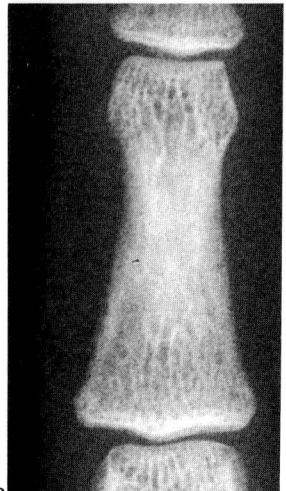

Fig. 2.2. *Secondary hyperparathyroidism.* This 24-year-old woman was an immigrant from India and developed osteomalacia by adhering to a vegetarian diet. **a** In addition to Looser zones in the obturator rings, hyperparathyroid erosions were evident around the symphysis pubis and **b** in their earliest stages, in some of the phalanges of the fingers.

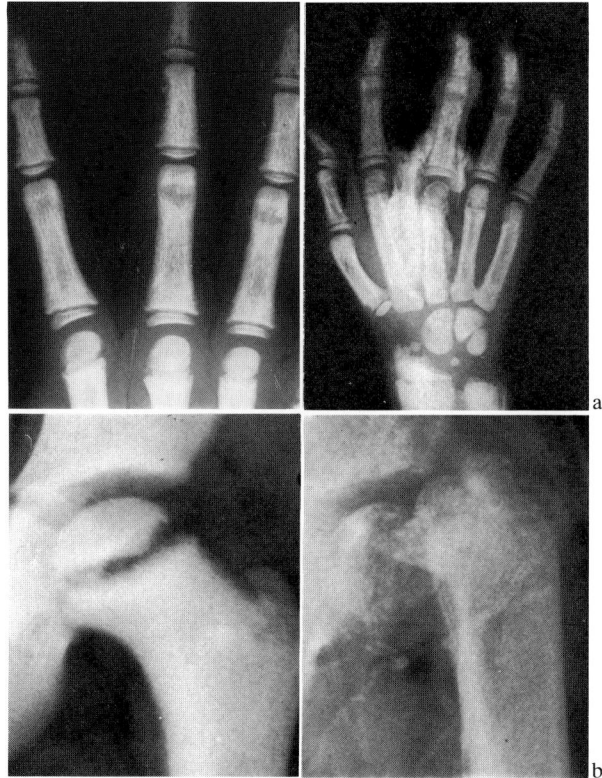

Fig. 2.4. *Secondary hyperparathyroidism in renal failure.* This 8-year-old boy presented with pain in the hips and knees. Gross rachitic changes deteriorated during the survival period of 22 months and were accompanied by massive calcification of vessels and soft tissues. At autopsy the kidneys were extremely atrophic and massive parathyroid hyperplasia was found. These serial studies demonstrated progression of the disease. **a** *Hands.* Typical erosions enlarged and massive calcification occurred in the soft tissues. **b** The left hip initially displayed rickets by failure of ossification of the proximal femoral metaphysis. The later film illustrates extreme destruction, likened to 'a post rotting within the earth', and such severe demineralisation that the calcified circumflex artery can be identified through the femur. All these abnormalities were symmetrical and the remainder of the skeleton was similarly affected.

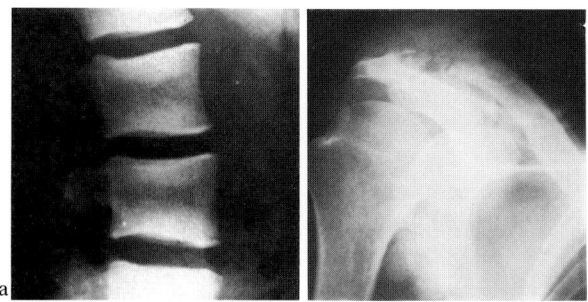

Fig. 2.3. *Secondary hyperparathyroidism.* **a** The 'rugger jersey' spine or 'sandwich vertebra' which occurs in this disorder presents a characteristic appearance. It is encountered only rarely in the primary form of the disease. The extreme density of the upper and lower portions of the vertebral bodies is not completely explained, but may be associated with a calcitonin effect. **b** Massive soft tissue calcification occurred in this man while undergoing prolonged renal dialysis, a recognised complication of this procedure. Observe gross absorption of the outer end of the clavicle.

Q1. A 19-year-old nurse presented complaining of pain in the left shoulder and upper arm which had been present since she started nursing 6 months previously. She was aware of weakness in the left arm when lifting patients.

On examination, movement of the cervical spine was limited and spasm of the left trapezius muscle was evident. Routine physiotherapy failed to relieve these symptoms and signs.

Radiological examination, undertaken after symptoms had persisted for 9 months, revealed this large lytic lesion in the proximal end of the humerus. The endosteal margin is densely sclerosed and the zone of transition is narrow. Organised periosteal reaction has developed around the shaft, being more prominent on the lateral aspect.

The lesion was explored.

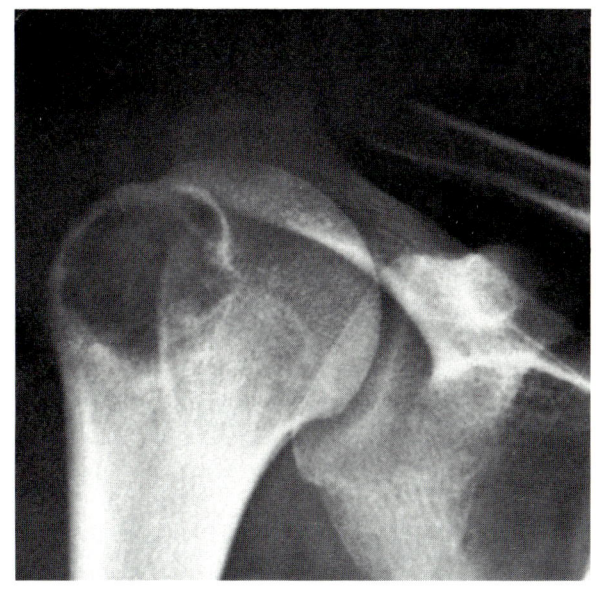

Q1a.

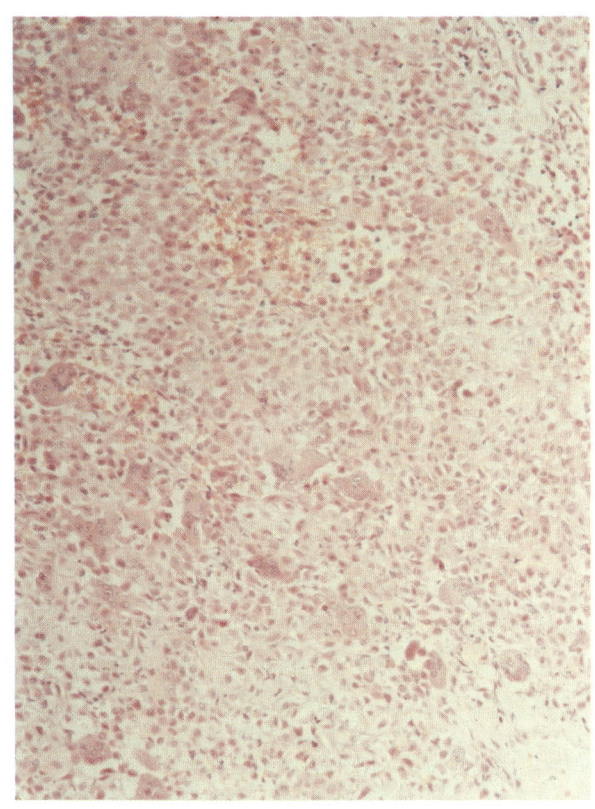

Q1b. (×140)

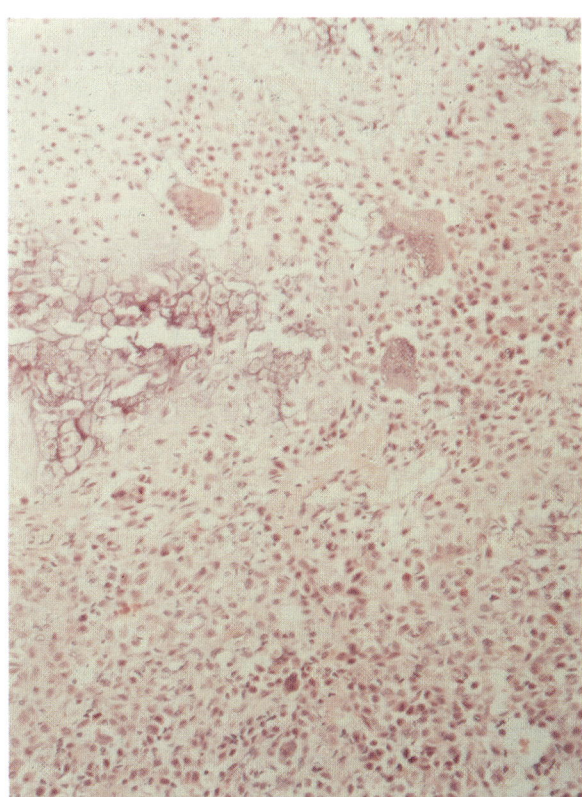

Q1c. (×140)

A1. Benign chondroblastoma of head of humerus

The clinical history of mild generalised discomfort in the shoulder and upper arm could have a number of explanations, including pain referred from the cervical spine, low-grade infection, synovitis, rotator cuff lesions and neoplasms.

The radiological appearance strongly suggested a benign neoplasm, particularly in view of the clearly defined and sclerotic peripheral margin with a narrow zone of transition. The site of the lesion corresponds to a former growth plate, from which structures these benign cartilaginous lesions are considered to originate. This pattern, in fact, is so characteristic of a benign chondroblastoma, particularly at this age, that no other diagnosis received serious consideration before the operation was undertaken.

The histological pattern also is characteristic of this benign tumour. The tissue is highly cellular, containing many, rather small, rounded cells with scattered and larger multinucleate giant cells (Q1b). In some areas (Q1c) these cells are separated by chondroid intercellular material, of which some is calcified.

Benign Chondroblastoma

This benign skeletal neoplasm is relatively uncommon, representing less than 1% of all benign bone tumours.

Approximately two males are affected for every female, and the lesion is most likely to occur in the first or second decade of life.

Clinical Features

The clinical manifestations of mild pain and tenderness, common to so many entities, are accompanied frequently by limitation of movement of an adjacent joint.

Radiological Features

1. Site. These tumours originate in growth plates, including those of apophyses. A predilection exists for the proximal ends of the humerus and femur and the area around the knee. Flat bones, such as the scapula, pelvis and even the patella are affected occasionally, but the spine and skull appear to be spared.

2. Appearance. The lesions are essentially osteolytic, with sclerotic endosteal margins and a narrow zone of transition. Characteristically the epiphysis is involved more extensively than the metaphysis. Associated organised periosteal reactions may be present. As the tumours mature, punctate calcification is likely to develop within them, emphasising their cartilaginous nature. Larger tumours may extend to the articular surface, consequently simulating, in the absence of calcification, a giant cell tumour (see Exercise 15). Equally, in some instances, cortical expansion and thinning may cause an aneurysmal bone cyst to be suggested (see Exercise 22). In such cases the definitive diagnosis is likely to depend on histological assessment.

Pathological Features

The present case illustrates the characteristic histological features of benign chondroblastoma, consisting of small-celled chondroblastic tissue, scattered giant cells and foci of chondroid matrix with calcification. The presence of giant cells sometimes causes diagnostic confusion with giant-cell tumour, but the age of the patient and the site of the lesion, as well as the absence of the spindle-celled stromal tissue of a giant-cell tumour, should help to avoid this diagnostic error.

Chondroblastomas are almost invariably benign, although, as an extreme rarity, instances of metastasis have been recorded.

Treatment

Curettage is usually curative, recurrence being rare if the procedure is performed thoroughly.

References

Diddell RJ, Louis CJ, Bromberger NA (1973) Pulmonary metastases from chondroblastoma of the tibia. J Bone Jt Surg 55B: 848–853

Jaffe HL, Lichtenstein L (1942) Benign chondroblastoma of bone. A reinterpretation of the so-called calcifying or chondromatous giant cell tumour. Am J Pathol 18: 969–978

McLeod RA, Beabout JW (1973) The roentgenographic features of chondroblastoma. Am J Roentgenol 118: 464–471

Schajowicz F, Gallardo H (1970) Epiphyseal chondroblastoma of bone. A clinico-pathological study of 69 cases. J Bone Jt Surg 52B: 205–226

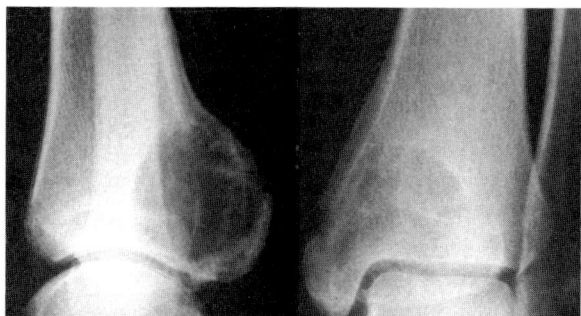

Fig. 1.3. *Chondroblastoma of tibia.* This 16-year-old boy had complained of chronic pain in the ankle. The large expansile lesion in the posteromedial portion of the distal end of the tibia has a well-defined endosteal margin. Some peripheral periosteal reaction had developed. The joint itself is unaffected. The appearance was considered before operation to be due to an aneurysmal bone cyst, but at operation solid tissue was found. The correct diagnosis should have been indicated by the peripheral bony shell being much thicker than the slender and atrophic shell surrounding an aneurysmal bone cyst.

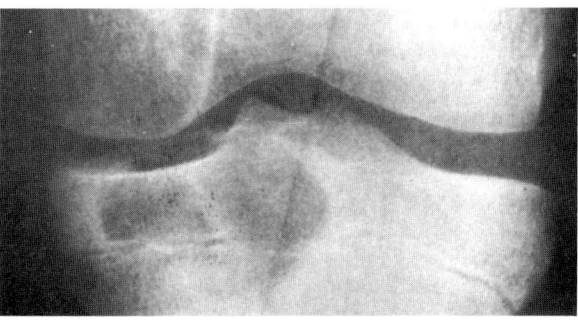

Fig. 1.1. *Chondroblastoma of tibia* in a 12-year-old boy presenting with moderately severe pain for several weeks. The lytic lesion traverses the growth plate, but has involved the epiphysis much more extensively than the metaphysis. Observe the clearly defined endosteal margin.

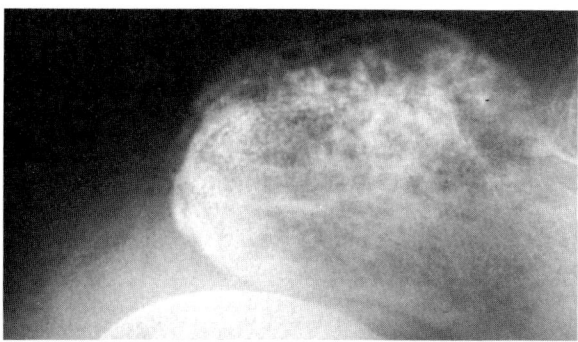

Fig. 1.4. *Chondroblastoma of acromion process.* This lesion illustrates involvement of an apophysis in a 14-year-old girl with discomfort in the shoulder of several months' duration. Some calcification is present.

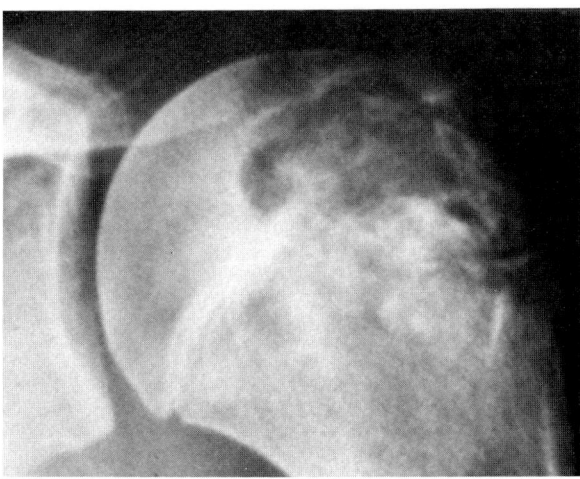

←

Fig. 1.2. *Chondroblastoma of humerus* in a 14-year-old girl who had complained of mild pain for several months. Again, the epiphysis is affected to a greater degree than the metaphysis. Punctate calcification indicates the tumour to be more mature. An organised periosteal reaction surrounds the proximal end of the humeral shaft.

Q1. This 42-year-old man complained of weakness of the right wrist and intermittent aching over a period of 5 years. These symptoms he attributed to a former injury for which a radiological examination 3 weeks later had revealed no abnormality.

Mild tenderness was elicited clinically, with minimal restriction of movement.

The radiographs at this time revealed a lucency within the lunate surrounded by diffuse increase of density in the remainder of this bone.

In view of the persistent symptoms the lunate was excised.

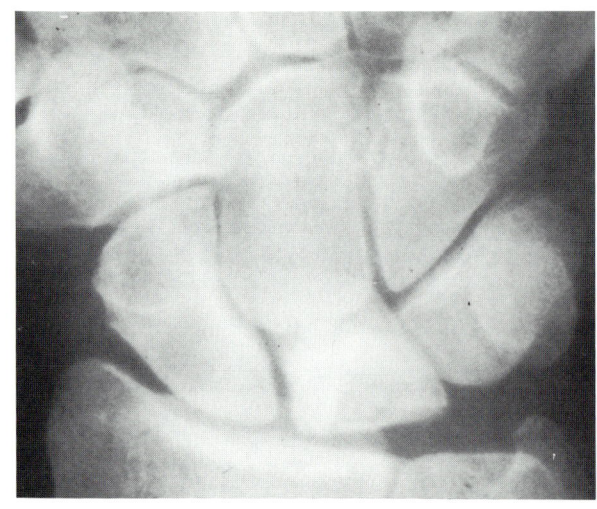

Q1a.

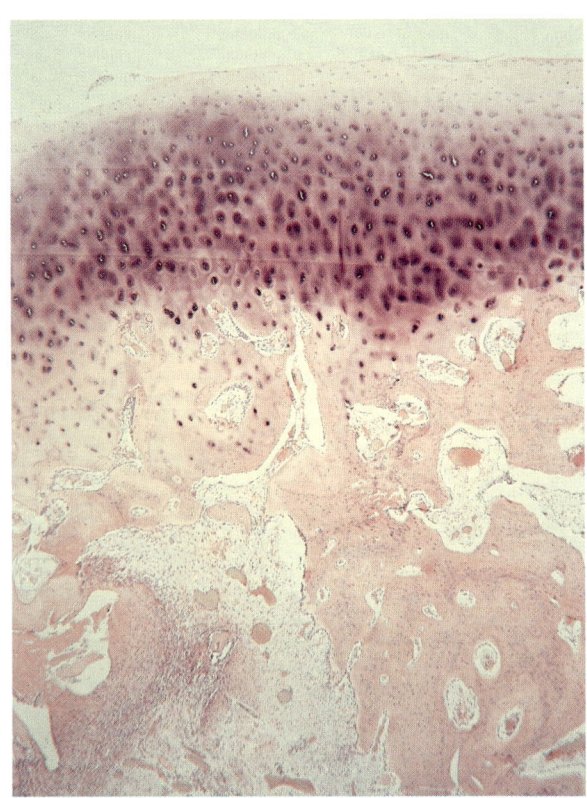

Q1b. (×26)

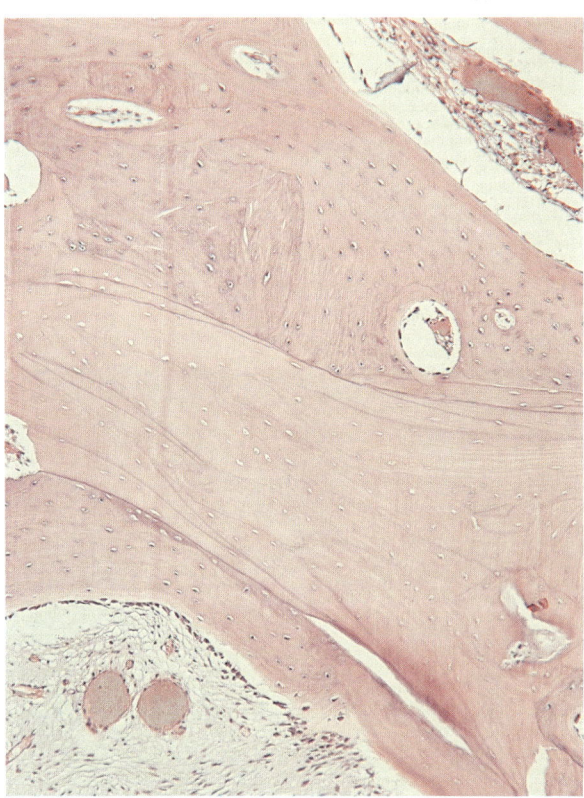

Q1c. (×70)

Q2. Pain and stiffness of the right elbow for 3 months caused this 13-year-old boy to seek medical advice, since discomfort was affecting his bowling at cricket.

On specific enquiry he admitted to a skateboard injury of this elbow, which had been incurred 2 years previously.

Clinical examination revealed no abnormality other than limitation of movement, especially pronation and supination. No history of locking of the joint was obtained.

Radiologically a lytic lesion with a sclerotic margin and a narrow zone of transition was shown in the former epiphysis for the capitulum, which had fused prematurely. Within this defect the presence of a central density was confirmed by tomography.

Surgical exploration was performed.

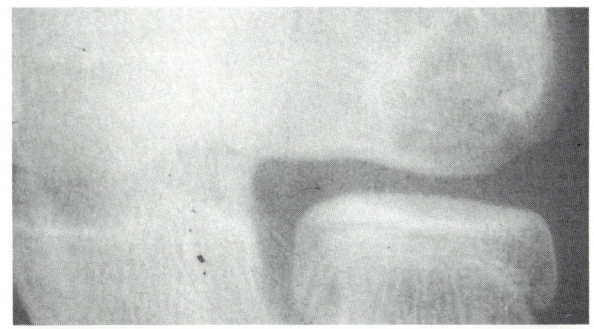
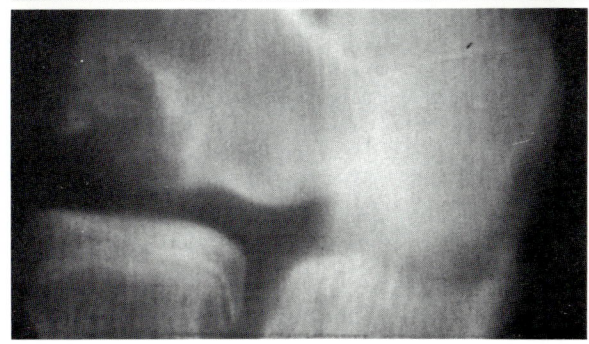

Q2a.

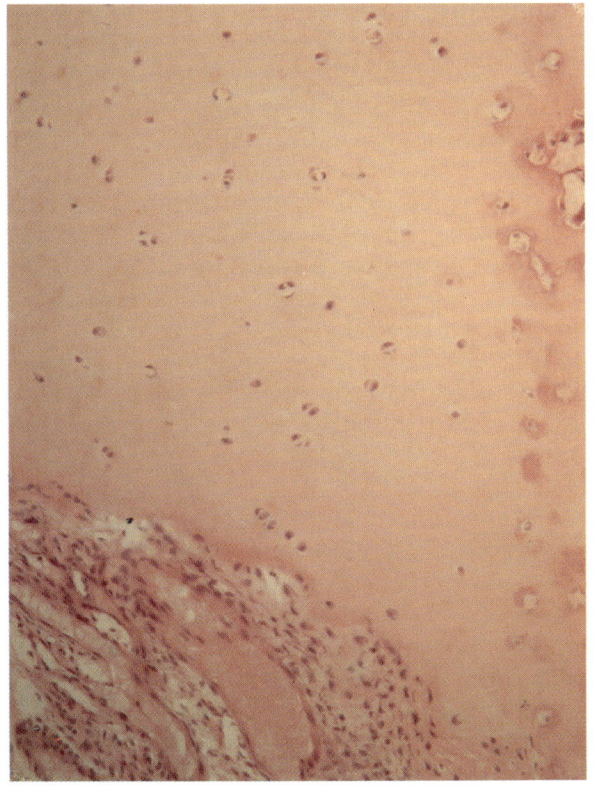

Q2b. (×100)

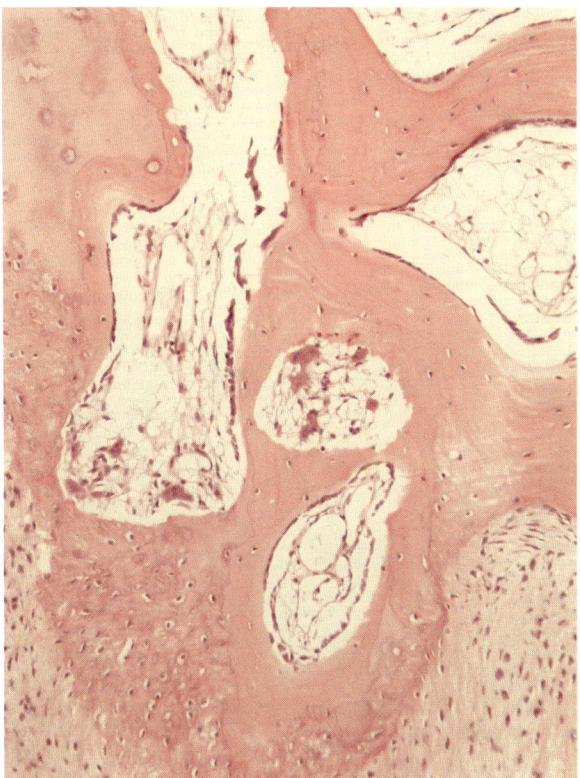

Q2c. (×100)

A1. Post-traumatic necrosis of lunate (Kienböck's disease)

The clinical history and the radiographic appearance are both typical of this entity, to which general reference has been made already in Exercise 7. The condition usually is encountered in young adults. It may be associated with congenitally short ulna, causing excessive stress at the apex of the carpal arch with consequent compromise of the vascular supply.

Q1b and c, from the excised bone, show widespread, patchy necrosis with newly formed viable bone covering the surfaces of the original dead trabeculae. The total amount of bone, as opposed to marrow space, is increased, accounting for the accentuated radiographic density. The area of radiographic lucency corresponds to a site where necrotic trabeculae have been resorbed and replaced by vascular fibrous tissue. The articular cartilage is normal, being intact and viable. In Q1c the viable newly formed bone, with nucleated osteocytes, is being produced by the surface of darkly staining osteoblasts. Its appearance contrasts with that of the deeper necrotic bone with its empty osteocyte lacunae.

Post-traumatic Necrosis of Individual Bones ('Osteochondritis')

Impairment of vascular supply to certain individual bones of growing epiphyseal centres may result in bone death. These lesions have been described in the past by the historical and somewhat inexact term. 'osteochondritis' with a variety of eponyms.

Clinical Features

Most of these abnormalities are recognised when radiological examination is undertaken on account of mild, localised pain of months' or even years' duration associated with restricted movement. Such symptoms may be very minor or possibly entirely absent so that the abnormalities may be detected incidentally. A history of a previous acute injury is obtained only seldom.

Radiological Features

1. Site. Individual bones affected include the lunate (Kienböck's disease), the navicular (Köhler's disease), the patella and, among others, even the sesamoids of the hallux. Certain epiphyseal centres, during the years of growth, are peculiarly liable to become necrotic, usually as a result of chronic stress. Reference to such change in the femoral head in children (Perthes' disease) has been made in Fig. 1.8 in Exercise 5. Similarly affected commonly may be the head of the 2nd metatarsal (Freiberg's disease) and the capitulum.

2. Appearance. As has been emphasised before, the development of radiographic evidence of bone death depends on secondary changes. No immediate alteration in the appearance of a bony segment affected by avascular necrosis can be recognised, although radionuclide scanning will show failure of uptake of the tracer. These secondary radiographic changes are attributable to collapse and fragmentation of a weakened bone structure, often associated with lucent areas due to resorption of the damaged trabeculae, or revascularisation. The former may result in permanent residual deformity, while the latter is indicated by progressive increase of sclerosis, reflecting the process of repair. Apparent density of a necrotic bone may be attributable to disuse osteoporosis of adjacent bones.

Pathological Features

On the rare occasions when histological study of these lesions is possible, the characteristic appearance of bone necrosis with revascularisation and repair is evident.

Treatment

Subject to the provision of appropriate protective measures, in the absence of actual damage to the affected bone, complete reconstitution may be expected, with relief of symptoms and restoration of a normal radiological pattern. When residual deformities have developed, however, surgical intervention may be indicated, as was the case in the patient illustrated in Q1.

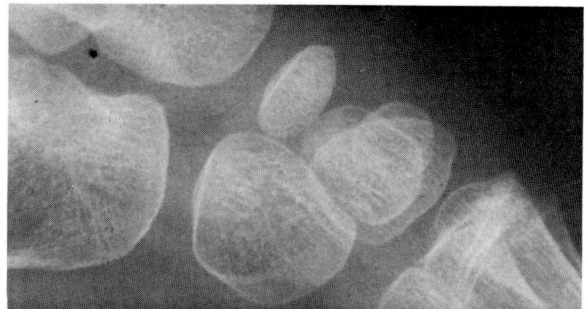
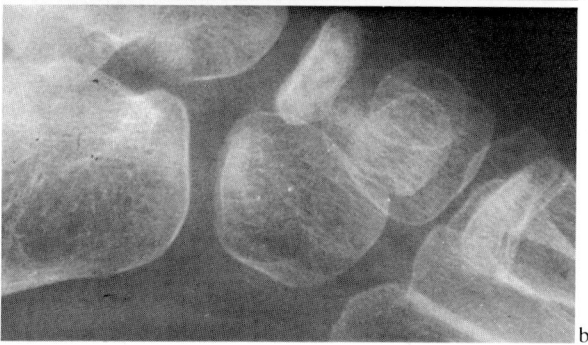

Fig. 1.1. *Köhler's disease.* This 8-year-old boy had complained of mild pain in the left foot for several weeks. The early film **a** showed diffusely increased density in the navicular, indicating revascularisation. Nevertheless, this bone was still fragile and 5 months later **b** it had undergone collapse and fragmentation.

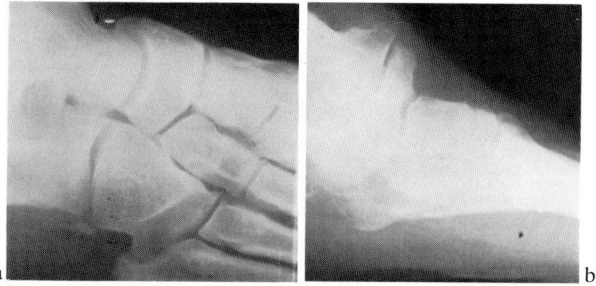

Fig. 1.2. *Post-traumatic necrosis of navicular ('adult osteochondritis').* At the age of 15 this girl had complained of chronic pain in the foot which had begun after a prolonged walking tour 6 months before. **a** No radiological abnormality was evident, but even then the navicular must have been necrotic, since pain continued and 5 years later **b** this bone was grossly flattened and deformed. Triple arthrodesis was necessary. Histologically the bone was dense, but no longer necrotic.

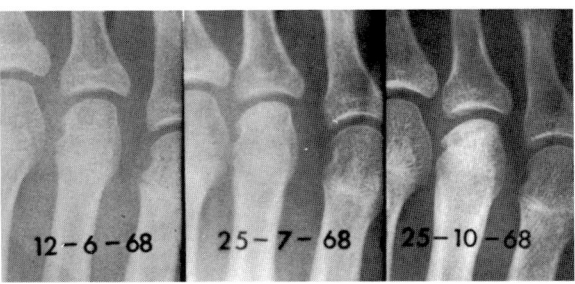

Fig. 1.3. *Freiberg's disease.* Serial studies of a necrotic 3rd metatarsal head in a 12-year-old girl, showing diffuse increase of density as revascularisation progressed. Nevertheless, this weakened bone underwent some degree of collapse and the shaft of the affected metatarsal developed stress thickening.

A2. Post-traumatic subarticular necrosis of capitulum ('osteochondritis dissecans')

Although the pre-operative radiological diagnosis of this condition was confident, concern was expressed clinically with regard to the possibility of chrondoblastoma (see Exercise 24). Premature fusion of the growth plate was attributable to associated hyperaemia.

The specimen removed at operation consisted of articular cartilage (Q2b) and bone (Q2c), which are being eroded by vascular connective tissue. The articular cartilage is viable. The bone shows increased remodelling, with active osteoblasts and osteoclasts (Q2c), but no necrotic bone tissue can be identified. Accepting the radiological diagnosis, these findings indicate that the originally necrotic bone has been removed, over a long period, by the remodelling process.

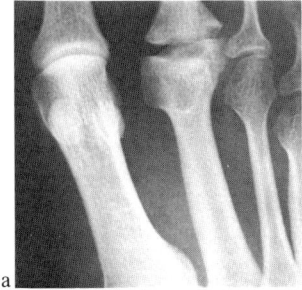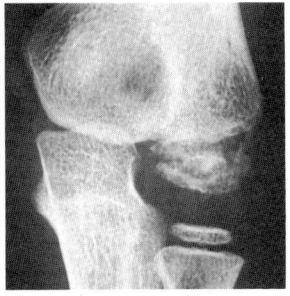

Fig. 1.4. a *Freiberg's disease.* A typical residual deformity of the second metatarsal head in a middle-aged woman, with reactive widening of the proximal phalangeal base and stress thickening of the metatarsal shaft. **b** *Post-traumatic necrosis of capitulum* in a 6-year-old boy with pain in the elbow for 3 months. This structure regenerated completely in follow-up examinations.

Post-traumatic Subarticular Necrosis ('Osteochondritis Dissecans')

These lesions are essentially stress fractures of articular surfaces and affect particularly adolescent and young adult males, usually being associated with athletic activity.

Clinical Features

Chronic discomfort in the affected joint is the usual cause of presentation, sometimes with a history of transient locking. Occasionally an acute injury will cause sudden pain, swelling and limitation of movement, but more commonly symptoms and signs are less severe. The patient usually has been exposed to chronic stress of contact sports or long-distance running. In the weight-bearing joints of the lower limbs the lesions may be symmetrical. When joints are congenitally abnormal, as in dysplasia epiphysealis multiplex, multiple lesions may be observed.

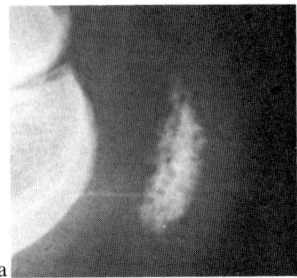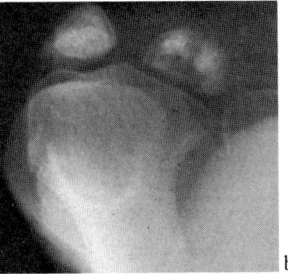

Fig. 1.5. *Post-traumatic necrosis—unusual sites.* **a** *Patella* in a child with chronic pain in the left knee and **b** *lateral sesamoid of the hallux* in an adult with pain in the forefoot. The latter bone clearly became fragile and developed a vertical stress fracture.

Radiological Features

1. Site. The knee is much the most common site to be involved, especially the lateral side of the medial femoral condyle. Other joints affected by particular stresses include the ankle (proximal surface of talus) in high and long jumpers, the elbow (capitulum) in the throwing arm ('little-leaguer's elbow') and the heads of the 1st metatarsals in ballet dancers. Involvement of the femoral head does occur, but is unusual.

2. Appearance. A crescentic articular defect is characteristic, involving almost invariably a *convex* surface. In long-standing lesions the margin of the defect becomes sclerotic and dense. The dissected fragment may be contained in the defect. Occasionally it may reincorporate spontaneously. Often, however, it separates into the joint as a 'loose body' or 'joint mouse'. Serial studies showing actual alteration in position are necessary to establish actual mobility of the displaced fragment as it may reattach to synovium. Since symptoms may be due to a fragment which is entirely cartilaginous or contains only a very small bony element, arthrography, preferably with air rather than an opaque contrast medium, may be rewarding. Any fragment which actually remains loose is liable to damage other portions of the articular surfaces, so that ultimately a number of loose bodies may be present. They may grow considerably and be of varying size, unlike the opacities observed in synovial chondromatosis, an entity discussed elsewhere in this volume.

Pathological Features

The opportunity to examine a recent articular fracture is rare. The separated fragment can be expected to have undergone necrosis as far as the bone and bone marrow are concerned, although the articular cartilage remains viable because of its nourishment by synovial fluid. At a later stage, as in Q2, revascularisation and remodelling can progressively remove any necrotic bone tissue. Alternatively, with renewed viability, it may enlarge in the same way as the intra-articular portions of bone observed in advanced degenerative joint disease.

Treatment

Certain osteochondral fragments may be repositioned with Smillie's pins. Reincorporation, however, usually depends not only on excellent apposition but also on the presence of some continuity of the articular cartilage and lack of significant displacement of the fragment from the parent bone. If reactive sclerosis around the articular defect has developed, indicating the lesion to be of considerable standing, the procedure is unlikely to succeed. A fragment which lies loose within the joint should be removed, in order to avoid further damage to the articular surfaces.

References

Aichroth P (1971) Osteochondritis dissecans of the knee. J Bone Jt Surg 53B: 440–447

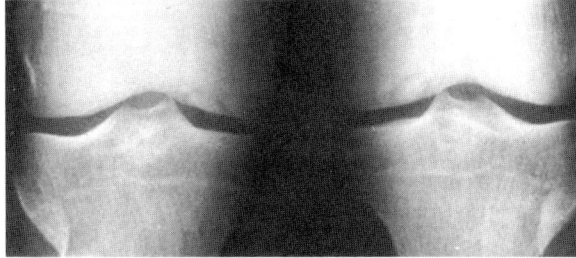

Fig. 2.1. *Post-traumatic subarticular necrosis of medial femoral condyles.* This young adult athlete with pain in the knee was found to have typical and symmetrical lesions of this type on the lateral aspects of both medial femoral condyles. The separated bony fragments are still contained within the concave articular defects.

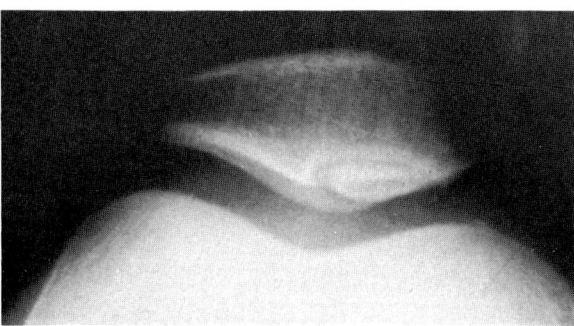

Fig. 2.2. *Post-traumatic subarticular necrosis of patella.* A similar lesion, in another 15-year-old boy with pain in the knee, is situated, as almost always, on the convex ridge of the patella and also contains the separated bony fragment. Abnormal stresses were probably due to the hypoplastic lateral femoral condyle, causing a tendency towards lateral subluxation of this sesamoid bone. (Note that, in the axial projection, the patella 'points' to the lateral side of the knee).

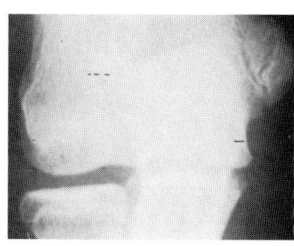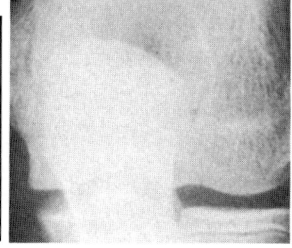

Fig. 2.3 *Post-traumatic subarticular necrosis of capitulum.* Another example in a 14-year-old boy, an expert tennis player, who had complained of right elbow pain. This well-defined articular defect in the capitulum was demonstrated. The sclerotic margin indicated the lesion to be of some standing, but the separated fragment had been resorbed. Reactive hyperaemia was responsible for accelerated growth, causing the radial head to be larger than its counterpart and to be nearer to epiphyseal fusion. Equally enlargement of the apophysis for the right medial epicondyle was evident.

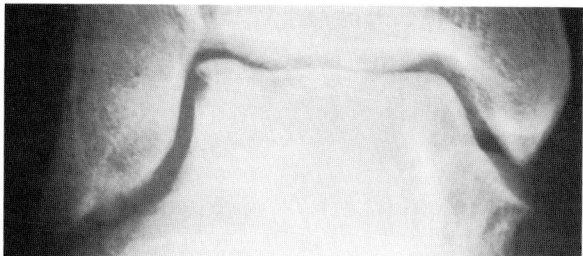

Fig. 2.4. *Post-traumatic subarticular necrosis of each talus.* This 25-year-old man had complained of pain in the right ankle **a** for 2 years following a mild injury. The dissected fragment on the supero-lateral aspect of the talus is in a typical site. **b** The symmetrical lesion in the left talus was asymptomatic and was discovered incidentally. The separated fragment had incorporated spontaneously.

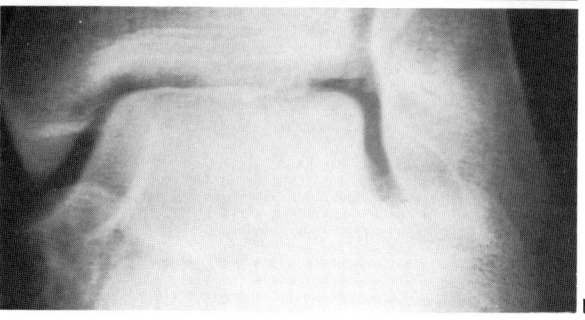

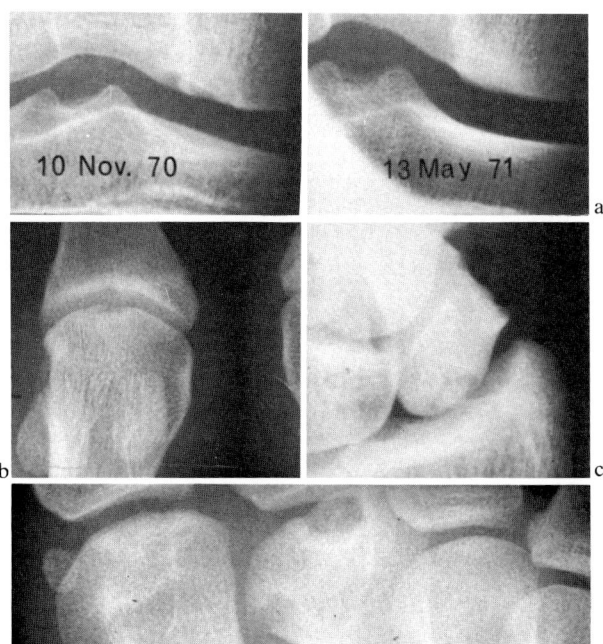

Fig. 2.5. *Post-traumatic subarticular necrosis—unusual manifestations.* **a** *Medial femoral condyle.* This typical lesion caused pain in a 10-year-old girl dancing pupil. Rather unusually, the dissected fragment reincorporated spontaneously within 6 months, with total relief of symptoms. **b** *1st metatarsal head* in another young ballerina. **c** *Scaphoid* and **d** *2nd and 3rd metacarpal heads* in a 16-year-old youth with generalised dysplasia epiphysealis multiplex. Observe the abnormal shape of these metacarpal heads. The other hand was similarly affected.

Q1. This 35-year-old man had complained of intermittent back pain for 3 years. More recently, weakness of the lower limbs had developed with consequent difficulty in walking.

Clinical examination confirmed weakness of both legs, with increased muscle tone. Reflexes were brisk, with sustained ankle and patellar clonus. Cutaneous sensation was decreased below the level of T7. The liver was enlarged.

Radiological studies revealed multiple abnormalities in the spine and pelvis. Increased density was evident in the bodies of T10, T11 and L2. Marked collapse of the body of T11 had taken place. Large osteolytic lesions with poorly defined margins were present in the left ilium, together with areas of sclerosis in the remainder of the pelvis.

A biopsy of the iliac lesion was performed.

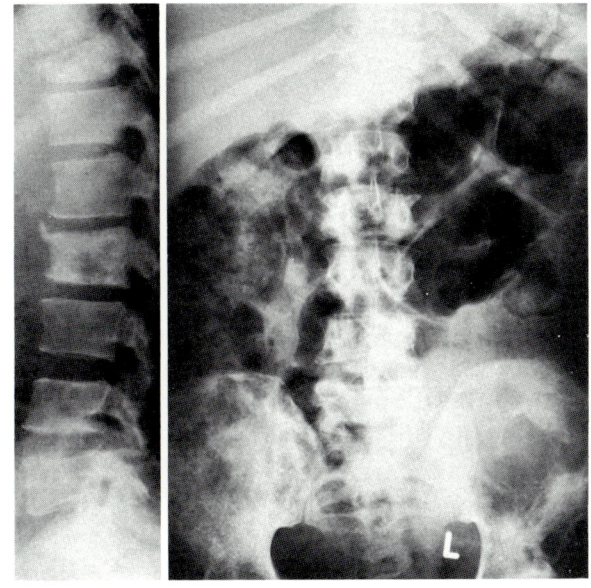

Q1a.

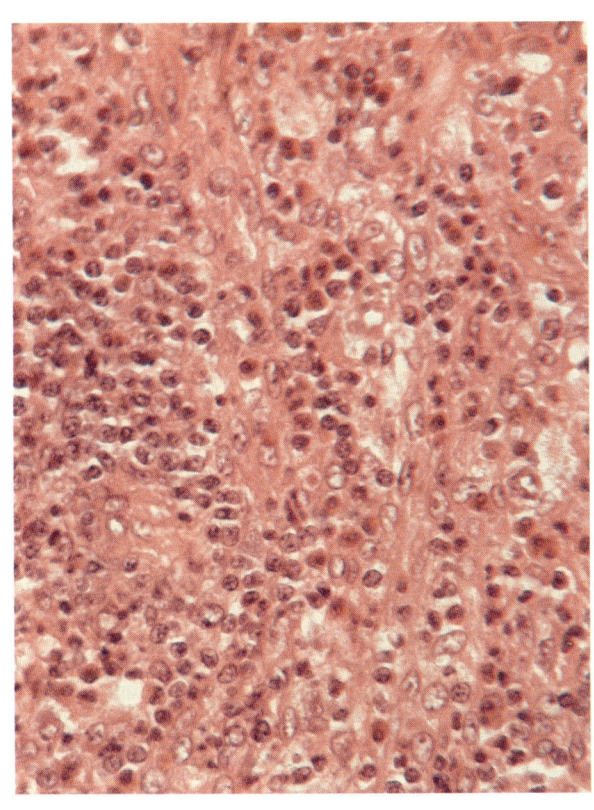

Q1b. (×450)

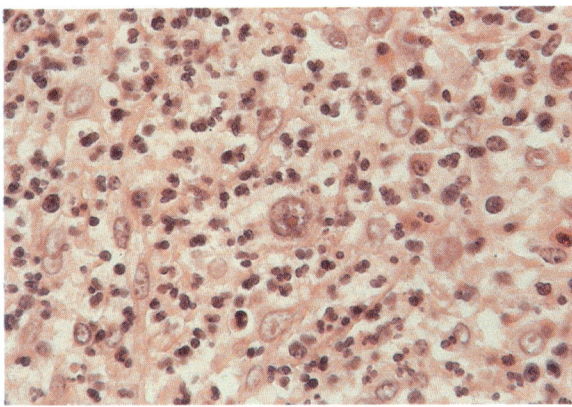

Q1c. (×450)

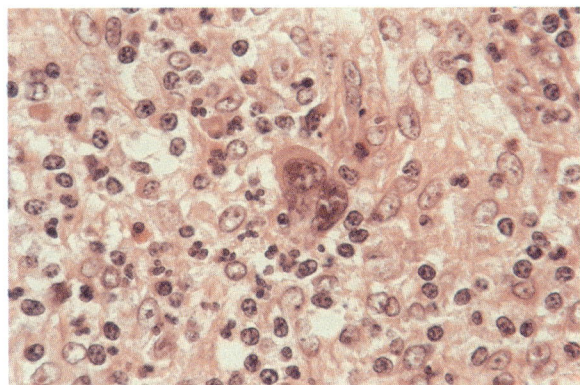

Q1d. (×450)

A1. Hodgkin's disease of spine and pelvis

The clinical findings and the multiplicity of the bone lesions demonstrated radiologically in areas of persistent haemopoietic activity suggested a marrow disorder of a lymphoma type. The early neurological signs and symptoms were attributable to spinal cord compression.

Transthoracic decompression of T6 was carried out, and the lesion of the ilium also was biopsied. Material was taken for culture, but this investigation proved to be negative. The histological studies revealed the presence of a large number of lymphocytes (Q1b) and of polymorphonuclear leucocytes (Q1c and d). At first sight this appearance suggested the possibility of an inflammatory disorder; however, this diagnosis was made unlikely by a negative culture. But in addition to the seemingly inflammatory cells, the tissue contains many large mononuclear cells and scattered giant cells. Some of these have very large single nuclei (Q1c), while others have deeply indented or multiple nuclei (Q1d), and all have prominent nucleoli. Many of the polymorphonuclear leucocytes are eosinophils. The lesion has, in fact, the features of Hodgkin's disease, and some of the giant cells have the morphological appearance of Sternberg-Reed cells.

The histological diagnosis of Hodgkin's disease was confirmed by the subsequent development of the case. After the spinal decompression operation, the patient developed postoperative pneumonia and ileus, and died 4 days later. At autopsy, lesions of Hodgkin's disease were found in thoracic lymph nodes and in the liver and spleen, as well as in bone marrow.

Hodgkin's Disease

Hodgkin's disease is a variety of lymphoma. It typically involves lymph nodes and lesions are also found commonly in the spleen and liver. Bone marrow involvement is not unusual as a terminal manifestation, but it is rare for cases of Hodgkin's disease to present on account of a bone lesion.

Clinical Features

Hodgkin's disease most commonly involves individuals from 20 to 30 years of age, often presenting as an asymptomatic cervical lymphadenopathy. Two males are affected for every female. Enlargement of lymph nodes may cause a wide spectrum of symptoms, particularly a chronic cough. Systemic symptoms and signs include anorexia, lassitude, loss of weight and intermittent and unexplained febrile attacks. Pruritus and other skin lesions are not uncommon. The liver and spleen are enlarged in half the patients and blood investigations commonly reveal anaemia, a raised ESR and an elevated γ-globulin. Involvement of the skeleton is detected in approximately 15% on presentation, but much more frequently in postmortem examinations. For some unexplained reason these lesions are especially liable to develop transient pain following the ingestion of alcohol. In most cases, the bone lesion develops in a patient with recognised lymph node involvement; in rare instances, however, such as the case in this Exercise, bone disease may be the presenting feature of the patient's illness. Occasionally such lesions, especially in the spine, may present with established secondary infection, obscuring the primary diagnosis.

Radiological Features

1. Site. Lymph node involvement may be shown, in the case of the common hilar lymphadenopathy, by orthodox chest films. Elsewhere lymphangiography is rewarding, but radionuclide scanning is a particularly sensitive procedure. Bone lesions are detected in the marrow cavities of the axial skeleton, the areas of persistent haemopoiesis in the adult, which include also the proximal ends of the femur and humerus. The spine, pelvis and sternum are particularly susceptible. Localised pressure erosions may develop in relation to enlarged lymph nodes.

2. Appearance. In half the cases the lesions are essentially osteolytic with a diffuse infiltrating pattern as shown in the left ilium in Q1a. In 10%–15% they are purely osteoblastic and in the remainder a mixture of these types is observed, as illustrated by the body of L2 in Q1a. Differentiation from metastatic disease (see Exercise 2) usually is influenced by the age of the patient. Mixed lesions in the pelvis, particularly of a young adult, always should arouse diagnostic suspicion of a lymphoma of this type.

Pathological Features

The diagnosis of Hodgkin's disease and its distinction from other types of lymphoma are based on the histological appearance of the lesions. A variety of cell types, including lymphocytes, eosinophil cells and large mononuclear cells may be present. The definitive diagnosis, however, depends on the recognition of the characteristic Sternberg-Reed giant cells, which are shown so clearly in Q1c and d. The current 'Rye' classification divides Hodgkin's disease into four subtypes: (a) lymphocyte predominant, (b) nodular sclerosis, (c) mixed cellularity, (d) lymphocyte depleted.

Prognosis is, to some extent, related to histological structure, the lymphocyte predominant type having the best, and the lymphocyte depleted type the worst prognosis. The characteristic histological appearances of Hodgkin's disease, in lesions of lymph nodes, are illustrated in Figs. 1.1 and 1.2.

Treatment

Without treatment Hodgkin's disease is fatal, survival often being limited to 2 years after presentation. The prognosis becomes more sinister in the presence of established bone lesions.

In recent years, however, treatment methods have enjoyed a considerable measure of success. Radionuclide scanning has permitted identification of major areas of involvement so that laparotomy and tissue sampling is undertaken less frequently.

Radiotherapy, employing megavoltage equipment and linear electron accelerators, is now a standard method of treatment. Delivery of around 4400 rads, at the rate of 1100 rads per week, is capable of eradicating all involved lymph chains and other lymphatic tissue within the body with a probability of cure in 95% of cases.

Chemotherapy began with the introduction of the first alkylating agents and antifolates. In the past decade a cyclically administered combination of nitrogen mustard, oncovin (vincristine), procarbazine and prednisone (MOPP) has been used in the treatment of advanced disease. Such multidrug combinations have proved to be of value in conjunction with radiotherapy in reducing the relapse rate. In children affected by the disease low dose radiotherapy followed by six cycles of MOPP has given a relapse-free survival rate of 90%, without impairment of bone growth. The benefits of chemotherapy must be balanced against their morbid effects, including azoospermia in males, occasional acute leukaemia and secondary non-Hodgkin's lymphoma. Its indiscriminate use should be avoided with milder forms of the disease which may be expected to respond well to radiotherapy alone.

References

Desforges JF (1979) Hodgkin's disease. N Engl J Med 301: 1212–1222

Granger W, Whitaker R (1967) Hodgkin's disease in bone, with special reference to periosteal reaction. Br J Radiol 40: 939–948

Horan FT (1969) Bone involvement in Hodgkin's disease. A survey of 201 cases. Br J Surg 56: 277–281

Kaplan HS (1980) Hodgkin's disease. Unfolding concepts concerning its nature, management and prognosis. Cancer 45: 2439–2474

Lukes RJ et al. (1966) Natural history of Hodgkin's disease as related to its pathologic picture. Cancer 46: 838–843

Scully RE (1978) Case records of the Massachusetts General Hospital (Case 8, 1978). N Engl J Med 298: 501–505

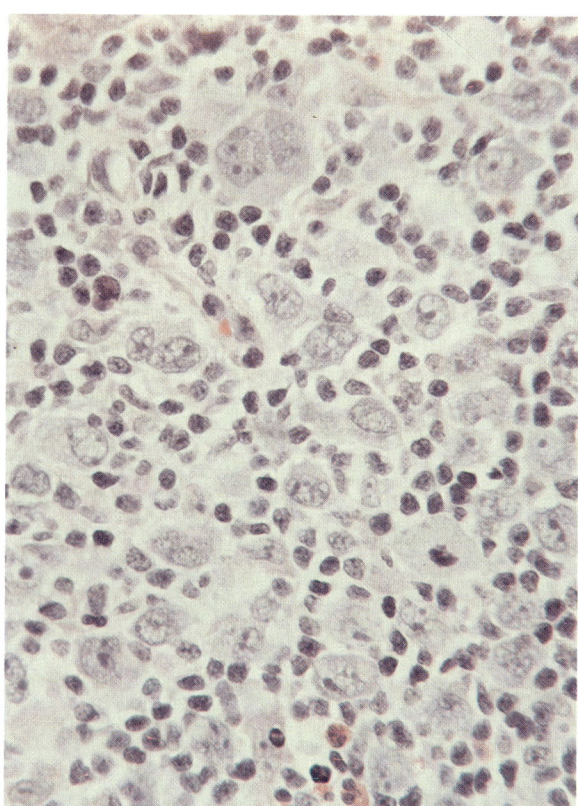

Fig. 1.1. *Hodgkin's disease: lymph node.* Tissue from a lesion of mixed cellularity, showing lymphocytes, large mononuclear cells, giant cells and eosinophils. (×650)

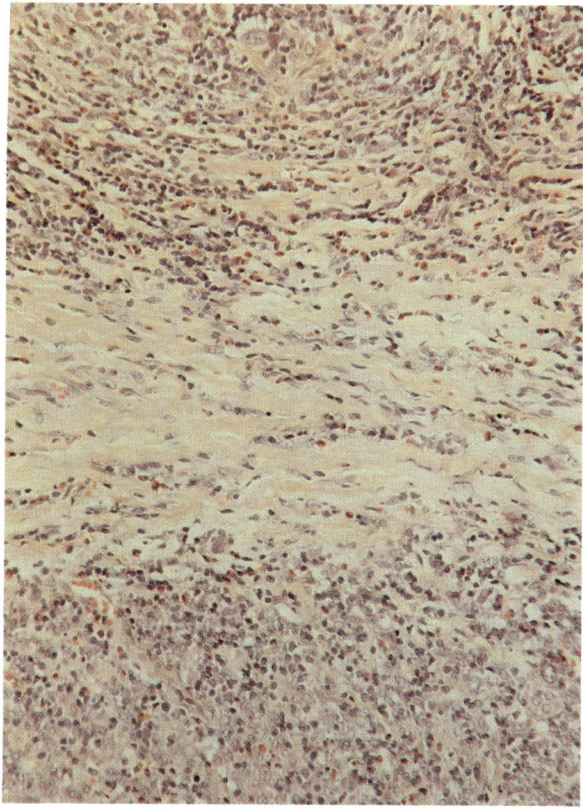

Fig. 1.2. *Hodgkin's disease: lymph node.* Tissue from a lesion showing nodular sclerosis. A band of dense fibrous tissue separates two nodules of more cellular tissue. (×145)

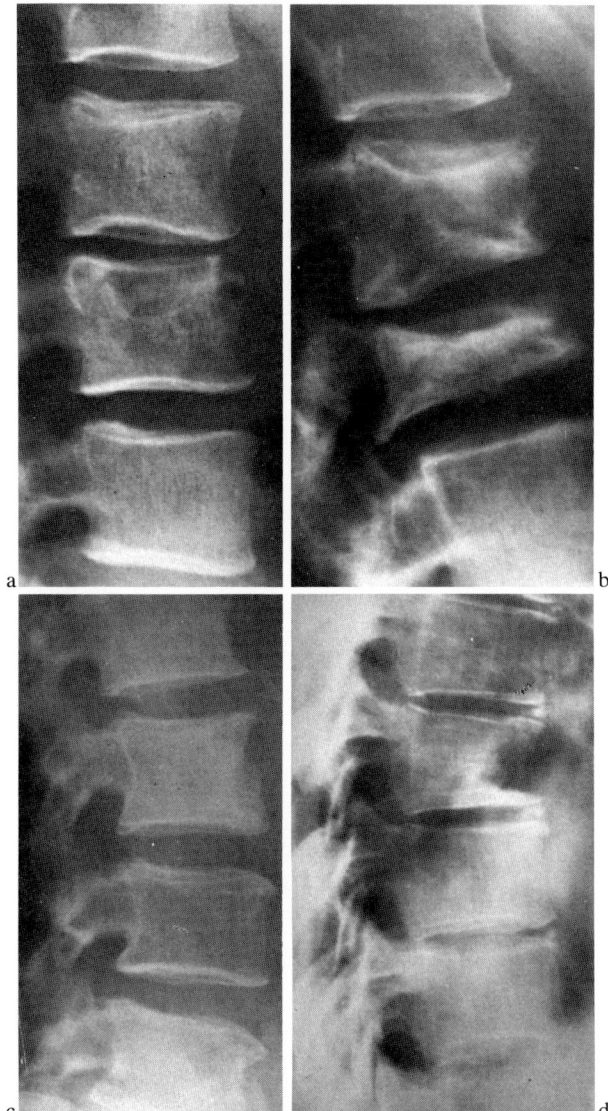

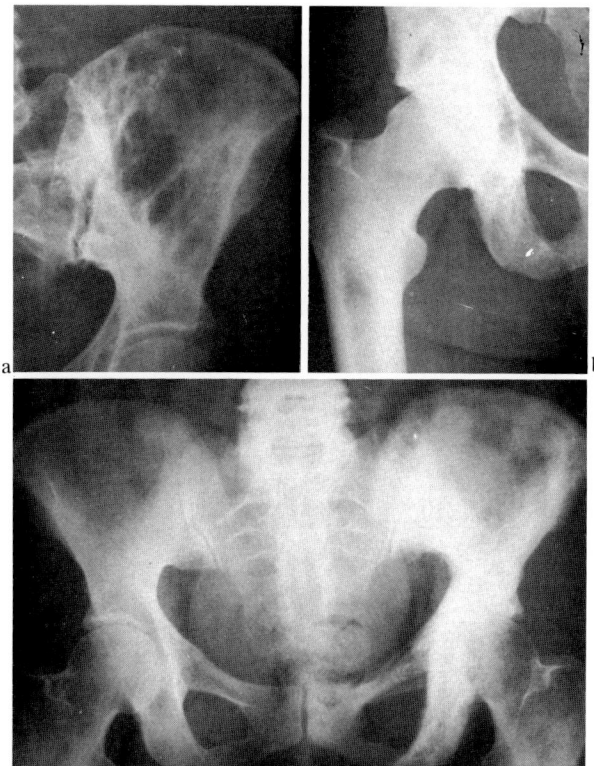

Fig. 1.4. *Hodgkin's disease—pelvis.* **a** *Osteolytic type.* Extensive destruction in left ilium in a young adult with pelvic pain. **b** *Mixed type* in obturator ring in another young man. A purely lytic medullary lesion is present in the femur. **c** *Osteoblastic type.* Widespread sclerosis throughout the left innominate bone of this woman with pain in the left hip was at first considered to be Paget's disease with the lytic area in the superior pubic ramus representing sarcomatous change. This diagnosis was influenced by the age of the patient—62 years—but Hodgkin's disease *can* develop late in life.

Fig. 1.3. *Hodgkin's disease—spine.* **a** *Osteolytic type.* Poorly defined bony destruction occurred in the bodies of L2 and 3 in a 35-year-old man with back pain for 1 year. The upper table of L3 has collapsed with consequent, but unusual, narrowing of the L2/3 disc space. An associated and widespread lymphadenopathy was present and the patient survived only 1 year. These changes were regarded initially as being infective. **b** *Mixed type.* Some sclerosis is present in addition to the areas of osteolysis in the bodies of L2 and 3. **c** *Osteoblastic type.* Diffuse increase of density is evident in the bodies of L1, 2 and 4. **d** *Pressure erosion* of anterior aspect of T8 by an enlarged lymph node.

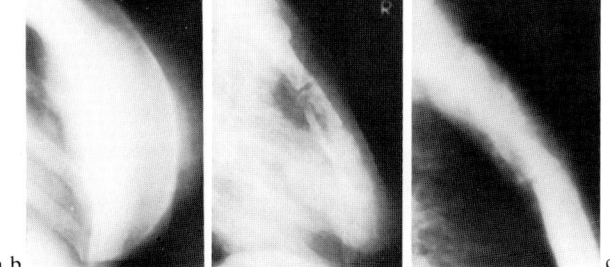

Fig. 1.5. *Hodgkin's disease—sternum.* **a** *Osteolytic type* in a young woman. Observe the retrosternal mass. **b** *Mixed type* in a young adult with a painful swelling. **c** *Osteoblastic type* in a 60-year-old man with sternal tenderness—another example of the disease presenting in later life.

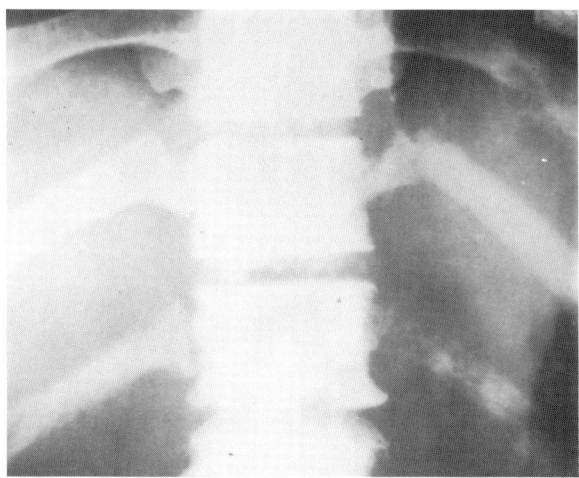

Fig. 1.6. *Hodgkin's disease—advanced.* Osteoblastic lesions in the vertebral bodies are accompanied by sclerotic and destructive changes in the left lower ribs with pathological fractures. Such an appearance in a young adult is virtually diagnostic. Isolated rib lesions usually cause considerable diagnostic difficulty.

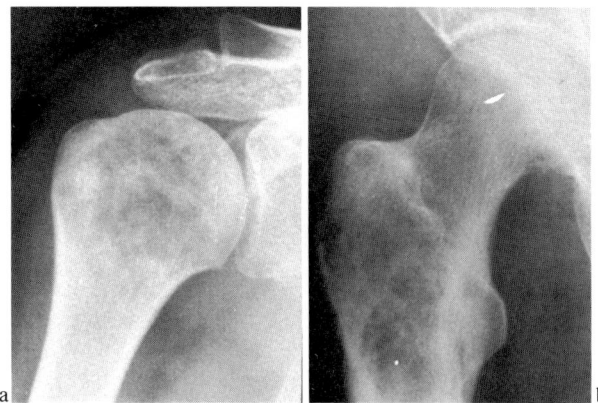

Fig. 1.9. *Hodgkin's disease—long bones.* Haemopoiesis persists in adult life in the proximal ends of the humerus and femur. Infiltrating lesions in **a** humerus, not an uncommon site, and **b** femur.

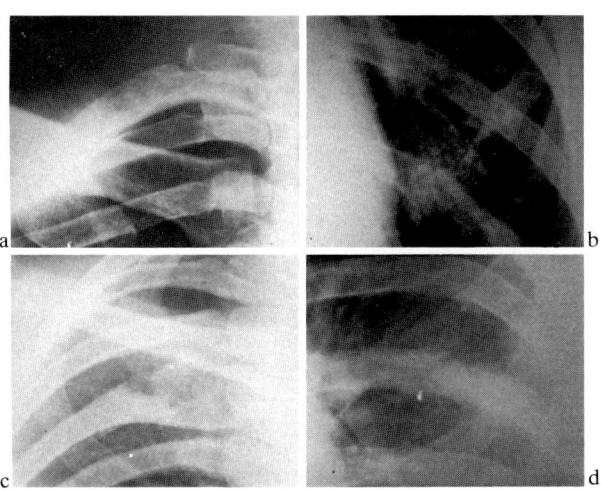

Fig. 1.7. *Hodgkin's disease—ribs.* Examples of isolated lesions. **a** *Infiltrating destruction* of 1st rib. **b, c** Osteolytic foci with expansion. **d** Osteoblastic lesion.

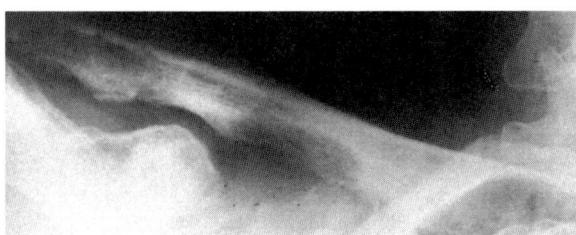

Fig. 1.8. *Hodgkin's disease—pressure erosion* of clavicle and scapula by an enlarged and fungating lymph node in a 20-year-old man.

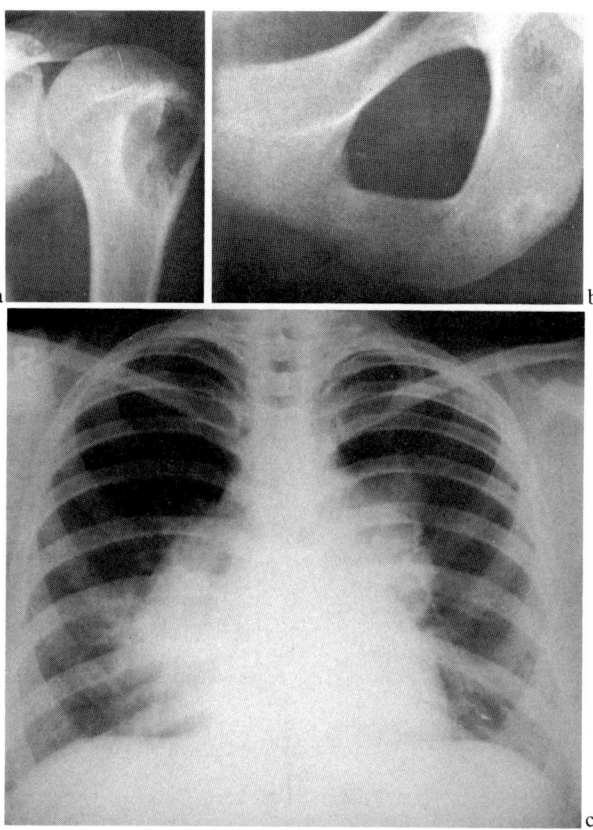

Fig. 1.10. *Generalised Hodgkin's disease.* This 22-year-old woman complained of pain in the left shoulder which was aggravated by alcohol—even a glass of sherry. **a** Although this lytic area with a mild periosteal reaction appeared benign and an eosinophil granuloma was suspected, skeletal survey revealed a similar lesion **b** in the left ischium and the chest film **c** demonstrated a classical hilar adenopathy. All these lesions responded well to radiotherapy.

Q1. This 53-year-old man complained of a recurrent swelling of the right leg, which had caused some discomfort for 5 months. Similar episodes had occurred in the past and on one occasion 20 years previously an operation had been performed, concerning which no details were available.

On clinical examination a tender swelling was observed on the anteromedial surface of the tibia, approximately 12.5×7.5 cm in size. No other abnormality was detected. Laboratory investigations, including serum calcium and phosphorus estimations, were normal.

Radiographs showed a large, expanding osteolytic lesion in the mid-shaft of the tibia, with a suggestion of central loculation. The endosteal margin was clearly defined by a narrow zone of sclerosis and the bulging cortex was greatly attenuated.

A biopsy was performed.

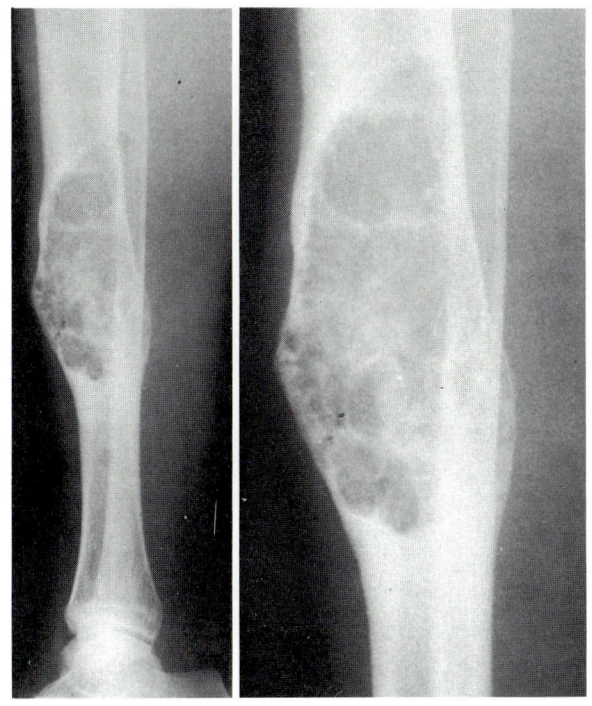

Q1a.

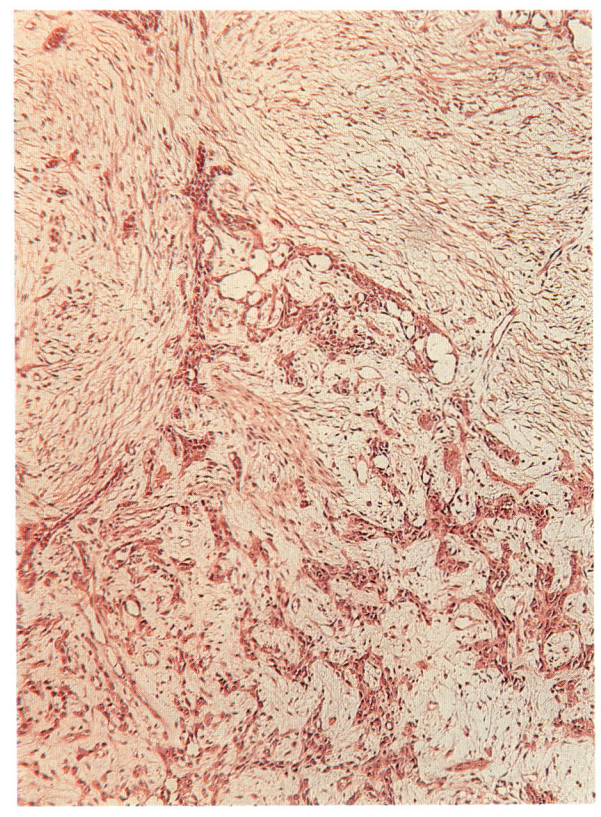

Q1b. (×75)

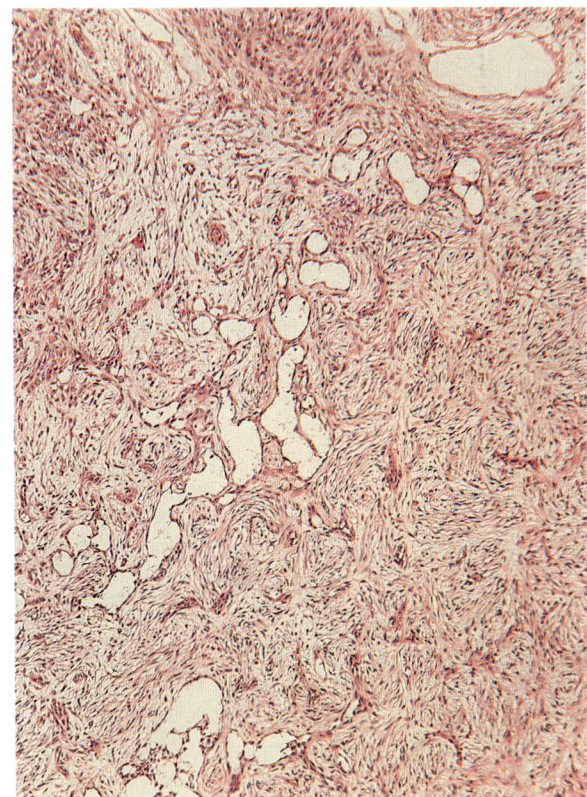

Q1c. (×75)

A1. Adamantinoma of tibia

The unusually long history, including the report of a previous operation, gave support to the pre-operative diagnosis of a benign lesion. Monostotic fibrous dysplasia or even an exceptionally aggressive and persistent non-ossifying fibroma were considered. An aneurysmal bone cyst was thought to be very unlikely in view of the history and the age of the patient. The normal biochemical findings permitted exclusion of a 'brown tumour' of hyperparathyroidism. The radiological features, and the location in the mid-shaft of the tibia, however, did raise the possibility of adamantinoma, an extremely rare, locally malignant tumour.

Q1b and c show a lesion made up of loosely arranged fibrous tissue containing clusters and strands of cells which differ in size and staining characteristics from the cells of the surrounding fibrous tissue and which appear to be epithelial in nature. Some of the epithelial cell clusters are solid, while in others small cystic spaces are present. At first sight, the presence of these apparently epithelial structures might suggest the possibility of metastatic cancer. In fact the histological findings are typical of the rare type of primary bone tumour usually referred to as 'adamantinoma of long bones'.

The patient was treated by local resection of the tumour, with plating and packing with cancellous bone. No evidence of local recurrence or of a metastasis had developed 2 years after this operation.

Adamantinoma of Long Bones

These rare tumours almost always involve the tibia, although they have been reported in other long bones, including the femur, humerus and ulna. They usually are locally malignant and grow slowly. Symptoms may have been present for many years before the patient seeks medical attention. In consequence the majority of patients are at least middle-aged on presentation, although a few have become symptomatic earlier, even in adolescence. An association with fibrous dysplasia has been the subject of a few reports. On rare occasions metastases have developed, as a late complication, usually to lymph nodes and lungs.

Clinical Features

Mild and long-standing pain and swelling at the affected site is the usual cause of presentation, but occasionally attention to the presence of the tumour is drawn by a pathological fracture. Laboratory investigations are unrewarding.

Radiological Features

1. Site. As indicated above, the vast majority of these tumours arise in the tibia, usually in its middle third. Involvement of other long bones is exceptional.

2. Appearance. Characteristically a central or eccentric area of osteolysis, often with a loculated pattern, is present. The overlying cortex is expanded and thinned or even totally destroyed. Pathological infractions may be evident.

The endosteal margin is sclerotic, with a narrow zone of transition. Satellite lesions may be present, resembling, and occasionally due to, fibrous dysplasia. Serial studies confirm a very slow rate of growth.

Pathological Features

The nature, and the histogenesis, of these tumours is still undecided. The name 'adamantinoma of long bones' was prompted by the presence of the apparently epithelial structures and by the histological similarity to the well-recognised adamantinoma (ameloblastoma) of the jaw, a tumour originating from dental epithelium. The occurrence of epithelial structures in a primary bone tumour is something of a puzzle. Some authorities have suggested, because of the cystic structures lined by flattened cells, that these tumours are not epithelial in nature, but vascular. Despite some ultrastructural studies, the matter is not yet resolved. The uncertainty with regard to histogenesis, however, does not give rise to any problem as far as the practical identification of the tumour is concerned.

In adamantinoma, the tumour tissue, or the adjacent bone, sometimes contains areas of fibrous tissue and bone trabeculae resembling fibrous dysplasia (see Exercise 1).

Treatment

Since symptoms are often so mild, the possibility of maintaining a conservative approach often deserves consideration. When more radical measures are required, total excision and packing with bone chips or a replacement bone graft is necessary, although recurrences are common. Particularly with established non-union of a pathological fracture, amputation may be unavoidable. These lesions are virtually insensitive to radiation therapy.

References

Changus GW, Speed JS, Stewart FW (1957) Malignant angioblastoma of bone. A re-appraisal of adamantinoma of long bone. Cancer 20: 540–559

Cohen DM, Dahlin DC, Pugh OG (1962) Fibrous dysplasia associated with adamantinoma of the long bones. Cancer 15: 515–521

Moon NF (1965) Adamantinoma of the appendicular skeleton. A statistical review of reported cases and inclusion of 10 new cases. Clin Orthop 43: 189–213

Stoker DJ (1977) Adamantinoma of tibia. Case report 22. Skeletal Radiol 1: 187–189

Unni KK, Dahlin DC, Beabout JW, Ivins JC (1974) Adamantinoma of long bones. Cancer 34: 1796–1805

Yoneyama T, Winter WG, Milsow L (1977) Tibial adamantinoma. Its histogenesis from ultrastructural studies. Cancer 40: 1138–1142

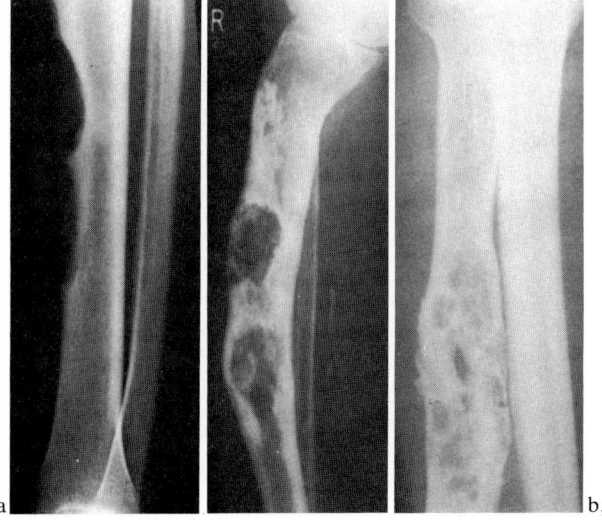

Fig. 1.1. *Adamantinoma of long bones.* **a** *Tibia*, showing an eccentric area of destruction, with total loss of the overlying cortex and a sclerosed endosteal margin. **b** *Tibia* in a 73-year-old woman with pain for 1 year. The tumour was situated in the large lytic area in the proximal portion of the bone, with typical thinning of the cortex. The lesions elsewhere were due to fibrous dysplasia, presumably the cause of a fracture sustained at the age of 11 years. **c** *Radius*. This extremely rare site was involved in a 62-year-old woman with pain and swelling for 1 year. Many recurrences followed curettage, grafting and ineffective radiotherapy. Amputation was refused. The patient survived for 20 years before dying of unrelated disease.

Q1. An athletic 12-year-old boy developed progressively severe pain below the left knee over a period of a few weeks.

The physician became concerned by persistence of the symptoms and questioned slight swelling of the proximal end of the tibia. No other clinical abnormality was detected.

Radiological examination revealed a diffuse periosteal reaction, apparently well organised, surrounding almost completely the proximal end of the tibia. This reaction was especially prominent on the posterior aspect of the bone.

A biopsy was performed.

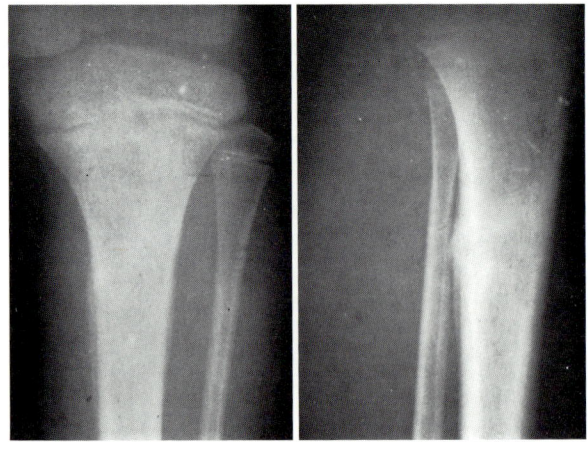

Q1a.

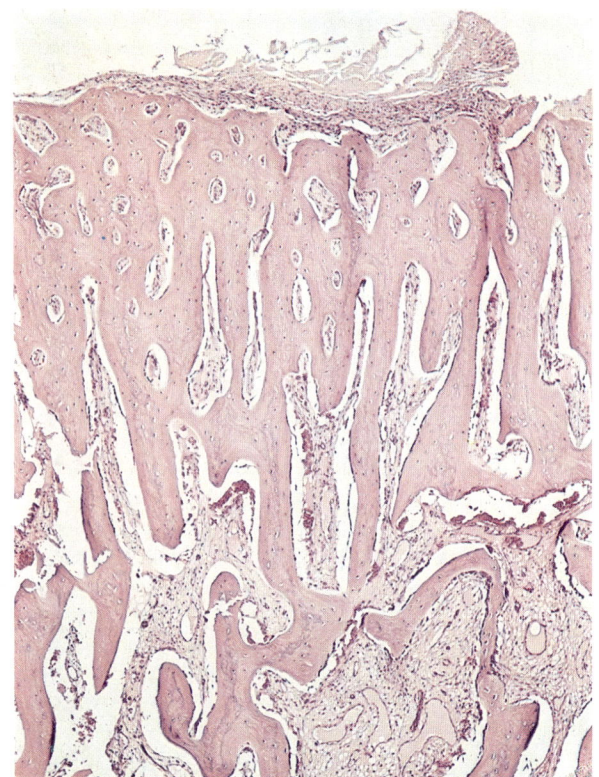

Q1b. (×45)

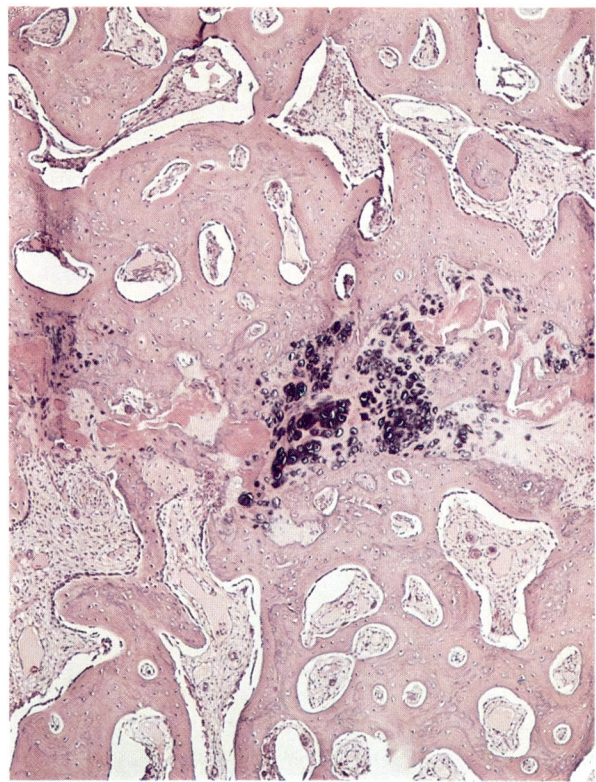

Q1c. (×50)

Q2. This 25-year-old man presented on account of mild, but increasing pain below the right knee.

On clinical examination localised tenderness was elicited on palpation of the proximal end of the tibia and the extremes of movement of the joint were painful.

The radiographs showed the proximal end of the tibia to be significantly increased in density, particularly on the lateral side, where an overlying periosteal reaction was evident.

The lesion was biopsied.

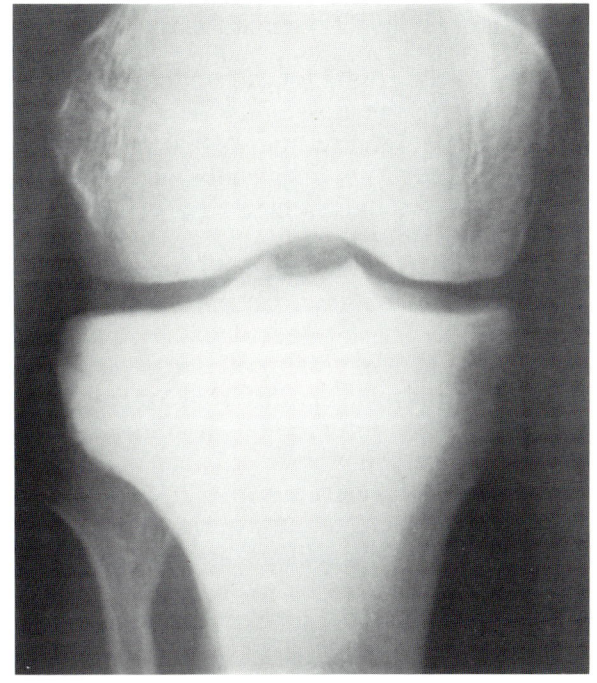

Q2a.

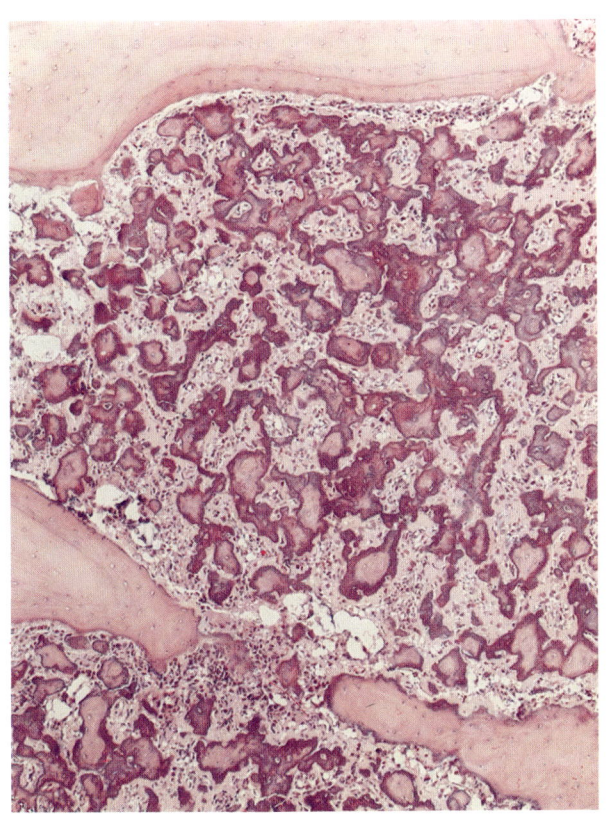

Q2b. (×50)

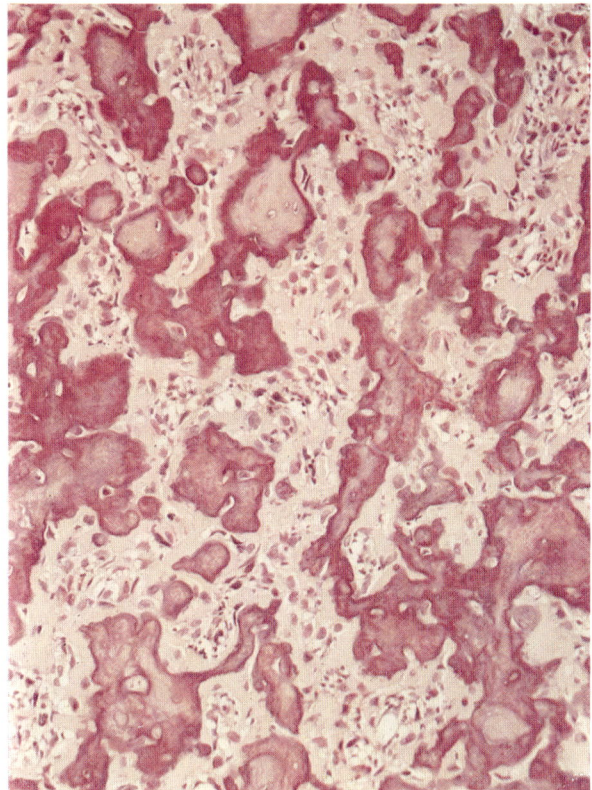

Q2c. (×120)

A1. Stress fracture of tibia

Although the radiological appearance did raise initially the possibility of a malignant tumour, the organised periosteal reaction at this particular site, especially in an active child, was strongly suggestive of a stress fracture. The histological findings were indisputable. Q1b shows vertical trabeculae of reactive periosteal bone on the surface of the tibial cortex. These trabeculae have a mature structure and a regular pattern of arrangement. They have a very different appearance, as does also the intervening vascular connective tissue, from that observed in an osteoblastic tumour, as illustrated in Q2. In Q1c the reactive periosteal tissue ('periosteal callus') includes areas of cartilage as well as bone. With conservative treatment symptoms regressed completely and a normal radiological appearance ensued.

Stress Fractures

Clinical Features

Minor and repeated mechanical insults, usually associated with athletic or occupational activity in healthy adolescents and young adults, induce these lesions, causing localised pain and tenderness. Elderly osteoporotic patients also are affected (see Exercise 3). Osteomalacia always should be excluded, particularly in elderly females. Stress fractures may complicate other pathological conditions, including Paget's disease (see Exercise 8), Cushing's syndrome (see Exercise 3) and various congenital disorders, such as osteopetrosis. They are liable also to occur when bone vitality has been impaired by previous irradiation (upper ribs, pelvis, femoral necks) (see Exercise 7).

Radiological Features

1. Site. The most common areas of the skeleton to be affected are the metatarsal necks, particularly the 2nd, representing the classical 'march' fracture, observed frequently in military recruits. Other bones often affected include the proximal end of the tibia, as in long-distance runners and male dancers, and the pars interarticularis in lumbar vertebrae, causing spondylolysis and spondylolisthesis. The latter abnormalities are observed occasionally as a result of occupational stress incurred by work on the hands and knees (carpet-layers and miners) and by female ballet dancers. Less common sites are the lower ribs, as a result of chronic coughing, the first rib, associated with carrying a heavy pack, and such areas as the obturator ring, the neck of the femur and the calcaneus.

2. Appearance. Recognition of the fracture line itself may be difficult, even with tomograms. Radionuclide scans are positive before typical radiological changes develop in days or weeks. The earliest radiological sign is formation of a peripheral sheath of callus, which may be so abundant that the appearance may be confused with infection or even a malignant bone tumour. As this callus grows and organises in serial studies a hazy zone of increased density develops across the fracture site (by which time symptoms may have resolved spontaneously). Such follow-up examinations are of value in differential diagnosis, particularly from an osteosarcoma.

Pathological Features

The histological appearance of a stress fracture is the same as that of other fractures. The reactive tissue of which it is made up, termed callus, consists of fibrous tissue, together with bone and cartilage. It may be an actively proliferating and highly cellular tissue which can be mistaken for a sarcoma, but the presence of mature bony structures, as in Q1b, or of mature cartilage, the latter often undergoing endochondral ossification, indicates its non-neoplastic nature. As in other fractures, the callus tissue undergoes progressive remodelling and conversion to mature bone.

Treatment

Premature biopsy should be avoided in favour of an expectant attitude, despite occasional demonstration radiologically of florid callus formation. Rest and reassurance are often adequate. Immobilisation in a plaster cast occasionally is necessary to relieve pain and limit activity, particularly with pars interarticularis fractures in adolescents. Fractures of the femoral neck may require prophylactic pinning.

References

Daffner RH (1978) Stress fractures: Current concepts. Skeletal Radiol 2: 221–229
Levin DC, Blazina ME, Levine E (1967) Fatigue fractures of the shaft of the femur: simulation of malignant tumor. Radiology 89: 883–885
Murray IPC (1980) Bone scanning in the child and young adult. Part II. Skeletal Radiol 5: 65–76
Sevitt S (1981) Bone repair and fracture healing in man. Churchill Livingstone, Edinburgh
Wilson ES, Katz FN (1969). Stress fracture. An analysis of 250 consecutive cases. Radiology 92: 481–486

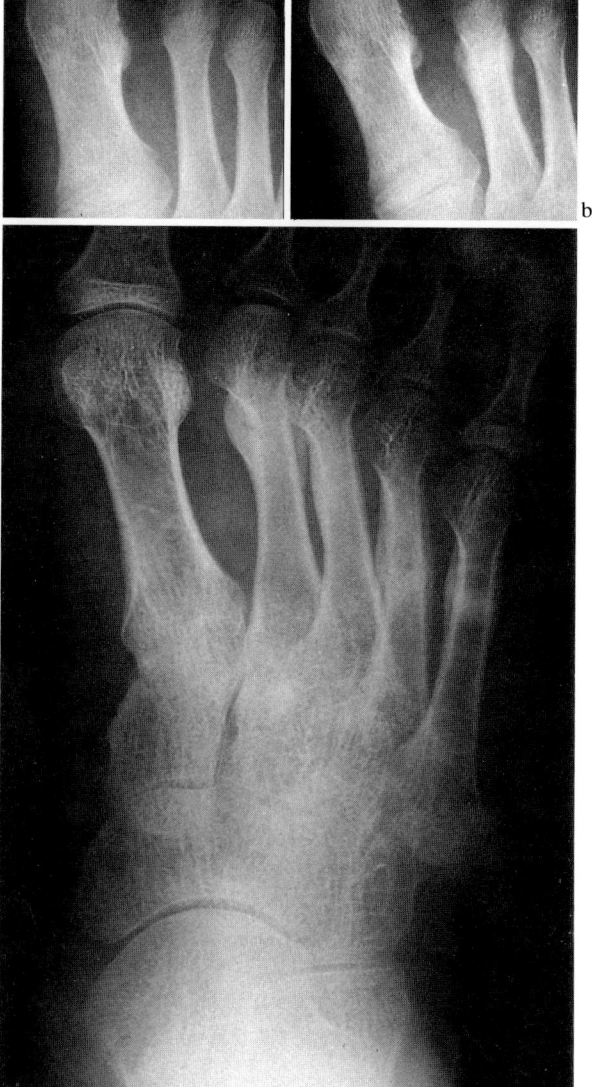

Fig. 1.1. *Stress fractures of metatarsals*—the bones most commonly affected by these lesions. **a** *2nd metatarsal.* This 12-year-old boy had complained of pain in the right forefoot since taking part in a cross-country run a week before. The initial radiograph showed only a minimal periosteal reaction on the medial side of the metatarsal neck. At this stage a radionuclide scan would have been positive. **b** Further examination 3 weeks later, after a period of rest, showed the development of a surrounding sheath of organised callus. By this time the patient was asymptomatic. **c** *2nd to 5th metatarsals.* These multiple fractures, in varying stages of repair, were found in a 22-year-old man with mild pain in the feet. He had been ambulant for 3 months following 2 years prolonged recumbency during conservative treatment for spinal tuberculosis. Similar fractures were present in the other foot. Observe generalised disuse osteoporosis.

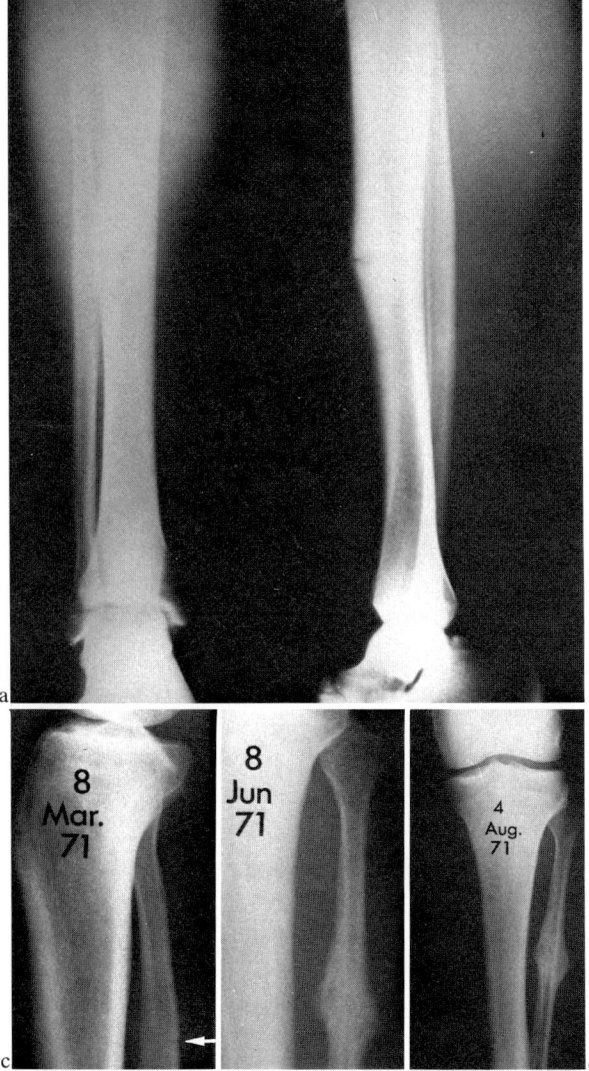

Fig. 1.2. *Stress fractures in athletes.* **a** *Tibia.* This 20-year-old man, a long-distance runner, complained of pain in the right leg. The cortical thickening on the anterior aspect of the tibia is a common response to this form of activity, the consequent pain being described as 'shin splints'. The lucent defect represents a stress fracture and should not be confused with an osteoid osteoma (see Exercise 21). Lesions of this type have become more common, especially in middle-aged individuals, as a result of the increased popularity of jogging. **b** *Fibula.* The minute infraction in the fibula (*arrow*) of this 30-year-old professional footballer with pain in the leg was not appreciated. **c** Pain persisted and 3 months later a localised swelling was palpable. The sheath of callus at the site of the fracture caused the radiographs to be referred for a second opinion to exclude an osteosarcoma. In view of the typical radiological appearance no further action was taken. **d** Complete consolidation of the lesion had taken place by the beginning of the following football season, when the patient was asymptomatic.

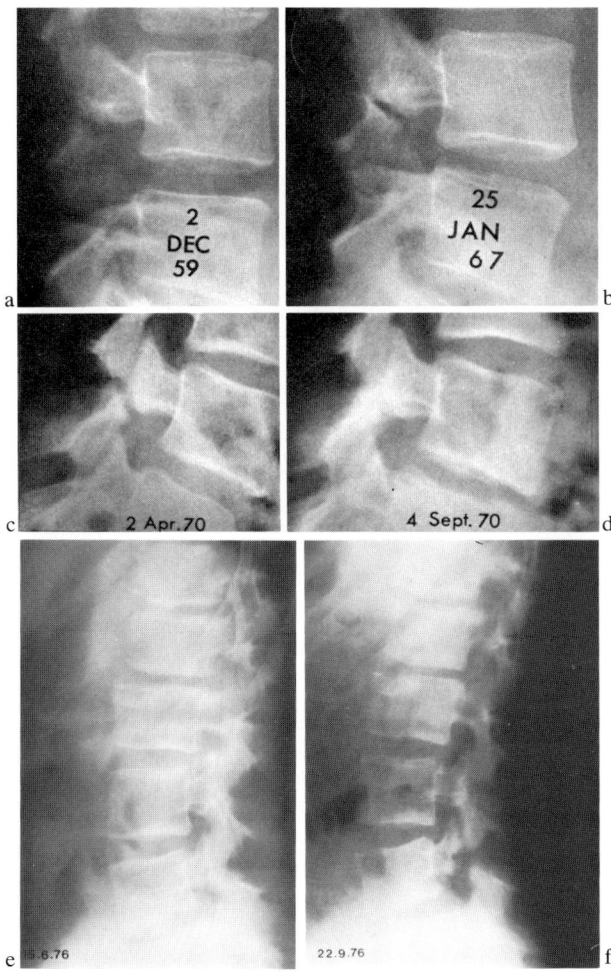

Fig. 1.3. *Stress fractures of the spine.* The pars interarticularis of the neural arch represents a site of particular frailty of the human skeleton, rendering it liable to stress fractures. Such lesions are common, and usually bilateral, but often are accompanied by such trivial symptoms that they may be recognised only as incidental abnormalities later in life. The vast majority occur in the 4th and 5th lumbar vertebrae. **a** This 20-year-old man developed low back pain in the course of occupational stress in carrying heavy loads. Defects in the neural arch of L4 were due to stress fractures with bone absorption causing the margins to be irregular. Symptoms resolved with rest. **b** Seven years later the fracture margins had become sclerotic, indicating established non-union to persist, a common result. Serial studies of this type exclude a congenital abnormality. At this time the patient was still asymptomatic. **c** Similar lesions in this 12-year-old girl united soundly **d** after 4 months' immobilisation in a plaster cast. **e** This 16-year-old boy complained of backache after putting the shot. Typical changes of Scheuermann's disease were present, with a particularly large prolapse of the nucleus pulposus into the body of L2 (see Exercise 5). The stress fracture of the neural arch of L5 was not recognised. **f** Six months later gross absorption of the fracture margins had developed, with a mild L4/5 spondylolisthesis. Despite this appearance symptoms had resolved completely.

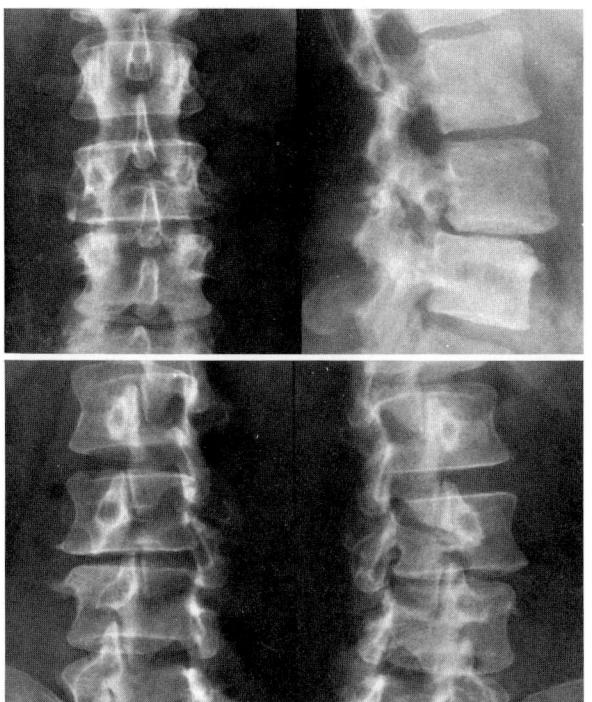

Fig. 1.4. *Bilateral pars interarticularis fractures of L3 with secondary derangement of L3/4 intervertebral disc and grade I L3/4 spondylolisthesis.* These lesions, clearly of considerable standing, were found in a middle-aged woman with chronic back pain. She had been a ballet dancer of distinction, so that the fractures were undoubtedly attributable to occupational stress. Their sclerotic margins again indicate established non-union. Oblique projections may be of great value in demonstrating pars interarticularis fractures, especially in their early stages.

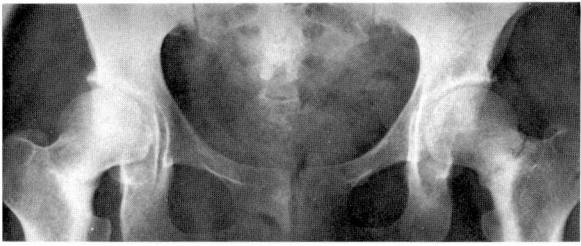

Fig. 1.5. *Stress fractures of femoral necks.* This 32-year-old African woman had been a leading performer in native dances, involving much stamping of the feet. Radiological examination on account of recent pain in the left hip disclosed not only a frank fracture of the left femoral neck, but also an infraction of the right femoral neck.

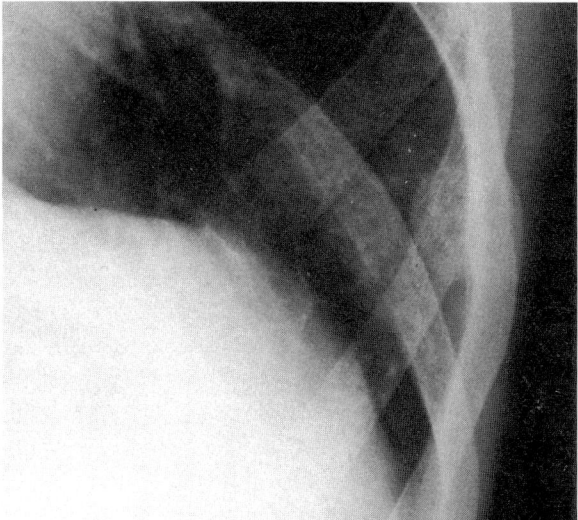
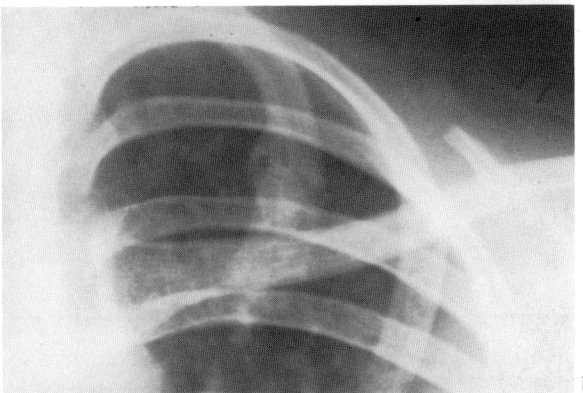
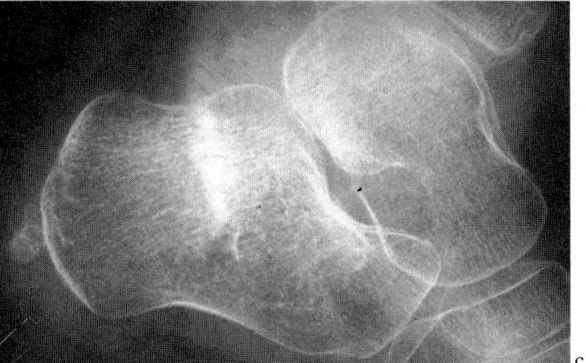

Fig. 1.6. *Stress fractures—less common locations.* **a** *8th and 9th ribs.* Fractures of this type may be caused by chronic coughing. In this elderly man the lesions were symmetrical and were surrounded by organising callus. **b** *1st rib.* This stress fracture shows characteristic callus formation at a site not uncommonly affected as a result of carrying a heavy pack. **c** *Calcaneus.* The oblique line of density indicated this unusual lesion. It occurred in a 6-year-old girl whose ankle had been immobilised for non-specific synovitis with consequent disuse atrophy.

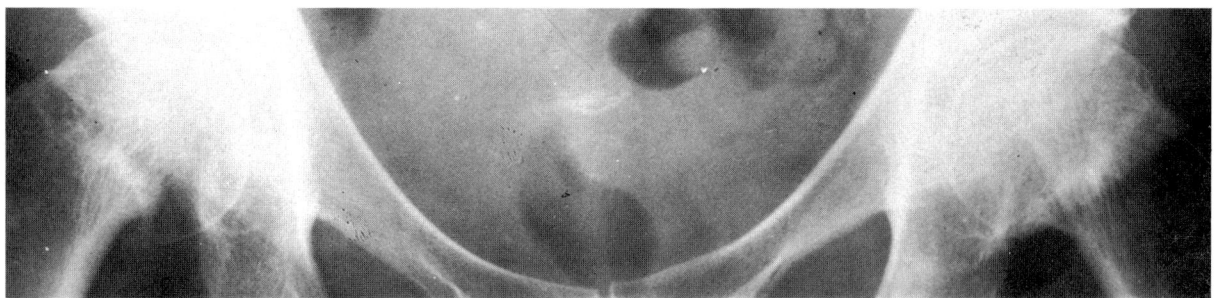

Fig. 1.7. *Stress fractures of femoral necks following irradiation.* This 33-year-old woman complained of pain in the hips. She had been treated for gynaecological cancer by radiation therapy 3 years before. Therapy of this type impairs vitality of bone, rendering it abnormally brittle. In larger doses it may cause actual necrosis of bone (see Exercise 7).

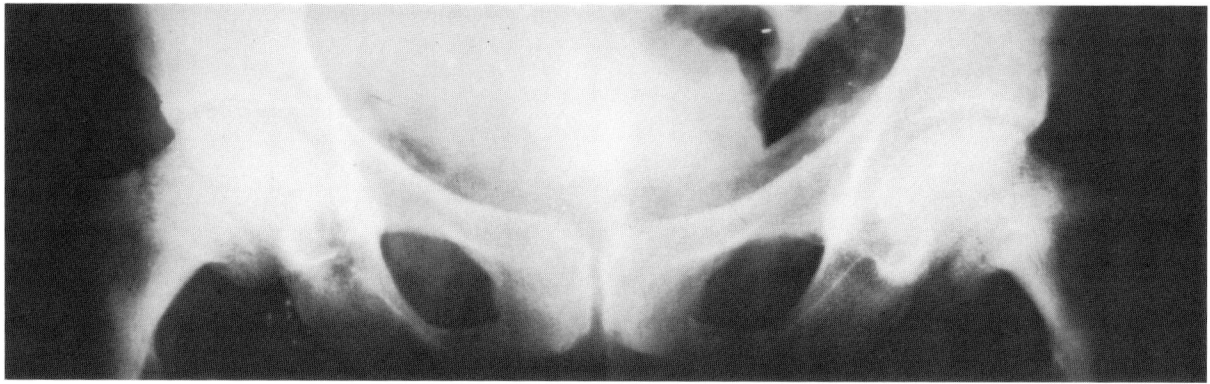

Fig. 1.8. *Looser's zones (stress fractures) in femoral necks in osteomalacia.* The bilateral zones of lucency are typical of these stigmata of osteomalacia. In this instance the cause was dietetic deficiency in a 22-year-old woman. The diagnosis of osteomalacia always deserves consideration when a lesion of this type is observed, particularly in elderly women (see Exercise 3).

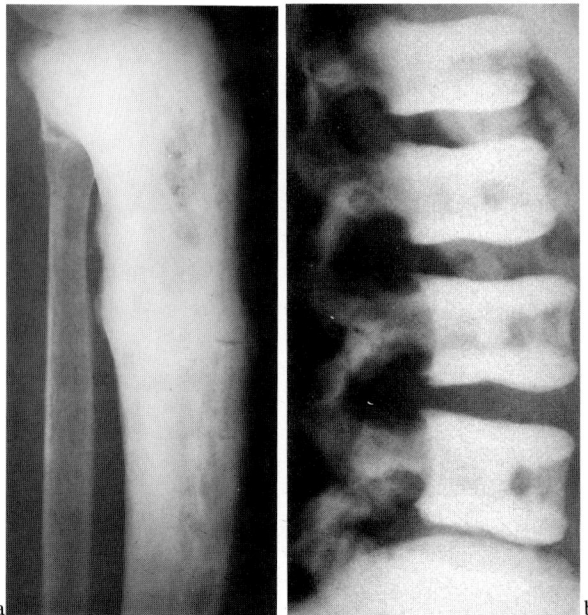

Fig. 1.9. *Pathological stress fractures.* **a** *Paget's disease.* The convex aspects of the femur and tibia in bone softened and bowed by this disease commonly display minute increment fractures in various stages of healing (compare Fig. 1.3c in Exercise 8). **b** *Osteopetrosis.* Despite the extreme density exhibited in this hereditary dysplasia, the affected bone is brittle, so that spontaneous pathological fractures are often responsible for recognition of its presence. This example illustrated stress fractures in the neural arches of L3 and L4 in a 13-year-old boy who presented with a stiff and painful back. Observe the classical 'sandwich' appearance of the vertebral bodies.

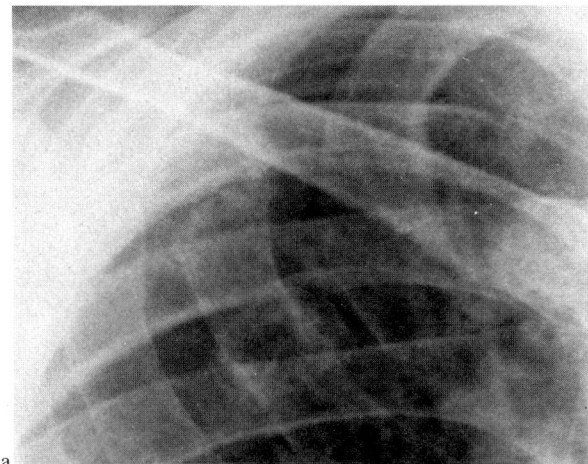
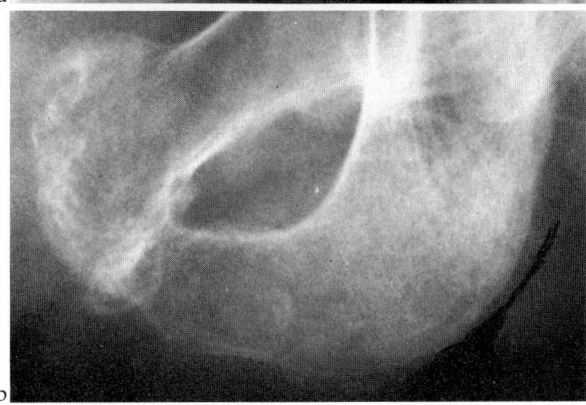

Fig. 1.10. *Cushing's syndrome.* Stress fractures involving the osteoporotic bone in this metabolic disease (see Exercise 3), whether of natural origin or due to steroid therapy, are not uncommon and frequently are asymptomatic owing to suppression of pain sense. **a** Rib and **b** obturator ring in a 26-year-old woman with advanced disease. These lesions were detected in a skeletal survey.

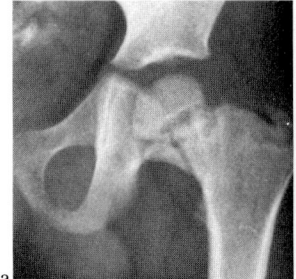
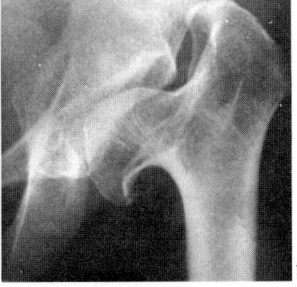

Fig. 1.11. *Coxa vara of childhood.* This peculiar condition may be congenital or acquired and is usually bilateral, the presenting abnormality being a waddling gait early in life. **a** The vertical defect in the medial portion of the proximal femoral metaphysis represents a stress fracture. **b** The typical residual adult deformity, again usually bilateral and often totally asymptomatic.

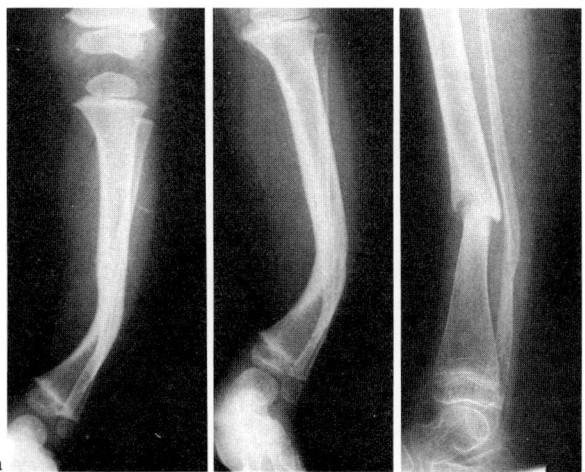

Fig. 1.12. *Neurofibromatosis.* Pseudarthrosis of the tibia is a well recognised manifestation of this familial disorder, as illustrated by these serial studies extending over 3 years in a young girl. The initial bowing culminates in a stress fracture and pointing of the bone ends, a complication very difficult to treat. Short-curve scoliosis, abnormalities of bone texture and asymmetrical growth represent other orthopaedic features of this entity.

A2. Osteosarcoma of tibia

In this case also doubt was expressed concerning the diagnosis. The periosteal reaction overlying the area of increased bone density was regarded initially as indicating either a response to mechanical stress or a low-grade inflammatory lesion, such as subacute osteomyelitis. The histological appearance of the biopsy specimen (Q2b and c), however, demonstrated the unmistakable pattern of a malignant bone-forming tumour – an osteosarcoma. The marrow spaces are occupied completely by cellular tissue with an irregular network of bone structures, entirely different from the trabeculae of reactive bone illustrated in Q1b. The more magnified view (Q2c) shows that these structures are surrounded by cellular tumour tissue (compare Q1b and c in Exercise 14). In this case biopsy was imperative in order to establish the correct diagnosis. In contrast, biopsy of the stress fracture in Q1 might have been avoided had clinical and radiological assessment been more accurate.

Q1. This 45-year-old woman had been aware of discomfort in the region of the left pubis for 8 months. She presented on account of a sudden acute exacerbation causing severe localised pain.

Clinical examination confirmed the presence of localised tenderness on the left side of the symphysis pubis, but no other abnormality was detected. Routine blood investigations were normal.

A radiograph of the pelvis (Q1a) demonstrated a large osteolytic lesion in the medial portion of the left pubic bone with poorly defined endosteal margins. A pathological fracture was evident, without significant displacement, but accounting for the acute pain. At this age the first diagnostic consideration was an osteolytic metastasis. No other bony abnormality was detected on skeletal survey and radionuclide scanning. To exclude a solitary metastasis from renal cancer an intravenous urogram was performed, but was negative. This study, however (Q1b), showed the osteolytic lesion more clearly and revealed extensive cortical destruction.

A biopsy was performed.

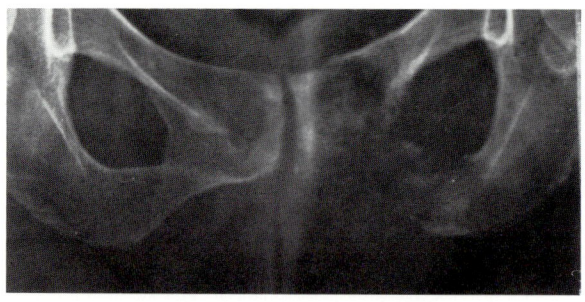

Q1a.

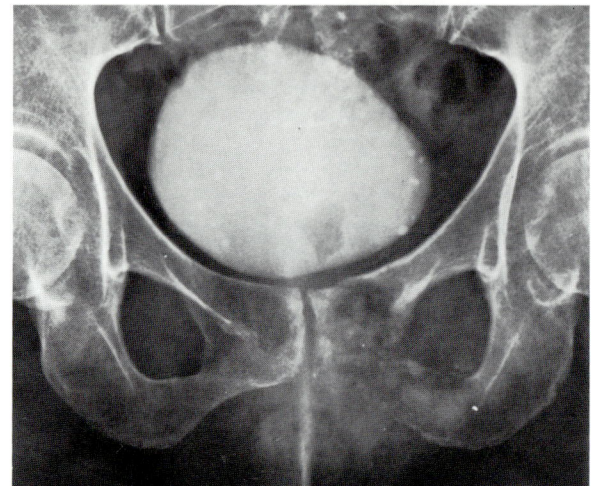

Q1b.

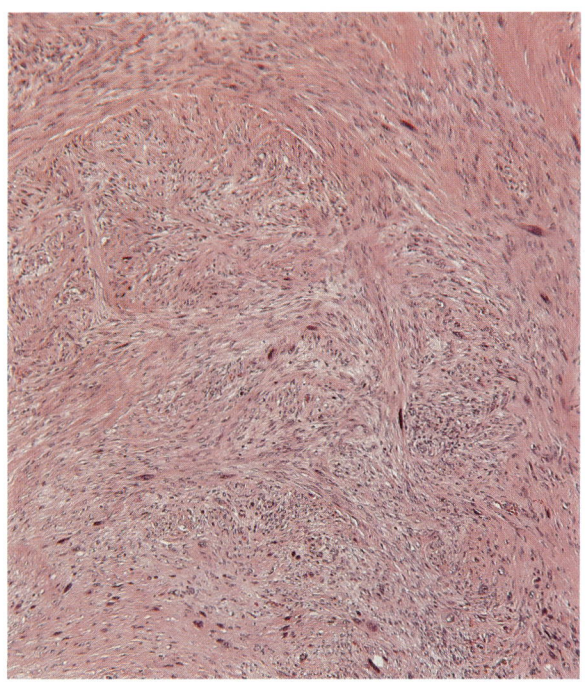

Q1c. (×55)

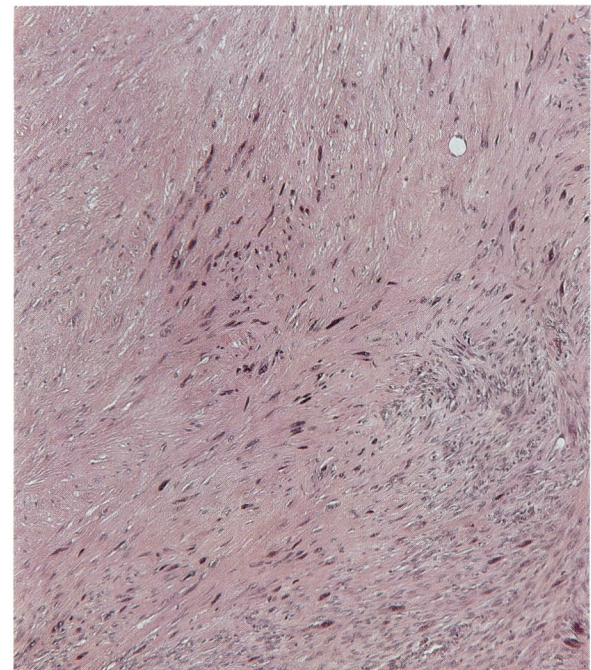

Q1d. (×55)

Q2. This 53-year-old woman had been aware of discomfort above the right knee for 2 years. During the preceding few weeks actual pain had developed, interfering with sleep and associated with a swelling on the outer side of the thigh.

On clinical examination the swelling was palpated easily. It was hard and tender on pressure. No other physical abnormality was detected. Apart from an elevated ESR all routine haematological and biochemical investigations were negative.

Radiographs of the affected limb showed a diffuse area of poorly defined medullary destruction in the femur, with erosion and fragmentation of the lateral cortex. Some bony fragments were displaced laterally within a soft tissue mass. Another lucent area situated more proximally in the femur was regarded as a satellite lesion and also had eroded the lateral cortex. Films of the chest were normal and skeletal survey revealed no other skeletal lesions. Only localised uptake of the tracer was evident on a radionuclide scan.

A biopsy was performed.

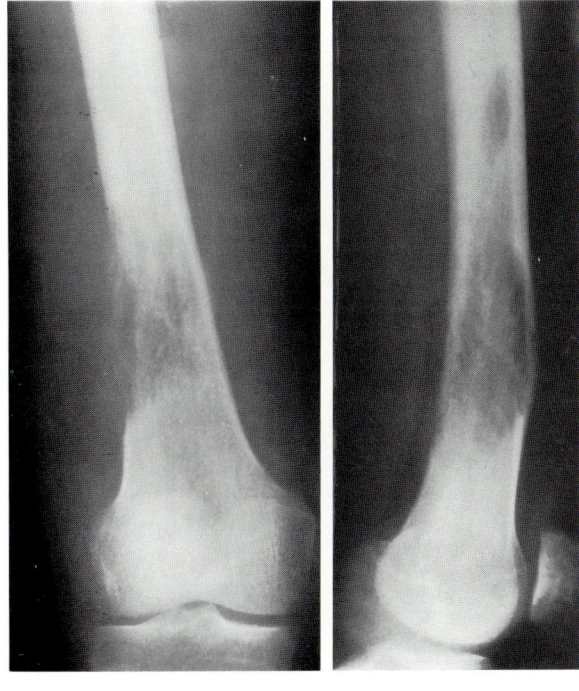

Q2a.

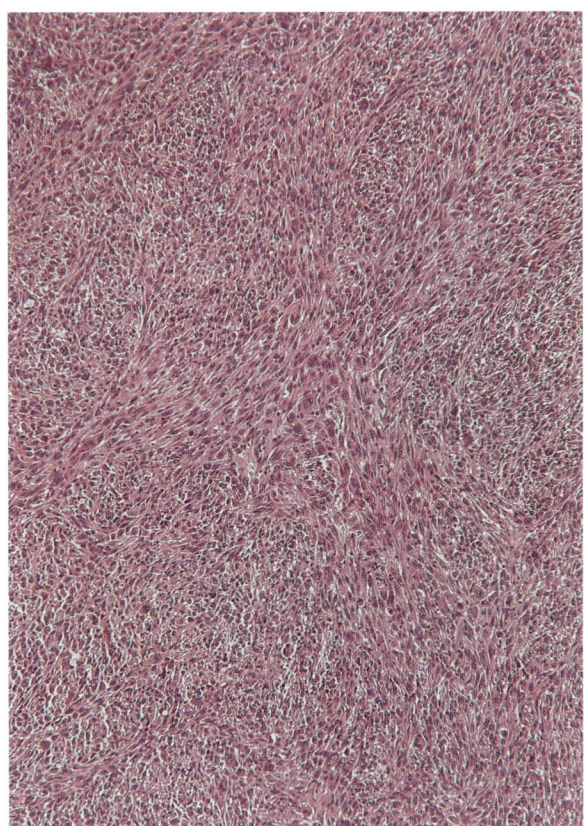

Q2b. (×60)

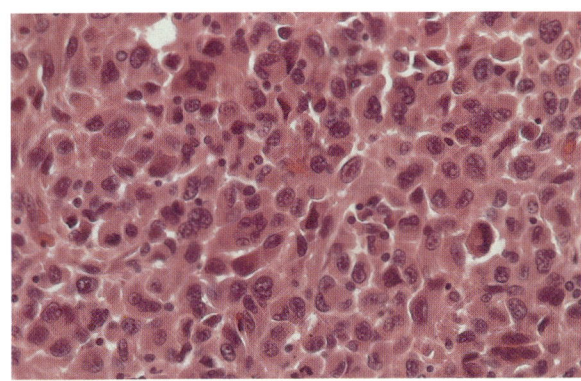

Q2c. (×220)

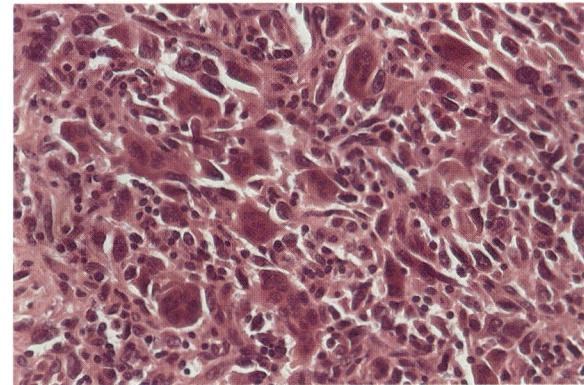

Q2d. (×220)

A1. Fibrosarcoma of pubis

The preliminary investigations appearing to have excluded metastatic disease, the possibilities of a primary tumour or some other localised lesion were considered pre-operatively.

The histological appearance is that of a fibrosarcoma (Q1c, d). The lesion consists of spindle-celled tissue. Some areas contain a considerable amount of intercellular collagen which can be recognised as strands of pink-staining material. Most of the cells have slender elongated nuclei, the appearance of which does not suggest malignancy. Other nuclei (Q1d) are large and irregular in outline, and stain darkly. These pleomorphic and hyperchromatic cells indicate that the lesion is a sarcoma. This is confirmed by the presence of scattered mitoses, some of them abnormal. The intercellular collagen lacks the trabecular pattern that would be expected in an osteosarcoma. The abundance of this intercellular collagen, the regularity of many of the nuclei and the relative infrequency of mitoses, establish the diagnosis of well-differentiated fibrosarcoma. These histological features bear no resemblance to a metastasis.

A wide local resection of the tumour was undertaken. Examination of the resected specimen showed extension of the tumour tissue through the cortex into the immediately adjacent soft tissue.

Fibrosarcoma

The term fibrosarcoma is applied to malignant tumours with a spindle-celled structure and showing production of collagen.

Fibrosarcomas are among the rarest of primary malignant tumours of bone, representing less than 4% of such neoplasms. Although any age in adult life may be affected, they occur predominantly between 30 and 50 years of age. Males and females are affected equally. Occasionally fibrosarcomas have been observed to arise in the fibrous tissue surrounding a bone infarct.

Clinical Features

As in the case of other primary malignant neoplasms of the skeleton, localised pain and swelling are the dominant presenting complaints. Although considerable variation exists in the duration of these symptoms and signs, according to the degree of malignancy, the history rarely exceeds a year. Their infiltrating and destructive nature makes them especially prone to pathological fracture, which may be the cause of presentation in as many as a quarter of cases.

Radiological Features

1. Site. The majority arise in the diametaphyseal portions of long bones, especially around the knee. Their occurrence in flat bones, such as the pelvis and ribs, is far less common. They may originate within the medullary cavity or have a periosteal location. Rarely, a fibrosarcoma originating in the soft tissues may erode adjacent bones.

2. Appearance. Fibrosarcomas are classically permeative and invasive, spreading widely in medullary bone with no clear marginal definition, consequently resembling often a malignant round cell tumour. The cortex frequently is destroyed to permit the development of moderately large extensions of the tumour into adjacent soft tissues. Calcification may be present within the abnormal tissue, especially when the site of origin is extraskeletal, so that a cartilaginous abnormality may be suspected.

In all these tumours a valuable diagnostic feature is the virtual absence of reactive or of tumour bone. Periosteal reactions, when they do develop, are slight or minimal. Vascular studies usually demonstrate a pathological circulation and CT is especially helpful in assessment of soft tissue extensions.

Pathological Features

Fibrosarcomas show a rather wide range of histological structure. Some are relatively benign lesions characterised by well-differentiated mature fibrous tissue, while others are highly malignant tumours consisting of undifferentiated tissue with extremely pleomorphic cells and relatively little intercellular collagen. Some well-differentiated tumours may mimic benign conditions such as desmoplastic fibroma or even fibrous dysplasia (see Exercise 1). Poorly differentiated osteosarcomas with relatively little bone formation can be misdiagnosed as fibrosarcomas, particularly on the basis of a limited biopsy sample.

Some tumours, previously regarded as fibrosarcomas, are now recognised as malignant fibrous histiocytomas (see Q2 of this Exercise).

Treatment

Since these tumours do not respond satisfactorily to radiation therapy, surgical removal is the treatment of choice. As a palliative measure, internal splinting of pathological fractures with metallic implants may be justified. Chemotherapy in general has proved to be unsuccessful, although occasionally a satisfactory response has been reported. Metastatic dissemination to the lungs is the usual terminal event. The prognosis clearly depends on the degree of histological differentiation, but is somewhat better, on the whole, than that of osteosarcoma.

References

Eyre-Brook AL, Price CHG (1969) Fibrosarcoma of bone. Review of 50 consecutive cases from the Bristol Bone Tumour Registry. J Bone Jt Surg 51B: 20–37

Dahlin DC, Ivins JC (1969) Fibrosarcoma of bone. A study of 114 cases. Cancer 23: 35–41

Huvos AG, Higinbotham NL (1975) Primary fibrosarcoma of bone. A clinico-pathological study of 130 patients. Cancer 35: 837–847

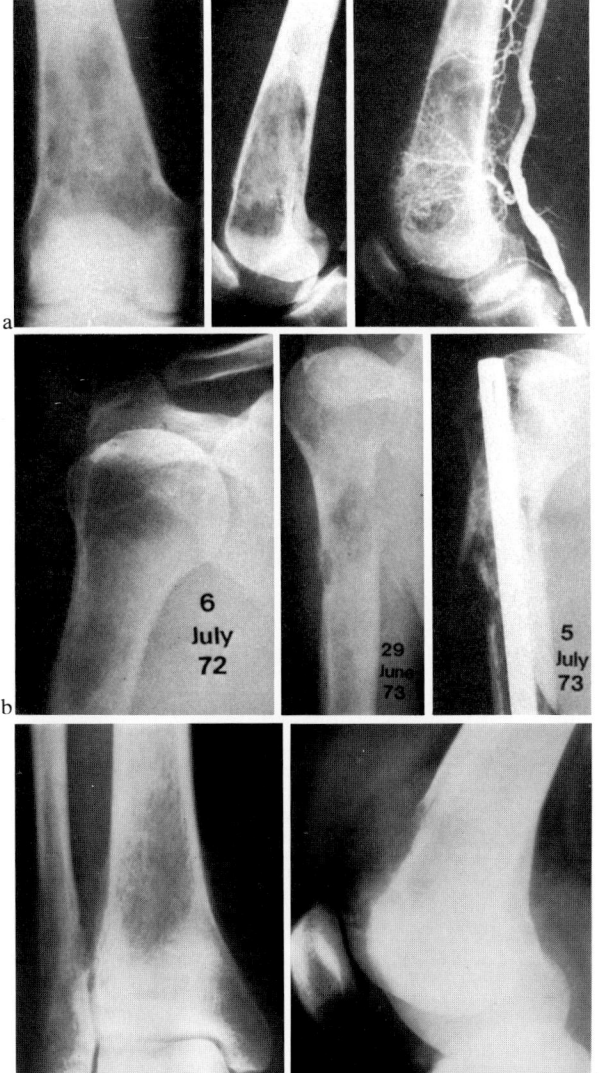

Fig. 1.1. *Fibrosarcoma—classical examples.* **a** This middle-aged man presented with a painful swelling above the knee which had developed within several months. The permeating destructive lesion in the medulla has poorly defined margins and has eroded the cortex. Hypervascularity is shown by the arteriogram, with displacement of the femoral artery by an extension of the tumour. **b** A similar destructive lesion in the proximal end of the humerus of this 61-year-old man had caused pain for 1 year. On presentation its significance was not appreciated. A year later a pathological fracture caused an acute exacerbation of pain and it was evident that gross extension of the tumour had taken place. Transient relief was obtained by internal fixation, but metastases had developed already. **c** In this instance the area of diffuse osteolysis in the distal end of the tibia was found in a 46-year-old man, who had complained of pain and swelling for only 6 months. Some periosteal reaction has occurred. Differential diagnosis from other malignancies, especially a reticulum cell sarcoma, or even infection, is difficult. **d** This parosteal lesion on the anterior aspect of the femur had developed within 1 year in a 23-year-old woman. The soft tissue mass contains no calcification. Extensive cortical destruction is evident. Observe the predilection for these tumours to arise around the knee.

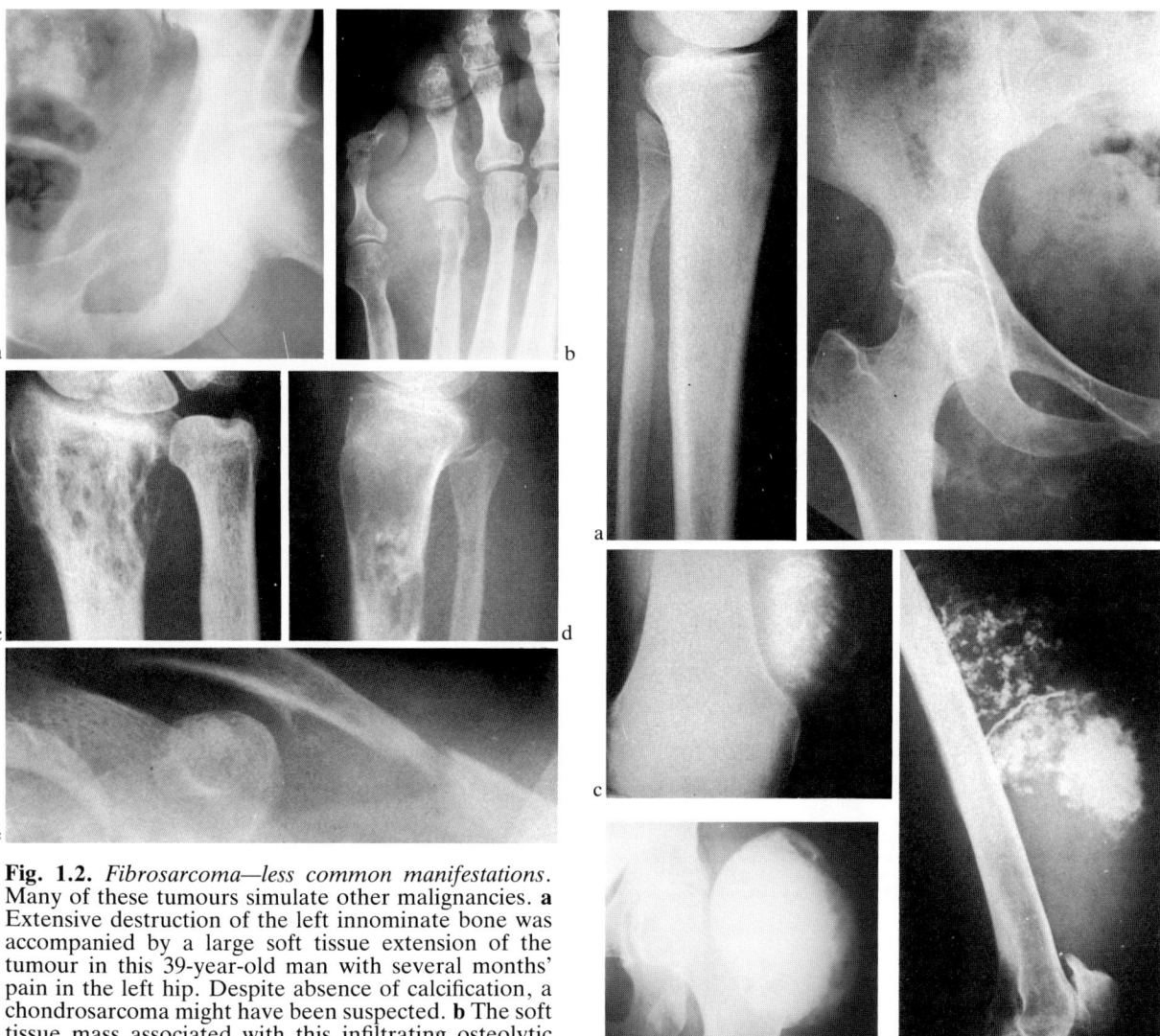

Fig. 1.2. *Fibrosarcoma—less common manifestations.* Many of these tumours simulate other malignancies. **a** Extensive destruction of the left innominate bone was accompanied by a large soft tissue extension of the tumour in this 39-year-old man with several months' pain in the left hip. Despite absence of calcification, a chondrosarcoma might have been suspected. **b** The soft tissue mass associated with this infiltrating osteolytic lesion of the 4th metatarsal caused separation of the 4th and 5th toes. The appearance is remarkably similar to a malignant round cell tumour, a diagnosis made much less likely by the age of this man (55 years). **c** Irregular destruction of bone in the distal end of the radius in this elderly man was regarded as being definitely malignant, but was interpreted initially as a metastasis. The diagnosis was established only by biopsy. **d** The oval area of osteolysis in the tibial shaft of this 23-year-old woman was regarded pre-operatively as a chondrosarcoma because of central foci of calcification. The possibility of calcification developing in a fibrosarcoma of bone must be appreciated, although this feature is more common when these tumours originate in soft tissues. **e** Sudden onset of pain in a swelling of the clavicle which had developed during the previous year in a 31-year-old man drew attention to this pathological fracture. The soft tissue mass is clearly defined and again the appearance at this age would suggest first a malignant round cell tumour. In all these cases, however, observe the paucity of reactive bone formation.

Fig. 1.3. *Fibrosarcoma—originating in soft tissue.* These tumours may cause pressure erosion of an adjacent bone and are liable to undergo varying degrees of calcification. CT and ultrasound studies may be of value. In cases of this type, malignancy may be suggested strongly, but the definitive diagnosis depends on histological assessment. Possibilities include osteosarcoma, chondrosarcoma, liposarcoma and, especially, malignant fibrous histiocytoma. It appears probable that the last of these entities has been confused often with fibrosarcoma in the past. **a** This scalloped erosion of the fibula was associated with a painful but uncalcified swelling in the calf of a 22-year-old woman. **b** Another fibrosarcoma near the right hip of a middle-aged woman showed diffuse whorls of calcification. **c**, **d** and **e** illustrate more heavily calcified fibrosarcomas in the soft tissues of the thigh.

A2. Malignant fibrous histiocytoma

Both the clinical and radiological findings suggested, in a woman of this age, a malignant tumour. Since other investigations had failed to disclose a primary neoplasm, the first consideration of metastatic disease was excluded. Equally the possibility of a plasmacytoma was made unlikely by several factors, including a normal albumin–globulin ratio, absence of Bence-Jones protein in the urine and a positive radionuclide scan. The radiological diagnosis of this aggressive, infiltrating lesion was considered to lie between reticulum cell sarcoma, fibrosarcoma and malignant fibrous histiocytoma.

As in Q1, the biopsy established the presence of a malignant spindle-celled tumour (Q2b–d). In the present case the tumour tissue is more cellular and pleomorphic, and very little intercellular collagen is present; bizarre cells and mitoses are numerous. A conspicuous feature is the arrangement of the tissue in interweaving bundles (Q2b), giving what is referred to as a 'storiform' pattern. The adjective 'storiform' is derived from the Latin word *storia*, meaning a mat constructed of straw or rope. As in Q1, no evidence of tumour bone formation is present. Some areas of the tumour (Q2d) contain scattered osteoclast giant cells and smaller rounded lymphocytic cells.

All these histological features characterise a group of tumours now referred to as malignant fibrous histiocytoma. Some indication of a storiform pattern, indeed, is evident in the case illustrated in Q1 (Q1c), but that lesion lacks the other histological features of a histiocytic tumour.

Following biopsy the clinical situation was complicated by a typically transverse pathological fracture. Prosthetic replacement was considered to be hazardous and disarticulation through the hip was performed, the patient remaining in good health during the following years. The ultimate prognosis, however, could only be guarded.

Malignant Fibrous Histiocytoma

The characteristics of malignant fibrous histiocytoma have not yet been agreed generally. Some authorities are hesitant to accept it as a separate and specific type of bone tumour, although it is well recognised as a variety of soft tissue neoplasm. The term is usually applied to a spindle-celled tumour, generally resembling a fibrosarcoma, both histologically and radiologically.

Clinical Features

As with so many soft tissue tumours, the presenting complaint is usually of a painful soft tissue swelling. Involvement of bone is distinctly less common than of soft tissues. The majority of reported bone lesions have occurred in the later years of adult life, but a few involve children and adolescents. Males are affected more frequently than females.

Radiological Features

1. Site. The metaphyseal regions at the ends of the long bones are the commonest location for this tumour, but lesions in the axial skeleton, including the pelvis, spine and ribs, have been described.

2. Appearance. The lesions are essentially osteolytic, and frequently expansile. Erosion of the overlying cortex is common, with extension of the tumour into the adjacent soft tissues, often with a clearly defined margin. Foci of calcification within the mass may be detected. A periosteal reaction may be stimulated, but endosteal reactive sclerosis tends to be absent. Such an appearance simulates a fibrosarcoma so closely that radiological differentiation is virtually impossible. Radionuclide scanning is positive.

Pathological Features

The tumours consist of spindle-celled tissue, often with a considerable degree of pleomorphism and mitotic activity. There is a general resemblance to fibrosarcoma, although most areas contain relatively little intercellular collagen. Features which usually are absent in fibrosarcoma, and which indicate a diagnosis of malignant fibrous histiocytoma, are (i) the so-called 'storiform' pattern produced by interweaving strands of tumour cells, (ii) the presence of histiocytic cells, distinguished from fibroblasts by their rounded outline, foamy cytoplasm and phagocytic activity, (iii) the presence of multinucleated giant cells and (iv) lymphocytic infiltration. The more conspicuous these features, the more likely the tumour is to be regarded as a malignant fibrous histiocytoma.

Histological distinction from benign lesions, and particularly from non-ossifying fibroma (see Exercise 6), occasionally presents a diagnostic problem.

Treatment

To judge from reported cases, these tumours are highly malignant. Surgical measures such as block resection or amputation are not always effective. Local recurrence and spread to lymph nodes, lungs and other parts of the body are common. Metastases sometimes develop within months of the initial presentation, and survival rarely exceeds 2 years. A large proportion of the malignant bone tumours developing in association with bone infarcts prove to be malignant fibrous histiocytomas.

References

Dahlin DC, Unni KK, Matsuno T (1977) Malignant fibrous histiocytoma of bone. Fact or fancy? Cancer 39: 1508–1516
Feldman F, Lattes R (1977) Primary malignant fibrous histiocytoma (fibrous xanthoma) of bone. Skeletal Radiol 1: 145–160
McCarthy EF, Matsuno T, Dorfman H (1979) Malignant fibrous histiocytoma of bone: a study of 35 cases. Hum Pathol 10: 57–70
Spanier SS, Enneking WF, Enriquez P (1975) Primary malignant fibrous histiocytoma of bone. Cancer 36: 2084–2098
Weiss SW, Enzinger FM (1978) Malignant fibrous histiocytoma. An analysis of 200 cases. Cancer 41: 2250–2266

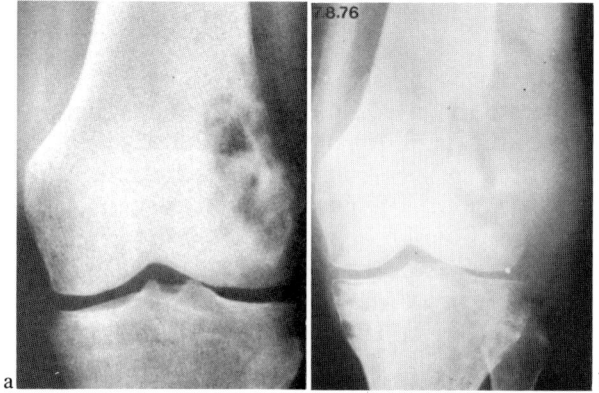

Fig. 2.1. *Malignant fibrous histiocytoma*. **a** This osteolytic lesion in the lateral femoral condyle was found in a 23-year-old woman who had complained of pain in the knee for only 3 months. The endosteal margin was poorly defined and the lateral cortex had been breached, with stimulation of a faint periosteal reaction. Preoperatively a fibrosarcoma or a reticulum cell sarcoma was suggested, but the correct diagnosis was established only by biopsy. Amputation was refused. **b** Two months later the tumour had enlarged greatly, with cortical fragmentation and a clearly delineated extension into the soft tissues. The patient died within a few months from pulmonary metastases.

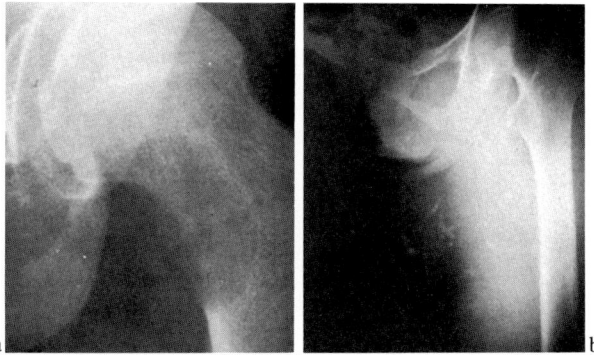

Fig. 2.2. *Malignant fibrous histiocytoma—further examples*. **a** This 15-year-old girl presented with mild pain in the left hip attributed to a fall 3 months earlier. The osteolytic lesion in the medial portion of the femoral neck had destroyed the cortex, but the endosteal zone of transition was narrow. The definitive diagnosis only was established histologically. At operation the lesion had not spread outside the bone and prosthetic replacement was performed. Somewhat exceptionally, this patient was alive and well 5 years later. **b** *Soft tissues*. This huge soft tissue mass, which had been present for some years in this 53-year-old woman, had enlarged and restricted movement during the previous few months. It contains strands of calcification and resembles a liposarcoma. Once again biopsy revealed the true nature of the lesion. The vast majority of these tumours originate in soft tissue.

Exercise 30

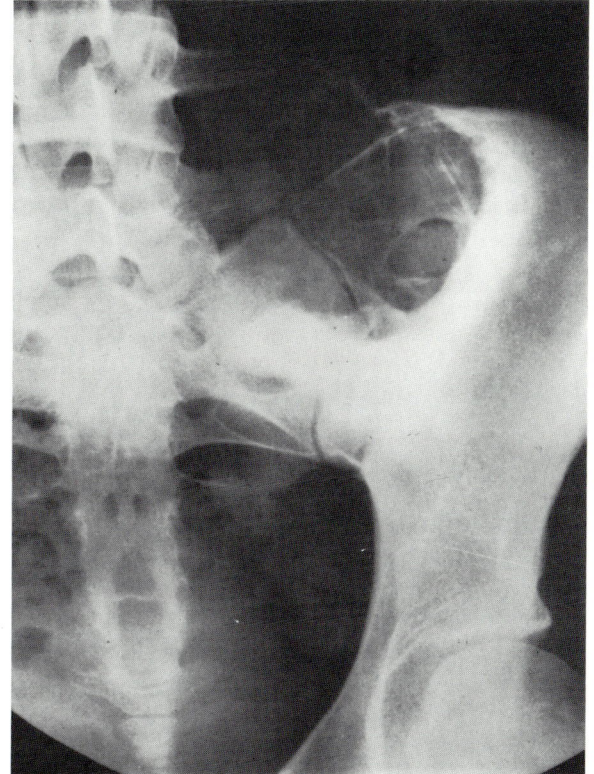

Q1a.

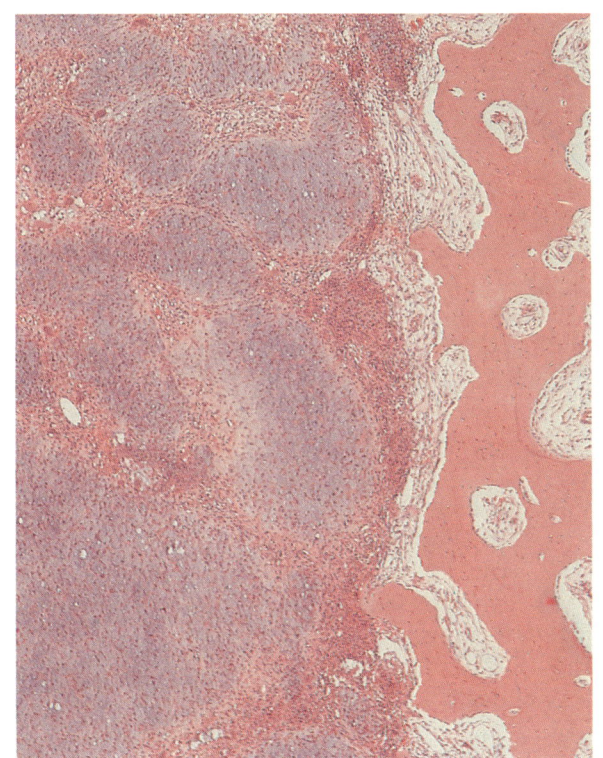

Q1b. (×40)

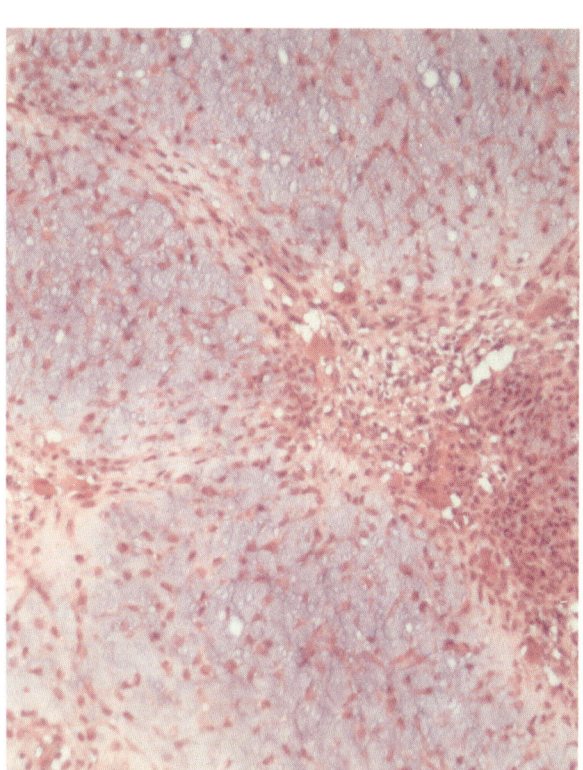

Q1c. (×135)

A1. Chondromyxoid fibroma of ilium

The clinical and radiological features favoured a benign neoplasm, but the possibility of malignancy was suspected on account of its extension into the adjacent soft tissues. A pre-operative diagnosis of a chondrosarcoma had been suggested.

At operation, the lesion was found to consist of a solid mass of firm cartilaginous tissue. The biopsy established a diagnosis, not of chondrosarcoma, but of chondromyxoid fibroma.

The histological appearance, as shown in Q1b and Q1c, is quite characteristic. The tumour consists of lobulated blue-staining chondroid tissue, separated by strands of more cellular tissue containing occasional multinucleated giant cells. Q1b shows the sharp margin of bone at the edge of the tumour. Bone trabeculae have been completely destroyed within the tumour itself, but outside it the trabeculae are increased in thickness, accounting for the extreme density apparent in the radiograph.

In Q1c the elongated and stellate appearance of the tumour cells is typical of chondromyxoid fibroma and aids the distinction from chondroma or chondrosarcoma, where more sharply outlined rounded cell spaces would be expected (see Exercises 12 and 16).

Following biopsy a local resection of the lesion was performed. The patient was alive and well, without evidence of local recurrence, 10 years later.

Chondromyxoid Fibroma

Before the description of this entity by Jaffe and Lichtenstein in 1948, cases had probably been regarded as low-grade chondrosarcomas. It is now recognised that these tumours are benign. The sexes are affected with equal frequency and most of the patients are adolescents or young adults. Chondromyxoid fibroma is a relatively rare type of tumour and is much less common than some other cartilage tumours such as chondroma or chondrosarcoma.

Clinical Features

These are essentially non-specific, the localised pain and swelling which chondromyxoid fibroma may cause being common to the majority of other skeletal neoplasms.

Radiological Features

1. Site. Long bones are most commonly affected, especially diametaphyseal areas. A predilection exists for the proximal end of the tibia, although other parts of the skeleton—as in the present case—can be involved. Lesions, for example, have been recognised in ribs, pubis and the small bones of the hands and feet. Serial studies show these tumours to grow extremely slowly.

Radiological diagnosis in such unusual areas is sufficiently difficult to make histological examination imperative.

2. Appearance. The lesions are essentially lytic, being rounded or oval, in the long axis of the affected bone, with eccentric expansion and thinning of the overlying cortex. The endosteal margin usually is sharply defined and sclerotic, with a narrow zone of transition. As in other cartilaginous lesions, central flecks of calcification may develop in time, but this feature, owing to the large fibrous element, is less usual.

Pathological Features

The typical chondromyxoid fibroma is made up of spindle-shaped or stellate cells, separated by abundant fibrous or chondroid matrix that contains numerous vacuoles. Lobules of this chondroid tissue are separated by more cellular vascular spindle-celled tissue containing scattered osteoclast giant cells (Fig. 1.1a and b). Chondromyxoid fibromas are occasionally confused with chondrosarcoma, but, as already noted, the absence of the round-celled cartilaginous tissue that is such a feature of low-grade chondrosarcoma usually permits easy distinction. The highly malignant spindle-celled type of chondrosarcoma, while lacking this recognisable round-celled cartilage, also lacks the lobulated pattern of chondromyxoid fibroma.

Treatment

Chondromyxoid fibromas sometimes recur locally, and this may require more extensive surgery than the simple curettage that is usually adequate to remove them. None have been reported to metastasise.

References

Jaffe HL, Lichtenstein L (1948) Chondromyxoid fibroma of bone. Arch Pathol 45: 541–555

Rahimi A, Beabout JW, Ivins JC, Dahlin DC (1972) Chondromyxoid fibroma. A clinicopathologic study of 76 cases. Cancer 30: 726–736

Schajowicz F, Gallardo H (1971) Chondromyxoid fibroma (fibromyxoid chondroma) of bone. Clinicopathological study of 32 cases. J Bone Jt Surg 53B: 198–216

Turcotte B, Pugh DC, Dahlin DC (1962) The roentgenologic aspects of chondromyxoid fibroma of bone. Am J Roentgenol 87: 1085–1095

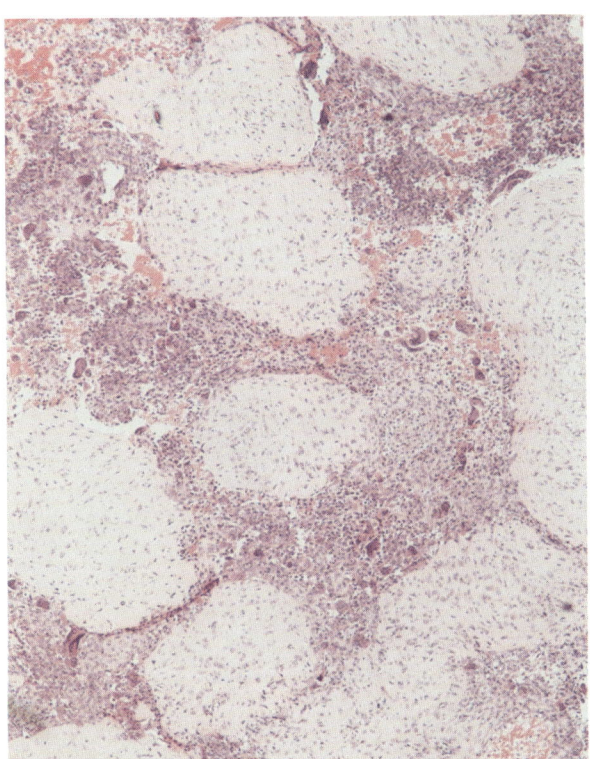

Fig. 1.1a. Another chondromyxoid fibroma, showing the characteristic lobules of chondroid tissue separated by strands of cellular tissue containing giant cells. (×44)

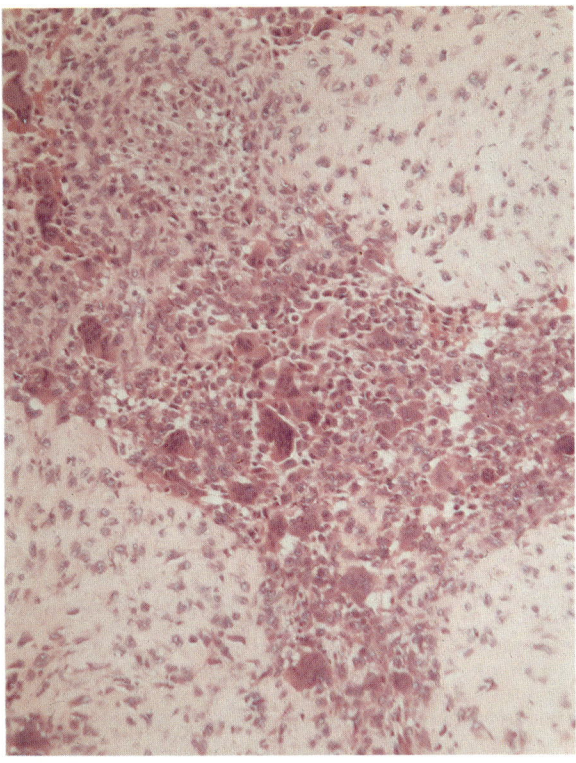

Fig. 1.1b. A more magnified view of the lesion in Fig. 1.1a, showing the appearance of the two types of tissue present. (×85)

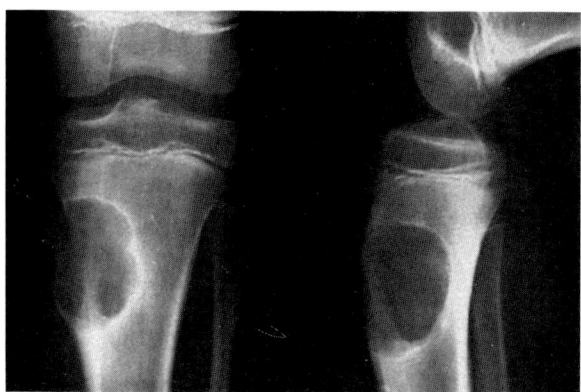

Fig. 1.2. *Chondromyxoid fibroma of tibia.* This 11-year-old girl had a tender swelling below the knee, which she declared to have developed in only 6 weeks. The large destructive and expanding lesion has a serpiginous, sclerotic, endosteal margin. The appearance and the location at this most common site were classical for this benign tumour. In view of the short history, however, a pre-operative diagnosis of aneurysmal bone cyst was suggested. At operation the tumour was unusually vascular, raising the concept that such cysts may be secondary to a variety of pathological precursors (see Exercise 22).

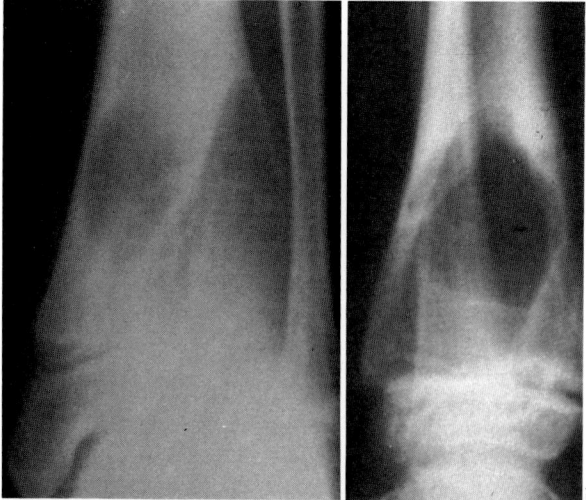

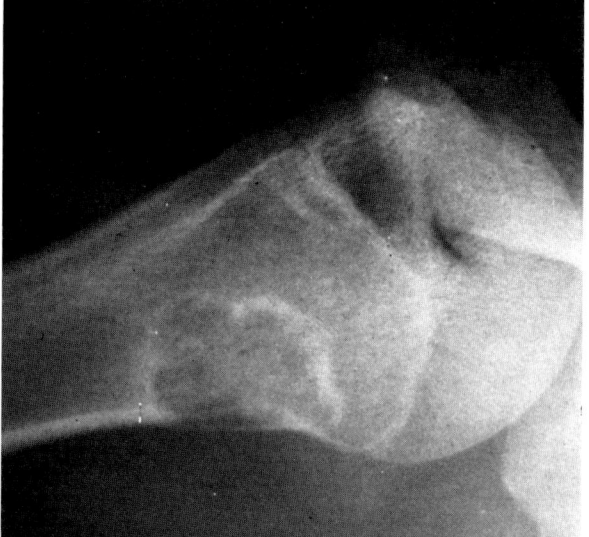

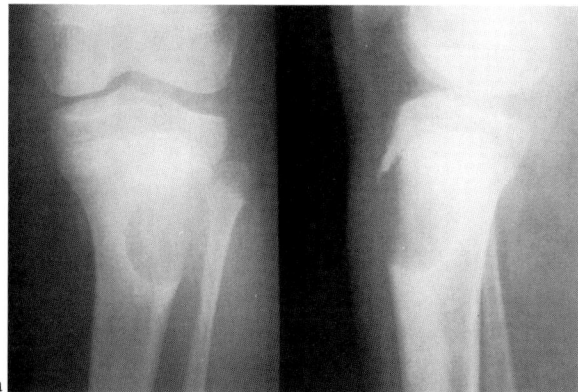

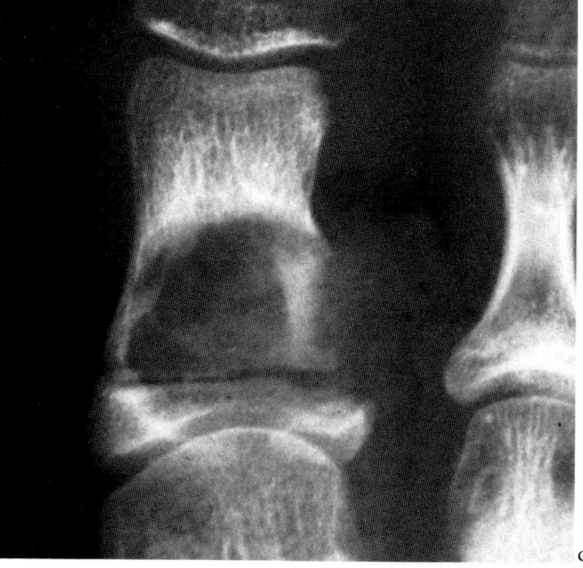

Fig. 1.3. *Chondromyxoid fibroma in children* **a** *Tibia.* Another similar eccentric lesion at the classical location in a 10-year-old boy with mild pain for many months. **b** *Tibia.* This more distal lesion shows the same features of an expanding, slightly lobulated area of bone destruction in a 12-year-old boy with discomfort for 5 months. The resemblance to an aneurysmal bone cyst is striking. **c** *Humerus.* This 14-year-old girl had mild shoulder pain, accentuated by physical activity, for 6 months. Although the typical diagnostic criteria are present, the appearance simulates a benign fibrous lesion. Biopsy was necessary. **d** *1st proximal phalanx of foot.* Foot pain in this 11-year-old girl was caused by this tumour in an unusual site. Again, the diagnosis depended on histological study.

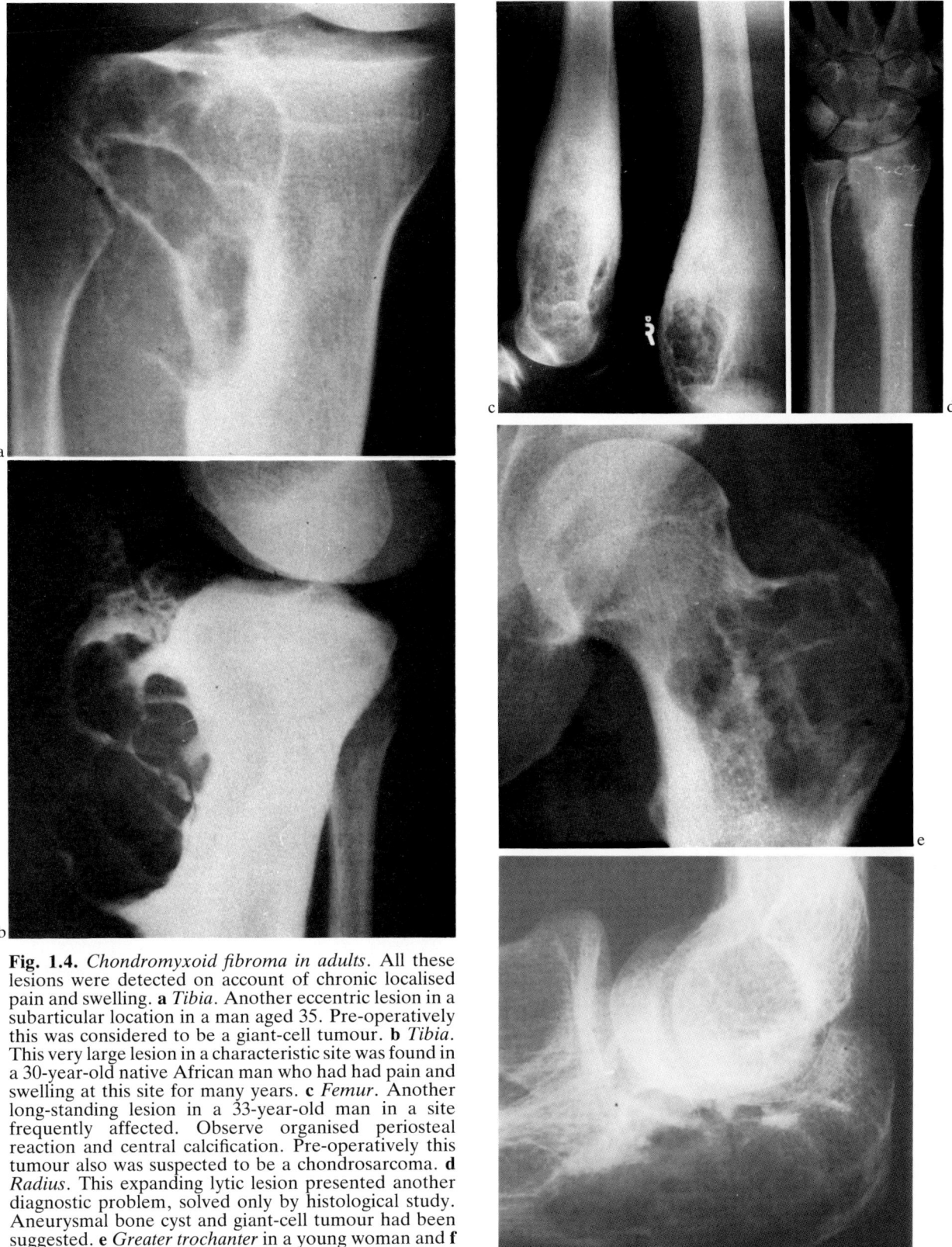

Fig. 1.4. *Chondromyxoid fibroma in adults.* All these lesions were detected on account of chronic localised pain and swelling. **a** *Tibia.* Another eccentric lesion in a subarticular location in a man aged 35. Pre-operatively this was considered to be a giant-cell tumour. **b** *Tibia.* This very large lesion in a characteristic site was found in a 30-year-old native African man who had had pain and swelling at this site for many years. **c** *Femur.* Another long-standing lesion in a 33-year-old man in a site frequently affected. Observe organised periosteal reaction and central calcification. Pre-operatively this tumour also was suspected to be a chondrosarcoma. **d** *Radius.* This expanding lytic lesion presented another diagnostic problem, solved only by histological study. Aneurysmal bone cyst and giant-cell tumour had been suggested. **e** *Greater trochanter* in a young woman and **f** *olecranon process* in a 39-year-old man. Both represent unusual sites and emphasise again the need for biopsy.

Q1. This 14-year-old boy had complained of intermittent pain in the right shoulder for 2 months with a recent exacerbation.

On clinical examination a firm swelling was palpable around the proximal end of the humerus. Pressure on this swelling elicited acute pain. All movements of the shoulder were restricted. A low-grade fever of 38°C was present. Laboratory investigations disclosed the ESR to be 28 mm/h and the leucocyte count to be 14 000 per mm^3, but otherwise were normal.

Radiologically a large osteolytic lesion was demonstrated in the diametaphysis of the humerus. The overlying cortex was eroded on its internal aspect and the zone of transition was wide. A minimal infraction was evident, with a mild periosteal reaction on its lateral side.

The lesion was explored.

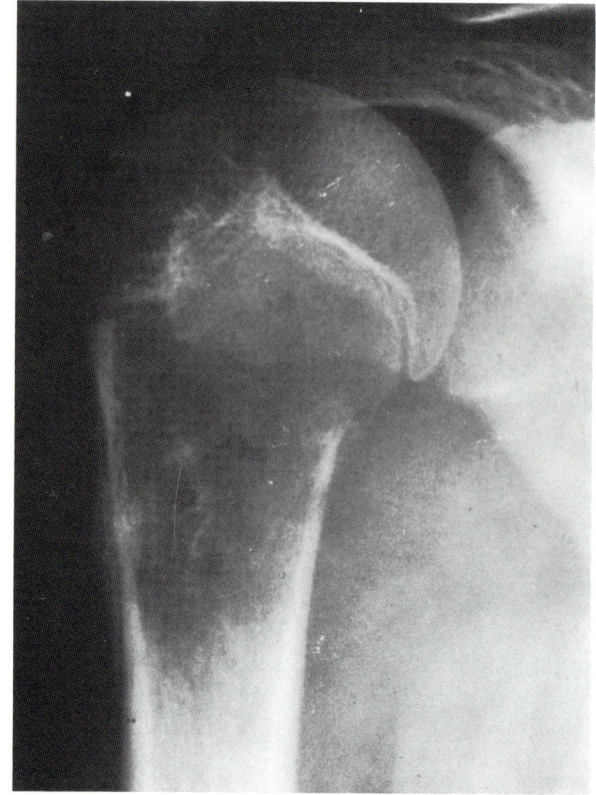

Q1a.

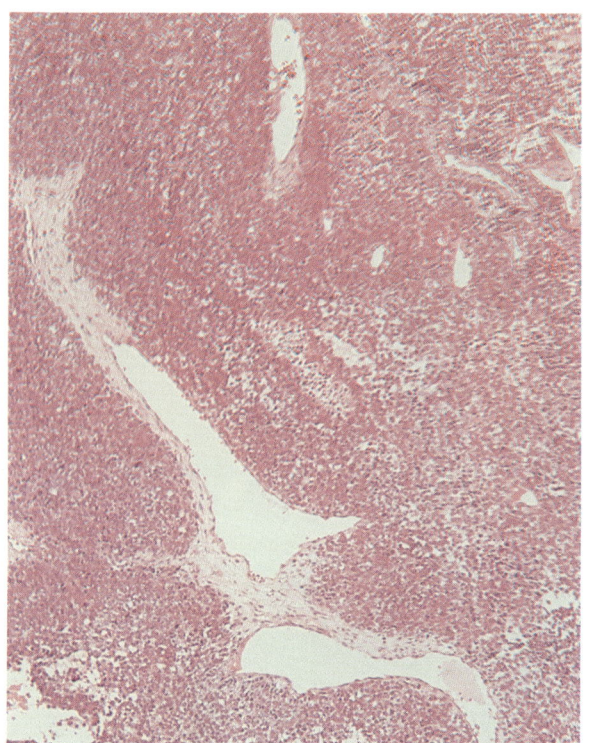

Q1b. (×80)

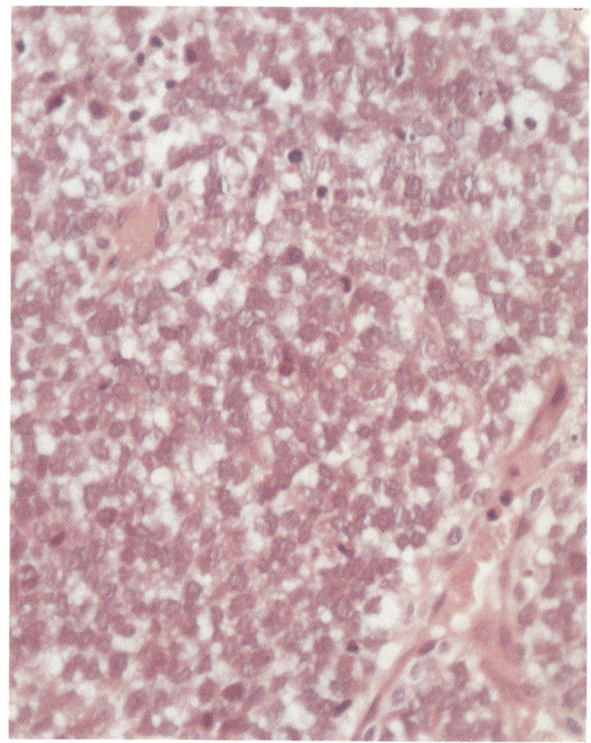

Q1c. (×390)

Q2. This 48-year-old man had experienced mild discomfort in the right forearm for 9 months. During the previous few weeks frank pain had developed, accompanied by a localised swelling.

On clinical examination the swelling was found to be tender and to lie within the deep tissues of the forearm. No other clinical abnormality was detected and routine laboratory investigations were normal.

Radiographs of the forearm confirmed swelling of the soft tissues on its volar aspect, with diffuse and irregular bone destruction within the central third of the medullary cavity of the radius. In the lateral projection it was evident that a portion of the anterior cortex had been destroyed. Skeletal survey revealed no other abnormality.

A biopsy of the lesion was performed.

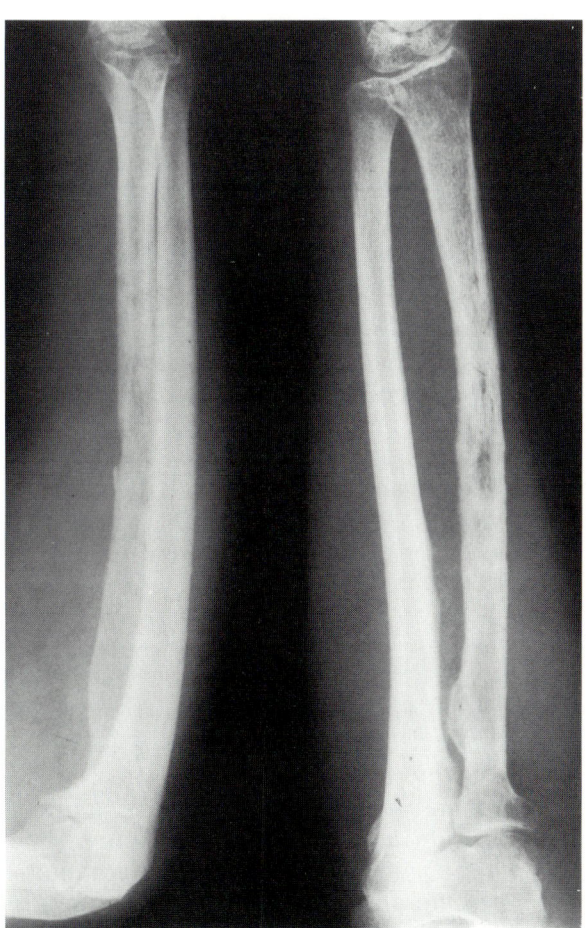

Q2a.

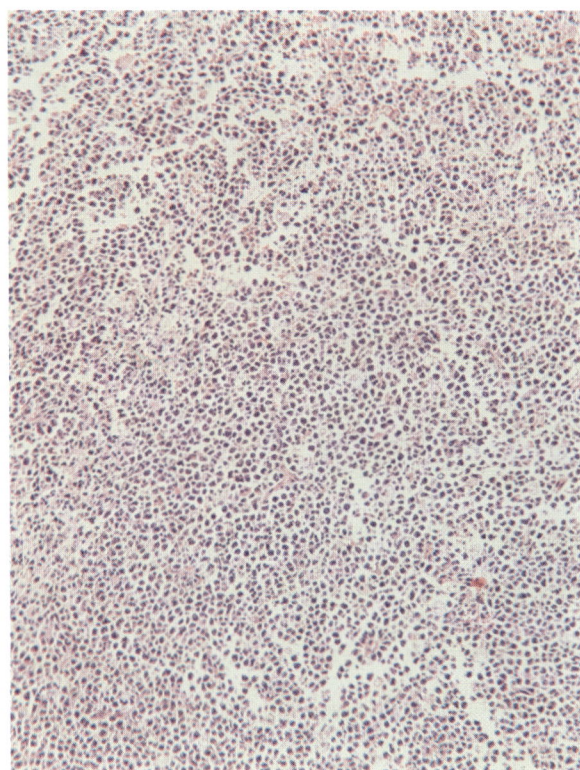

Q2b. (×80)

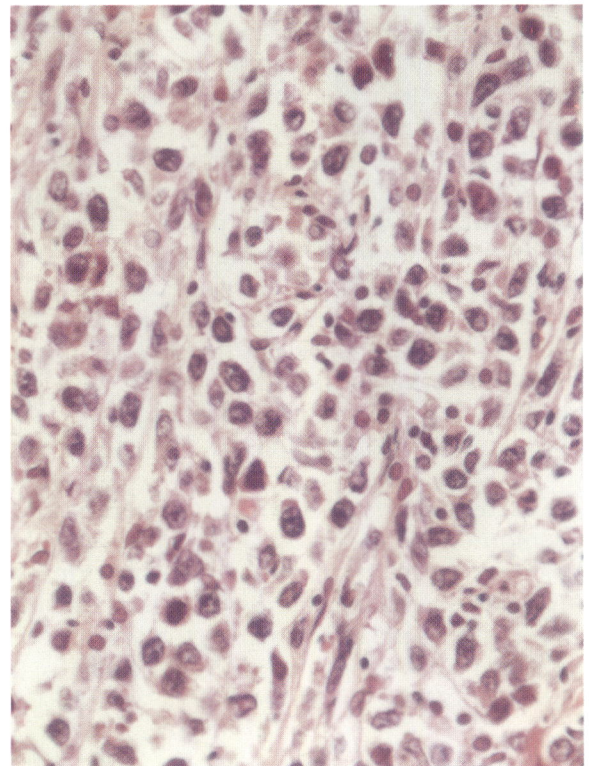

Q2c. (×390)

A1. Ewing's sarcoma of humerus

Both the clinical and radiological findings in this case caused a malignant neoplasm to be suspected, rather than infection or histiocytosis. Absence of bone formation favoured a malignant round-cell tumour, rather than an osteosarcoma.

At operation, the lesion consisted of pale tissue which extended through the cortex to the adjacent soft tissue. A rapid frozen section showed the presence of highly cellular tumour tissue. No micro-organisms were found on examination of a stained smear and no growth was obtained on culture. The appearance of the lesion, in the definitive paraffin sections, is shown in Q1b and Q1c, and confirmed the diagnosis of a malignant neoplasm. The tumour consists of cells with round nuclei and indistinctly outlined cytoplasm. This appearance is typical of a 'malignant round-cell tumour' of bone. Further investigations are necessary to reach a more specific diagnosis. The age of the patient, the site of the lesion and the radiological appearance had suggested Ewing's sarcoma. This diagnosis was supported by the presence, in appropriately stained sections, of intracellular glycogen (Fig. 1.1a), indicated by dark red material within the tumour cells. It was supported further by the absence of intercellular reticulin fibres (Fig. 1.1b). These features permitted differentiation from other types of 'malignant round-cell tumour', which include lymphoma, reticulum-cell sarcoma, metastatic neuroblastoma and metastatic carcinoma. Histological evidence of any of these entities was lacking in the biopsy specimen. A diagnosis of neuroblastoma, in particular, was excluded by absence of catecholamines in the urine.

The patient was treated with radiotherapy and chemotherapy. Despite an initially favourable response by the primary tumour, pulmonary metastases developed and the patient died 2 years after presentation. Metastases were present in the lungs and in other bones.

Ewing's Sarcoma

The term "Ewing's sarcoma" is used to designate a group of non-osteogenic round-celled tumours of bone, usually involving a long bone in a young patient. Clinically, radiologically and even histologically, distinction from other types of round-cell tumour, such as metastatic carcinoma, lymphoma, reticulum-cell sarcoma and metastatic neuroblastoma, sometimes can be difficult.

This tumour is relatively uncommon, being responsible for approximately 5% of all primary malignant bone neoplasms. It is a disease of childhood and early adult life. The tumour is rarely encountered under the age of 5 years and is uncommon after the age of 30 years. A slight male predominance has been recorded.

Clinical Features

A fundamental consideration is that these patients frequently show evidence of a generalised illness. In addition to localised symptoms and signs they are lethargic, anaemic and often febrile, with an elevated ESR. Such patients may mislead the clinician; not infrequently patients with Ewing's sarcomas have been diagnosed as having acute osteomyelitis and treated accordingly. The tumour itself, as was the case in Q1, causes localised pain and tenderness and the affected bone enlarges relatively rapidly, usually to become more prominent than is the case in other bony malignancies.

Radiological Features

1. Site. Locations of these tumours are divided almost equally between the flat bones and the shafts of the major bones of the limbs. The innominate bones are affected more commonly than other flat bones, but these tumours sometimes are found in the scapula, ribs and spine. Very rarely a lesion in a vertebral body may undergo such collapse that the 'silver dollar' vertebra appearance may result, being comparable to eosinophil granuloma (see Fig. 1.2a in Exercise 20). Involvement distal to the wrist and ankle is somewhat exceptional.

2. Appearance. Since these lesions originate in marrow, they cause an infiltrating destructive pattern within medullary cavities. Overlying periosteal reactions develop, and may be multilaminar or 'onion-peel' in type, possibly representing intermittent attempts to contain growth of the neoplasm. When the cortex is eroded and the tumour perforates the laminated periosteum it extends into adjacent soft tissues, producing an opacity with a clearly demarcated edge. The marginal periosteal remnants are described as Codman triangles. Such a pattern, indeed, may be evident at the first presentation of the patient, at which time a smooth scalloped erosion of the lateral cortex ('saucerisation') may be evident as a valuable diagnostic sign. Apart from the reactive new bone which is formed by the periosteum, these tumours are almost entirely osteolytic. As a response to treatment, however, considerable sclerosis may develop, with an eventual reversion to normal bone architecture.

As mentioned above, the disease culminates finally in metastatic dissemination. Radiological differentiation from the secondary deposits of a neuroblastoma then may be difficult, since multiple lesions of this type individually bear resemblance to Ewing's tumours (see Fig. 1.8g in Exercise 2).

Pathological Features

Ewing's tumours consist of indistinctly outlined cells with rounded nuclei, showing relatively little nuclear pleomorphism but numerous mitoses. The tumour cells usually contain abundant glycogen, a feature absent in other round-cell tumours.

Ewing's sarcoma lacks the intercellular network of reticulin fibres which is characteristic of reticulum-cell sarcoma (see Q2 of this Exercise). Histological distinction between Ewing's sarcoma and metastatic neuroblastoma may be difficult or impossible. The presence of a rosette pattern of the tumour cells is a distinctive histological feature of neuroblastoma. This appearance, however, while often present in the primary tumour, is found only rarely in bone metastases. In cases of neuroblastoma positive evidence for such a diagnosis may be provided by demonstration of catecholamines in the urine, a feature lacking in Ewing's sarcoma.

The precise histogenesis of Ewing's sarcoma is not known, but these tumours are generally believed to originate from the cells of the bone marrow rather than from the connective tissue of bone itself.

Treatment

In the past, radical surgery with ablation of limbs rarely succeeded in delaying widespread dissemination of a disease which is essentially systemic. Surgical intervention in the present era is confined virtually to biopsy procedures and local eradication.

Ewing's sarcomas, however, are particularly sensitive to radiation therapy and chemotherapy. Because of the primary involvement of the marrow, emphasis has been placed on radiotherapy being administered to the entire bone which is affected. An adjacent joint should be included in the field of treatment. A lesion in such a site as the pubic bone demands irradiation of the whole pelvis. Similarly, the entire hemithorax should be treated in the case of rib involvement. In later phases of the radiotherapeutic programme more localised fields should be employed, including only the focus demonstrated radiologically and adjacent portions of apparently normal bone. Supplementary whole-body irradiation by low dosage has been advocated, but is not generally accepted. Radiotherapy alone greatly improved the prognosis for this malignant condition, but its efficacy has been enhanced considerably by the introduction of adjuvant systemic chemotherapy. The agents employed include vincristine, cyclophosphamide, methotrexate and actinomycin D. Chemotherapy should be continued for a minimum of 2 years. A survival period of approximately 5 years may be expected in 50% of cases. Despite some survivals for even longer periods, the ultimate fate of many of these patients is still sudden dissemination of the tumour to cause multiple and fatal metastases in the lungs and occasionally in other parts of the skeleton.

References

Ball J, Freedman L, Sissons HA (1977) Malignant round-cell tumours of bone: an analytical histological study from the Cancer Research Campaign's Bone Tumour Panel. Br J Cancer 36: 254–268.

Llombart-Bosch A, Blanche R, Peydro-Olata A, (1978) Ultrastructural study of 28 cases of Ewing's sarcoma: typical and atypical forms. Cancer 41: 1362–1373

MacIntosh DJ, Price CHG, Jeffree GM (1975) Ewing's tumour. A study of behaviour and treatment in forty-seven cases. J Bone Jt Surg 57B: 331–340

Marsden HB, Stewart JK (1964) Ewing's tumours and neuroblastomas. J Clin Pathol 17: 411–417

Pritchard DJ, Dahlin DC, Dauphine RT, Taylor WF, Beabout JW (1975) Ewing's sarcoma. A clinicopathological and statistical analysis of patients surviving 5 years or longer. J Bone Jt Surg 57A: 10–16

Razek A, Perez CA, Tefft M et al. (1980) Intergroup Ewing's sarcoma study. Local control related to radiation dose, volume, and site of primary lesion of Ewing's sarcoma. Cancer 46: 516–521

Rosen G, Wollner N, Ten C et al. (1974) Disease-free survival in children with Ewing's sarcoma treated with radiation therapy and adjuvant four-drug sequential chemotherapy. Cancer 33: 384–393.

Schajowicz F (1950) Ewing's sarcoma and reticulum-cell sarcoma of bone. J Bone Jt Surg 41A: 344–356

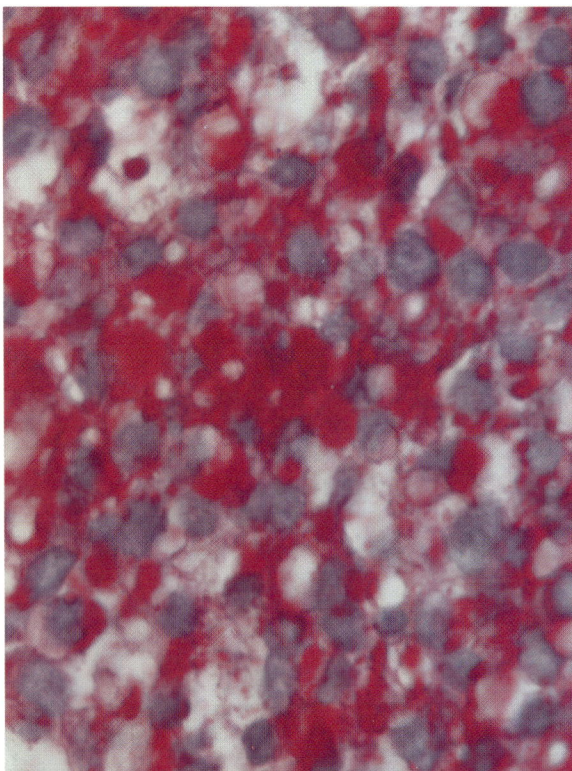

Fig. 1.1a. A section stained by the periodic-acid–Schiff technique to show the presence of glycogen. This takes the form of rounded collections of dark red material within the tumour cells. (×630)

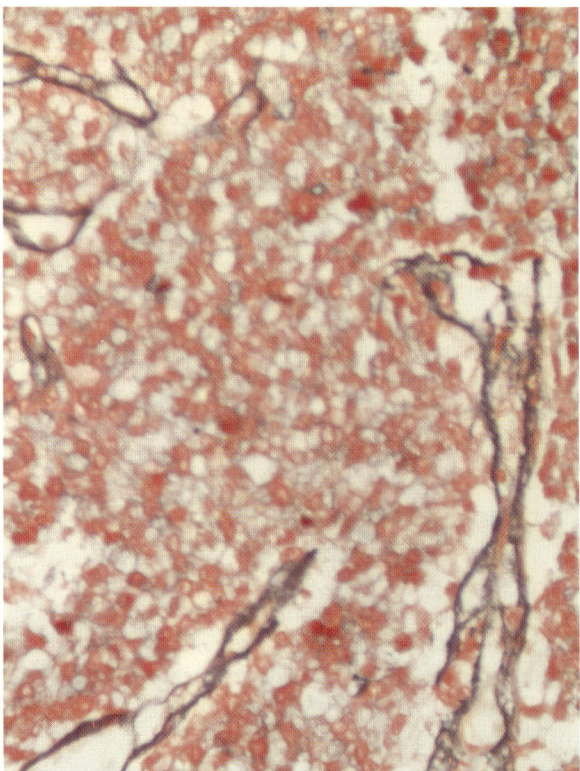

Fig. 1.1b. A section stained to show reticulin fibres, which appear black. No intercellular reticulin is present, the only positively staining fibres being located in the walls of small blood vessels, of which they are a normal component (see Fig. 2.1b for a positive reaction). (×360)

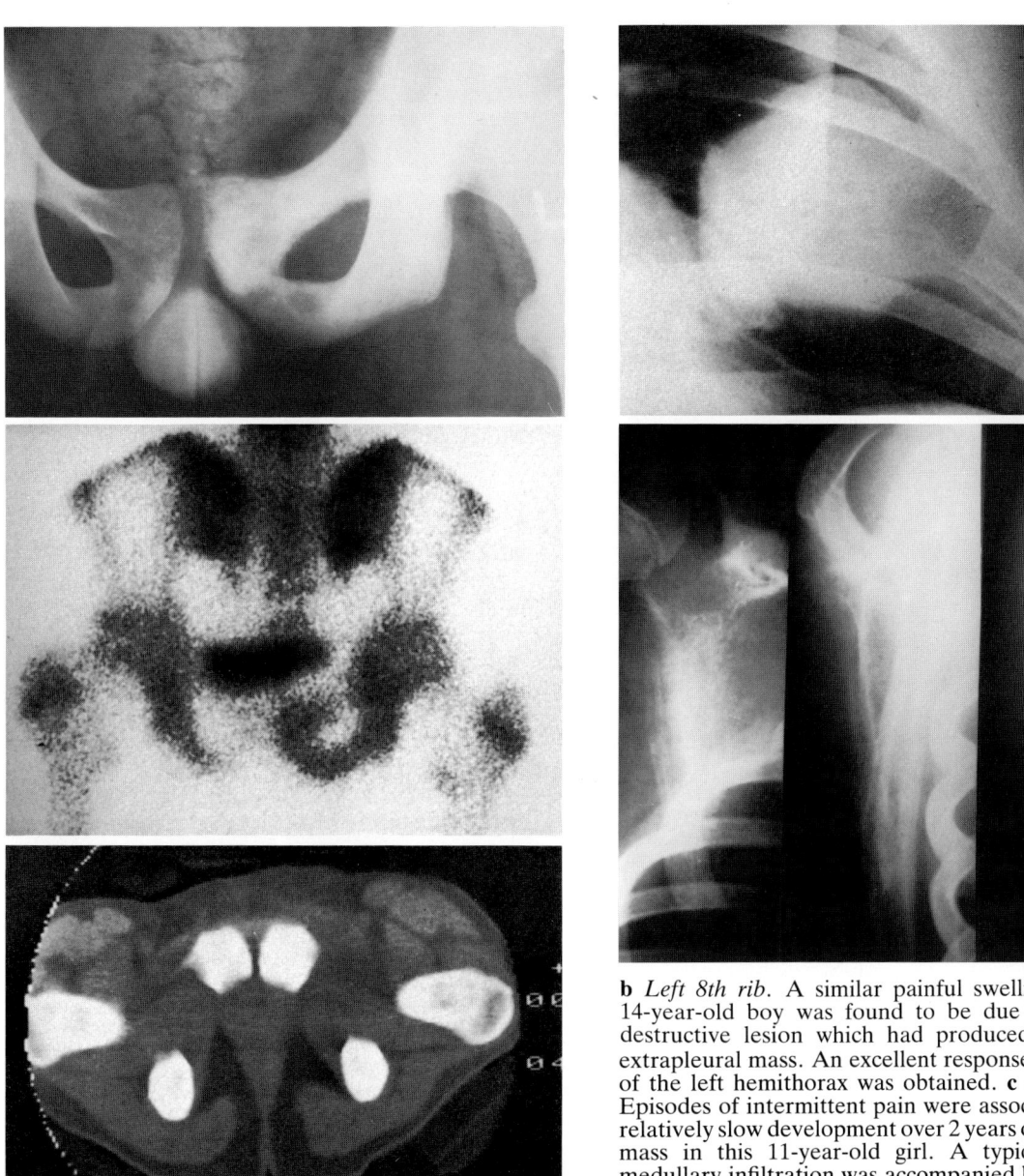

Fig. 1.2. *Ewing's sarcoma—flat bones.* **a** *Left ischium.* This destructive and infiltrating lesion had caused localised pain and swelling in a 14-year-old boy. A well-defined soft tissue extension and periosteal reactions had developed. Radionuclide scanning showed increased uptake of the tracer and a CT scan revealed the true size of the soft tissue mass. The lesion was treated by radiotherapy, followed by total excision and chemotherapy. He was alive and well 4 years later.

b *Left 8th rib.* A similar painful swelling in another 14-year-old boy was found to be due to this highly destructive lesion which had produced a very large extrapleural mass. An excellent response to irradiation of the left hemithorax was obtained. **c** *Right scapula.* Episodes of intermittent pain were associated with the relatively slow development over 2 years of a firm tender mass in this 11-year-old girl. A typical pattern of medullary infiltration was accompanied by a laminated periosteal reaction. The extent of the mass was shown by a soft tissue exposure. This child was debilitated and slightly pyrexial. The lesion responded well to radiation therapy and chemotherapy, but survival was limited to 4 years.

Ewing's Sarcoma

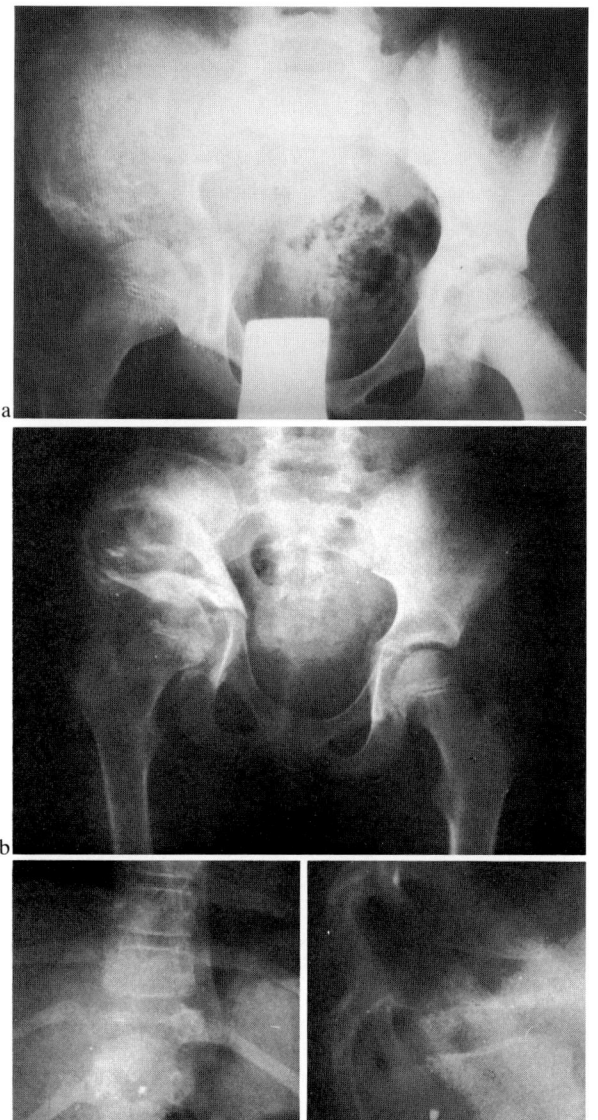

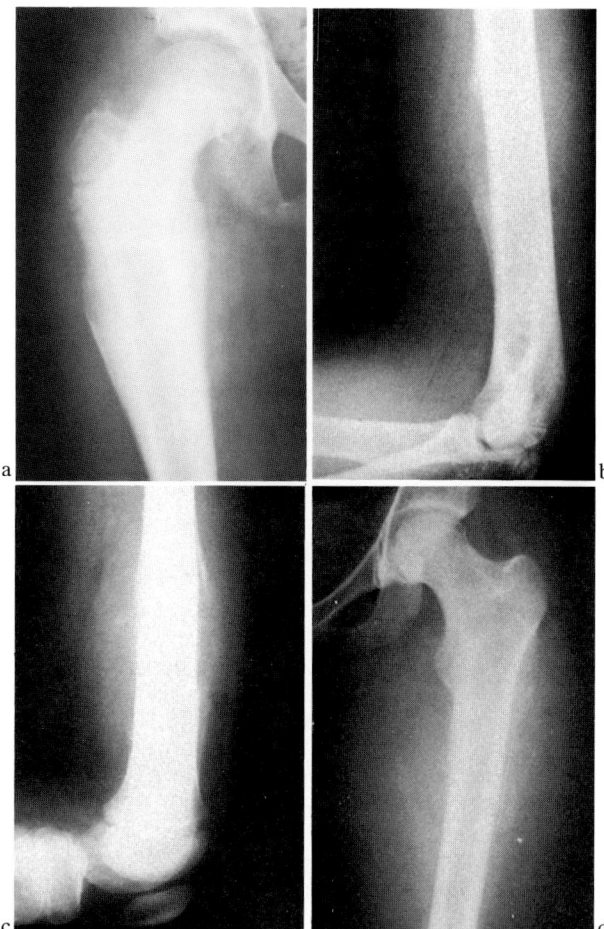

Fig. 1.3. *Ewing's sarcoma—metastasis from pelvis.* **a** This tumour in the right ilium of a 5-year-old boy with symptoms of only a few weeks' duration **b** sclerosed with irradiation but in less than a year **c** a metastasis in the body of T11 had undergone complete collapse to resemble the 'silver dollar' vertebra observed often with an eosinophil granuloma (see Exercise 20). Bilateral paravertebral opacities were attributed to haematomas rather than extensions of the tumour. Gross cord pressure signs had ensued and death occurred shortly afterwards. Exceptionally a primary Ewing's sarcoma may arise in a vertebral body.

Fig. 1.4. *Ewing's sarcoma—long bones.* These cases illustrate the extent of the tumour which may be evident at the time of presentation and its predilection for the diaphyseal portions of long bones. **a** *Femur* in a 9-year-old boy, showing medullary infiltration with some reactive sclerosis and a typical lamellated or 'onion-peel' periosteal reaction. A biopsy defect is evident on the lateral side of the bone. **b** *Humerus* in an 11-year-old girl. In this case poorly defined medullary osteolysis is associated with a distinct soft tissue extension. The periosteal reaction has been penetrated by the tumour to leave the adjacent periosteal remnants known as Codman's triangles. **c** *Femur* with a circumferential extension into the soft tissues in a 12-year-old boy. More displacement of the periosteum has occurred and a characteristically shallow erosion of the anterior cortex demonstrates the diagnostic feature of 'saucerisation'. **d** *Femur.* An even larger tumour mass was present in this 18-year-old girl. The displaced periosteum has attempted to maintain continuity.

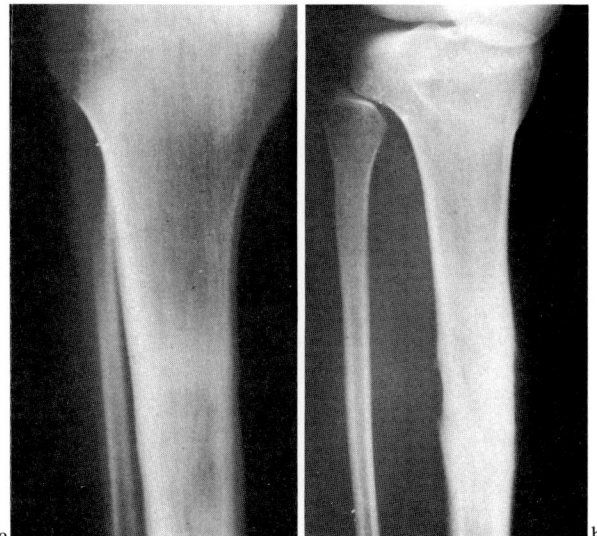

Fig. 1.5. *Ewing's sarcoma—evolution.* **a** This 16-year-old boy had complained of a constant ache in the right leg for 3 months. This radiograph, showing diffuse medullary osteoporosis of the mid-shaft of the tibia and an overlying and well-organised periosteal reaction, was interpreted as being due to low-grade pyogenic infection. Symptoms persisted despite treatment with antibiotics. **b** Ten weeks later classical 'saucerisation' defects on both sides of the bone, with Codman triangles and soft tissue extensions, indicated the nature of the lesion. This diagnostic pitfall is well recognised (see Exercise 10).

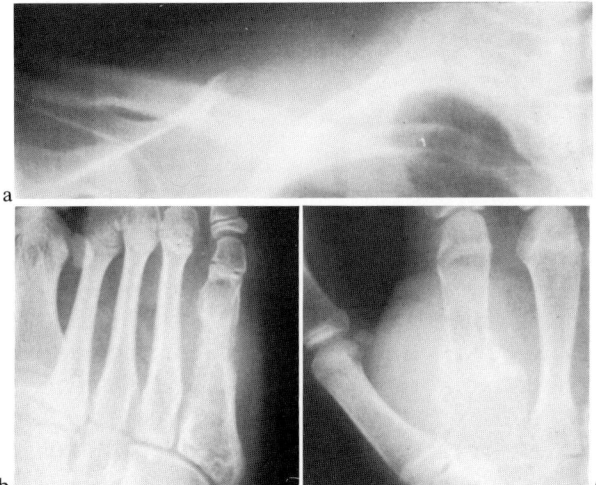

Fig. 1.6. *Ewing's sarcoma—unusual locations.* **a** *Clavicle.* This lesion in a young adult shows the typical diagnostic features of diffuse medullary infiltration, periosteal reaction, 'saucerisation' defect and a clearly defined soft tissue mass. **b** *5th Metatarsal.* Identical features are present in relation to this tumour in a child. As in the case of Fig. 1.5, the diagnosis offered in error was pyogenic infection. Subsequent biopsy established the correct diagnosis. **c** *2nd metacarpal.* This lesion in a 14-year-old boy exhibited similar characteristics, but in addition was complicated by a pathological fracture.

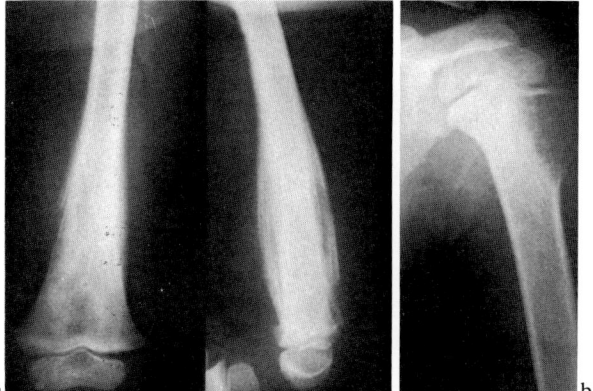

Fig. 1.7. *Ewing's sarcoma—metastatic dissemination* is the fate of many patients with this highly malignant tumour. **a** At an unusually early age this neoplasm, exhibiting a classical lamellated periosteal reaction and a Codman's triangle, was found in a 4-year-old boy with a painful swelling above the knee. Despite an excellent initial response to radiotherapy, metastases in the lungs and remainder of the skeleton, including **b** the proximal end of the humerus, developed soon after, with a fatal outcome.

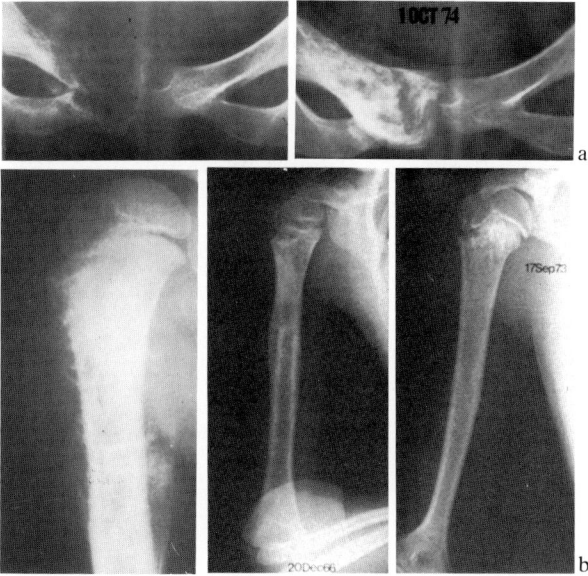

Fig. 1.8. *Ewing's sarcoma—response to treatment.* **a** *Pubis.* This expanding osteolytic lesion, causing localised pain and swelling in a 19-year-old girl, was interpreted initially as an aggressive aneurysmal bone cyst (see Exercise 22). At operation the lesion consisted of solid neoplastic tissue and the diagnosis was established histologically. With radiotherapy the tumour contracted and sclerosed, but the patient succumbed to multiple metastases within 14 months. **b** *Humerus.* By contrast, this typical and histologically confirmed Ewing's tumour, which was treated by a combination of radiotherapy and chemotherapy, reverted to a normal appearance 7 years later and the patient was alive and well 17 years after the original presentation. Such a long-term survival is indeed exceptional.

A2. Reticulum-cell sarcoma of radius

In this patient also the pre-operative findings, as in Q1, suggested a malignant tumour—either a solitary metastatic deposit or one of primary origin.

At operation, the lesion consisted of pale tissue which had extended through the cortex into the adjacent soft tissues. As in the previous case (Q1), investigations at the time of operation confirmed the presence of a malignant tumour and not an inflammatory lesion. The general appearance (Q2b and c) is, once again, that of a 'malignant round-cell tumour' of bone. In the present case, however, the cells and their nuclei are less uniform in their appearance than those illustrated in Q1b and c. Some of the nuclei stain relatively darkly with haematoxylin. These features, together with the absence of intracellular glycogen (Fig. 2.1a) and the presence of intercellular reticulin fibres (Fig. 2.1b), establish a diagnosis of reticulum-cell sarcoma.

The patient was treated by amputation, and was alive and well 10 years later.

Reticulum-Cell Sarcoma of Bone

The term 'reticulum-cell sarcoma' has been applied, since the paper of Parker and Jackson in 1939, to a group of non-osteogenic round-cell tumours of bone with cytological features which are different from those of Ewing's sarcoma. As with Ewing's sarcoma, the precise histogenesis of reticulum-cell sarcoma is not known, but a relationship to tumours of lymphoid tissue has been suggested and reticulum-cell sarcomas are sometimes referred to as 'malignant lymphoma' or 'histiocytic lymphoma'.

Unlike Ewing's tumour, the majority of these neoplasms are detected in middle life, usually between the ages of 30 and 50 years. Two males are affected for every female.

Cases of generalised lymphoma tend to occur in an older age group and affect primarily lymph nodes. The skeleton ultimately may be involved, the resulting lesions exhibiting individually a radiological appearance which may be identical to a primary reticulum-cell sarcoma of bone.

Clinical Features

The usual presenting complaint is of vague and intermittent pain. Episodes of such discomfort may be separated by intervals of several months. A diffuse and tender swelling usually reflects infiltration of soft tissues. In a surprisingly large proportion of patients, however (as many as 25%), development of the tumour is so silent that its presence is heralded by a pathological fracture through an extensive zone of osteolysis. In contrast to these relatively mild symptoms, patients with the rare sclerotic form of the disease often experience severe and disabling pain, commonly associated with an unexplained peripheral neuropathy.

Radiological Features

1. Site. A distinct predilection exists for the diametaphyseal portions of the long bones to be affected, particularly in relation to the knee. The proximal end of the humerus is another common site. In the axial skeleton the tumour may develop in such bones as the pelvis, ribs, clavicle and scapula. Vertebral involvement is unusual. The peripheral bones and the calvarium are affected only rarely.

2. Appearance. Permeating destruction of medullary bone is almost constant, resulting in a poorly defined area of osteolysis with a wide zone of transition. Pathological fractures are typically transverse. Owing to the relative well-being of many of these patients the neoplasm may be extensive before its presence is appreciated. In due course the overlying cortex is destroyed, probably coincidentally with the onset of symptoms. As the tumour grows, extensions into adjacent soft tissues become increasingly apparent and clearly defined, but usually are smaller than those observed with Ewing's tumour. Periosteal and endosteal reactive bone then is likely to develop, but such bone is relatively sparse, being much less abundant than with the majority of other malignant bone neoplasms. The rare sclerosing type of reticulum-cell sarcoma, mentioned above, may simulate Paget's disease.

Pathological Features

Within the group of round-cell tumours of bone, reticulum-cell sarcoma is recognised, and is distinguished from Ewing's sarcoma, by the pleomorphism of the tumour cells and their nuclei and by the more distinct cytoplasmic outlines of the cells and the darker nuclear staining with haematoxylin (Q2b, Q2c). A characteristic feature is the presence of a network of intercellular reticulin fibres (Fig. 2.1b), from which the tumour takes its name. In contrast to Ewing's sarcoma, intracellular glycogen is not present (Fig. 2.1a). There are, however, often problems of specific histological identification with malignant round-cell tumours of bone. The distinction between Ewing's sarcoma and reticulum-cell sarcoma usually can be made by employing the criteria outlined (cytological features, glycogen, reticulin), but occasional cases show both types of tissue. Sometimes the histological distinction between reticulum-cell sarcoma and Hodgkin's disease can be difficult or uncertain.

Treatment

All patients in whom the diagnosis is established should be subjected to isotope and radiological scans to exclude multifocal lesions. If the lesions are multifocal then treatment by radiotherapy and cytotoxic drugs on a regime similar to that for Ewing's tumour is indicated. Unifocal lesions, where accessible, as for example in the proximal end of the femur, may be treated by prosthetic replacement followed by local low dosage radiotherapy. Peripheral tumours with widespread tissue infiltration are best treated by amputation or limb ablation. In principle, as with Ewing's tumours, the object of treatment is the surgical reduction of the bulk of the primary tumour, local radiotherapy to prevent dissemination and the subsequent use of systemic cytotoxins. The prognosis is better than that of Ewing's tumour. Orthodox therapy achieves a 25% 10-year survival. Whether cytotoxic therapy will improve this figure has yet to be determined.

References

Ball J, Freedman L, Sissons HA (1977) Malignant round-cell tumours of bone: an analytical histological study from the Cancer Research Campaign's Bone Tumour Panel. Br J Cancer 36: 254–268

Boston HC, Dahlin DC, Ivins JC, Cupps RE (1974) Malignant lymphoma (so-called reticulum-cell sarcoma) of bone. Cancer 34: 1131–1137

Francis KC, Higinbotham NL, Coley BL (1954) Primary reticulum-cell sarcoma of bone. Report of 44 cases. Surg Gynecol Obstet 99: 143–146

Parker F, Jackson H (1939) Primary reticulum-cell sarcoma of bone. Surg Gynecol Obstet 68: 45–53

Wilson TW, Pugh DG (1974) Primary reticulum-cell sarcoma of bone, with emphasis on roentgen aspects. Radiology 65: 343–351

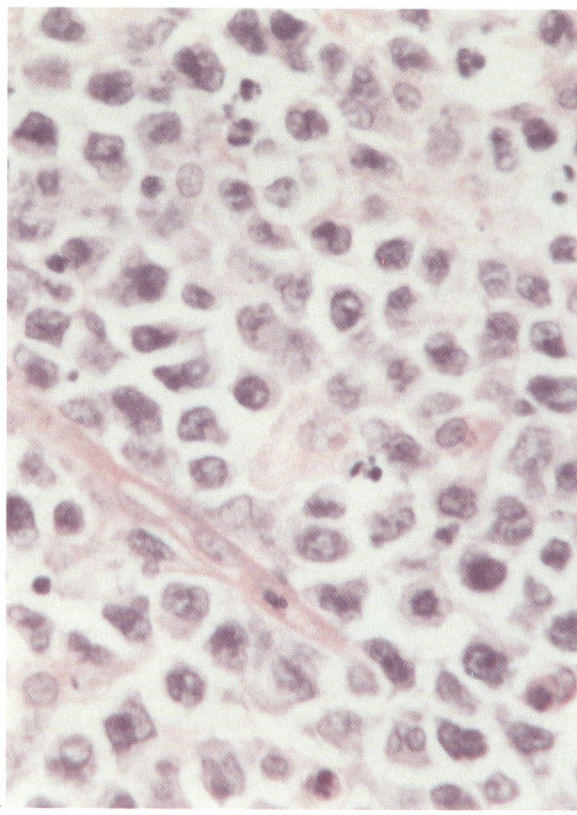

Fig. 2.1a. A section stained by the periodic-acid–Schiff technique showing the absence of glycogen (see Fig. 1.1a for a positive reaction). (×630)

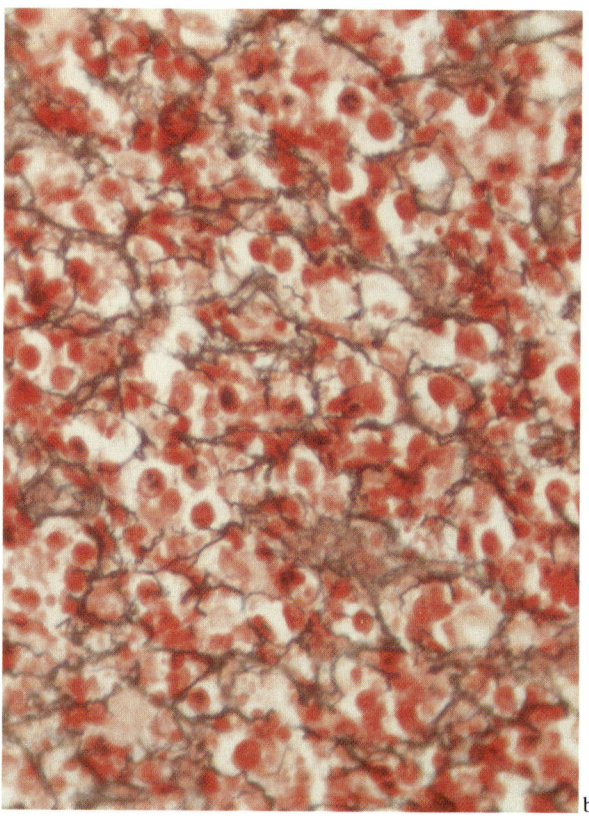

Fig. 2.1b. A section stained to show reticulin fibres, which appear black. Note the uniform network of fibres, passing between individual cells or surrounding small groups of cells. (×360)

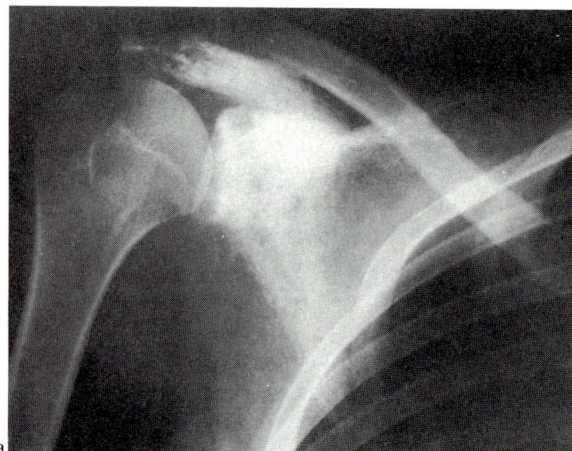

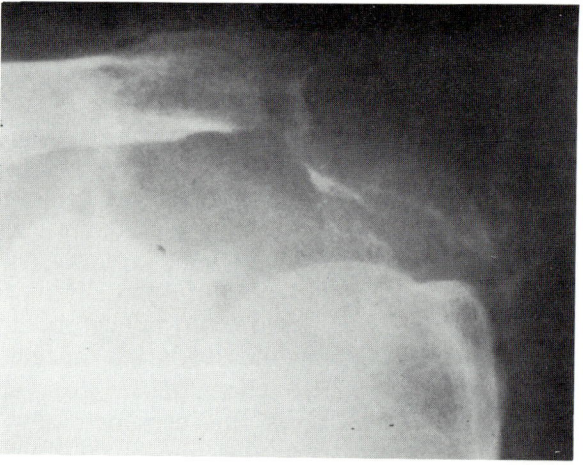

Fig. 2.2 *Reticulum-cell sarcoma—flat bones.* All these primary malignant tumours of bone exhibit a diffuse infiltrating pattern in medullary cavities comparable to the changes observed with Ewing's tumour. They occur, however, in older patients. **a** *Scapula.* The entire bone was affected in this 43-year-old man. Observe periosteal reactions and interspersed strands of sclerosis.

b *Acromion process of scapula* This 32-year-old man complained of a painful swelling, attributed by him to an injury 7 months previously. The gross expansion of the osteolytic lesion caused an aneurysmal bone cyst to be diagnosed, but at operation it was found to consist of solid grey material. **c** *Pubis and ischium.* This lesion was encountered in a younger patient, a woman aged 23 who

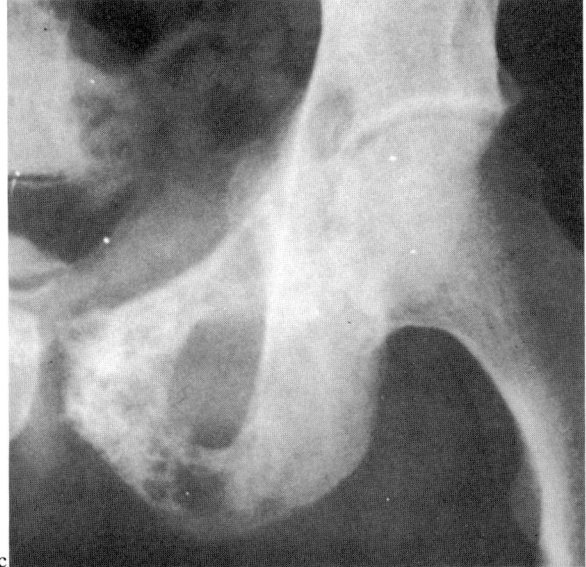
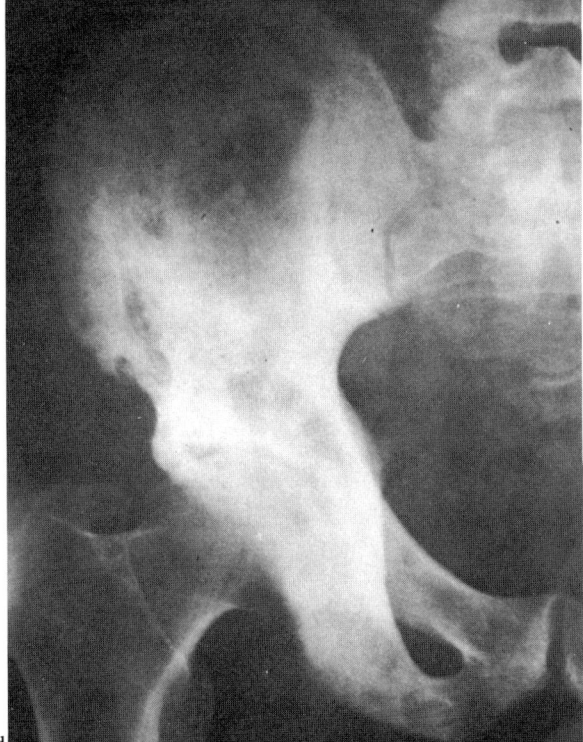

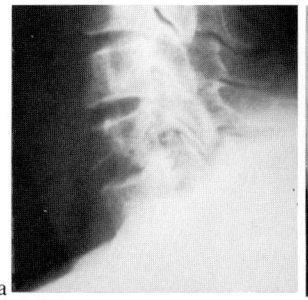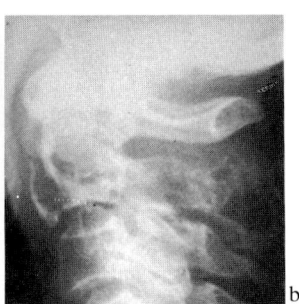

Fig. 2.3. *Reticulum-cell sarcoma—spine.* **a** *Body of C6.* This 56-year-old man presented with symptoms and signs of spinal cord pressure. Permeating osteolysis and partial collapse of this vertebral body were evident. A metastasis was suspected, but biopsy, establishing the diagnosis, was performed during an operation for posterior spinal fusion. Symptoms were relieved entirely for 6 months. **b** *Body and neural arch of axis.* This bizarre lesion with gross expansion of the spinous process in an elderly patient caused diagnostic difficulty.

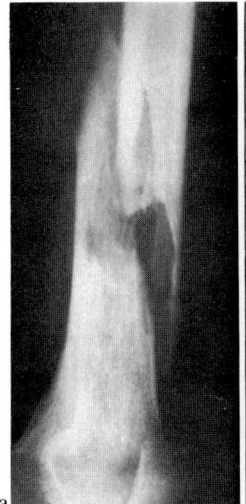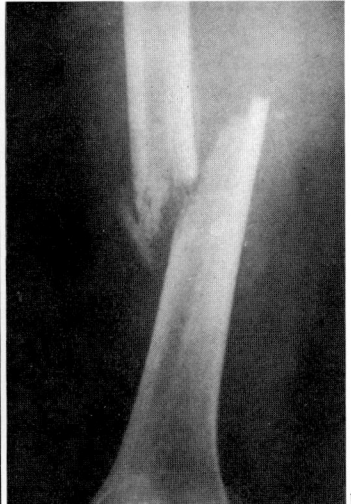

Fig. 2.2. *(continued)*
had developed localised pain. Once again this permeating destructive process is associated with sclerotic elements. **d** *Right innominate bone.* This 69-year-old man died of intercurrent disease. This diffuse sclerotic lesion had been suspected to be a Paget's sarcoma (see Exercise 14). This is a most unusual radiological appearance for reticulum-cell sarcoma, and the diagnosis was established only by histological examination.

Fig. 2.4. *Reticulum-cell sarcoma—pathological fractures.* These tumours are frequently so silent in their development that their presence is recognised only by a spontaneous fracture. These examples occurred **a** in a 25-year-old man, with a typically destructive lesion in the femur, and, by contrast, in **b** the femur of a 73-year-old woman. In the latter case the histological diagnosis caused some surprise, as a metastasis had been suspected.

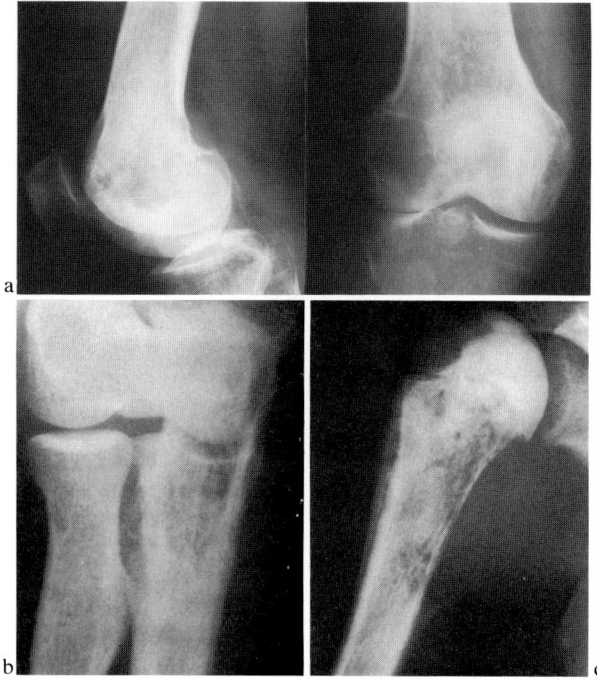

Fig. 2.5. *Reticulum-cell sarcoma—long bones.* As indicated in Fig. 2.4, the femur is affected frequently. These lesions tend to arise towards the ends of long bones, particularly near the knee, as illustrated in Q2 and **a** in this 32-year-old man with localised pain. At this age the subarticular involvement of the distal end of the femur might suggest a giant-cell tumour (compare Fig. 1.1b in Exercise 15). **b** The appearance of this infiltrating tumour in the proximal end of the ulna is more characteristic. It was found on account of mild pain in the elbow of a 31-year-old man. **c** This example in the proximal end of the humerus of an adolescent girl shows periosteal reaction and a Codman's triangle and emphasises the sclerosis which may be observed in these neoplasms, together with marked similarity to a Ewing's sarcoma.

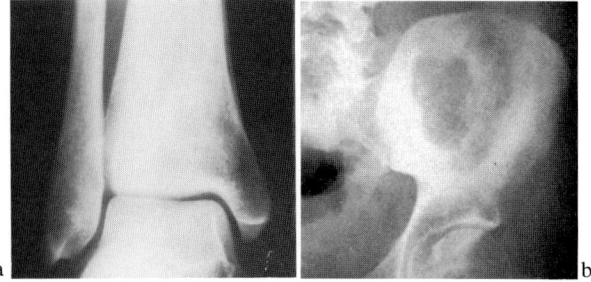

Fig. 2.6. *'Malignant round cell' tumour.* Even histological study can fail on occasion to permit definitive typing of these medullary neoplasms. This was the case in **a** this tumour in the distal end of the tibia in a 30-year-old woman with mild pain in the ankle. Medullary involvement was minimal, but a periosteal reaction had developed. **b** The same histological diagnosis was made after biopsy of this irregular lytic lesion in the ilium of this 28-year-old man. Observe peripheral sclerosis, especially on the medial side of the tumour.

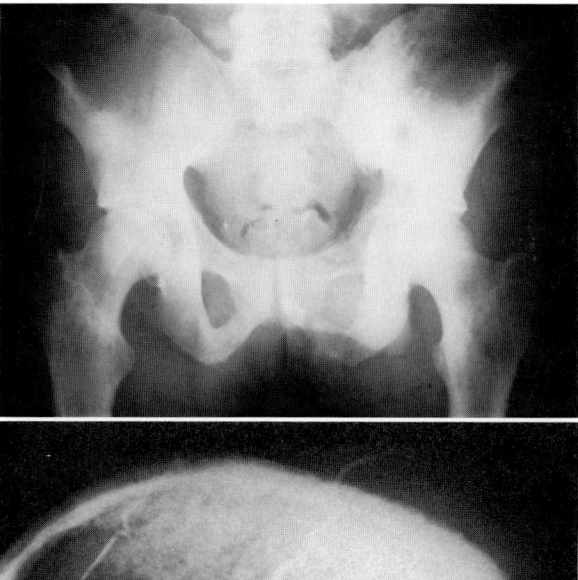

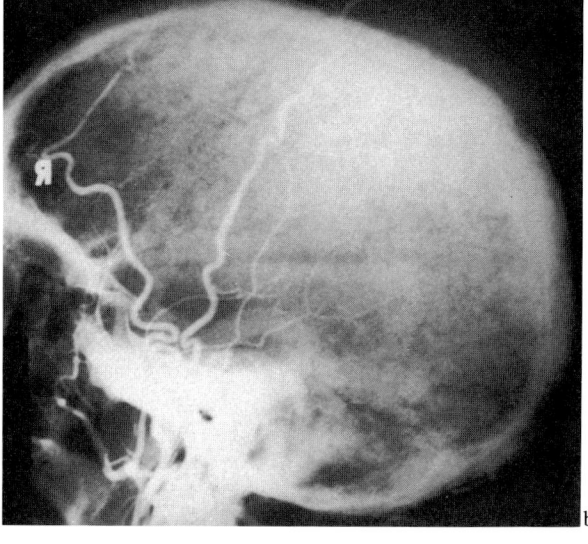

Fig. 2.7. *Reticulum-cell sarcoma of lymph nodes— metastatic spread to skeleton.* Lesions of this type are described as 'secondary' reticulum-cell sarcoma of bone, as opposed to the 'primary' form illustrated above. The individual lesions are radiologically similar to those of the primary form. **a** *Pelvis.* Multiple lytic areas developed in the skeleton in this 49-year-old man 10 years after treatment for a generalised lymphadenopathy had been begun. This film shows a typical lesion in the left superior pubic ramus and others in the remainder of the pelvis and in the proximal ends of the femora. **b** *Skull.* This 66-year-old man slowly developed a relatively painless swelling on the vertex of the skull. Radiologically it was shown to be associated with disseminated areas of bone destruction, resembling metastases. A generalised lymphadenopathy had been diagnosed histologically as reticulum-cell sarcoma 6 years before.

Exercise 32

Q1. This patient, a 52-year-old man, gave a history of severe pain in the region of the sacrum for 1 year.

On clinical examination, a palpable mass was felt per rectum, but no neurological or other abnormalities were detected.

Radiological examination showed a large, expanding osteolytic lesion in the central portion of the sacrum. The sigmoid colon was observed to be displaced forwards by a soft tissue mass during a barium enema.

A biopsy was performed.

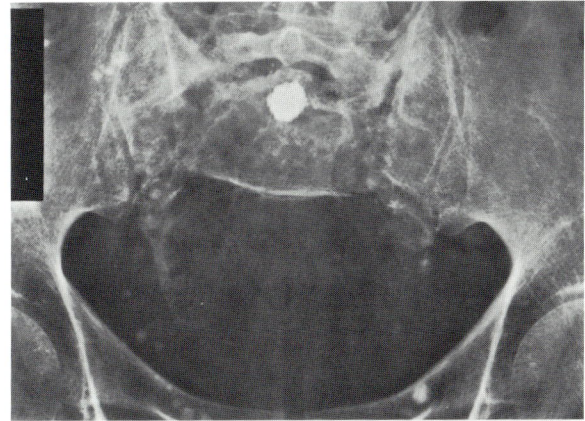
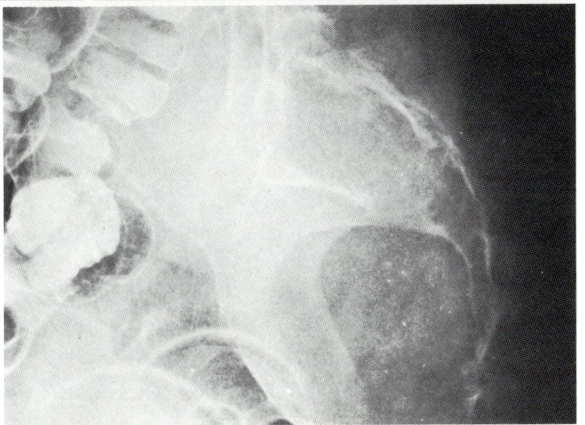

Q1a.

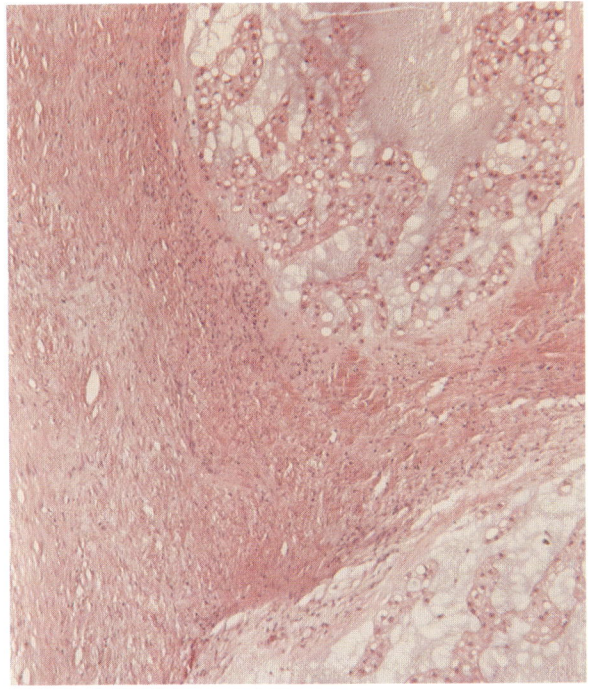

Q1b. (×65)

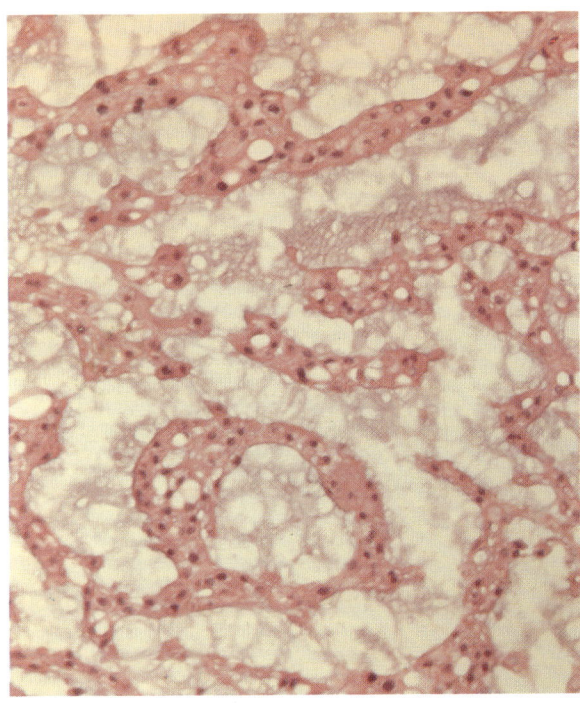

Q1c. (×160)

A1. Chordoma of sacrum

The radiological appearance of this destructive lesion strongly suggested this diagnosis, largely on account of its symmetrically central position and the smooth and regular outlines of its margins. Other diagnostic considerations had included a metastasis, a plasmacytoma and a giant-cell tumour. At operation, the mass was found to consist of greyish gelatinous tissue. The biopsy confirmed the clinical and radiological diagnosis of chordoma, and an attempt was made to carry out a local resection of the lesion. Removal of the tumour, however, was incomplete, and surgery was followed by radiotherapy to the sacral area. Two years later there was a massive local recurrence.

The illustrations (Q2b and c) show the characteristic histological structure of chordoma. The tumour is lobulated, and the tumour cells are arranged in strands and masses which are separated by blue-staining mucinous material. The tumour cells, sometimes referred to as 'physaliphorous cells', appear highly vacuolated. In routine paraffin sections, however, it is difficult to distinguish between vacuolation of the cell cytoplasm and vacuolation of the adjacent intercellular material.

Chordoma

Chordoma is a tumour which occurs only in the axial skeleton. It is believed to develop from remnants of notochordal tissue, to which it shows a morphological resemblance. Chordomas usually occur in middle aged or elderly individuals and are more common in males than in females.

Clinical Features

Localised chronic pain is the usual presenting symptom, but, according to the portion of the axial skeleton involved, corresponding neurological deficits may occur. Since these tumours usually grow slowly, these deficits may be equally slow to develop, but ultimately paraplegia may ensue. In the case of the more common involvement of the sacro-coccygeal area, the extension of the tumour into the pelvis frequently causes chronic constipation, which may, indeed, be the presenting complaint. If the clivus and the base of the skull are affected, the symptoms and signs may resemble those of pituitary adenoma, a cranio-pharyngioma or a naso-pharyngeal tumour. Although chordomas usually remain localised and progressive, often over periods of years, metastases do occur on rare occasions.

Radiological Features

1. Site. Over half of these tumours occur in the sacro-coccygeal area. Another third occur in the clivus and base of the skull and the remainder may affect any other portion of the spine.

2. Appearance. The sacro-coccygeal lesions are situated in the mid-line and almost always are evident as lytic, expanding areas of the type illustrated, together with soft tissue extensions. These masses frequently contain areas of calcification. The margins are sharply defined. These tumours may spread proximally into the lower lumbar vertebrae. Those at the base of the skull are also destructive. On the other hand, in the remainder of the spine, wide discrepancies in these patterns may be observed. Some are lytic, with a peculiar affinity for C2, whereas others may show massive formation of tumour bone, even resembling an osteosarcoma.

Pathological Features

The tissue of a chordoma is typically gelatinous, and is characterised histologically by a large amount of mucoid intercellular material in which the strands and masses of tumour cells are scattered. The intercellular material can sometimes have a chondroid appearance, but distinction from chondrosarcoma can be made because of the absence, in chordoma, of rounded cells and distinct cell spaces (see Exercise 16). More typical cartilage is sometimes encountered in chordomas of the skull base, and its presence may complicate histological diagnosis and lead to an erroneous diagnosis of chondrosarcoma.

Treatment

These tumours usually fail to respond to radiotherapy or chemotherapy, although these procedures are not infrequently used in inoperable cases. Radical surgical ablation is the only successful treatment, but is applicable only to tumours in accessible sites, such as the sacrum. Even then, it is associated with high morbidity. Persistent sinuses often develop, and indicate inadequate ablation.

References

Dahlin DC, MacCarty CS (1952). Chordoma. A study of fifty-nine cases. Cancer 5: 1170–1178

Higinbotham NL, Philips RF, Farr HW, Husta HO (1967) Chordoma. Thirty-five year study at Memorial Hospital. Cancer 20: 1841–1850

Utne JR, Pugh DG (1955) The roentgenologic aspects of chordoma. Am J Roentgenol 74: 593–608

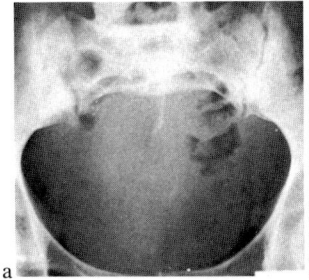
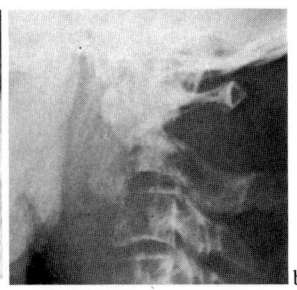

Fig. 1.1. *Chordoma.* **a** *Sacrum.* A typical lesion in an elderly woman with long-standing pain and chronic constipation. **b** *Body of C2.* This frankly aggressive tumour developed relatively rapidly, within a year, in a 28-year-old man with increasing neck pain. A very large retropharyngeal mass is present.

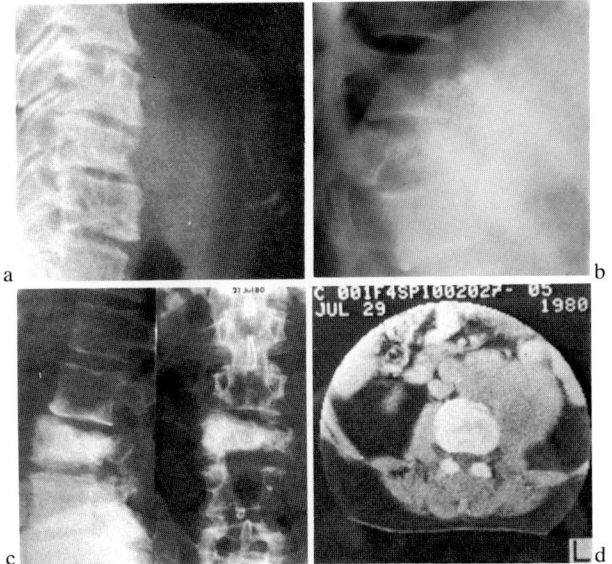

Fig. 1.2. *Chordoma.* Other spinal lesions in which the diagnosis only was established histologically. **a** *Body of C5* in an elderly woman with chronic pain in the neck. A barium swallow confirmed oesophageal displacement by the huge soft tissue mass. A radionuclide scan was positive. **b** *Body of T12* with collapse and massive ossification in the adjacent soft tissue extension, resembling an osteosarcoma, in a middle-aged man with back pain. **c** *Body of L3* in a 45-year-old man. Collapse and sclerosis had developed during the previous 2 years. **d** The soft tissue extension is shown in the CT scan.

Q1. This 49-year-old man complained of chronic pain and swelling of the left third toe. The swelling had developed during the previous 3 months, but no history of an antecedent injury was obtained.

Clinical examination confirmed the affected toe to be swollen and slightly tender, but it was not inflamed.

Radiological examination revealed a large, expanding osteolytic lesion in the 3rd middle phalanx, with expansion and thinning of the overlying cortex.

The toe was amputated.

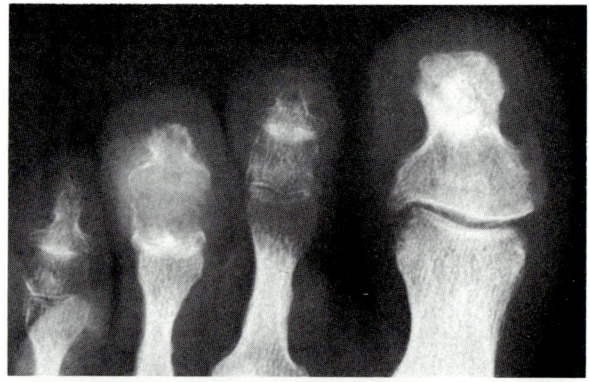

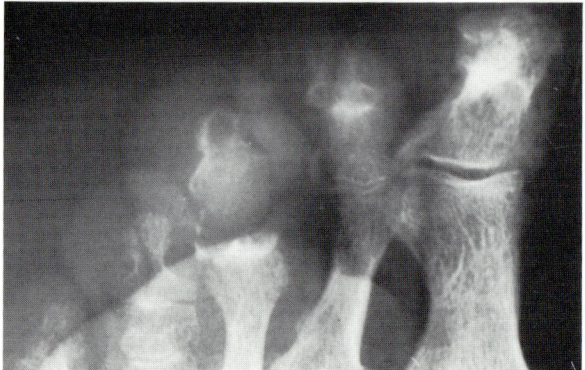

Q1a.

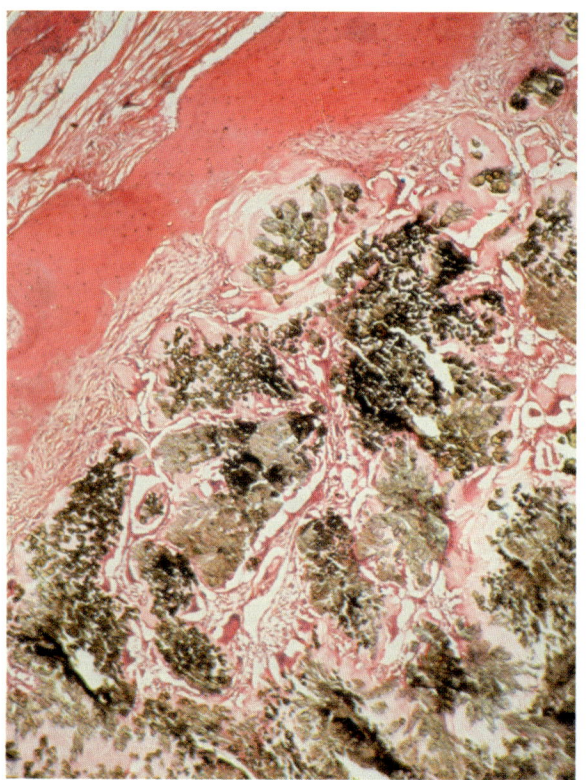

Q1b. (×30)

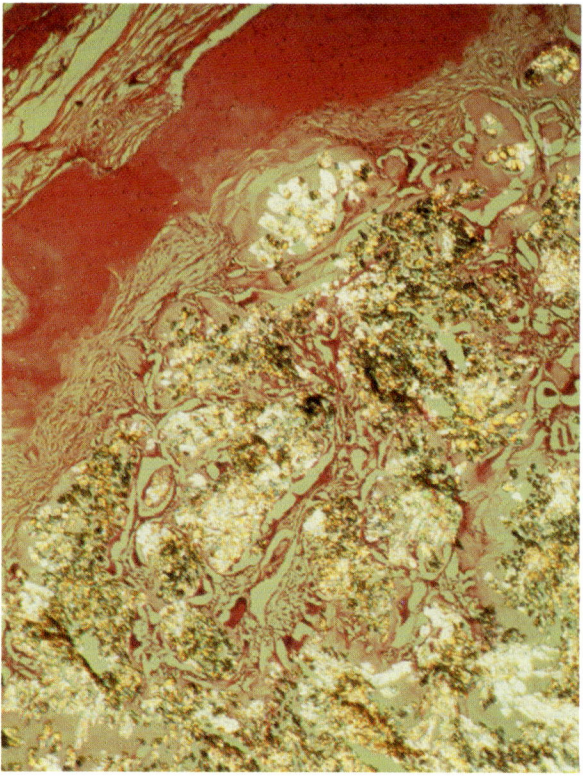

Q1c. (×30) Polarised light

Q2. This 69-year-old woman had complained of increasing pain in both knees for 10 years The pain affected the right knee especially severely and limited greatly her ability to walk, even with the support of a cane.

Physical examination revealed a bilateral genu valgum deformity, more marked on the right than the left. The right knee was distinctly unstable with valgus stress. Passive movement produced crepitus, especially in the right knee. This clinical picture indicated bilateral osteoarthritis or degenerative joint disease.

The radiographs confirmed the clinical diagnosis. The lateral compartments of both knees were significantly narrowed, with moderate osteophyte formation. The most striking abnormality was extensive eburnation of the right medial tibial condyle, which clearly had caused the valgus deformity.

Prosthetic replacement of the joint was undertaken. Q2a and Q2b illustrate the microscopic appearance of the menisci.

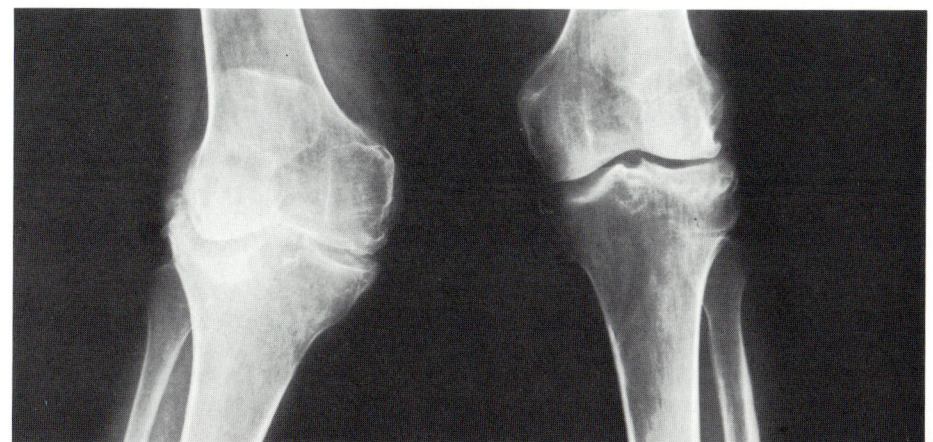

Q2a.

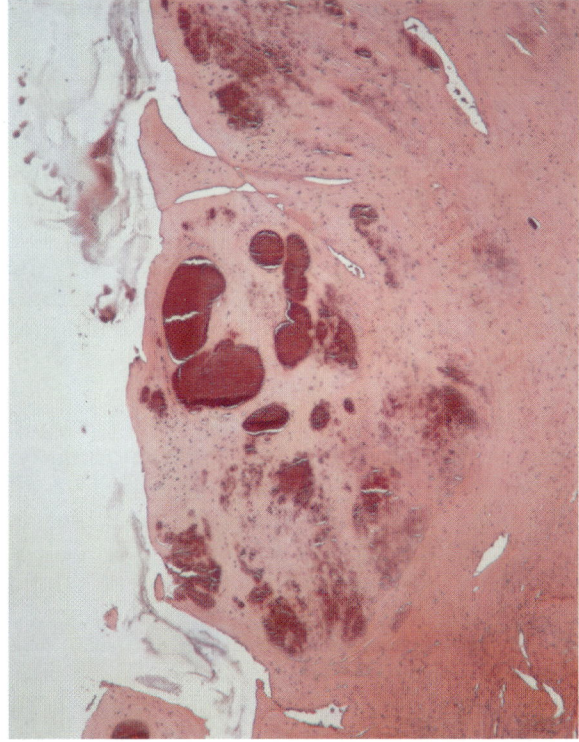

Q2b. (×32)

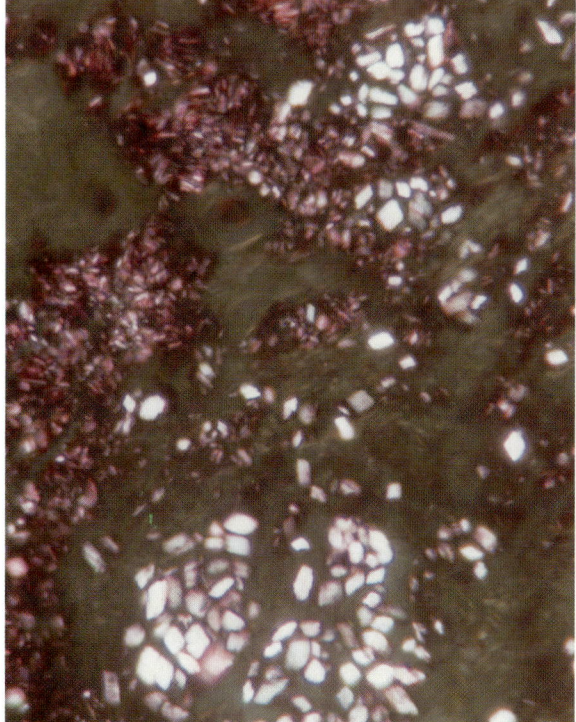

Q2c. (×400) Polarised light

A1. Gouty tophus of 3rd middle phalanx

The radiological appearance of this lytic lesion at first aroused suspicion of an osteolytic metastasis, particularly from a pulmonary primary neoplasm (cf. Fig. 1.8c in Exercise 2). Radiographs of the chest, however, were normal, and the possibility of a benign or even malignant synovial lesion was considered. Biopsy was advised, but the surgeon decided to amputate the toe.

Histological examination of the specimen showed involvement of the bone and adjacent soft tissues by a mass of vascular fibrous tissue containing conspicuous crystalline deposits (Q1b). When examined in polarised light the crystals are birefringent (Q1c). In fact they show the needle-like appearance and negative birefringence characteristic of urate crystals, establishing a diagnosis of gout. This was confirmed by the finding of a greatly elevated serum uric acid.

The clinical and radiological errors in diagnosis deserve emphasis. Solitary lesions caused by this metabolic disease can present misleading diagnostic features.

Gout

Gout is a disorder of purine metabolism, characterised by hyperuricaemia, in which crystals of sodium urate are deposited in a variety of tissues, particularly those of joints. It affects ten males for every female, usually over the age of 40 years, with no ethnic predilection. It is characterised by attacks of joint pain, often extremely acute, but sometimes subacute or even mild. The aetiology is unknown, but there is often evidence of familial liability to the disease. Diagnosis depends on the demonstration of persistently elevated values for serum uric acid, or on the identification of urate crystals in the joint tissues or synovial fluid.

Secondary hyperuricaemia, sometimes with symptoms of gout, may occur in association with a variety of other diseases, including some rare hereditary disorders (glycogen storage disease; Lesch-Nyhan syndrome), myeloproliferative disorders (particularly leukaemia), certain endocrine disorders and also following treatment with diuretics, salicylates or pyrazinamide.

Clinical Features

Asymmetrical and painful joint swellings of rapid onset usually draw attention to the disorder. The 1st metatarso-phalangeal joints are especially liable to be affected (podagra), causing warm, erythematous swellings which are acutely painful. Although such exacerbations may be associated with dietary indiscretions, more often they have been precipitated by exposure to alcohol, cold, minor injuries or medications, such as diuretics. In most instances, however, no clinical explanation is found.

Although gout may present as classical podagra, with transient episodes of acute crystal synovitis, it may become evident also as chronic tophaceous gouty arthritis associated with soft tissue deposits. These manifestations are due to the deposition of crystals of monosodium urate from supersaturated serum and tissue fluid. For confirmation of the clinical diagnosis a prerequisite is the demonstration of hyperuricaemia. Normal serum concentrations vary from 360 to 450 μmol/litre (60–75 mg/litre), and some overlap exists between gouty and non-gouty patients. For practical purposes, hyperuricaemia may be regarded as being present at concentrations above 420μmol/litre in men and 360 μmol/litre in women.

The majority of patients with primary gout do not manifest an isolated genetic abnormality. Hyperuricaemia is due to variations in both metabolic and renal function, resulting in increased formation or decreased excretion of uric acid. To these variables must be added the effects of a high calorific diet, elevated purine content foods and alcohol.

All patients with gout, either primary or secondary, should be examined fully for disorders of the cardiovascular and renal systems, as mild degrees of hypertension or impaired renal function are not uncommon. Preliminary investigations include serum uric acid, blood urea, a full blood count and urinalysis for protein. Estimations of plasma lipids should also be undertaken, although the association between hyperuricaemia and hyperlipidaemia is still not established.

Repeated and intermittent episodes culminate in the development of secondary degenerative changes in the affected joints, resulting in chronic pain and stiffness. Gross disorganisation and deformities may result. In severe cases uric acid calculi may form, causing renal colic and an obstructive nephropathy.

In addition to involvement of joints, soft tissue deposits of urates in para-articular areas eventually form large, nodular and usually painless swellings, which clinically are virtually diagnostic of the disease. They are observed most commonly in relation to the hands, feet, ears and elbows.

Radiological Features

1. Site. As indicated above, the radiological manifestations of gout are encountered most frequently in relation to the small joints of the hands and feet. Less commonly they are observed around major joints of the limbs, with a peculiar affinity for the olecranon process of the ulna. These areas of bone destruction due to urate deposits often are multiple, but even in their absence the diagnosis may be indicated by swellings in soft tissues.

2. Appearance. The typical gouty tophus is evident as a clearly circumscribed and rounded osteolytic area near, but often remote from, an articular surface. Unlike the para-articular erosions of the chronic arthritides of the rheumatoid type, which correspond to synovial attachments, these lesions have no such anatomical correlation. The associated deposits of urates which develop in the later stages of the disease also tend to be clearly defined and frequently contain amorphous calcifications. Even in established disease, peri-articular demineralisation due to hyperaemia or dense atrophy is rarely present, a feature of value in differentiation from rheumatoid arthritis (see Exercise 18). In the final stages of the most severe forms of the disease the degree of joint disintegration and deformity may be so gross that diagnostic recognition of the original abnormalities becomes impossible.

For the clinician and the radiologist the solitary tophus presents the greatest diagnostic hazard, as in Q1 of this Exercise. In the vast majority of cases of gout the diagnosis has been established on clinical and chemical grounds long before radiological studies become positive. Nevertheless, such solitary tophi do occur without a classical clinical onset and it is wise, when such abnormalities are demonstrated, to consider this diagnostic possibility. Lesions of this type have been described as pseudotumours and have been observed to affect not only small bones of the hands and feet, but also such structures as the olecranon process and the patella.

Pathological Features

In the acute stage the involved tissues show changes of acute inflammation. Crystals of sodium urate are present in the joint tissues and in the synovial fluid. They are birefringent, and can be recognised by scanning tissue sections, or aspirated joint fluid, in polarised light.

In Fig. 1.1a the birefringent urate crystals appear as bright structures against a dark background. In Fig. 1.1b, using a first order red compensator, the positions in which the same crystals appear blue or yellow establish that they are negatively birefringent. This, together with their needle-like shape, enables them to be distinguished from the positively birefringent, and much more angular, crystals of calcium pyrophosphate that are present in chondrocalcinosis. Urate deposits can be identified also by a variety of chemical reactions, including that with methenamine silver (Fig. 1.2).

In the more chronic stage of tophaceous gout, large deposits may develop in the juxta-articular tissues (including bones, tendons and ligaments) and in the soft tissues of the ear. These gouty tophi consist of masses of urate crystals surrounded by fibrous tissue containing numerous foreign body giant cells (Fig. 1.3). As the lesions become chronic, progressive destruction of the adjacent bone may occur, and changes of secondary osteoarthritis frequently develop. Calcification of the gouty tophi may occur, but is unusual.

Treatment

Colchicine still has a role in the management of acute gout in conjunction with more recently introduced drugs such as phenylbutazone and indomethacin. Following an acute attack, the decision to lower the level of serum uric acid is critical because, if commenced, such treatment must be continued regularly and indefinitely. The indications are a high serum concentration, suggesting progressive disease; recurrent acute attacks; joint destruction and tophi formation, and, finally, evidence of renal damage. The most commonly used drug is allopurinol. It competitively inhibits the enzyme xanthine oxidase which oxidises xanthine and hypoxanthine to uric acid and also suppresses purine biosynthesis. Acting rapidly, it may precipitate acute attacks in the initial stages of treatment; consequently colchicine, phenylbutazone or indomethacin are used concurrently in the early months of treatment.

Because of the efficacy of allopurinol, uricosuric drugs are used less frequently. They lower the serum uric acid level by inhibiting renal tubular reabsorption. Those drugs in present use are probenecid, ethebenecid and sulphinpyrazone. In the treatment of early uncomplicated gout, there is little to choose between allopurinol and uricosuric agents. The suggestion that overproducers of uric acid should be treated with allopurinol and under-excretors with uricosuric drugs is attractive, but possibly specious.

Severe dietary restrictions are no longer necessary though moderation should be recommended with regard to alcohol and high protein containing foods. Gouty individuals tend to be overweight and weight reduction in itself corrects mild degrees of hyperuricaemia. Hypertension, if present, also should be treated.

References

Catto M (1973) Pathology of gout. Scott Med J 18 [Suppl 1]: 232–238
Currey HLF (1968) Examination of joint fluids for crystals. Proc R Soc Med 61: 969–971
Dodds WJ, Steinbach AL (1966) Gout associated with calcification of cartilage. N Engl Med J 275: 745–749
Jaffe HL (1972) In: Metabolic degenerative and inflammatory diseases of bones and joints. Lea and Febiger, Philadelphia
McCarty DJ, Hollander JL (1961) Identification of urate crystals in gouty synovial tissues. Ann Intern Med 54: 452–460
Murray RO (1977) Case report No. 15. Skeletal Radiol 1: 173–174
Scott JT (1980) Long term management of gout and hyperuricaemia. Br Med J 281: 1164–1166
Spilberg I (1975) Current concepts of the mechanism of acute inflammation in gouty arthritis. Arthritis Rheum 18: 129–134
Watt I, Middlemiss H (1975) The radiology of gout. Clin Radiol 26: 27–36

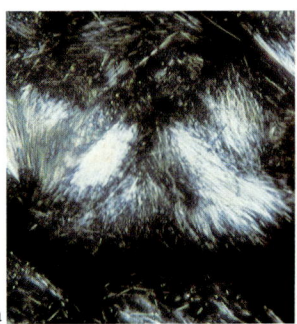 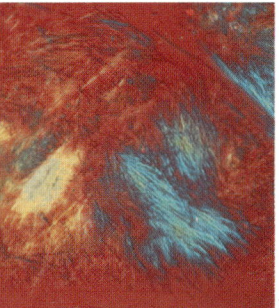

Fig. 1.1. a Urate crystals, viewed in polarised light. The needle-shaped crystals appear bright against a dark background. (×120) **b** The same crystals, viewed in polarised light, but with a first order red compensator. (×120)

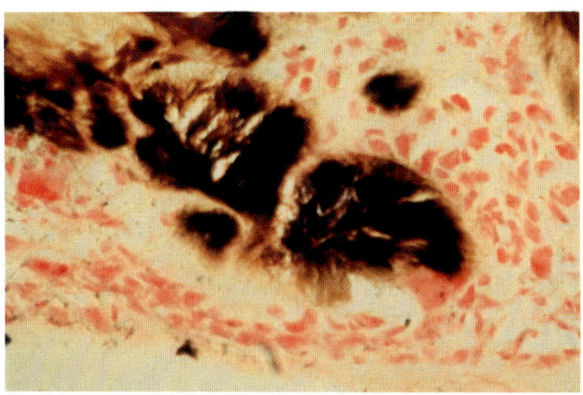

Fig. 1.2. From the case illustrated in Q1. An un-decalcified section stained with methenamine silver demonstrating the urate deposits, which are stained black. The crystals are surrounded by cellular reactive tissue. (×125)

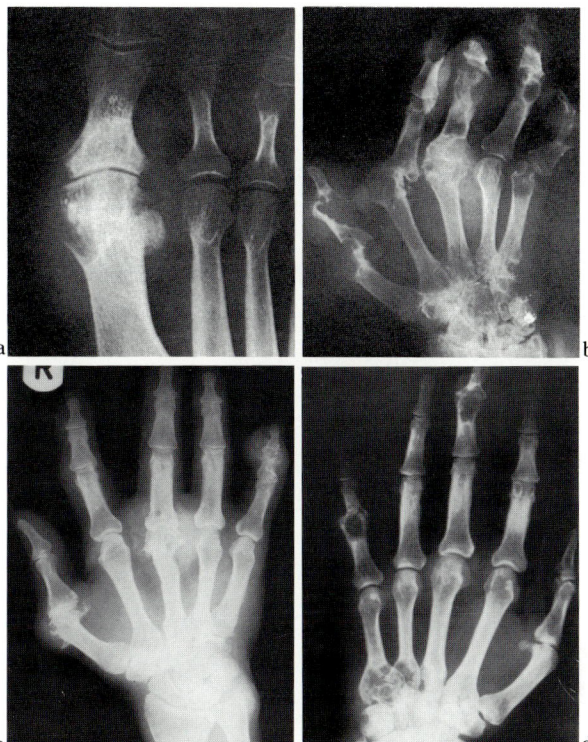

Fig. 1.4. *Gout—classical examples*, all in elderly men with long-established disease. **a** *1st metatarso-phalangeal joint (podagra)*. Clearly defined punched-out defects are evident in the metatarsal head, with a large soft tissue swelling. Normal bony density is maintained. **b** *Hand*. The ravages of advanced disease are accompanied by multiple deformities. Even in this case generalised demineralisation is not prominent. **c** *Hand*. Some of these lytic lesions are remote from joints. Amorphous calcifications lie within the gouty masses in the soft tissues. **d** *Hand*. Many lytic tophi are present. Observe bulbous expansion of the lesions, particularly those in the bases of the 4th and 5th metacarpals.

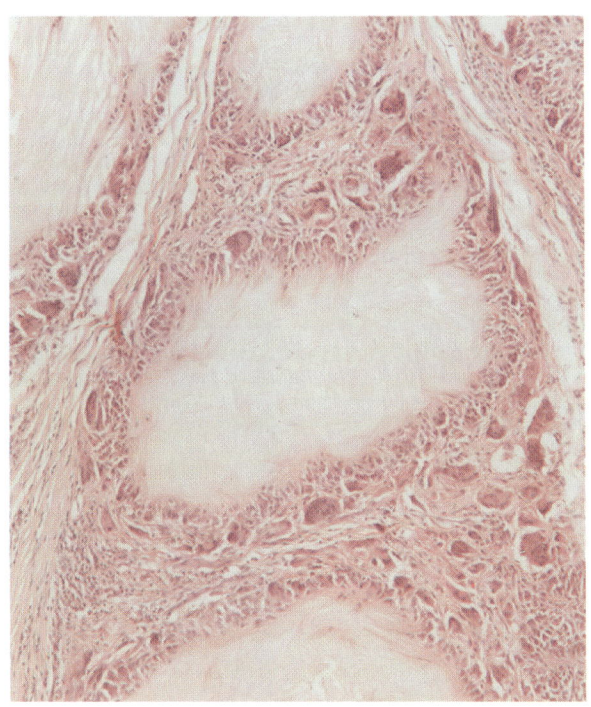

Fig. 1.3. Part of a gouty tophus as seen in a decalcified histological preparation. The crystalline urate material has been dissolved, but is surrounded by reactive tissue containing numerous giant cells. (×85)

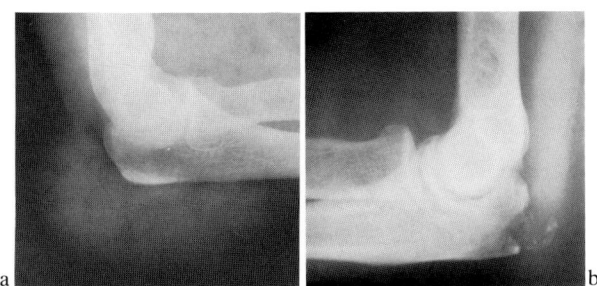

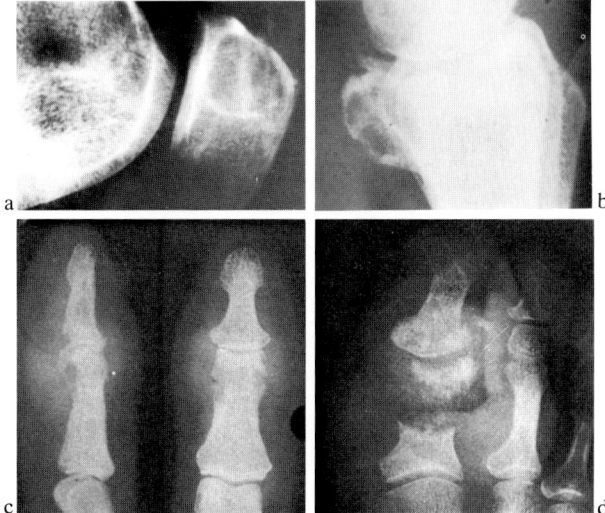

Fig. 1.5. *Gout—olecranon bursa.* Painful swellings over the point of the elbow, especially in men past middle age, always should arouse suspicion of this diagnosis. **a** This huge soft tissue mass, containing faint calcification, was a gouty tophus. The other elbow was similarly affected. **b** Another example with more obvious calcification.

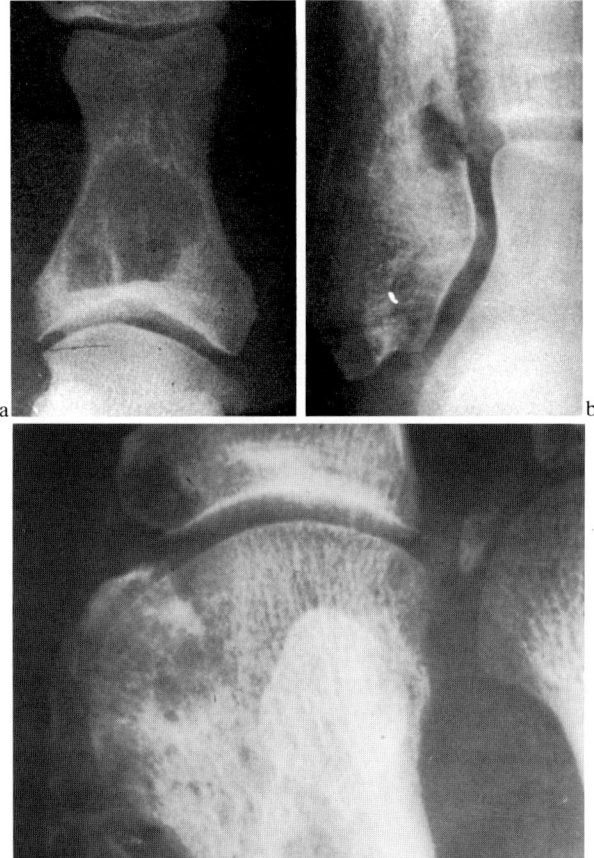

Fig. 1.6 *Gout—unusual manifestations.* **a** *Pseudotumour of 1st proximal phalanx.* This lytic and clearly defined lesion was found in a 62-year-old man with established gout for 18 years. It could easily be confused with a post-traumatic subarticular cyst. Other tophi were present, including those in the 1st metatarsal head. **b** *Ankle.* This 40-year-old man complained of intermittent pain in the right ankle. The lytic area in the fibula caused gout to be suspected. The foot was painless, but routine examination **c** revealed not only a huge destructive tophus in the medial sesamoid of the hallux with calcification in the adjacent soft tissues, but also another tophus in the base of the 1st proximal phalanx. When doubt exists, examination of both the hands and the feet is advisable.

Fig. 1.7. *Gout—further solitary lesions causing diagnostic difficulty.* **a** *Pseudotumour of patella.* This lytic lesion, associated with chronic pain in an elderly man, proved to be a solitary gouty tophus. **b** *Distal end of radius.* The nature of this expanding area of bone destruction in a middle-aged man complaining of pain in the wrist was established only by histological examination of biopsy material. **c** *Terminal interphalangeal joint of index finger.* Soft tissue swelling and erosions on the neck of the middle phalanx at first suggested pigmented villonodular synovitis in this patient—unusually a 48-year-old woman. Shortly afterwards calcified material was discharged and examination of the feet revealed gouty tophi. **d** *Proximal phalanx of hallux.* An example of a gouty pseudotumour due to hyperuricaemia associated with Fallot's tetralogy in a 33-year-old man—a recognised complication.

A2. Osteoarthritis with chondrocalcinosis

The clinical findings and the radiological appearance were typical of severe and long-standing osteoarthritis or degenerative joint disease. The extensive eburnation of the right medial tibial condyle is an appearance commonly encountered when the pain of the disorder has been suppressed partially by the prolonged administration of analgesics, such as indomethacin, phenylbutazone or steroids (see Exercise 5). In this patient, however, the radiographs did not reveal evidence of chondrocalcinosis, of which the presence was established only by the subsequent histological studies, a point of some diagnostic importance.

At operation, the diagnosis of osteoarthritis was confirmed. The articular cartilage of the joint was degenerate and the cartilage of the lateral tibial plateau extensively eroded. Deposits of white chalky material were present in the remaining articular cartilage and in the menisci. Q2b and Q2c show the microscopic appearance of the meniscal deposits. Collections of darkly staining material are present in the superficial part of the meniscal fibrocartilage. When examined in polarised light (Q2c) these darkly staining areas are seen to consist of small birefringent crystals, which, appearing as bright structures against a dark background, consist of calcium pyrophosphate dihydrate. The distinction from urate crystals, which are deposited in joint tissues in gout (Q1c) and which also are birefringent, depends on the fact that urate crystals show negative birefringence while calcium pyrophosphate crystals show weak positive birefringence.

Polyarticular Chondrocalcinosis (Pseudogout—Calcium Pyrophosphate Deposition Disease)

The term 'chondrocalcinosis' or 'pseudogout' usually is applied to a type of arthritis in which the presence of crystals of calcium pyrophosphate dihydrate in joint tissues is associated with acute episodes of joint pain simulating gout. Often, however, the condition is recognised in the absence of symptoms during incidental radiological examination.

Calcium pyrophosphate crystals frequently can be identified in aspirated joint fluid. The variation in incidence of these cases in certain populations and families has suggested the possibility of a genetically determined disease. It is clear, however, that calcium pyrophosphate crystals can be present in joint tissues in a variety of other diseases, including rheumatoid arthritis, osteoarthritis, haemochromatosis and hyperparathyroidism, and that they can be found in individuals without joint symptoms. In severe osteoarthritis, as in the present case, crystals of this type can be identified in approximately 10% of cases, involving the residual articular cartilage, the fibrocartilage of the knee joint menisci and the synovial tissues.

Clinical Features

Although, as indicated above, detection of this disease of unknown origin may be completely incidental, especially in elderly women, symptoms of joint pain are the common presenting complaint, usually affecting patients in later life. A slight female preponderance exists. Differentiation from gout, which affects males more commonly, depends on the demonstration of normal levels of uric acid. Hyperparathyroidism, in which calcified deposits in soft tissues also may be present (see Exercise 23), can be excluded equally by normal values for serum calcium, phosphate and alkaline phosphatase.

Radiological Features

1. Site. Articular cartilages of major joints are the sites of election for deposition of calcium pyrophosphate crystals. The menisci of the knee, the triangular cartilage of the wrist and the fibrocartilage of the symphysis pubis also are affected commonly. Bursae and tendon sheaths represent other areas in which the crystals may be deposited.

2. Appearance. The crystals are radiographically dense and often outline the structures affected very clearly, as, for example, by causing punctate or curvilinear opacities within the articular cartilages of femoral condyles or a vertical linear density within the symphysis pubis. This pattern is virtually diagnostic.

Pathological Features

The diagnosis is established most readily by demonstrating the presence of calcium pyrophosphate crystals in fluid aspirated from an affected joint, especially with the use of polarising light to assess their weakly positive birefringent nature. Confirmation may be obtained by the gross appearance and microscopic pattern of the affected tissues, as in the present case. Calcium pyrophosphate dihydrate is soluble in acids and is consequently removed during the decalcification process that usually precedes the preparation of histological sections of bone specimens.

In some cases of calcium pyrophosphate deposition disease (as it is sometimes termed) in association with osteoarthritis, the crystals appear to precede, and to induce, the degenerative changes in the affected joints. In other cases, such as that discussed above, it appears more likely that the crystal deposition is a secondary phenomenon.

Treatment

Treatment is essentially symptomatic with a variety of analgesics. Steroid therapy is to be deprecated. Aspiration of a painful and swollen joint usually provides at least transient relief. Operative intervention is indicated only where severe joint degeneration has developed.

References

Bocher J, Mankin HJ, Berk RN, Rodnan GP (1965) Prevalence of calcified meniscal cartilage in elderly persons. N Engl J Med 272: 1093–1097

Currey HLF (1968) Examination of joint fluids for crystals. Proc R Soc Med 61: 969–971

Hamilton EBD (1976) Diseases associated with CPPD deposition disease. Arthritis Rheum 19: 353–357

Jensen PSP, Putman CE (1975) Current concepts with respect to chondrocalcinosis and the pseudogout syndrome. Am J Roentgenol 123: 531–539

Lagier R (1981) L'approche anatomo-pathologique du concept de chondrocalcinose articulaire. Rheumatologie 33: 421–437

McCarty DJ (1976) Calcium pyrophosphate dihydrate crystal deposition disease. Arthritis Rheum 19: 275–285

Reginato AJ, Hollander JL, Martinez V, Valenzuela F, Schiapachasse V, Covarrubias E, Jacobelli S, Arinoviche R, Silcox D, Ruiz F (1975) Familial chondrocalcinosis in the Chiloe Islands, Chile. Ann Rheum Dis 34: 260–268

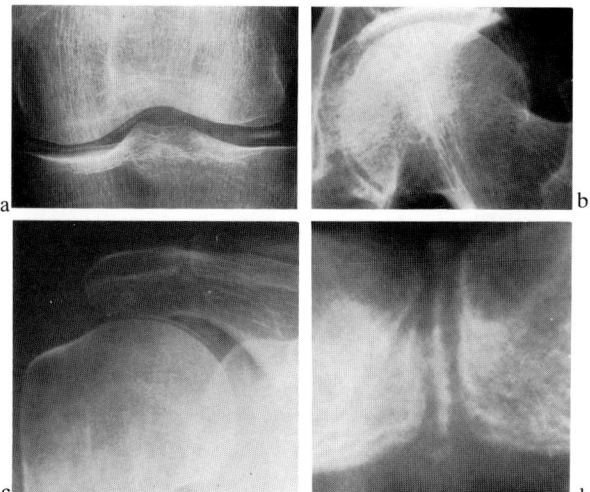

Fig. 2.1. *Chondrocalcinosis.* Typical calcifications associated with mild, but generalised, arthralgia were found in this 67-year-old woman in **a** knee, **b** hip, **c** shoulder and **d** symphysis pubis.

Other Metabolic Arthropathies

Two other generalised disorders of joints may give rise to attacks of articular pain and stiffness, thus entering into differential diagnosis of gout and chondrocalcinosis, the diseases which are the main subjects of consideration in this Exercise. Recognition of these entities often depends primarily on radiological findings rather than histological study.

Ochronosis (Alkaptonuria)

This rare hereditary disease is due to the absence of the enzyme homogentisic oxidase. The metabolism of phenylalanine-tyrosine is blocked, and homogentisic acid accumulates. Some is secreted by the kidney and imparts a black colour to the urine, if this is allowed to stand and oxidise. In mild forms the condition is asymptomatic, but in more severe forms it causes almost pathognomonic calcification of intervertebral discs and premature degenerative changes in major joints, producing symptoms of pain and stiffness. Treatment is symptomatic.

References

Detenbeck LD, Young HH, Underdahl LO (1970) Ochronotic arthropathy. Arch Surg 100: 215–219

Lagier R, Steiger U (1980) Hip arthropathy in ochronosis. Anatomical and radiological study. Skeletal Radiol. 5: 91–98

O'Brien WM, Banfield WG, Sokoloff L (1961) Studies on the pathogenesis of ochronotic arthropathy. Arthritis Rheum 4: 137–152

Wilson's Disease (Hepato-lenticular Degeneration)

Although this very rare inherited, autosomal recessive disorder is productive principally of neurological abnormalities, including tremor and dysarthria, secondary involvement of joints is characteristic. The basic metabolic error concerns copper, with a decrease in the serum copper binding protein, ceruloplasmin, so that the concentration of copper in soft tissues and cartilage is enhanced. Renal involvement may result in osteomalacia. Articular cartilage is affected, eventually being responsible for a most unusual 'fringe' appearance of joint surfaces, associated with pain and stiffness occurring in young adult life, much earlier than classical degenerative disease. As a result, irregularities of muscle attachments, as on the greater trochanters, commonly develop. Once again, treatment is symptomatic.

Reference

Kaklamanis P, Spengos M (1973) Osteoarticular changes and synovial biopsy findings in Wilson's disease. Ann Rheum Dis 32: 422–427

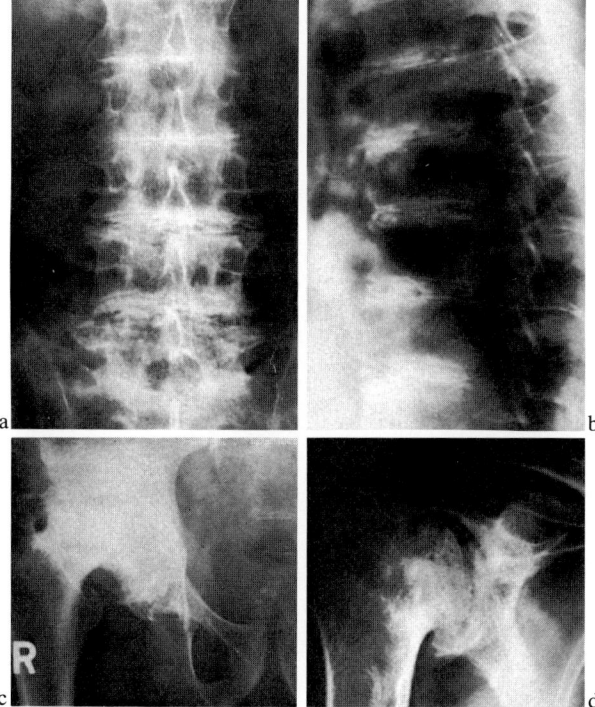

Fig. 3.1. *Ochronosis—typical features.* Calcification in intervertebral discs of **a** lumbar spine and **b** thoracic spine. Degenerative changes in major joints—**c** hip and **d** shoulder. Such changes may develop relatively early in life, but this patient was a 64-year-old man. Although he had complained of progressive stiffness of the spine, shoulders and hips for many years, he had sought medical advice on account of prostatic symptoms. Homogentisic acid was found in the urine.

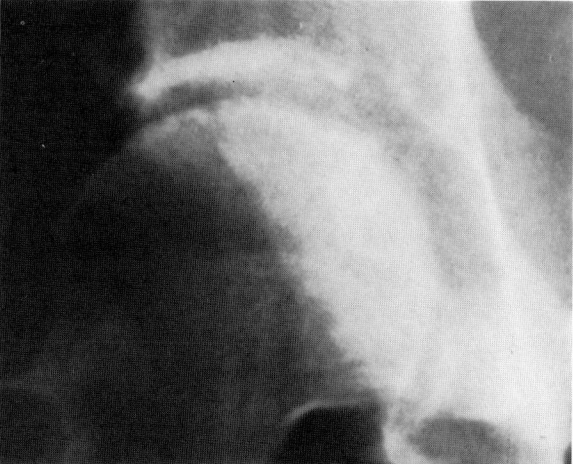

Fig. 4.1. *Wilson's disease.* In this 22-year-old man the diagnosis had been established on neurological grounds 4 years before, at which time radiographs had appeared normal. He developed increasing pain and stiffness in major joints, particularly the hips. The articular surface of the femoral head shows the unique 'fringing' which is typical of this disorder.

Exercise 34

Q1. This 14-year-old girl had complained of chronic and persistent low back pain for 2 years.

On clinical examination pain and tenderness were elicited over the dorsal aspects of the 2nd and 3rd lumbar vertebrae, associated with a mild scoliosis convex to the right and centred at this level. No other clinical abnormality was detected. Routine biochemical investigations were normal.

Radiographs, in addition to confirming the scoliosis, revealed an expanding osteolytic lesion involving the left pedicle and transverse process of L2.

This lesion was explored.

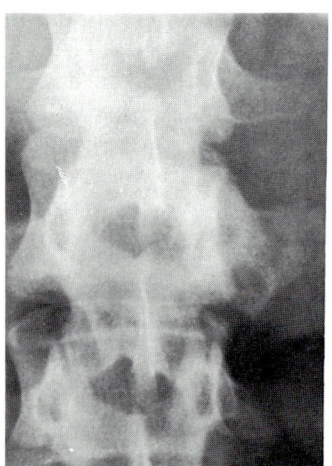
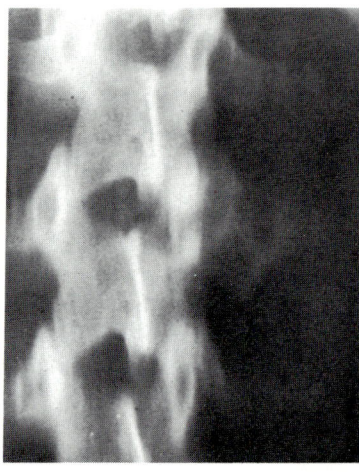
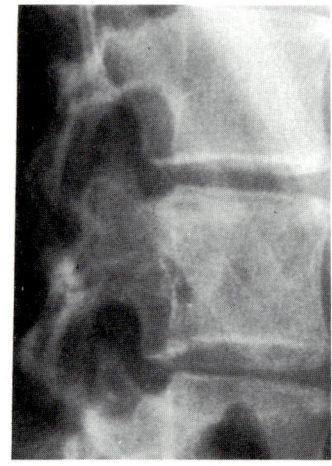

Q1a.

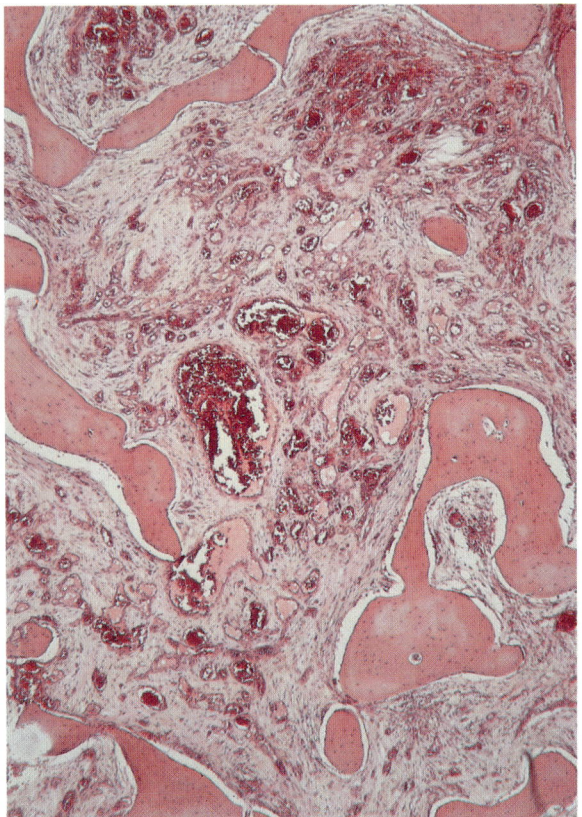

Q1b. (×38)

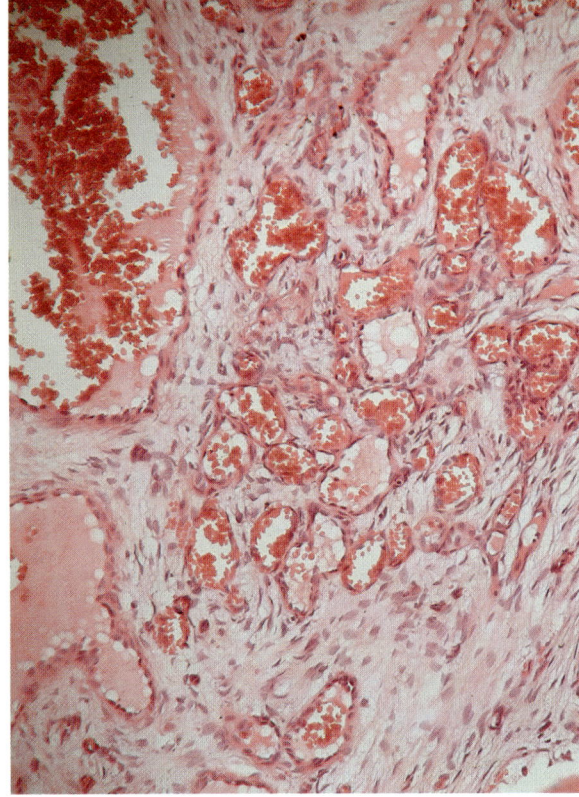

Q1c. (×104)

Q2. Intermittent attacks of back pain in this 61-year-old woman had been attributed to established ankylosing spondylitis.

During the 4 months prior to presentation, gradual onset of weakness and sensory loss in both legs, coupled with sphincteric involvement, had caused her to become bedridden. Neurological examination revealed an upper motor neurone lesion at the level of T11. All serological, haematological and biochemical investigations were normal, but the protein level in the cerebrospinal fluid was elevated.

Radiological examination of the spine demonstrated the classical changes of ankylosing spondylitis, with squaring of the vertebral bodies and extensive syndesmophyte formation. In addition, in the body of T11 a coarse honeycomb pattern was evident which extended into the neural arch. This lesion had destroyed the anterior cortex and had caused some posterior expansion. Bilateral and clearly defined soft tissue masses were present. Myelography then showed a complete extradural block at this level.

Surgical exploration was undertaken.

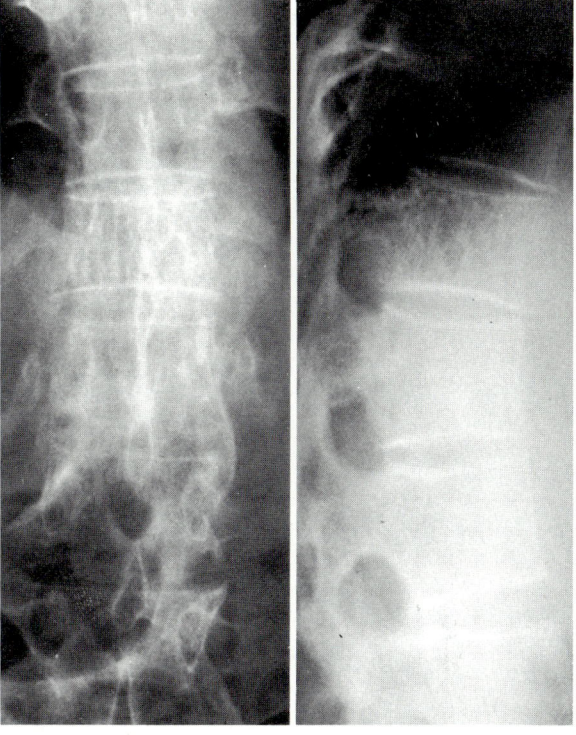

Q2a.

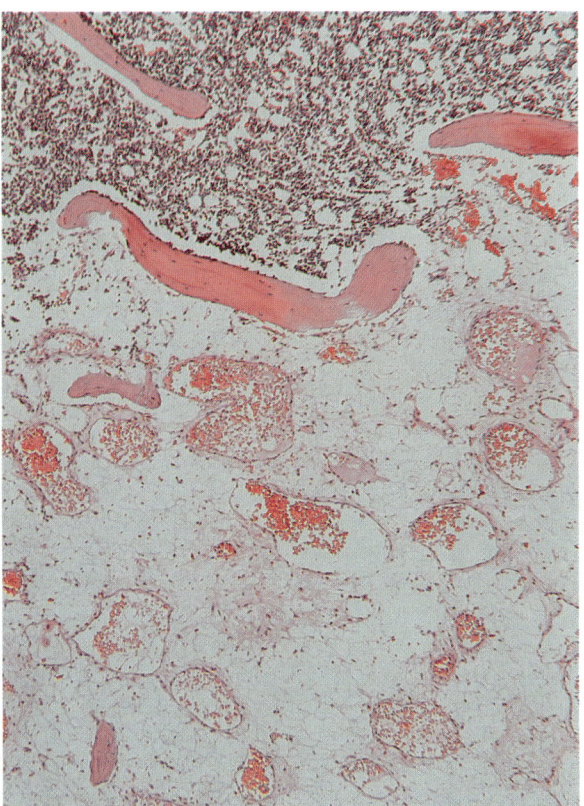

Q2b. (×48)

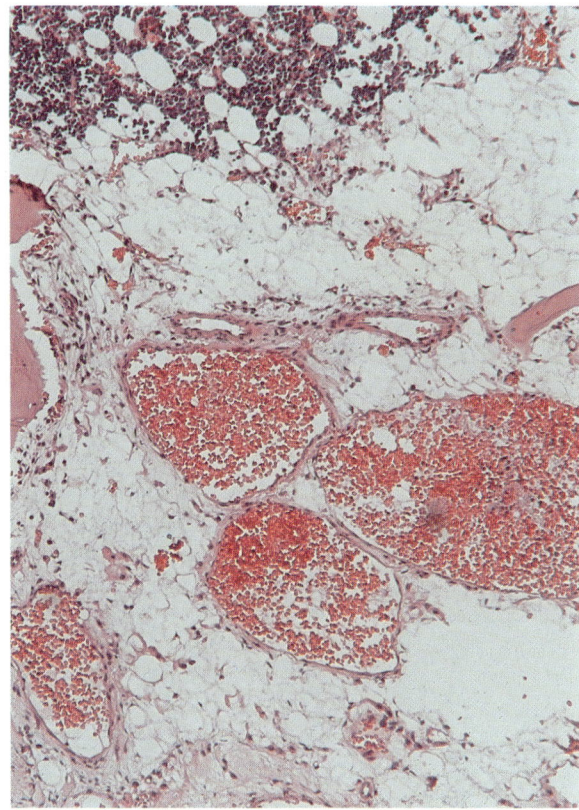

Q2c. (×94)

A1. Cavernous haemangioma of L2

The clinical finding of painful scoliosis in a child should suggest always the possibility of a unilateral lesion in the spine, usually situated at the apex of the scoliotic concavity. The commonest abnormality of this type is an osteoid osteoma (see Exercise 21), but others include benign osteoblastoma, aneurysmal bone cyst, eosinophil granuloma and localised infections. In this patient the radiological pattern was consistent with a benign neoplasm and the possibilities of both benign osteoblastoma and aneurysmal bone cyst were suggested pre-operatively.

At operation, however, the left side of the neural arch and the left transverse process were found to be expanded by a mass of vascular tissue which bled copiously. Partial excision was performed.

The histological sections (Q1b and c) showed the bone and bone marrow to have been replaced by fibrous tissue containing many thin-walled blood vessels, lined by a single layer of endothelium. The majority are small capillaries, but a few larger sinusoidal structures are also present. These findings establish the diagnosis of haemangioma.

This surgical procedure failed to relieve the pain completely. The tumour recurred and after 2 years more radical resection was undertaken, with the same histological findings. Following protection, for a few months with a corset, to avoid recurrence of scoliosis, healing by sclerosis took place and the patient was well and asymptomatic 4 years later.

A2. Capillary haemangioma of T11

This entity had been considered pre-operatively in the differential diagnosis, although certain radiological features were by no means typical. Even though the lesion clearly involved the neural arch, the classical vertical trabecular striations, usually present with this neoplasm, were absent. Moreover the bilateral soft tissue masses were distinctly misleading, contributing to an appearance more aggressive than that usually encountered in a spinal haemangioma. Furthermore, clinical experience with these tumours indicates that they are rarely responsible for symptoms and signs of spinal cord compression. In a patient of this age, indeed, the most probable diagnosis was a metastasis.

At operation, through an antero-lateral approach, the cord was decompressed. The consistency of the bone was remarkably normal. Unlike the case described in Q1, the bone was only moderately vascular.

The histological studies again established the diagnosis of a haemangioma, the sections demonstrating numerous thin-walled capillaries (Q2b) interspersed with large sinusoidal structures (Q2c), lined again by a single layer of endothelium. Many fat cells were present. The histological patterns in these two cases of haemangioma are essentially the same. Differentiation into cavernous and capillary types depends essentially on the degree of vascularity encountered during surgical intervention and is therefore a clinical rather than a radiological or histological decision.

The patient was treated by low dose radiotherapy and, 6 years later, was alive and asymptomatic, her paraplegia having disappeared completely. The ankylosing spondylitis was quiescent.

Haemangioma of Bone

Symptomatic haemangiomas of bone are relatively rare, representing only 1% of bone tumours. Clinically silent lesions, however, are recognised more commonly as incidental radiological findings and have been recorded in approximately 10% of autopsy material. These unimportant vascular malformations may be regarded as hamartomas. At the other end of the spectrum, haemangiomas of bone tend to present with a long history of pain at the affected site and may even, as in the cases of spinal involvement described in this Exercise, be responsible for significant secondary symptoms and signs. Malignant degeneration is virtually unknown. Occasionally more than one bone is affected. In such cases further vascular malformations often are encountered in soft tissues. It will be recalled that the association of haemangiomas of soft tissue with multiple enchondromas constitutes Maffucci's syndrome (see Exercise 16).

Haemangiomas must be distinguished from other benign vascular lesions, such as aneurysmal bone cyst (see Exercise 22) and haemangiomatosis, and from the more aggressive malignant vascular tumours, angiosarcoma and haemangio-endothelioma.

Clinical Features

As mentioned above, the diagnosis of these lesions is made most commonly by their incidental radiographic demonstration. Two females are affected for every male. The great majority are recognised in middle life. In the comparatively small number of cases which are symptomatic, chronic pain is the usual presenting complaint. For some reason unexplained, it has been observed that spinal lesions become more painful during pregnancy. Exceptionally, cord pressure symptoms may develop, possibly accentuated by vertebral collapse due to a pathological fracture.

When the tumours arise in the calvarium or appendicular skeleton, localised swelling is common, but often these swellings are painless. A clinical clue to their nature may be provided by the presence of vascular malformations of the skin.

It is of particular interest to the orthopaedic surgeon that these tumours may affect joints, especially the knee. Such lesions have been observed to present in childhood or adolescence on account of recurrent haemarthrosis. When they become sufficiently large to palpate they have a peculiar consistency akin to a wet sponge.

Radiological Features

1. Site. More than half these tumours arise in the skull, particularly the parietal and frontal bones, and are encountered rarely in orthopaedic practice. A quarter affect the spine, almost always as solitary lesions. The remainder involve the appendicular skeleton, the pelvis and the ribs.

2. Appearance. Lesions in the calvarium occur as clearly defined areas of osteolysis, often several centimetres in diameter and frequently containing stellate new bone formation, often described as 'spoke-wheel' or 'sunburst' patterns. Tangential views may show these spicules of reactive bone to project into an associated swelling. In vertebrae the classical appearance is coarsening of the vertical trabeculae within the affected body and a coarse trabecular texture of the neural arch. It is important to appreciate that these vertebral tumours usually cause little or no enlargement of the abnormal bone, a point of value in differentiation from Paget's disease. This relative absence of enlargement is in direct contrast to the tumours arising elsewhere in the skeleton, where bulbous expansions are frequent and often contain spicules of reactive new bone formation. Occasionally the lucent channel of an enlarged vessel leading to such a peripheral tumour may be identified. When a haemangioma arises in soft tissues, with or without associated bone involvement, it is characterised typically by a soft tissue mass containing numerous calcified phleboliths.

Pathological Features

Histologically, haemangiomas consist of a collection of vascular spaces, lined by a single layer of endothelium, with a capillary or cavernous pattern. The marrow may be fatty and some fibrous tissue may be present. Most of the bone trabeculae within the lesion are destroyed, although some residual thickened trabeculae can give the coarsely trabecular pattern and spicule formation which are radiological features of these lesions. Histological distinction between a benign neoplasm of blood vessels and a hamartomatous malformation may be difficult or impossible.

Treatment

Many of the hamartomas detected incidentally may require no treatment, or, at most, occasionally follow-up examinations. Painful symptoms usually respond satisfactorily to low-dose radiotherapy. More aggressive lesions may be treated by ligation or embolisation of the afferent vessels, often in conjunction with radiotherapy. Other manifestations of these tumours may require appropriate surgical measures such as spinal decompression and excision with grafting.

Fig. 1.2. *Haemangioma—spine*. **a** The extradural block, which was found in the patient in Q2, is a rare complication of this tumour. **b** Chronic pain in the neck in this 37-year-old woman was attributed to the obvious degenerative disc lesion (see Exercise 5) at the C5/6 level. The vertical and coarse trabecular striations in the body of C6 are typical of a haemangioma. These lesions, particularly the hamartomatous variety, frequently are asymptomatic, do not cause enlargement and usually are detected incidentally. **c** This example of another classical haemangioma of the body of L3, showing typical vertebral striation, was of particular interest. Localised pain had developed in this 35-year-old woman during a pregnancy which had terminated in a miscarriage 2 years before. The pain had persisted, but had become less severe. Aggravation of symptoms of a spinal haemangioma during pregnancy is well recognised.

References

Dorfman HD, Steiner GC, Jaffe HL (1971) Vascular tumors of bone. Human Pathol 2: 349–376

Sherman RS, Wilner D (1961) The roentgen diagnosis of hemangioma of bone. Am J Roentgenol 86: 1146–1159

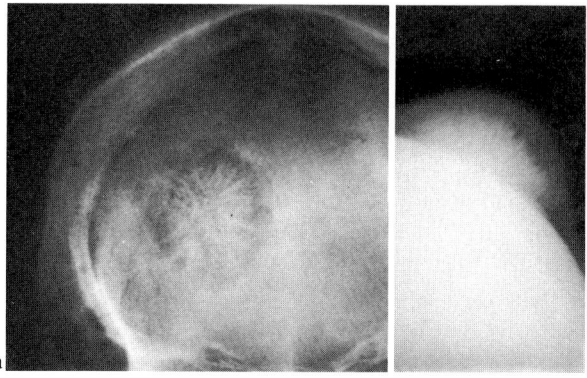

Fig. 1.1. *Haemangioma—calvarium*. This is the commonest site for these benign tumours. **a** This lytic lesion in the right frontal bone caused a slightly tender swelling in a middle-aged man. It has clearly defined margins and contains central spicules of new bone formation resembling the spokes of a wheel. **b** In this example of another tender swelling the radiating spicules of bone have a 'sun-burst' pattern.

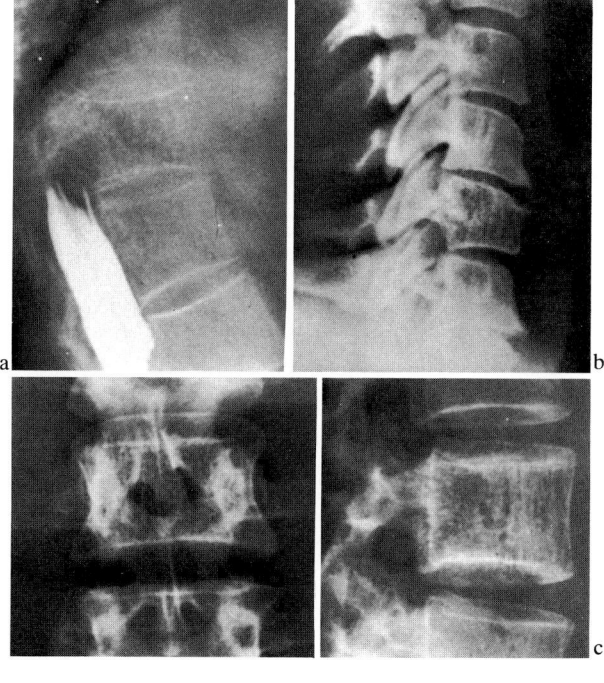

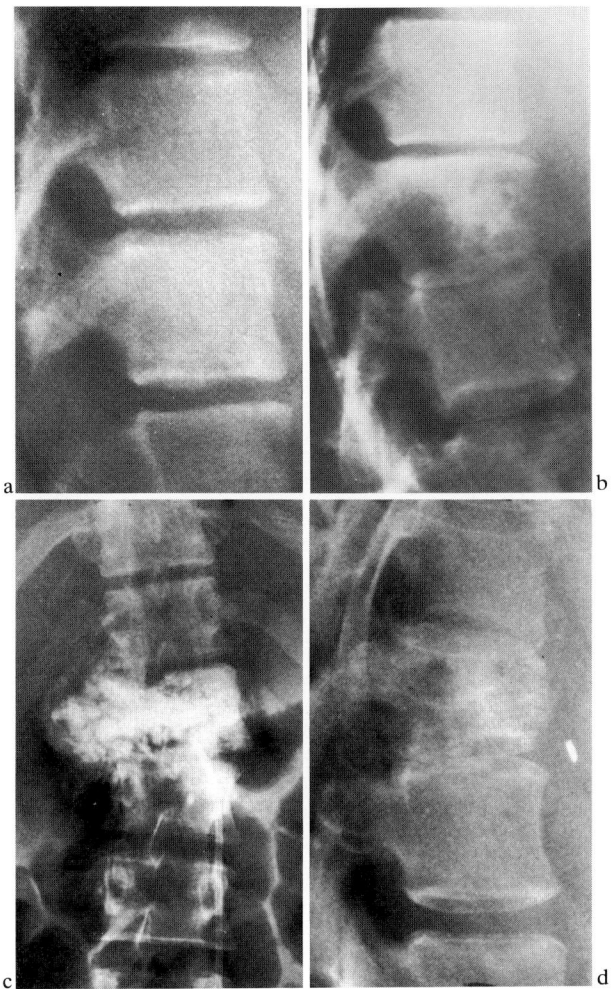

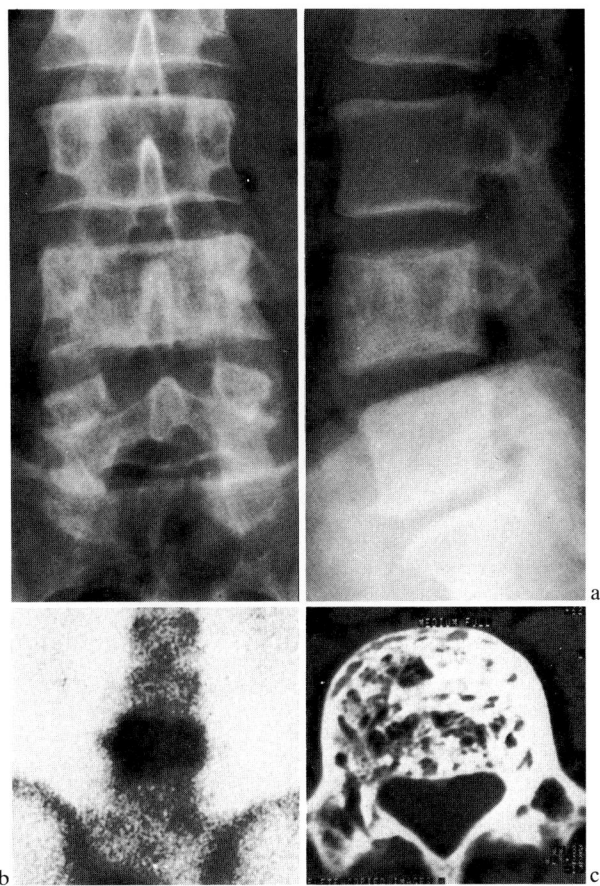

Fig. 1.3. *Haemangioma of T12—value of angiography.* This 29-year-old man had complained of intermittent backache for 6 years. **a** On presentation possible lucency of the posterior portion of the body of T12 was suspected to be due to this neoplasm, but no definitive treatment was given. **b** Two years later symptoms had persisted and increased. By this time multiple lucencies had developed, with partial collapse. At operation a large soft tissue mass, purple in colour, was found to arise from this vertebra. It had a well-defined capsule. When compressed it collapsed then re-expanded slowly, indicating its cavernous, vascular nature. **c** Segmental catheterisation of the afferent vessels outlined both the osseous and soft tissue components of the tumour. Subsequently these vessels were ligated and radiotherapy was administered, posterior fusion being undertaken at a later date. **d** A year later excellent consolidation had taken place and the patient was asymptomatic. This unusual case was reported in detail by Bucknill et al. in 1973 (J Bone Jt Surg 55B: 534–539).

Fig. 1.4. *Haemangioma of L4—investigation by other modalities.* **a** This 61-year-old man presented with intermittent claudication, attributable neither to the obvious degenerative change in the lumbo-sacral disc nor to the abnormal texture of the body of L4. The coarse vertebral striation suggested a haemangioma, but the slight enlargement of this vertebral body, unusual with an asymptomatic haemangioma, favoured Paget's disease (see Exercise 8). **b** Differentiation between these entities was not aided by the radionuclide scan, since both these conditions are likely to demonstrate increased uptake of the tracer. **c** In this case the definitive diagnosis was established only by the CT demonstration of the vascular malformation.

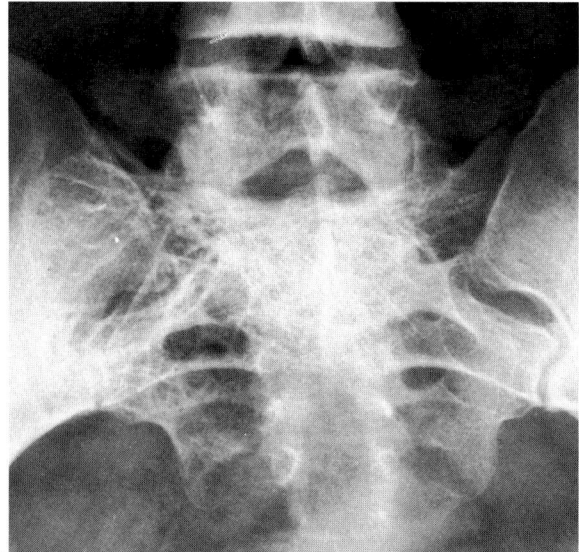

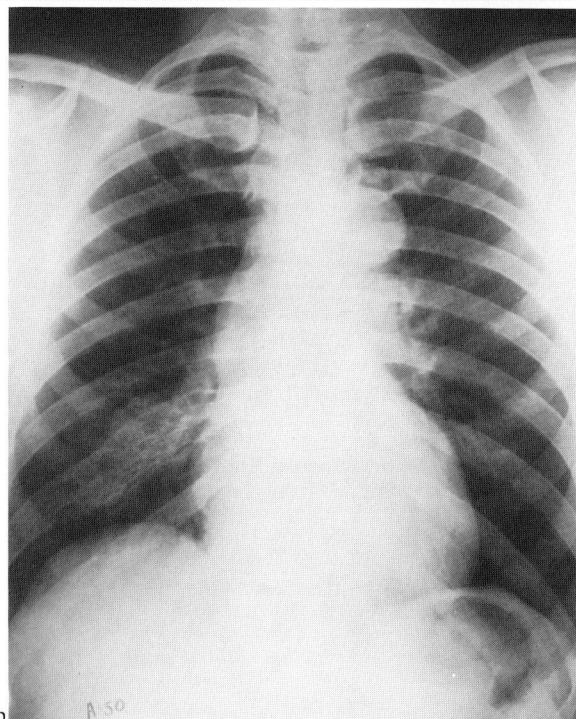

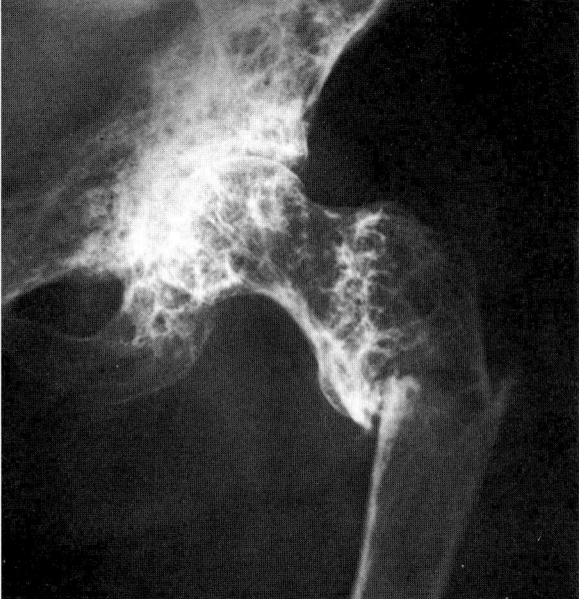

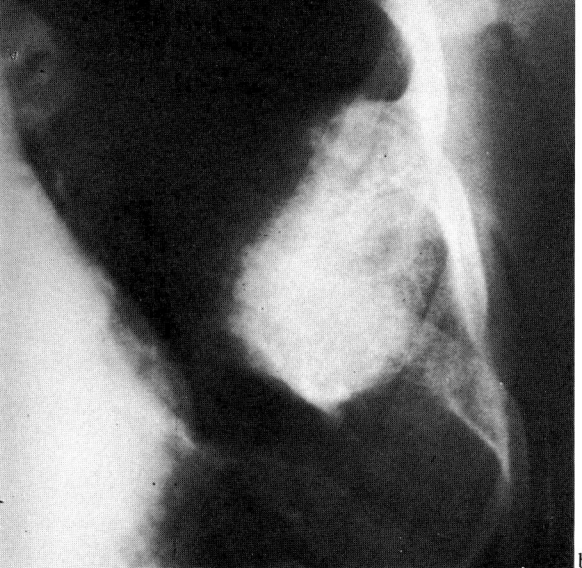

Fig. 1.5. *Haemangioma—flat bones.* **a** *Sacrum.* This young woman complained of mild pain over the right sacro-iliac joint. The coarse trabecular striation is typical of this neoplasm. No bony enlargement is evident. **b** *Rib.* The same pattern of coarse linear trabeculation is present in this lesion, which was demonstrated by chance on a routine chest film. The patient was asymptomatic and the appearance was considered to be sufficiently characteristic to permit biopsy to be avoided.

Fig. 1.6. *Haemangioma—multiple lesions.* Although these tumours are usually solitary and often asymptomatic, in rare instances numerous lesions can affect the skeleton. **a** This 48-year-old woman suffered a spontaneous fracture of the femur, having had no previous complaints. Its transverse location emphasised its pathological nature (see Q1 of Exercise 15). The mottled pattern of osteolysis involving the proximal portion of the femur was evident also in the right innominate bone. Skeletal survey disclosed several other haemangiomas, including one **b** in the anterior end of the left 6th rib, causing bulbous expansion. Biopsy of this rib confirmed the diagnosis.

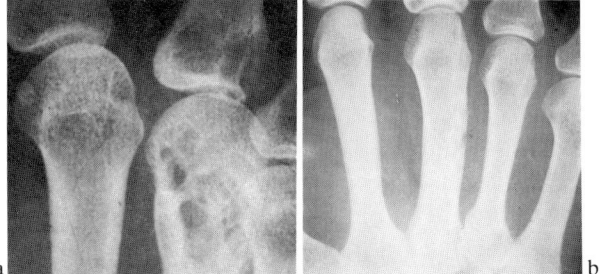

Fig. 1.8. *Haemangioma—short bones.* These locations for this tumour are distinctly rare, but when they are affected such lesions present diagnostic difficulty. **a** The lytic lesions in the base of the 3rd proximal phalanx and the head of the 3rd metacarpal were responsible for mild pain and swelling in this middle-aged physician. Both enchondromas and pigmented villonodular synovitis were considered before biopsy established the diagnosis. **b** The lytic lesion in the 3rd metacarpal shaft, which caused localised pain in a young woman, has, with hindsight, a vascular pattern. Before biopsy revealed its benign nature, a malignant tumour had been suspected.

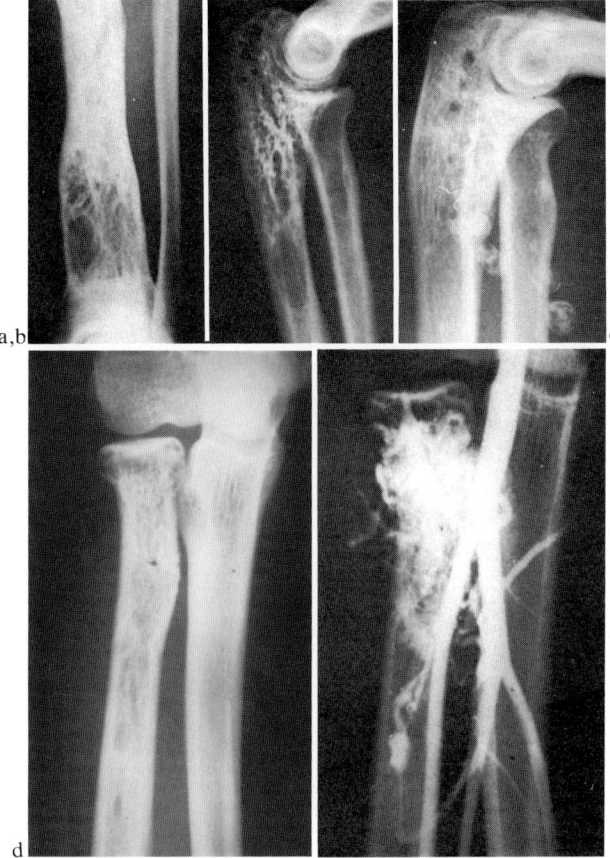

Fig. 1.7. *Haemangioma—long bones.* Such sites are relatively uncommon, but in our experience they arise particularly in close relationships to joints. They exhibit a pattern of vascularity similar to that already illustrated elsewhere in the skeleton. Most are mildly tender and slight expansion of the affected bone is common. Associated involvement of soft tissues may be indicated by the presence of a soft tissue mass which may contain calcified phleboliths. **a** *Tibia.* **b** *Ulna.* **c** Another *ulna* with phleboliths in the adjacent soft tissues. **d** *Radius.* This 14-year-old girl complained of chronic pain in the elbow, attributed to a mild injury several years previously. Not only is the radiological appearance typical, but the serpiginous lucency of an afferent vessel can be identified clearly. This vessel was clearly demonstrated by the arteriogram, which illustrates again the hypervascularity of the tumour.

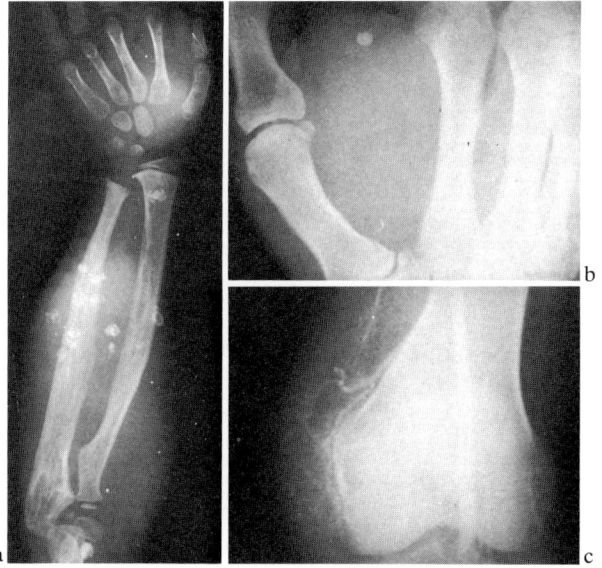

Fig. 1.9. *Haemangioma—involvement of soft tissues.* Generally dating from birth these hamartomatous malformations are accompanied frequently by cutaneous manifestations including the classical 'port-wine' stain. Bone may be affected by accelerated maturation and premature epiphyseal fusion due to hyperaemia, by pressure erosions and occasionally by periosteal reactions. **a** In this 4-year-old child vascular abnormalities are present in the radius and ulna. Huge soft tissue masses in the forearm and hand have caused pressure erosions on the radius and 2nd metacarpal. Multiple phleboliths are present. **b** This mass in the hyperthenar eminence contains a few calcified phleboliths, but that **c** overlying the medial side of the left knee required arteriography to confirm the vascularity which had been recognised clinically. This tumour was the cause of repeated haemarthroses in a young man.

Other Vascular Abnormalities of the Skeleton

At this point brief reference may be made to other, and even rarer, vascular abnormalities affecting the skeleton.

1. Haemangiomatosis (massive osteolysis; 'vanishing bone disease'; Gorham's syndrome)

This condition is characterised by slow but relentless absorption of bone. The process may begin in childhood or middle life. It may be confined to a single bone or affect a number of adjacent bones. Such cases present clinically with dull persistent pain at the site of disease, possibly complicated by deformity associated with a pathological fracture. When the spine and thorax are involved death may ensue through respiratory and cardiac embarrassment. The development of a chylous pleural effusion is a bad prognostic factor. Serial radiological studies show progressive resorption of bone, usually over a prolonged period of several years.

Pathologically the defective bone is derived either from blood vessels or lymphatic channels and replaced by angiomatous tissue comparable to that encountered in an unusually diffuse haemangioma.

Symptomatic treatment with radiotherapy has not proved successful, but spontaneous remissions have been recorded.

References

Gorham LW, Wright AW, Schultz HH, Maxon TC (1954) Disappearing bone. A rare form of massive osteolysis. Am J Med 17: 674–682

Ritchie G, Zeier G (1956) Hemangiomatosis of the skeleton and the spleen. J Bone Jt Surg 38A: 115–122

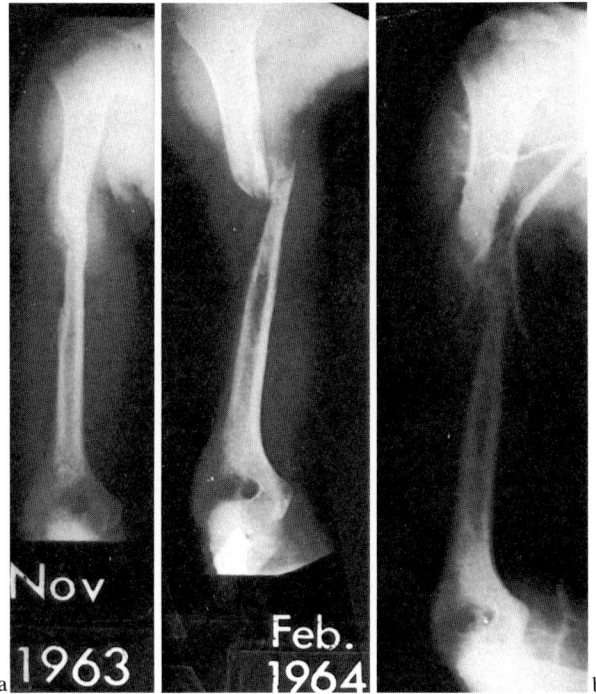

Fig. 2.1. *Haemangiomatosis—single bone involvement.* This 37-year-old man had complained of a constant ache in the region of the right shoulder for 2 years. **a** The lytic defect on the lateral aspect of the humerus was suspected initially to be a fibrosarcoma. A pathological fracture was followed by **b** absorption and pointing of the ends of the fragments within a few weeks—a characteristic feature of the disease. **c** Angiography was unrewarding, disclosing no excessive vascularity and only displacement of the brachial artery. Treatment by massive prosthetic replacement of the humerus was very successful, the patient being alive and well 15 years later. This interesting case has been reported in detail by Poirier [J Bone Jt Surg (1968) 50B: 158–160].

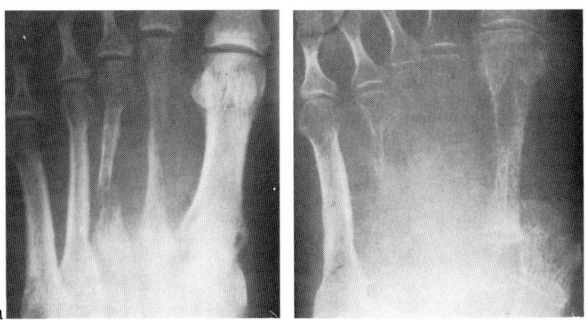

Fig. 2.2. *Haemangiomatosis—multiple bone involvement.* Increasing pain in the left foot caused this 38-year-old woman to seek medical advice. On presentation no radiological abnormality was detected, but symptoms persisted and became more severe. Only 5 months later extensive destruction **a** of the 2nd and 3rd metatarsal shafts had developed. Serial studies showed slow but inexorable progression of the disease, culminating **b** 18 months later in extensive loss of the 1st to 4th metatarsals inclusive and many of the distal tarsal bones. Amputation was necessary.

2. Cystic Angiomatosis

This unusual disease, of obscure origin, is recognised, in most cases, by the incidental radiological demonstration of numerous clearly defined lytic areas scattered throughout the axial skeleton and major long bones. These hamartomatous malformations appear to develop during childhood and adolescence, when attention to the entity may be drawn by pathological fractures. As in the case of haemangioma, a female predominance exists. Histological studies of affected bone show the majority of these cystic lesions to be curiously empty, although some have an endothelial lining and others are occasionally sufficiently vascular to permit comparison with diffuse and multiple haemangiomas. If the disorder is confined to the skeleton the prognosis is good, the lesions tending to remain static and relatively unimportant. A more serious outcome may be expected when similar hamartomas arise in soft tissues, particularly the spleen, liver and lungs.

References

Boyle WJ (1972) Cystic angiomatosis of bone. J Bone Jt Surg 54B: 626–636
Brower AC, Culver JE, Keats TE (1973) Diffuse cystic angiomatosis of bone. Am J Roentgenol 118: 456–463

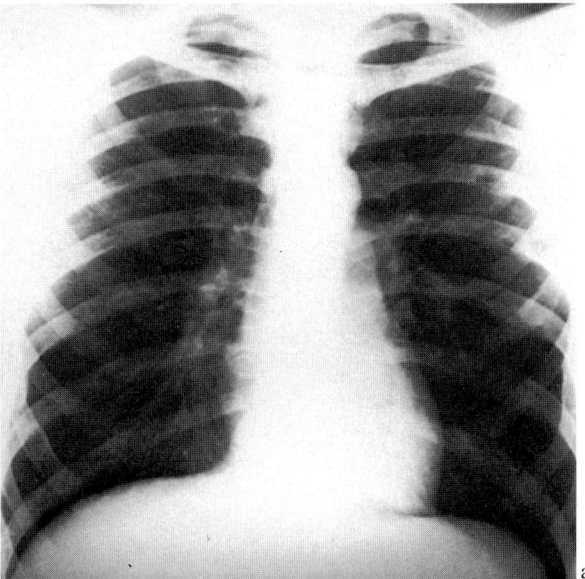
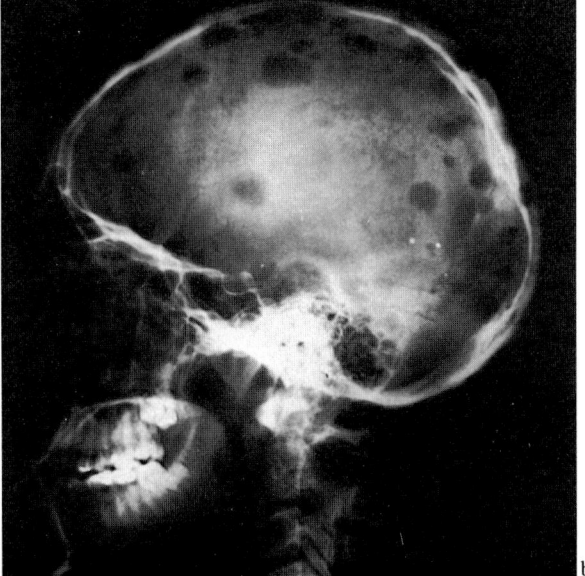
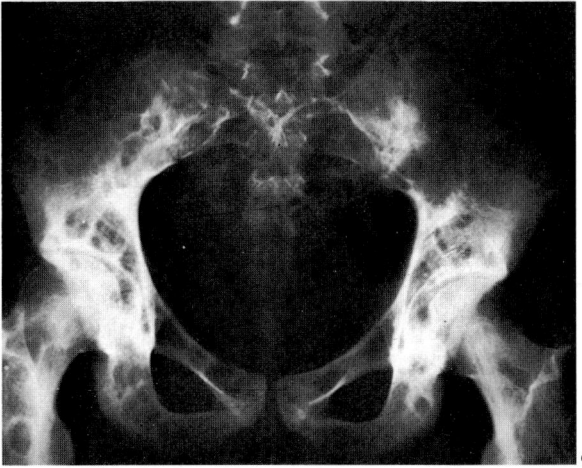

Fig. 2.3. *Cystic angiomatosis.* Numerous clearly defined lytic lesions in the ribs were detected in a routine examination of the chest **a** of a 19-year-old man who had been referred with a swelling in the hand, which was radiologically normal. The presence of these abnormalities prompted a skeletal survey. Many other areas of destruction were found, as shown in **b** the calvarium and **c** the pelvis and femora. The patient had no clinical symptoms. The diagnosis was established by biopsy, the lymphatic vessels being defective and in some areas showing lymphangiectasis, a feature observed also by lymphangiography.

3. Haemangiopericytoma

The vast majority of these unusual vascular tumours, derived from pericapillary pericytes, occur in soft tissues. Very rarely they have been recognised in bone, causing localised pain in young adults. The radiological appearance of an expanding lytic lesion in any part of the skeleton is non-specific, although simulation of an aneurysmal bone cyst is usual. The diagnosis depends on histological demonstration of elongated pericytes, which are related to the smooth muscle cells of vessel walls, and marked hypervascularity. A peculiar and unexplained secondary complication of these tumours has been described, hypophosphataemic osteomalacia. This condition has been observed to regress spontaneously after excision of the haemangiopericytoma.

Generally accepted as a variant of haemangiopericytoma is the *glomus tumour*, which is probably the most common manifestation of this neoplasm. These tumours affect particularly terminal phalanges, causing intermittent pain and swelling over periods of years. If arising in soft tissues they may produce a smooth pressure erosion, if in bone a clearly defined but non-specific area of bone resorption. This entity is discussed in greater detail elsewhere in this work.

References

Renton P, Shaw DG (1976) Hypophosphataemic osteomalacia secondary to vascular tumours of bone and soft tissues. Skeletal Radiol 1: 21–24

Unni KK, Ivins JC, Beabout JW, Dahlin DC (1971) Hemangioma, hemangiopericytoma and hemangioendothelioma (angiosarcoma) of bone. Cancer 27: 1403–1414

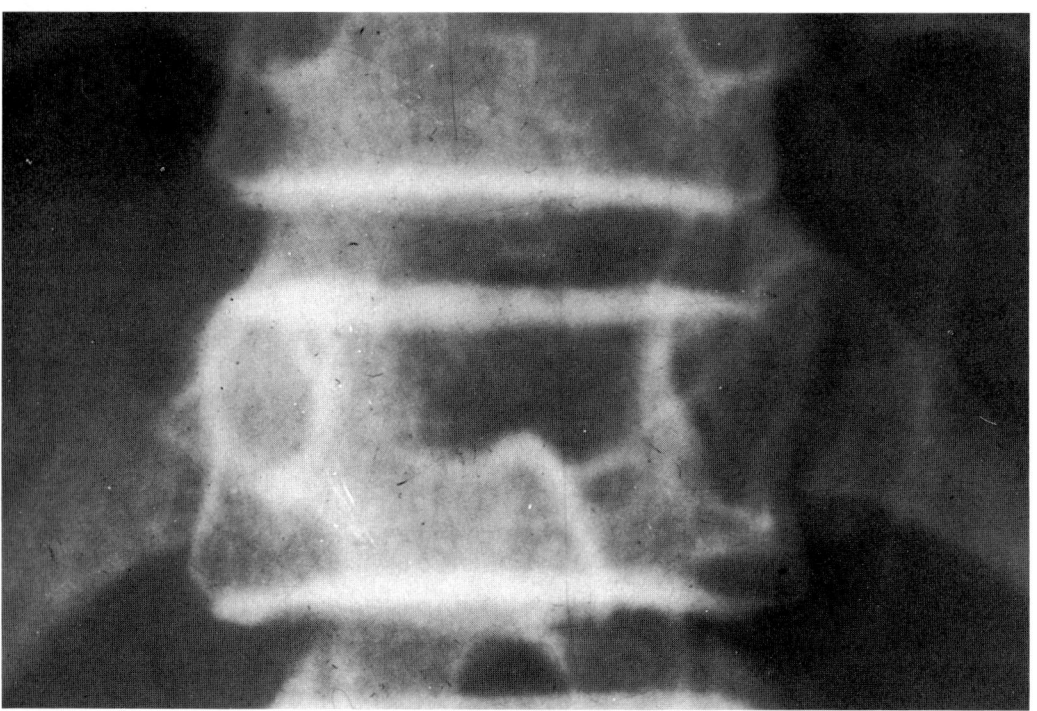

Fig. 2.4. *Haemangiopericytoma of T12.* The expanding lytic lesion which had destroyed the left pedicle of T12 has a clearly defined sclerotic margin. It was found in a young man complaining of chronic pain in this area. Pre-operatively, a confident diagnosis of aneurysmal bone cyst was offered. The correct diagnosis was established only by histological study of the biopsy specimen. Some authorities have postulated a malignant form of this tumour to exist, but others accept such malignancy as a variant of angiosarcoma.

4. Arteriovenous Aneurysms

Arteriovenous aneurysms may be congenital or traumatic. Congenital lesions of this type cause localised hyperaemia with consequent overgrowth of adjacent bones, being one of the causes of discrepancy in limb length. If a major long bone is affected, the vascular malformations in the surrounding soft tissues, demonstrated easily by clinical detection of a vascular bruit and also by angiography, should be corrected surgically to avoid a consequent cardiac overload later in life. Traumatic aneurysms may follow fractures or penetrating injuries and result in sharply delineated areas of bone resorption.

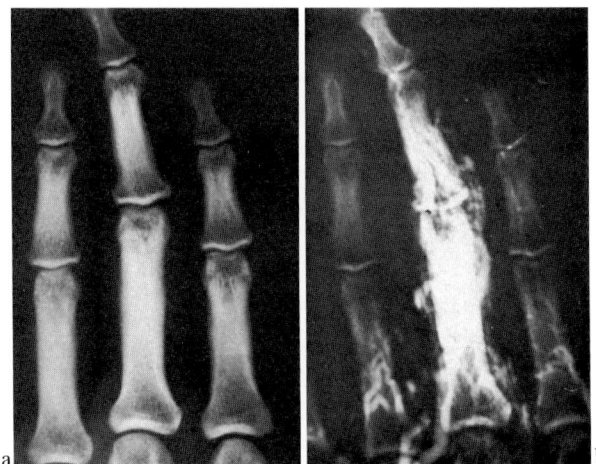

Fig. 2.5. *Congenital arteriovenous aneurysm.* **a** Marked enlargement of the bones and soft tissues of the left middle finger was demonstrated by arteriography **b** to be due to a congenital vascular malformation. Overgrowth was due to hyperaemia having been present during the years of skeletal development.

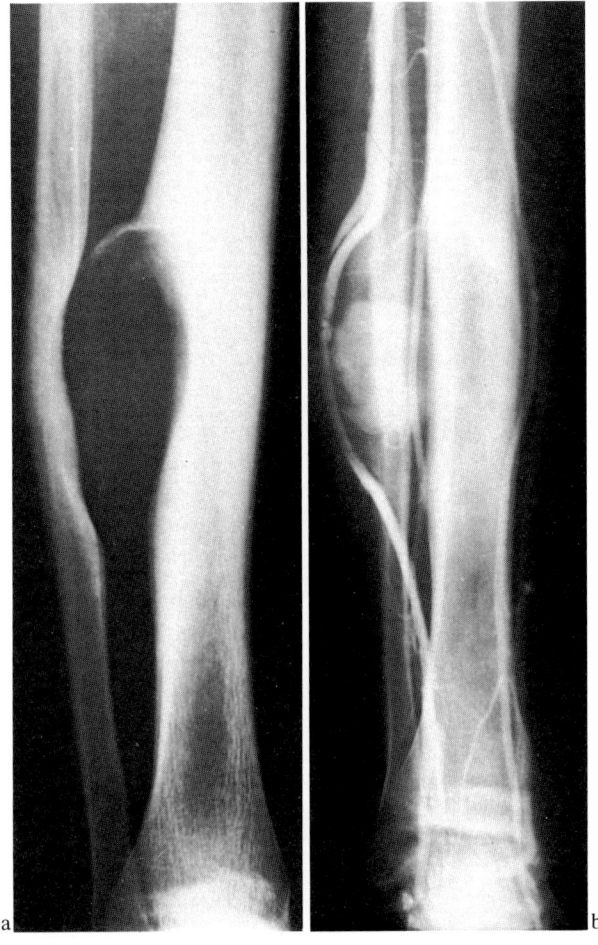

Fig. 2.6. *Traumatic arteriovenous aneurysm.* **a** This expanding lytic lesion in the tibia caused a painful swelling in the leg of a young man. Its long-standing nature was evident from secondary pressure erosion of the adjacent portion of the fibula. Clinically a vascular bruit was detected. This abnormality had resulted from a stab wound several years earlier. **b** Arteriography demonstrated the vascular abnormality. Similar lesions have been observed as a sequel to fracture.

Exercise 35

Q1. This 58-year-old American black woman had complained of pain in the right hip for 2 months, attributed to a fall.

Clinically a history was obtained of a myocardial infarct requiring hospitalisation a year before. All movements of the right hip were painful, with limitation of movement. No other abnormality was detected.

Radiological examination showed the texture of the upper portion of the right femoral head to be abnormal, with mixed areas of lucency and sclerosis. An infraction of its lateral margin was evident.

Total prosthetic replacement of this hip was undertaken.

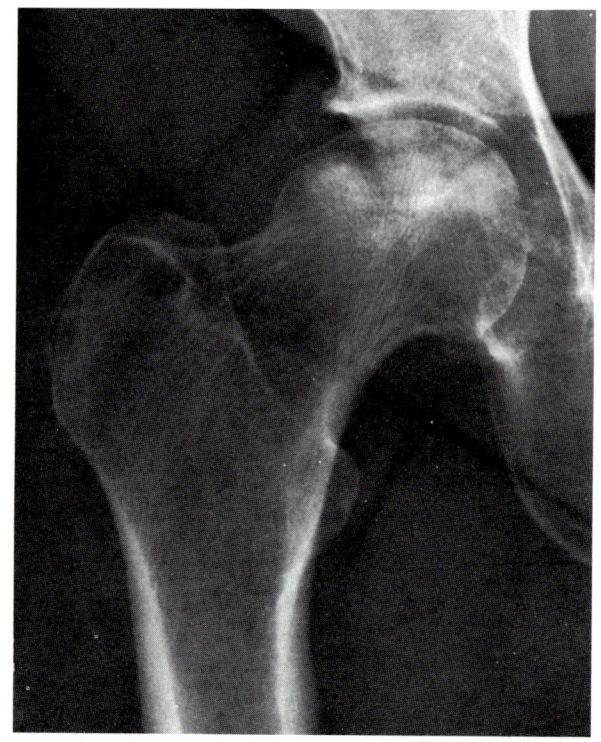

Q1a.

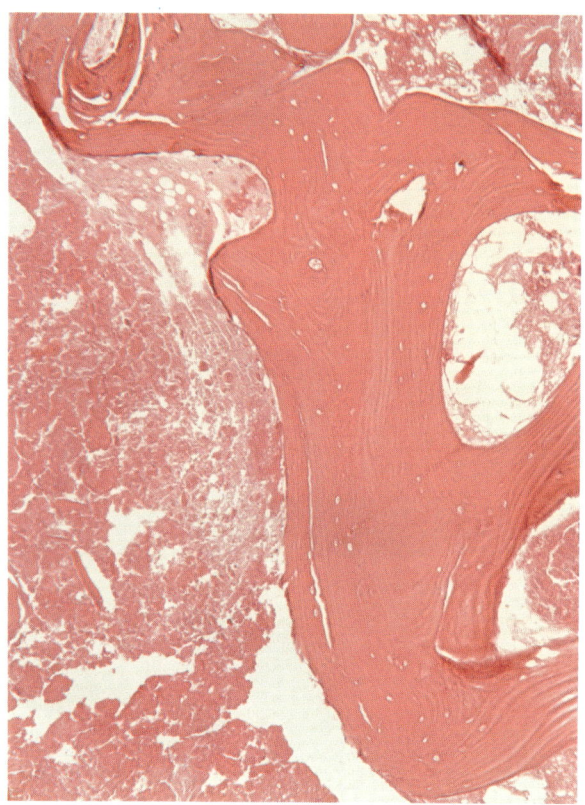

Q1b. (×85)

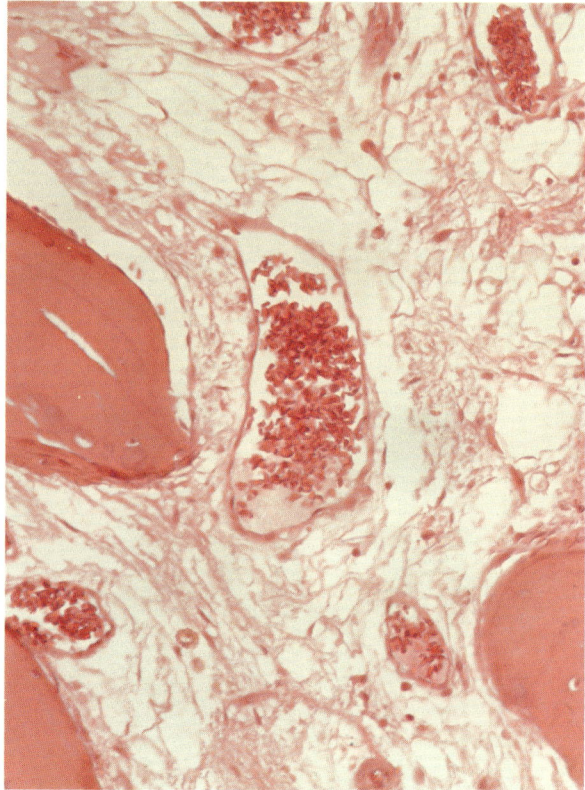

Q1c. (×190)

Q2. This patient, an American Jewish woman aged 24 years, complained of pain in the right hip, present for 3 years and recently increasing in severity.

At the age of 19 she had been involved in a motor accident and had sustained a fracture of the shaft of the right femur.

Clinical examination showed limitation of all movements of the right hip. Moderate enlargement of the liver and spleen was present. Haematological examination gave normal results.

The radiographs of the right hip revealed remarkable disintegration of the femoral head with collapse of its superior articular surface. An expanding lytic area was shown partially in the mid-shaft of the femur and a supplementary film of the distal end of this bone was obtained. Extensive sclerosis in the shaft appeared to be related to the former fracture, but osteolysis was evident in the supracondylar area with thinning and expansion of the cortex.

A total hip replacement operation was performed.

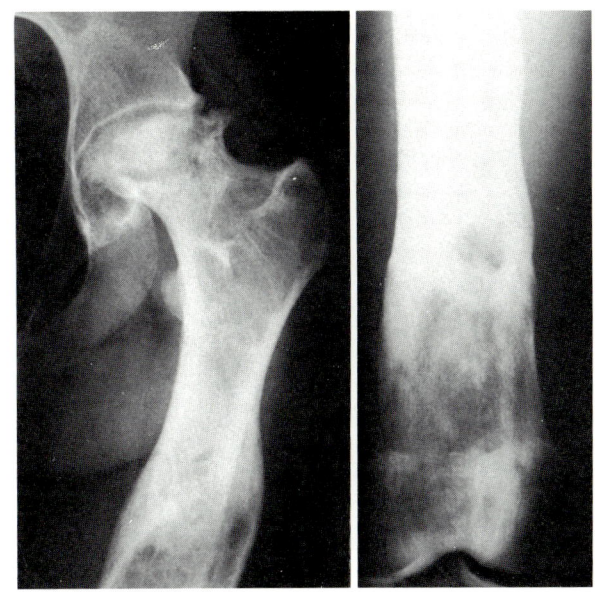

Q2a.

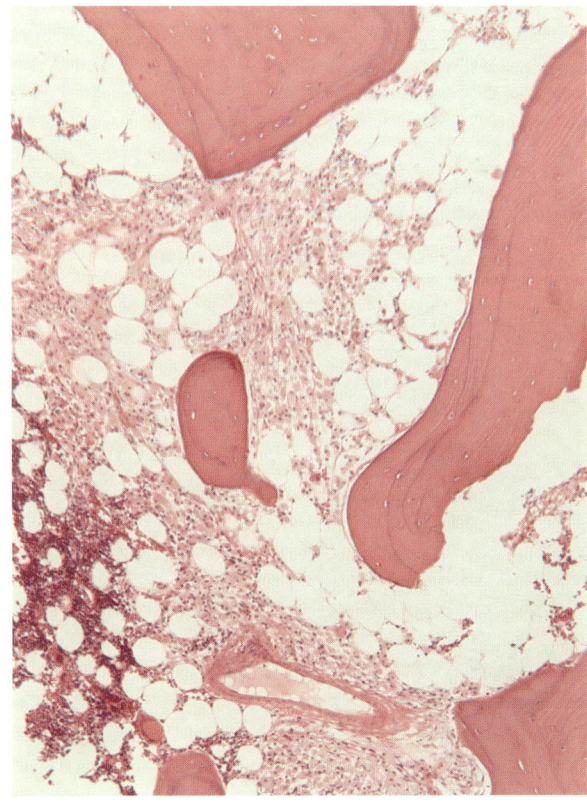

Q2b. (×75)

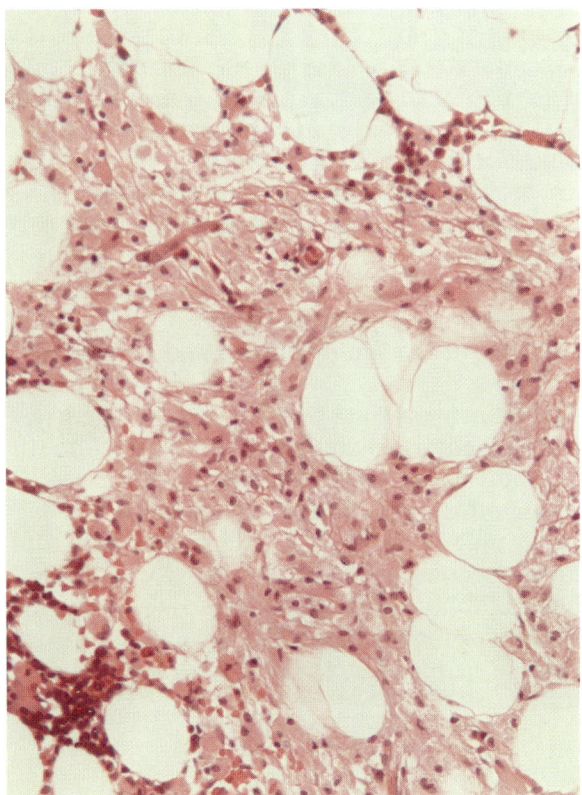

Q2c. (×190)

A1. Sickle cell disease with infarct of right femoral head

The radiological appearance of a lytic area in the femoral head, with an infraction of its lateral side, and the marginal sclerosis of a revascularisation front, is typical of an infarct.

These findings, in a black patient, at once suggested the diagnosis of sickle cell disease, and this was confirmed by a positive sickle cell test and by haemoglobin electrophoresis, which showed 55% haemoglobin S and 45% haemoglobin C. No normal haemoglobin A was present. Additional laboratory data were: Hb 12.5 g, haematocrit 38.5%, ESR 35 mm/h, reticulocytes 14%, bilirubin increased.

The histological illustrations (Q1b and c) are from the resected femoral head, which showed a localised area of infarction, taking the form of a wedge-shaped area of tissue immediately deep to apparently normal articular cartilage. In the infarcted area, bony trabeculae are devoid of osteocytes and the marrow spaces are filled with necrotic debris (cf. Fig. 1.2 in Exercise 7). At the margin of the infarcted area (Q1c) the marrow shows evidence of revascularisation. An interesting feature is the distorted appearance of the red blood cells within blood vessels. These cells are normally round, but in the present case they have an angular, crescentic ('sickle cell') appearance. This deformity of the erythrocytes is a response to anoxia and presumably occurred in the interval between the surgical removal of the femoral head and its fixation.

The laboratory data from the patient's earlier hospital admission indicated the occurrence of haemolysis, and a further haemolytic 'crisis' occurred during convalescence from the hip replacement operation. This patient was heterozygous for both haemoglobin S and haemoglobin C. This SC disease is usually less severe, as far as its haematological manifestations are concerned, than the homozygous SS form.

Sickle Cell Disease

Sickle cell disease is a genetically determined condition where an abnormal form of haemoglobin (haemoglobin S) is present. It is common in certain African populations and in their descendants, and also occurs in some Mediterranean peoples. When deoxygenated, the abnormal haemoglobin undergoes physical changes which lead to the distortion of erythrocytes, and ultimately to vascular stasis and haemolysis. The homozygous state (SS) is characterised by severe haemolytic anaemia, while the heterozygous state (AS) is revealed only by a positive sickle cell test (the in vitro distortion of erythrocytes when exposed to a low oxygen concentration) and by the occasional presence of haematuria, usually following physical stress or anoxia.

Many abnormal haemoglobins have been identified, not all of them associated with disease. A milder form of sickle cell disease is encountered in association with haemoglobin C, particularly in heterozygous individuals, where both haemoglobin S and haemoglobin C are present (SC).

Clinical Features

The clinical manifestations of sickle cell disease are many and varied. Mild or severe anaemia may be present. According to the degree of anaemia, the classical symptoms and signs of weakness, pallor, fatigue and dyspnoea will vary. In many instances of mild disease these features are totally absent or minimal, but in more serious cases jaundice may reflect excessive destruction of the abnormal erythrocytes. Prolonged anaemia stimulates compensatory extramedullary haemopoiesis with hepatosplenomegaly. As in all severe haemolytic anaemias, the ultimate hazard of secondary cardiac enlargement and congestive heart failure exists.

Vascular occlusion, causing infarcts, may involve a variety of organs, including the brain, the heart and the skeleton. Such episodes precipitate 'sickle cell crises'. Abdominal 'crises' are accompanied by fever, vomiting and leucocytosis and may simulate appendicitis or other abdominal emergencies. Infarction of the skeleton causes acute attacks of localised bone pain lasting for several days or even weeks, as in the present case. Bone infarcts, especially in young children, may become infected, particularly by organisms of the salmonella group, resulting in all the features of acute or chronic osteomyelitis (see Exercise 10). Commonly, the bone infarcts in childhood are diagnosed erroneously as being acute osteomyelitis.

Radiological Features

1. Site. This blood disease may stimulate compensatory marrow hyperplasia throughout the skeleton, although these manifestations are generally less severe and widespread than in the more dramatic forms of thalassaemia. In children these changes are evident especially in the small bones of the hands and feet and may be observed occasionally in the skull. In adults medullary bone is often affected. Infarcts in children may occur in the spine, long bone shafts and the bones of the hands and feet, but in adults they tend to be confined to the femoral and humeral heads and the vertebral bodies.

2. Appearance. Marrow hyperplasia causes coarsening of trabeculae. Eventually these structures become thickened and endosteal apposition of bone may result in the classical appearance of a 'bone within a bone'. In the skull mild degrees of diploic widening and 'sunray' spiculation may be observed.

Infarcts in the femoral and humeral heads are comparable to those described in Exercise 7. In the vertebral bodies, however, they produce the almost diagnostic sign of 'cupping', due to collapse of the necrotic central portions of the vertebral plates. It may be difficult to differentiate infection occurring in a phalanx of a young child from pre-existing medullary hyperplasia.

Pathological Features

Histologically, the bones in these various types of lesion can show changes of marrow hyperplasia, infarction or osteomyelitis.

Treatment

Acute crises are treated medically with analgesics, sedation and oxygen, though the last is ineffective in relieving pain and is of little therapeutic value if the arterial Po_2 is normal. Joint replacement in these patients is technically difficult and carries a greater risk of infection, particularly staphylococcal. Consequently antibiotic cover should be extended. Post-operatively the risk of loosening of prostheses due to further infarction is always present. The risk of fracture of the femoral shaft is increased because of the pre-existing bony abnormality.

References

Barton CJ, Cockshott WP (1962) Bone changes in hemoglobin SC disease. Am J Roentgenol 88: 523–532
Golding JSR, MacIver JE, Went LN (1959) The bone changes in sickle cell anaemia and its genetic variants. J Bone Jt Surg 41B: 711–718
Lehmann H, Huntsman RG (1966) Man's hemoglobins. Lippincott, Philadelphia
Pollen AG (1961) Bone changes in haemoglobin SC disease. Proc R Soc Med 54: 822–823
Reynolds J (1962) An evaluation of some roentgenographic signs in sickle cell anemia and its variants. South Med J 55: 1123–1128
Song J (1971) The pathology of sickle cell disease. Charles C. Thomas, Springfield, Ill.

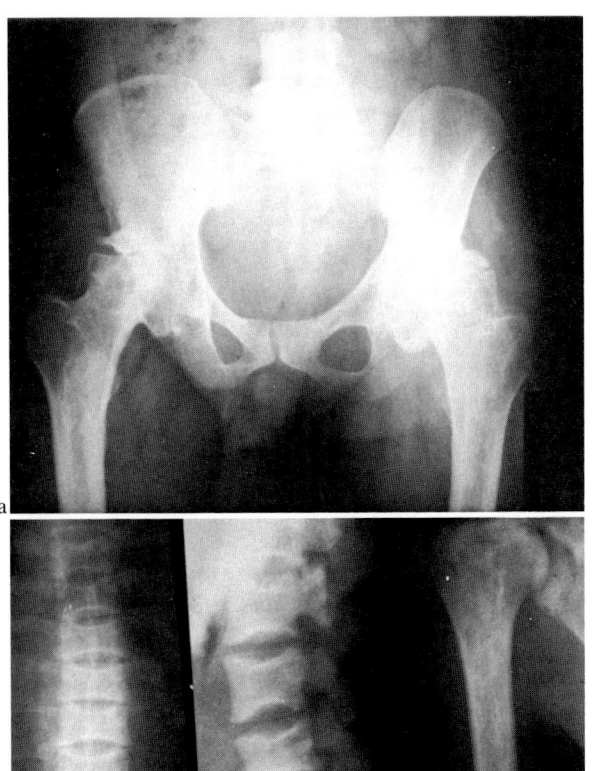

Fig. 1.1. *Sickle cell disease—classical features.* **a** Old infarcts of femoral heads in a 37-year-old black man complaining of severe pain in the left hip for 3 years. He gave a history of episodes of acute bone pain in childhood—clearly 'sickle cell crises'. Observe trabecular sclerosis in the femoral medullary cavities, which are narrowed by endosteal bony apposition, giving the appearance of a 'bone within a bone'. Note incidentally the lower pole of an enlarged spleen. **b** Another 29-year-old black man with 'cupping' of the vertebral bodies due to infarction. The density in the humeral head represents another infarct, an appearance not uncommon in affected individuals and discovered sometimes incidentally (the 'snow cap' sign). Endosteal bony apposition has narrowed the medullary cavity, within which a coarse, sclerotic trabecular pattern is evident.

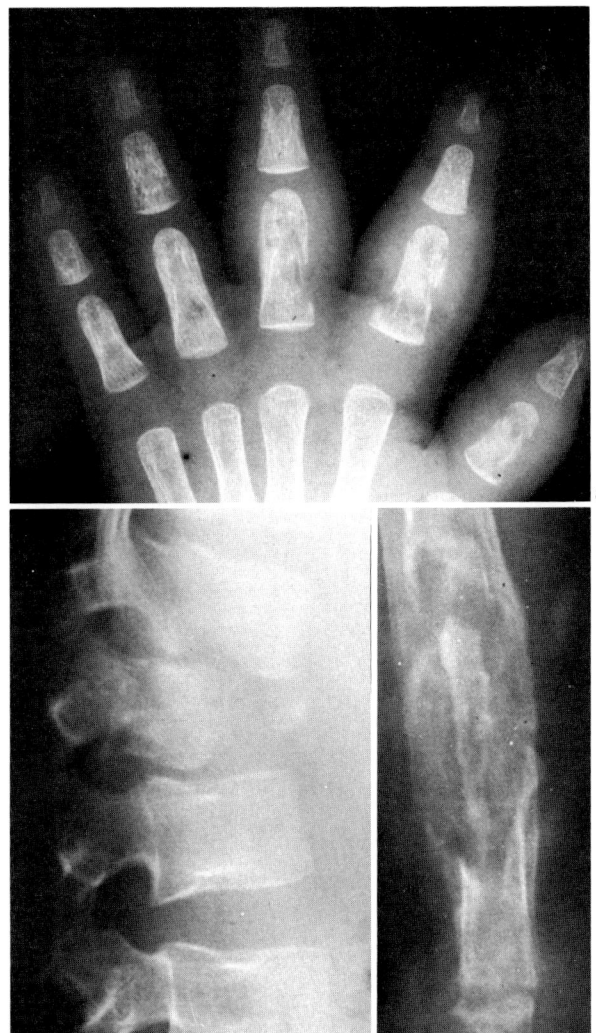

Fig. 1.2. *Sickle cell disease—infarcts complicated by salmonella infection.* **a** All these bones in the hand of a 2-year-old black child have coarse trabeculae, an appearance virtually diagnostic. The 2nd and 3rd proximal phalanges were infected with diffuse swelling of the adjacent soft tissues. **b** This 14-year-old black girl developed acute back pain. Sickle cell disease is indicated by 'cupping' of the vertebral bodies, and classical changes of osteomyelitis have affected the bodies of L1 and 2 with narrowing of the intervening disc space (see Exercise 13). The blood culture grew paratyphoid B organisms. **c** Massive infarction in the femur of a Nigerian child, with superadded salmonella osteomyelitis and sequestration. This was one of many infective lesions, all of which responded rapidly to antibiotics.

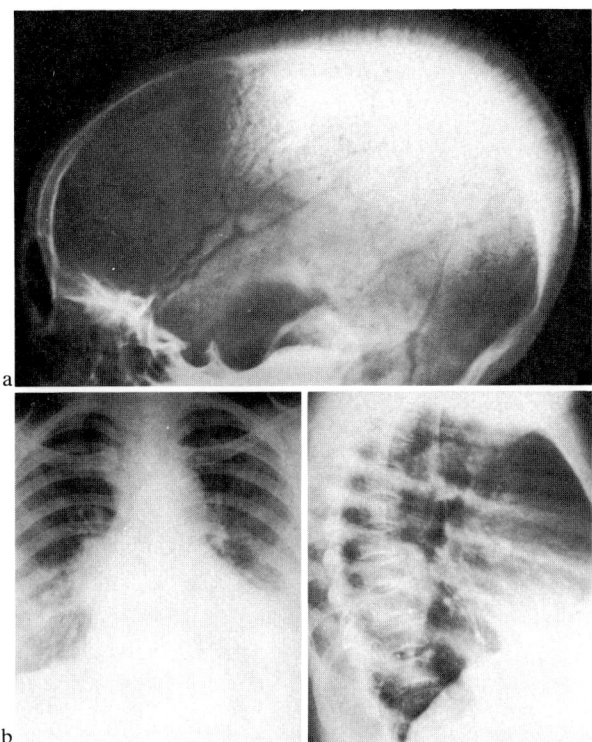

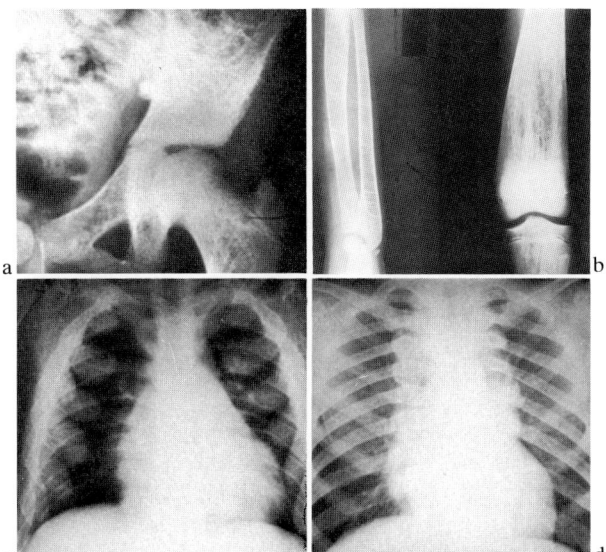

Fig. 1.3. *Sickle cell disease—less common manifestations.* **a** This 18-year-old black youth was asymptomatic, but the disease had widened the diploic spaces of the skull and, unusually, had provoked florid 'sunray' spiculation. **b** In this middle-aged black woman with severe disease, widespread skeletal involvement had produced typically coarse trabeculae in the haemopoietic areas, with some collapse of thoracic vertebral bodies. The rounded, opaque, paravertebral mass was due to extramedullary haemopoietic tissue.

Fig. 1.5. *Thalassaemia major.* These advanced manifestations of gross marrow hyperplasia were observed in a 15-year-old Chinese boy. **a** *Hip*, with coarse trabeculation and expansion of the superior pubic ramus. **b** *Long bones*, showing modelling abnormalities, including a flask-shaped femur. **c** *Chest*, with similar involvement of the ribs and cardiac enlargement. The youth died from cardiac failure, the usual outcome of such severe disease. **d** A Greek man aged 22, requiring repeated transfusions to maintain life, developed opaque paravertebral masses due to extramedullary haemopoiesis (cf. Fig. 1.3b in this Exercise), but exhibited only minimal evidence of bone involvement.

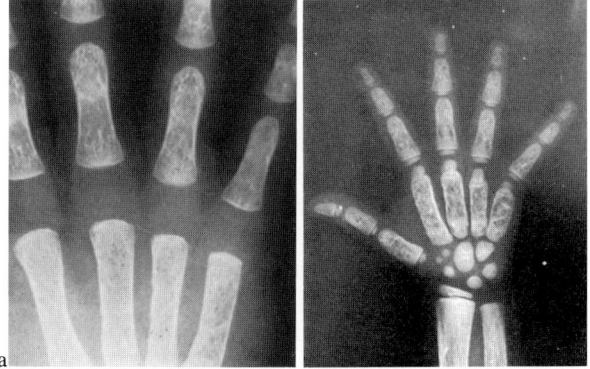

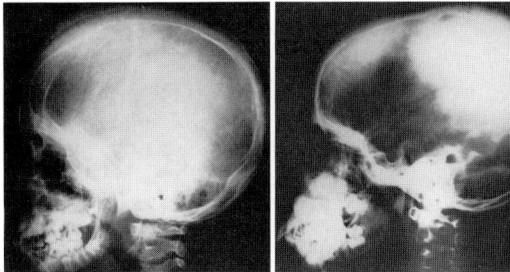

Fig. 1.4. *Thalassaemia (Mediterranean or Cooley's anaemia)* is another hereditary haemolytic anaemia, endemic in certain ethnic groups and varying greatly in severity. It also causes marrow hyperplasia, but is not associated with infarction or infection. These examples in the hands of Lebanese children show **a** the accentuated medullary trabeculation in early disease and **b** florid changes of the same type with expansion of the bones, including the radius and ulna.

Fig. 1.6. *Marrow hyperplasia in the skull in chronic haemolytic anaemias.* **a** *Thalassaemia.* Severe disease in a young Malayan child was accompanied by diploic thickening and the relatively rare, but well-known 'hairbrush' sign of sunray spiculation. Hyperplastic overgrowth may deform the sinuses, producing the clinical feature of a rodent facies. **b** *Iron deficiency (acquired) anaemia* in a Central African child who was fed on milk alone for the first 5 years of life caused similar changes, but the rest of the skeleton was reported to be normal.

A2. Gaucher's disease

The effects of obvious infarction with collapse of the femoral head (see Exercise 7) in a young Jewish patient at once suggested this diagnosis both clinically, on account of associated hepatosplenomegaly, and radiologically, because of the additional abnormality of the distal end of the femur. In this area the medullary osteolysis and expansion—giving the classical shape of an Erlenmeyer flask—were virtually diagnostic of this disorder of the reticulo-endothelial system.

The histological illustrations (Q2b and c) are from the resected femoral head. The head, as seen in a slab radiograph prepared from it (Fig. 2.1), has undergone destruction of most of the articular cartilage and of a large area of subchondral bone. The cancellous bone adjacent to the area of destruction shows (Q2b) occasional empty osteocyte lacunae, although evidence of widespread bone necrosis is lacking. The pattern of cement lines indicates that active bone remodelling has been in progress. Much of the fatty and haemopoietic bone marrow is replaced (Q2c) by an accumulation of large mononuclear cells, the cytoplasm of which contains granular or finely fibrillar material. These are 'Gaucher cells', and their presence is pathognomonic of Gaucher's disease.

The gross changes in the femoral head (Fig. 2.1) are completely consistent with the radiological diagnosis of a bone infarct, but the collapse and disintegration of the affected area of bone has resulted, at this late stage, in the disappearance of virtually all necrotic bone tissue.

Gaucher's Disease

Gaucher's disease is an autosomal recessive disorder, occurring particularly in Jews of European stock and characterised by a deficiency of the enzyme β-glucosidase responsible for the breakdown of the lipid material *kerasin* (a glucocerebroside). This material consequently accumulates in affected tissues, particularly the reticulo-endothelial cells of the liver, spleen and bone marrow. Bone infarcts occur more commonly in individuals with Gaucher's disease than in the rest of the population. The reasons for this are not fully understood.

Clinical Features

This familial condition commonly becomes symptomatic between the ages of 10 and 30 years.
Anaemia causes pallor, weakness and fatigue. Splenomegaly is a virtually constant finding, indicating a physiological response to anaemia. Simultaneous enlargement of the liver is not uncommon. Episodes of acute bone pain reflect the development of infarcts and may be the presenting symptom.

Radiological Features

1. Site. Haemopoietic marrow is primarily affected, so that the bony changes of Gaucher's disease are usually encountered throughout the skeleton in young patients. In adults, the areas of persistent haemopoiesis—the axial skeleton and the proximal ends of the femora and humeri—mainly are involved. Infarcts occur especially in the femoral and, less often, the humeral heads, but tend also to involve the diaphyses of long bones, particularly the femur and tibia. Occasionally the spine is affected by infarction.

2. Appearance. Initially, the abnormal bones only appear osteoporotic, but, as trabeculae are destroyed, progressively enlarging medullary lucencies develop. These lucencies eventually become confluent, resulting in a typical 'cross-hatched' pattern. At the same time medullary hyperplasia causes modelling abnormalities of long bones, with cortical thinning, as illustrated in Q2a, and culminating in the distal end of the femur in the classical deformity resembling the shape of an Erlenmeyer flask. As in the case of sickle cell disease, this disorder may provoke endosteal apposition of bone. Less commonly overlying periosteal reactions may be evident.

Infarcts in Gaucher's disease have no radiological features which permit their differentiation from those of other origin described in Exercise 7.

Pathological Features

The 'Gaucher cells' (Q2b and c) are large. They may contain more than one nucleus and their cytoplasm has a finely fibrillar appearance likened to crumpled tissue paper. β-Glucosidase, mentioned above as the deficient enzyme in Gaucher's disease, is a lysosomal enzyme, and electron microscopic study of Gaucher cells shows them to contain large numbers of lysosomes distended with lipid material.

Treatment

No specific therapy exists. Relief of bone pain has been reported with relatively small doses of radiotherapy and by corticosteroids. Abdominal symptoms due to hypersplenism may respond well to splenectomy, a procedure which does not appear to accelerate the bony manifestations of the disease. Infarcts of the femoral head in children should be protected from weight-bearing, but in adult life prosthetic replacement often is required. Such operations are compromised by a greater degree of blood loss and an increased liability to secondary infection. Long stem prostheses are advocated to counteract the greater risk of subsequent loosening. Perhaps the most hopeful aspect of treatment is the possibility of replacement of the enzyme deficient in this disease (β-glucosidase).

References

Amstutz HC, Carey EJ (1966) Skeletal manifestations and treatment of Gaucher's disease. J Bone Jt Surg 48A: 670–701

Brady RO et al. (1974) Replacement therapy for inherited enzyme deficiency. Use of purified glucocerebrosidase in Gaucher's disease. N Engl J Med 291: 989–993

Hibbs RG et al. (1970) Biochemical and electron microscopic study of Gaucher cells. Arch Pathol 89: 137–153

Katz JF (1967) Recurrent avascular necrosis of the proximal femoral epiphysis in the same hip in Gaucher's disease. J Bone Jt Surg 49A: 514–518

Law MM et al. (1981) Hip arthroplasties in Gaucher's disease. J Bone Jt Surg 63A: 591–601

Lee RE et al. (1977) Gaucher's disease. Clinical, morphological and pathogenetic considerations. Pathol Annu 12: 309–339

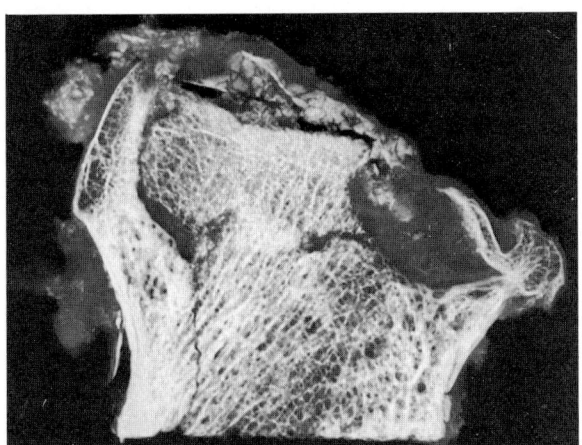

Fig. 2.1. Slab radiograph from resected femoral head, showing loss of articular cartilage and subchondral bone.

Gaucher's Disease

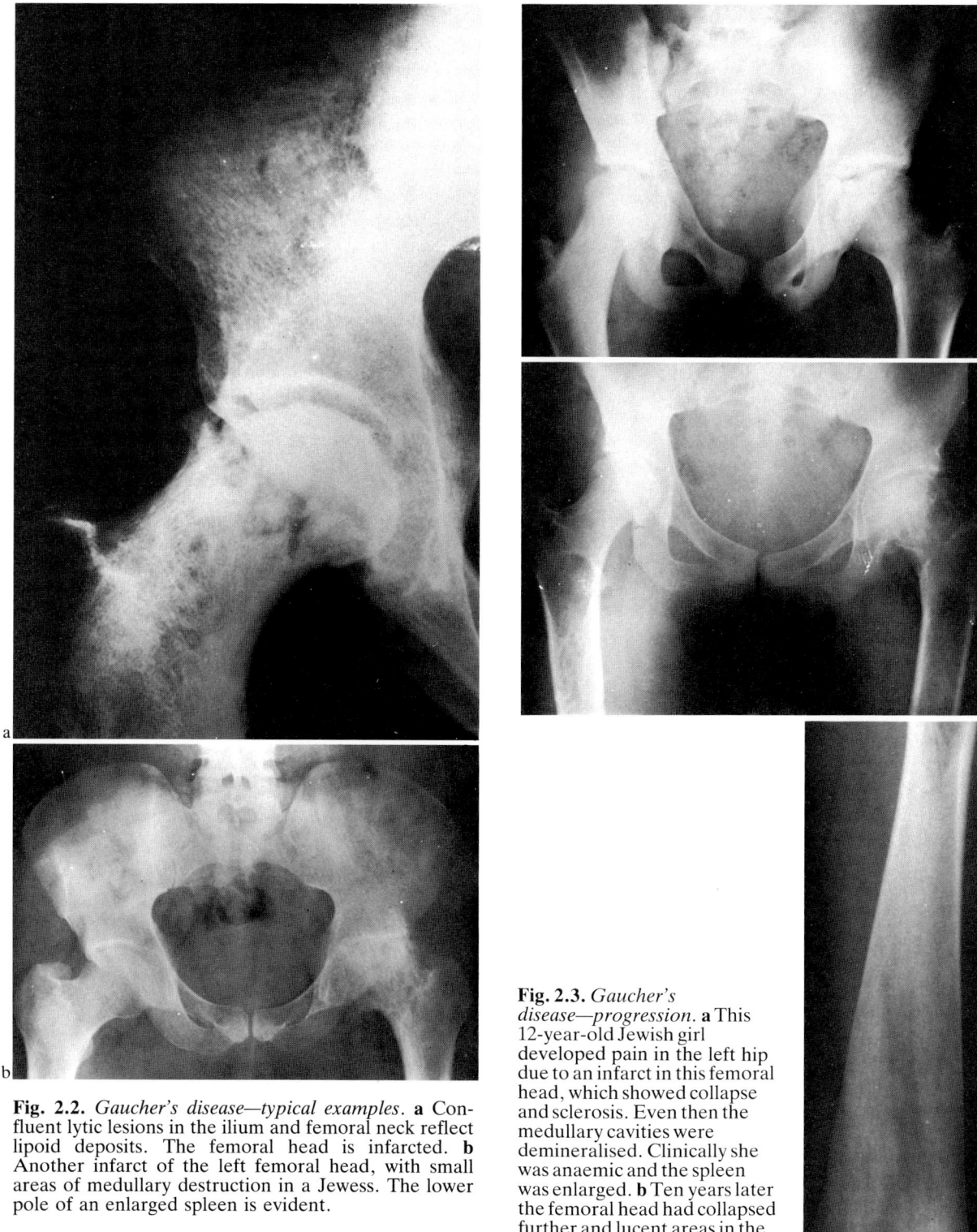

Fig. 2.2. *Gaucher's disease—typical examples.* **a** Confluent lytic lesions in the ilium and femoral neck reflect lipoid deposits. The femoral head is infarcted. **b** Another infarct of the left femoral head, with small areas of medullary destruction in a Jewess. The lower pole of an enlarged spleen is evident.

Fig. 2.3. *Gaucher's disease—progression.* **a** This 12-year-old Jewish girl developed pain in the left hip due to an infarct in this femoral head, which showed collapse and sclerosis. Even then the medullary cavities were demineralised. Clinically she was anaemic and the spleen was enlarged. **b** Ten years later the femoral head had collapsed further and lucent areas in the femora had a 'cross-hatched' pattern typical of the disorder. At this time **c** typical modelling deformities had affected the femora.

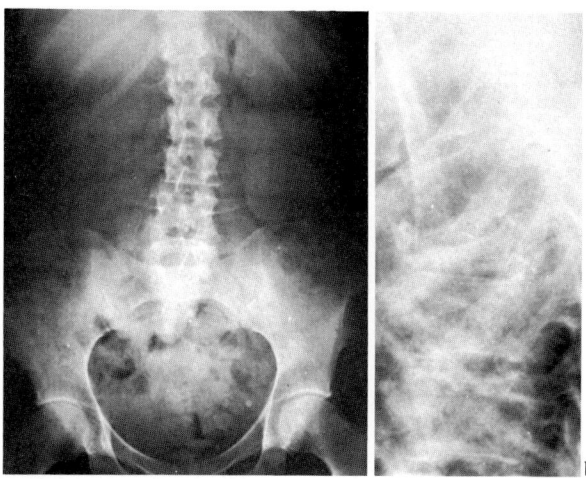

Fig. 2.4. *Gaucher's disease.* This 53-year-old woman had been treated empirically for anaemia for over a year. The development of dragging abdominal discomfort led to clinical recognition of a greatly enlarged spleen, which **a** was demonstrated also radiologically. Density of the left femoral head suggested infarction and the diagnosis was confirmed by marrow biopsy. Sudden onset of thoracic girdle pain while lifting a sick relative 2 years later led to the disclosure **b** of severe collapse of the body of T7. Vertebral infarcts are uncommon but well recognised in Gaucher's disease.

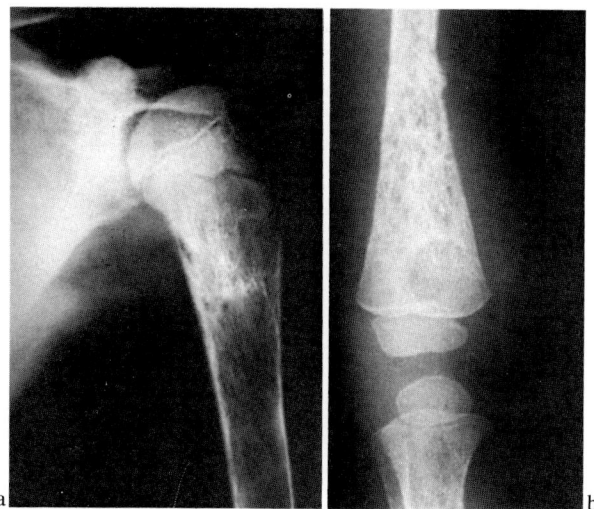

Fig. 2.6. *Gaucher's disease in early childhood* usually carries a graver prognosis. **a** Widespread areas of medullary osteolysis in the humerus of this 8-year-old Jewish child were typical of generalised skeletal involvement. **b** Even more severe changes were present throughout the skeleton of this 3-year-old girl. Modelling abnormalities had begun already to develop. This patient suffered numerous pathological fractures. She survived only a few months.

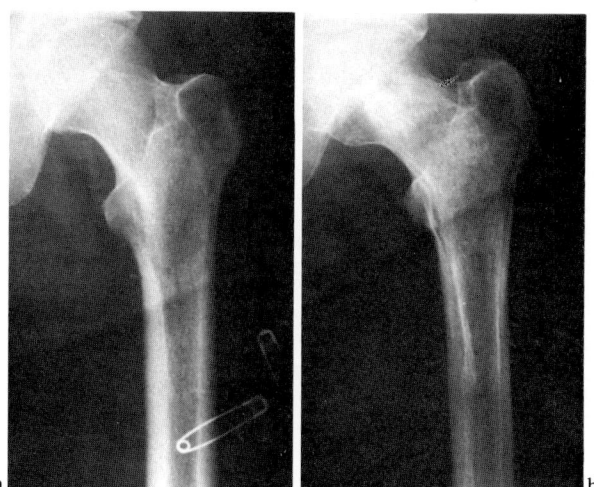

Fig. 2.5. *Gaucher's disease—endosteal apposition of bone.* The early film **a** of this 41-year-old man showed irregular medullary lucencies. Two years later **b** the classical appearance of a 'bone within a bone' had developed.

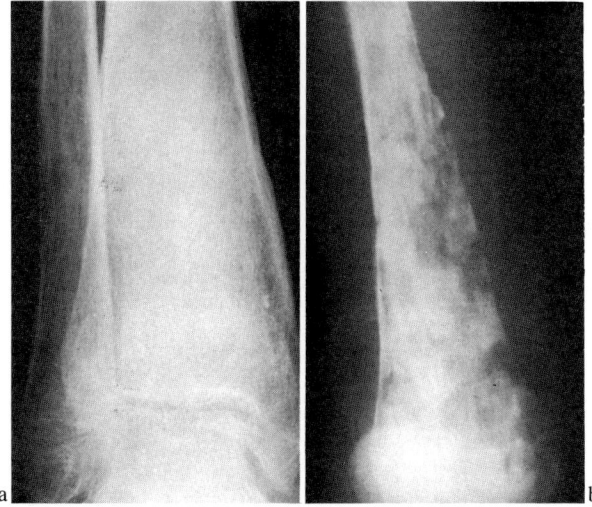

Fig. 2.7. *Gaucher's disease—less common manifestations.* **a** Medullary lucencies and modelling abnormalities in the distal ends of the tibia and fibula with relatively unusual periosteal reactions. **b** These destructive areas in the flask-shaped femur of a patient with established Gaucher's disease were due to superadded osteomyelitis—a well-recognised complication.

Exercise 36

Q1. This 29-year-old female complained of a swelling on the dorsal aspect of the right wrist. She had noticed this swelling for the first time 3 years before and stated that on several occasions it had become even more prominent and that other swellings also had appeared in this area. They had been painful, particularly at night. No other joints were affected.

Clinical examination revealed no abnormality apart from the tender swelling around the affected wrist.

Radiological examination revealed areas of bone erosion on both sides of the second and third carpometacarpal joints. These erosive lesions were clearly defined, with narrow sclerotic margins.

Laboratory investigations: ESR 9 mm/h; Hb 14.6 g; WBC 7700 per mm^3; serological tests for rheumatoid factor were negative

At operation a lobulated, homogeneous, pink mass was found to extend deep to the extensor tendons attached to the bases of the second and third metacarpals.

Histological sections of this mass are illustrated below.

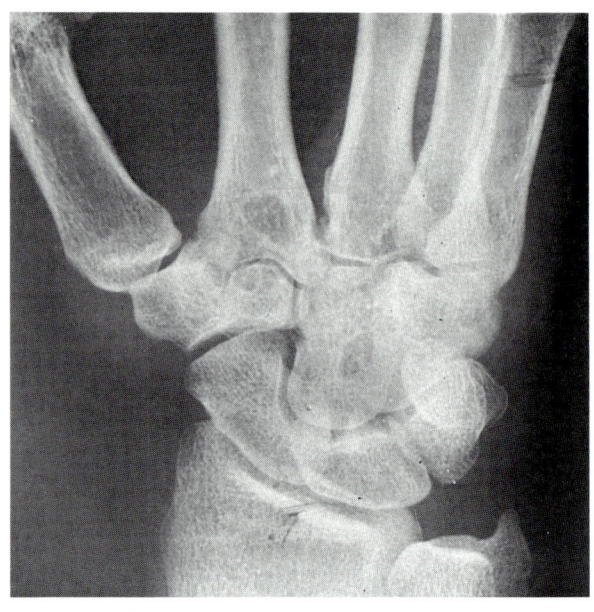

Q1a. (×300)

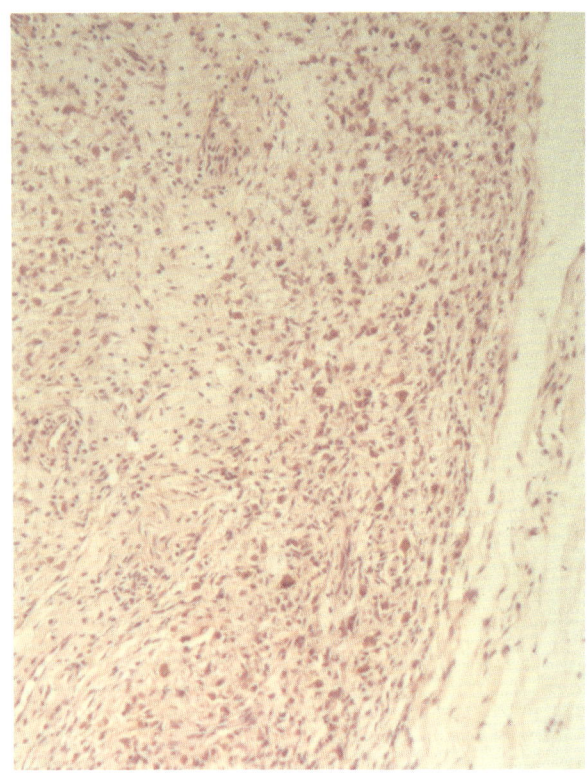

Q1b. (×120)

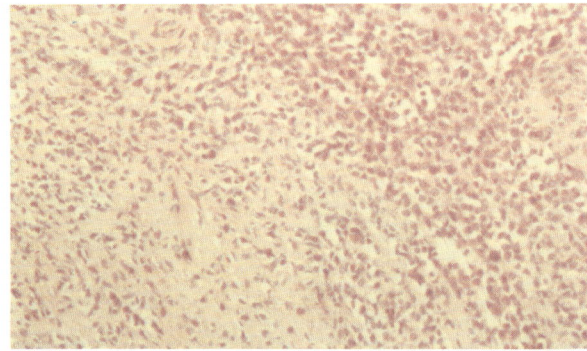

Q1c. (×120)

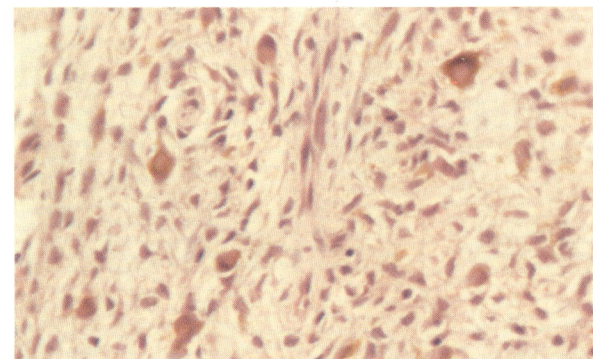

Q1d. (×300)

Q2. This 20-year-old woman complained of a mildly painful swelling around the right elbow.

This swelling had enlarged steadily during the preceding 2 years, causing increasing limitation of movement.

Radiological examination showed a soft tissue mass, clearly defined, on the anterior aspect of the joint. With this was associated extensive destruction of the proximal end of the ulna, with a slightly irregular zone of transition. Lesser erosions were evident on the radial tuberosity and below the medial epicondyle of the humerus. The joint space and its articular surfaces appeared normal.

Biopsy of the lesion was performed.

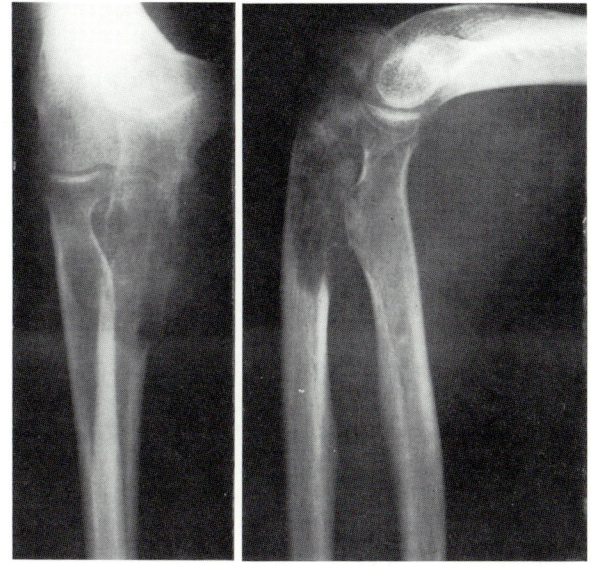

Q2a.

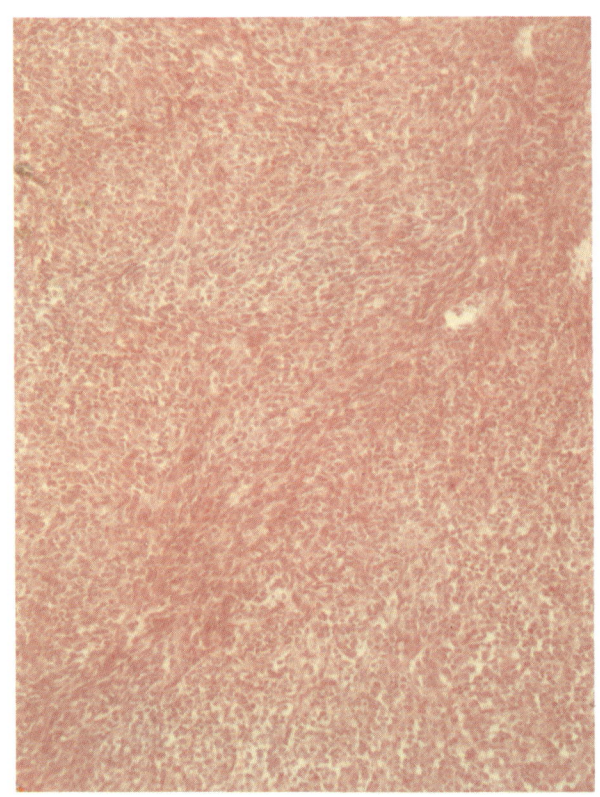

Q2b. (×125)

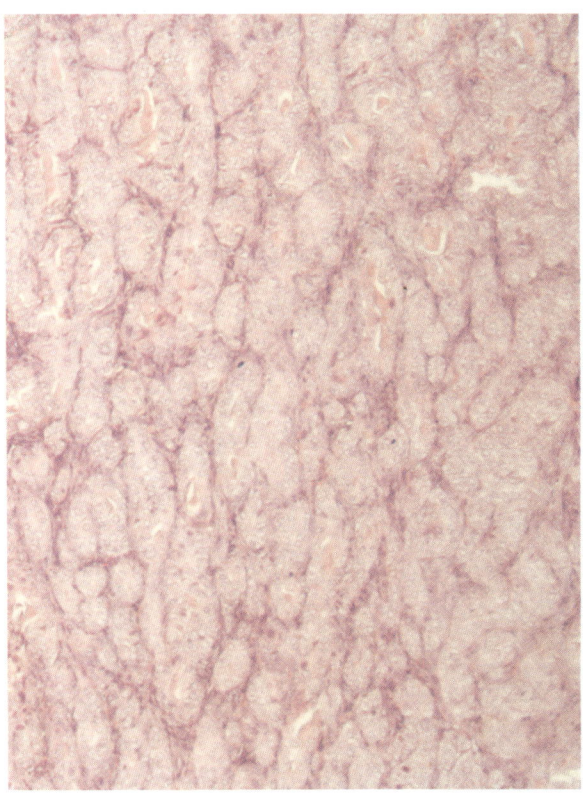

Q2c. (×125)

A1. Pigmented villonodular synovitis

The clinical symptoms and signs in this patient suggested that the swelling had originated in synovial tissue. The chronic nature of this swelling, and the relatively mild discomfort which it had caused, favoured a benign process. Diagnostic possibilities therefore included a low-grade inflammatory state, such as an indolent tuberculous infection (see Exercise 11) or, despite the normal serological findings, monarticular rheumatoid arthritis (see Exercise 18). Among benign synovial neoplasms requiring consideration were synovial chondromatosis (see Exercise 9) and pigmented villonodular synovitis. The last and correct diagnosis was supported by the radiological appearance. Para-articular erosions on both sides of a joint, as were evident in this case, tend to incriminate synovium. Preservation of the articular surfaces virtually excluded a tuberculous infection. Absence of surrounding hyperaemic osteoporosis made a localised rheumatoid arthritis unlikely. Erosions of this type, however, can occur in synovial chondromatosis before the pathognomonic calcifications of that disease develop.

The diagnosis was established finally by the characteristic appearance of the histological sections. Q1b, c and d show a variety of cell types to be present, including spindle-shaped cells, round cells (lymphocytes and plasma cells), histiocytes and giant cells. In Q1d some of these cells are seen to have phagocytosed brown pigment. This pigment is haemosiderin. Its presence within the proliferative nodules of affected synovium is responsible for a typical brownish discolouration which frequently can be recognised macroscopically during surgical exploration, accounting for the name of the disease. In this particular case relatively little pigment was present, as is apparent not only from the histological illustrations, but also from the description of the tissue as pink in colour. The haemosiderin content of the lesion, however, was demonstrated even more clearly by use of the special staining technique of Perls' reaction for iron, which proved positive by production of an intense blue reaction, as illustrated in Fig. 1.1a. Hyaline fibrous tissue, which also develops commonly in this condition, is shown in Fig. 1.1b.

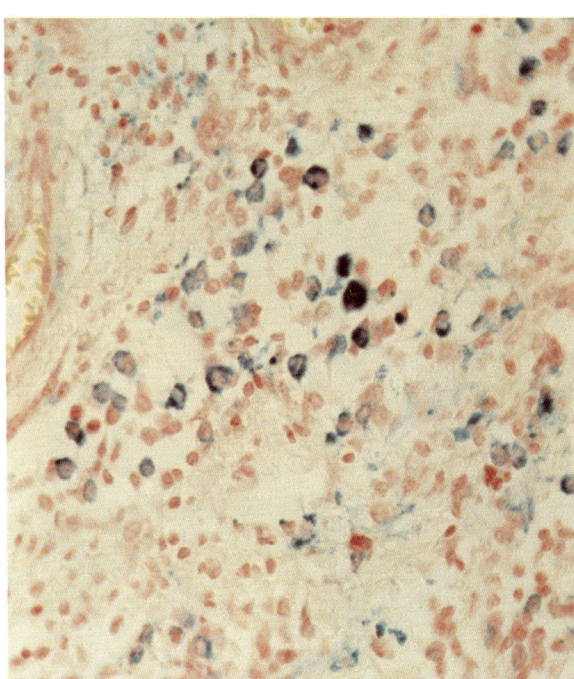

Fig. 1.1a. *Perls' reaction for iron.* Numerous phagocytic cells contain haemosiderin pigment which gives an intense blue reaction. (×300)

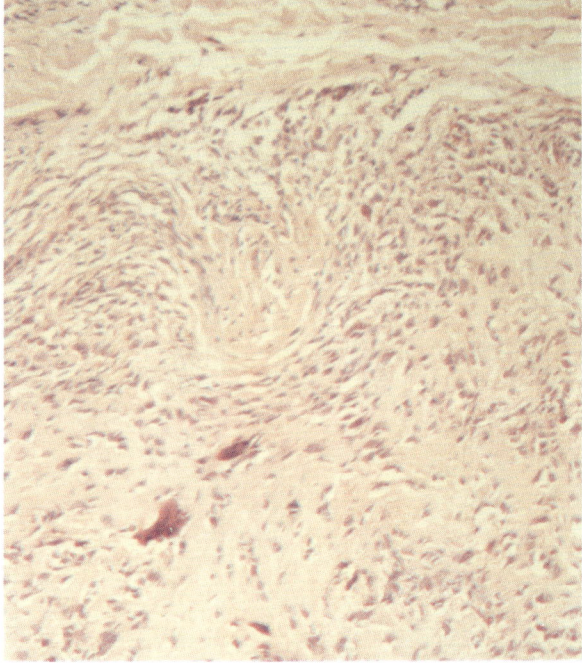

Fig. 1.1b. This field shows hyaline fibrous tissue, a common component of these lesions. (×120)

Pigmented Villonodular Synovitis

This disease is regarded generally as a benign neoplasm of the synovial lining of joints, tendon sheaths and bursae. The lesions usually are solitary and occur in adolescents and young to middle-aged adults. It is to be distinguished sharply from its malignant counterpart, the malignant synovioma (synovial sarcoma), which is described also in this Exercise and which occurs near, although not in, joints. Many confusing synonyms for the condition have existed in the past, so that the term pigmented villonodular synovitis is preferred to such descriptions as 'benign synovioma' or 'giant-cell tumour of the tendon sheath'.

Clinical Features

Mildly painful and chronic swellings, particularly around joints, are characteristic. They tend to limit movement only after they have existed for several years. Intra-articular effusions may be present, aspiration revealing haemorrhagic or xanthochromic fluid with a high content of cholesterol. All routine investigations are normal. Malignant change is virtually unknown.

Radiological Features

1. Site. The synovial tissue around major joints, especially the knee, hip, ankle and wrist, is affected most commonly. Involvement of small joints and tendon sheaths of the hands and feet and of bursae, however, is well recognised.

2. Appearance. The nodular soft tissue swellings often are defined clearly and tend to be somewhat dense owing to their haemosiderin content. As they enlarge, smooth pressure defects develop on adjacent bones, especially in relation to synovial attachments. These para-articular erosions become particularly large in relation to tightly encapsulated joints, such as the hip, ankle and small joints of the fingers and toes. Their presence on *both* sides of a joint of which the articular surfaces are normal provides a valuable diagnostic clue. The margins of the erosions generally are sharply defined by a narrow and dense zone of reactive sclerosis. Diagnosis becomes more difficult when the erosions are confined to one side of a joint, but arthrography may reveal nodular synovial swellings. Only with long-standing lesions do joint spaces become narrowed and irregularity of the articular surfaces develop. Even then normal density of the adjacent bone tends to be preserved. With such advanced disease, arthrography may demonstrate startling abnormality of the contour of the joint cavity, with huge diverticula corresponding to the sites of bony erosion.

Calcification within these soft tissue masses is a rarity and, if present, should prompt consideration of a malignant synovioma (synovial sarcoma).

Pathological Features

The lesion takes the form of diffuse villous or nodular involvement of synovial membrane, often with extension into adjacent soft tissue for bone. Gross pigmentation of the affected tissue usually is present, so that the lesions are coloured orange or brown on macroscopic examination. Although usually diffuse, involvement is sometimes limited to localised nodules of the same type. Histologically the condition is characterised by the presence of many different types of cell, including fibroblasts, histiocytes, lymphocytes, plasma cells and giant cells. Although the nature of the entity has long been disputed, it is widely accepted as a benign synovial tumour.

The nodular synovial lesions of rheumatoid arthritis are less bulky and consist largely of lymphocytes and plasma cells with relatively few giant cells and little or no haemosiderin.

Treatment

Synovectomy is the treatment of choice, even when symptoms are comparatively mild, since unnecessary amputations have been performed in the past in the belief that these neoplasms are malignant. In most cases excision of the synovium is necessarily incomplete, so that recurrences are not infrequent. Radiotherapy has not proved to be of value. In advanced lesions where joint destruction has become extensive, arthroplasty may be performed.

References

Byers PD et al. (1968) The diagnosis and treatment of pigmented villonodular synovitis. J Bone Jt Surg 50B: 290–305

Fraire AE, Fechner RE (1972). Intra-articular localized nodular synovitis of the knee. Arch Pathol 93: 473–476

Jaffe HL, Lichtenstein L, Sutro CJ (1941) Pigmented villonodular synovitis, bursitis and tenosynovitis. Arch Pathol 31: 731–765

Jones FE, Soule EH, Coventry MB (1969) Fibrous xanthoma of synovium (giant-cell tumour of tendon sheath, pigmented nodular synovitis); a study of one hundred and eighteen cases. J Bone Jt Surg 51A: 76–86

Schajowicz F, Blumenfeld I (1968) Pigmented villonodular synovitis of the wrist with penetration into bone. J Bone Jt Surg 50B: 312–317

Scott PM (1968) Bone lesions in pigmented villonodular synovitis. J Bone Jt Surg 50B: 306–311

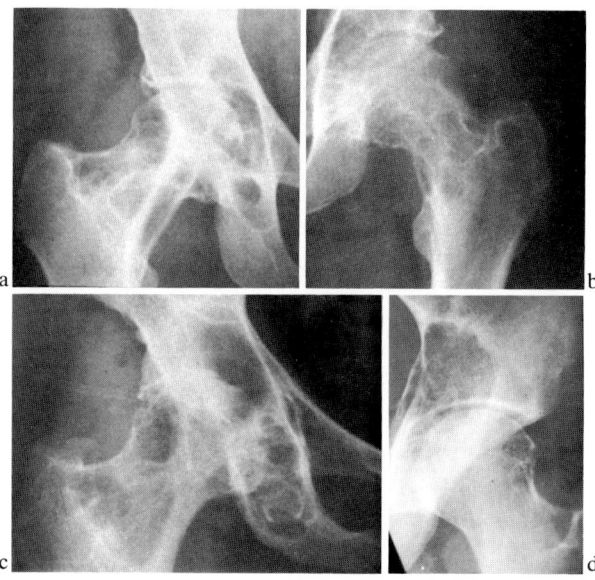

Fig. 1.2. *Pigmented villonodular synovitis—hip.* These examples illustrate increasing severe involvement of this tightly encapsulated joint by this synovial disease. Soft tissue proliferations tend to be somewhat dense owing to their haemosiderin content. Clearly defined para-articular erosions on both sides of the joint simplify diagnosis. **a** This 32-year-old man had complained of localised swelling and intermittent pain for 18 months. The joint space was reasonably well preserved, with intact articular surfaces. **b** Similar symptoms in this 29-year-old man were accompanied by numerous erosions on the femoral neck. Again, the joint space was virtually normal and no surrounding osteoporosis had developed. **c** Still larger erosions of the same type were present in this 35-year-old man, affecting both the acetabulum and the femoral neck. He had been aware of discomfort in this hip for several years. **d** An unusually large acetabular erosion was evident in this 28-year-old woman in whom a recent exacerbation of pain had followed discomfort in this hip for 5 months. Observe further erosions on the femoral neck. Even with this more aggressive lesion, integrity of the joint was maintained. Histological confirmation was obtained in all these cases.

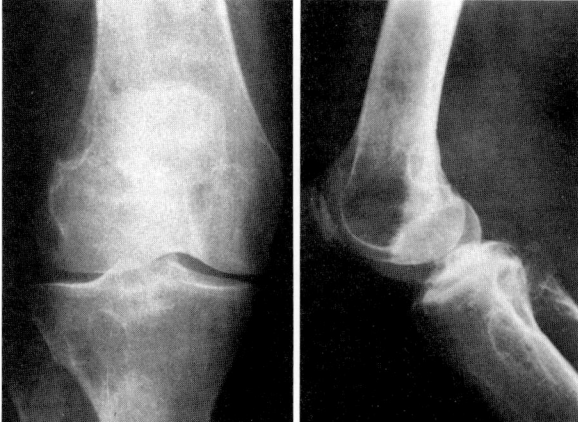

Fig. 1.3. *Pigmented villonodular synovitis—knee.* Since the knee is loosely encapsulated, erosions are usually smaller, as evident particularly on the lateral femoral condyle. This 61-year-old woman had a long history of pain and swelling. Observe also similar involvement of the tibio-fibular joint. Even so the articular surfaces, the joint space and bone density are all normal.

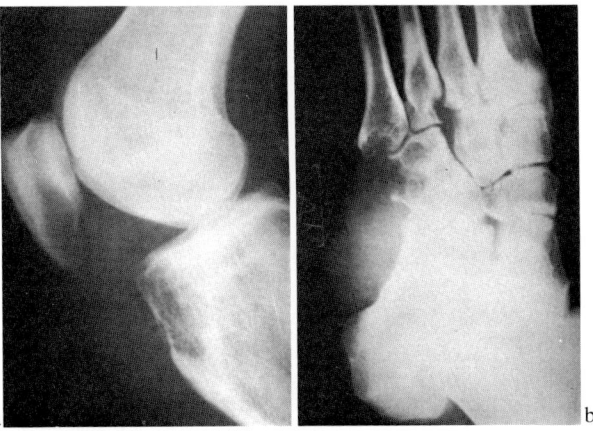

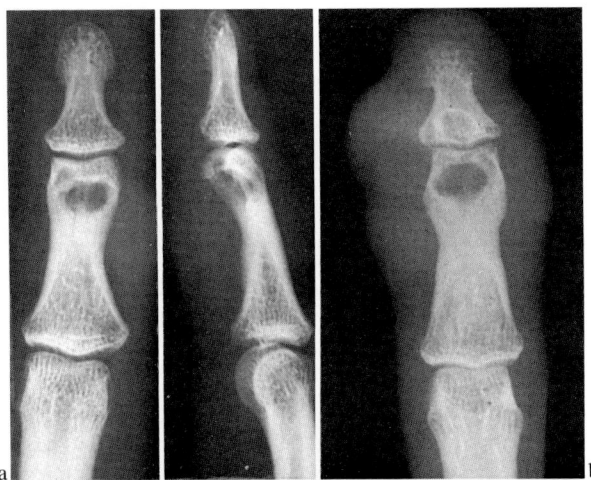

Fig. 1.4. *Pigmented villonodular synovitis—less common manifestations.* **a** The diagnosis of this solitary erosive lesion on the anterior side of the tibia was more difficult. It occurred in a 49-year-old man with a chronic and mildly painful swelling below the knee. A clue to the nature of the well-defined soft tissue mass was its relative increase in density caused by the haemosiderin component. **b** Localised pain and swelling on the lateral side of the foot of this 34-year-old man was associated with classical radiological features of this disorder. The swelling was outlined clearly and was dense. Precisely delineated erosions were present on both sides of the 5th tarso-metatarsal joint and on the bases of the 3rd and 4th metatarsals.

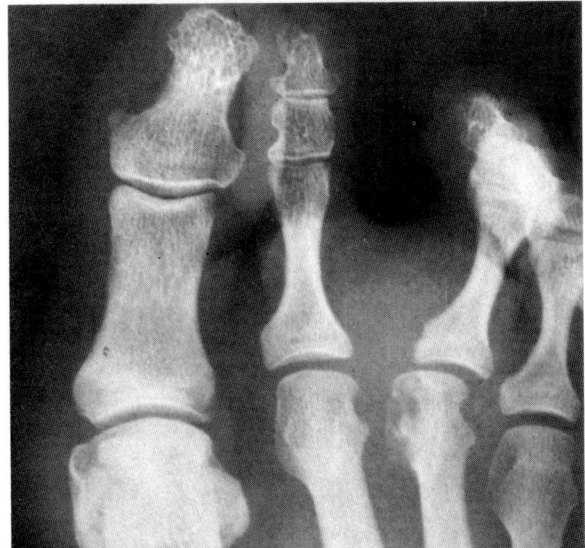

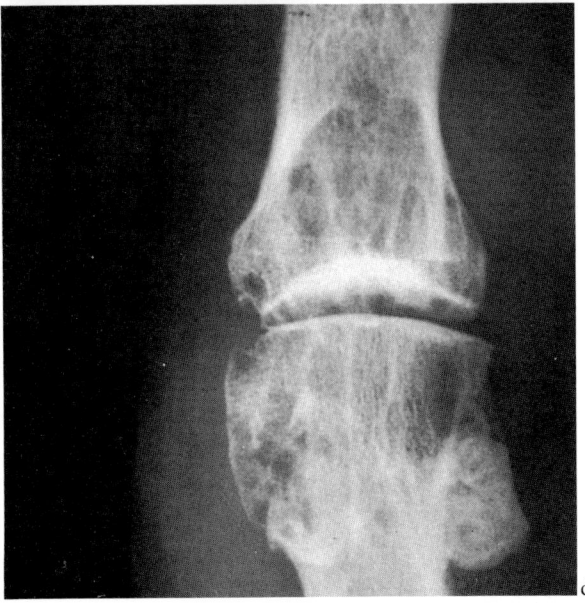

Fig. 1.5. *Pigmented villonodular synovitis—digital lesions.* Involvement of small joints of the hands and feet is not uncommon. Usually they cause persistent and mildly painful swellings and exhibit characteristic radiological appearances. **a** This erosion on the palmar aspect of the neck of the proximal phalanx of the left index finger corresponded to the synovial attachment of the joint capsule. The soft tissue was typically dense in this 23-year-old man. **b** A similar lesion, with erosions on both sides of this interphalangeal joint, was observed in a 22-year-old man and was associated with a lobular soft tissue mass. This swelling had continued to enlarge despite two previous attempts at total synovectomy, an indication of the frequency of recurrence after this therapeutic procedure. **c** In this instance the disease had caused a painful swelling between the 2nd and 3rd toes for 5 years. The patient was a 43-year-old woman, so that rheumatoid arthritis was suspected. Despite a para-articular erosion on the head of the 3rd metatarsal the joint space and the articular surfaces appeared normal, but the swelling had caused lateral subluxation of the 3rd proximal phalanx. **d** Typically well-defined erosions around an intact 1st metatarso-phalangeal joint with rather dense soft tissue swelling represent pathognomonic features of the entity. They were found in a young woman before the disease had been recognised. In the belief that the lesion was malignant, amputation was performed, with long-term survival of the patient. This iatrogenic tragedy has been repeated in more recent years.

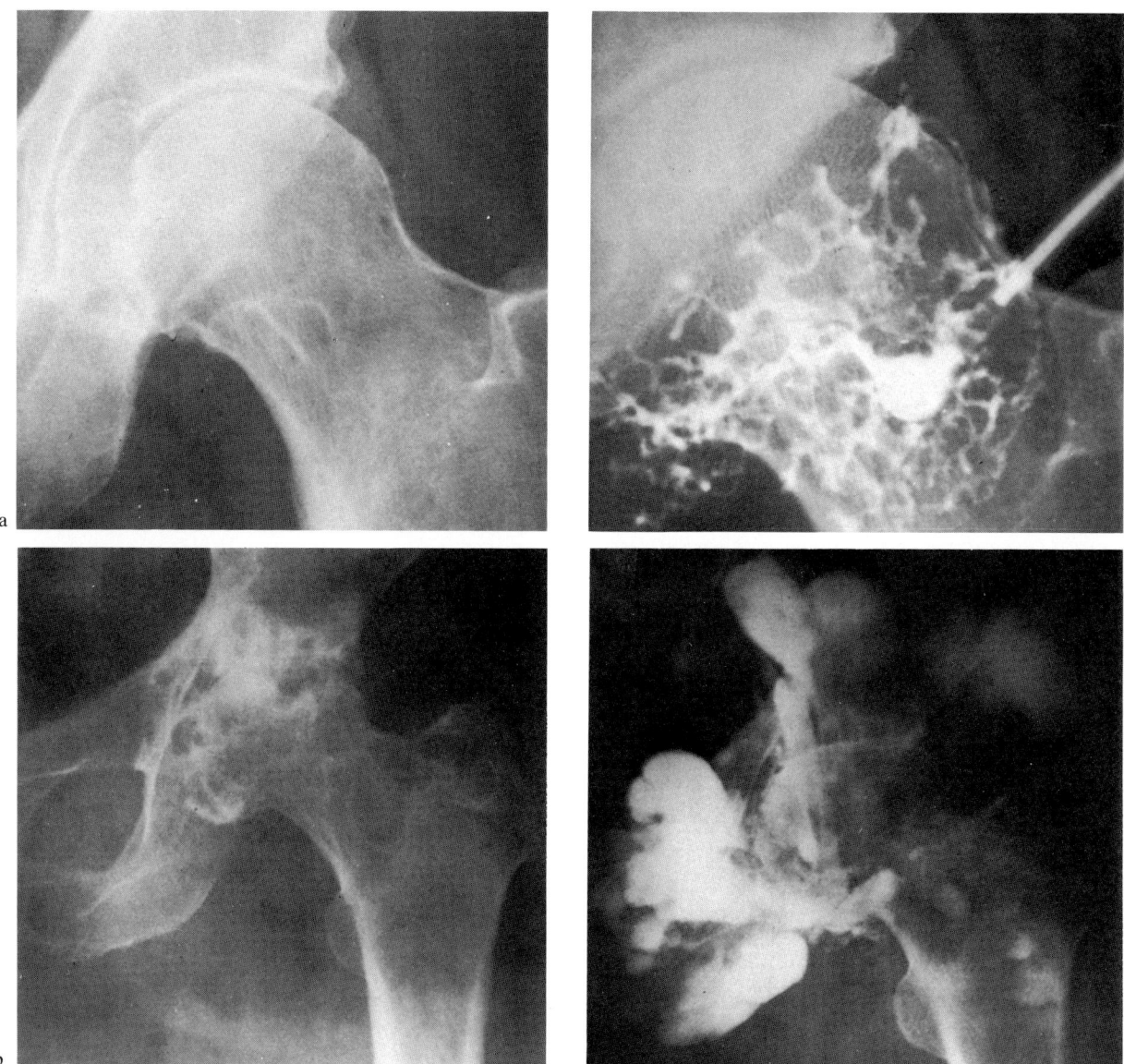

Fig. 1.6. *Pigmented villonodular synovitis—arthrographic appearances.* **a** This 44-year-old man had complained of mild discomfort in the left hip for 2 years, with a history of minor episodes of the same type throughout adult life. Physical examination revealed no abnormality, but minor erosions of the neck of the femur and an intact hip joint suggested the diagnosis. The arthrogram revealed the classical nodular pattern of the disease. Synovectomy was offered, but deferred at the request of the patient. **b** More advanced evidence of the disease was present in this 48-year-old woman who had complained of increasing pain in the left hip for 5 years. Not only were massive, but again clearly defined, para-articular erosions present on the femoral neck, greater trochanter and acetabulum, but they extended to the ischiopubic junction. The disease was sufficiently advanced to have caused narrowing of the joint space, but still no gross demineralisation had developed. A large and dense soft tissue mass was present. The arthrogram filled a greatly enlarged joint cavity, with classical diverticula extending to the sites of bony erosion.

A2. Malignant synovioma (synovial sarcoma) of elbow

The clinical and radiological findings suggested strongly a tumour of peri-articular soft tissues. Erosion of the bones on both sides of the joint indicated involvement of the capsule and synovium. Such a pattern may be observed with inflammatory lesions of synovium, such as tuberculosis (see Exercise 11), rheumatoid arthritis (see Exercise 18), and also in pigmented villonodular synovitis, as in Q1 of this Exercise. Malignancy was indicated by the wide zone of transition in the ulnar lesion.

The histological appearance of the two selected fields (Q2b and c) is remarkably different. In Q2b undifferentiated spindle-cell tissue is present, which, by its cellularity alone, suggests a malignant tumour. In contrast, Q2c shows elongated tubular structures. In a different context these appearances might indicate an epithelial neoplasm. This biphasic pattern of the tissue is, in fact, characteristic of malignant synovioma (synovial sarcoma) and distinguishes it from other types of soft tissue tumours, such as fibrosarcoma. Synovial sarcoma originates in soft tissues and the extensive osseous involvement, as in the present case, is to be regarded as a secondary feature. In this unfortunate patient routine examination of the chest revealed multiple 'cannon-ball' metastases. Survival was less than 2 years.

Malignant Synovioma

Malignant synovioma is a rare, highly malignant tumour, arising usually in the neighbourhood of joint capsules, bursae or tendon sheaths. The peak incidence is in the third decade and 75% present before the age of 40. No significant predilection for either sex has been recognised.

Clinical Features

Classically a soft tissue mass develops over a period of 2–3 years, increasing slowly in size. Localised pain and tenderness often is mild and in a quarter of patients such symptoms are surprisingly absent. The diffuse, palpable swelling may be accompanied by localised erythema and cause restriction of movement of an adjacent joint.

Radiological Features

1. Site. The knee, hip, ankle, elbow and wrist are, in that order, the joints most commonly affected, but the small joints of the feet and hands may be involved.

2. Appearance. Initially the only abnormality may be a rounded or lobulated soft tissue mass. Suspicion as to its nature may be aroused by its presence in the neighbourhood of joints or other synovial structures.

Secondary and irregular erosions of capsular attachments, however, particularly if observed on both sides of an intact joint, provide more valuable diagnostic information, which may be supported by calcifications within the mass in later stages. Such calcification may be the only clue in lesions remote from joints and even then a wide differential diagnosis exists.

Pathological Features

The characteristic biphasic histological structure illustrated in the present case is considered to reflect a synovial pattern of differentiation, the alveolar appearance corresponding to synovial spaces. These tumours usually originate in juxta-articular soft tissues, rather than in synovial membrane itself. As indicated above, they occur occasionally at sites remote from pre-existing synovial structures.

Malignant synovioma is to be regarded as being quite distinct from pigmented villonodular synovitis, with which it must not be confused.

Treatment

All simple ganglia should be examined histologically after their removal, because, although malignant synoviomas usually are firm and fibrous, they may be soft and mucoid and so be mistaken macroscopically for a more benign lesion.

Simple excision is associated with a high rate of local recurrence, diminished only slightly by post-operative radiotherapy. Amputation does not appear to reduce the occurrence of metastases to regional lymph nodes and the lungs. 45% survive 5 years and 30% 10 years.

Cytotoxic drugs have probably decreased the incidence of metastases, but their value as yet is unproven.

References

Bennett GA (1947) Malignant lesions originating in synovial tissues (synoviomata) J Bone Jt Surg 29: 259–291

Cadman NL, Soule EH, Kelly PJ (1965) Synovial sarcoma: an analysis of 34 tumours. Cancer 18: 613–627

Cameron HU, Kostuik JP (1974) A long term follow up of synovial sarcoma. J Bone Jt Surg 56B: 613–617

Haagensen CD, Stout AP (1944) Synovial sarcoma. Ann Surg 20: 826–842

Tillotson JF, McDonald JR, Janes JM (1951) Synovial sarcoma. J Bone Jt Surg 33A: 459–473

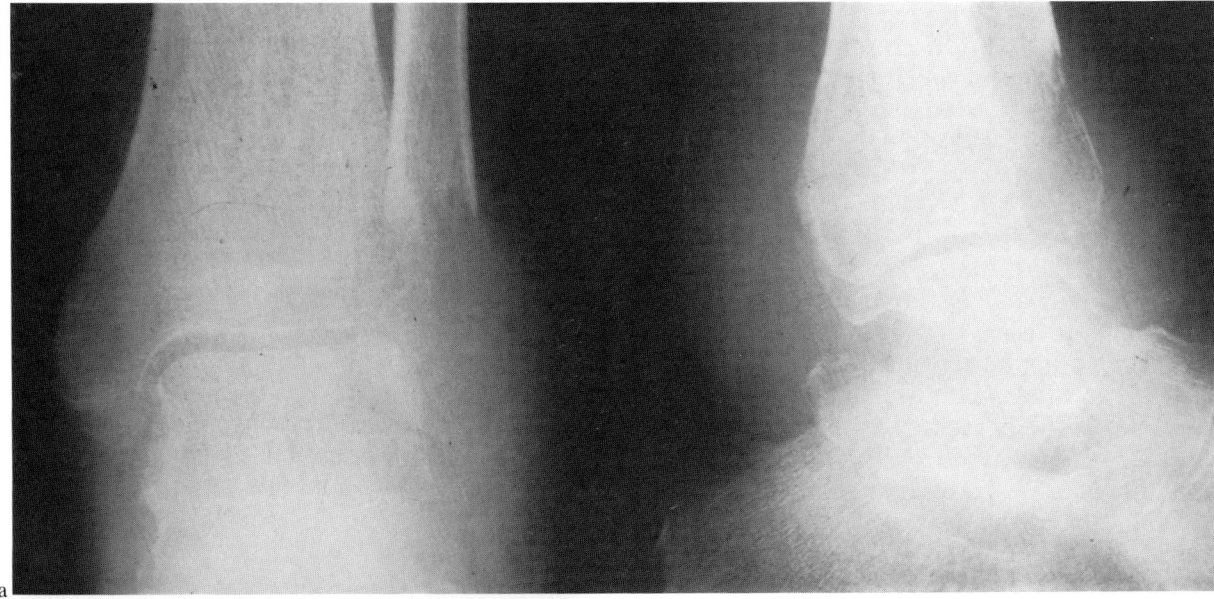

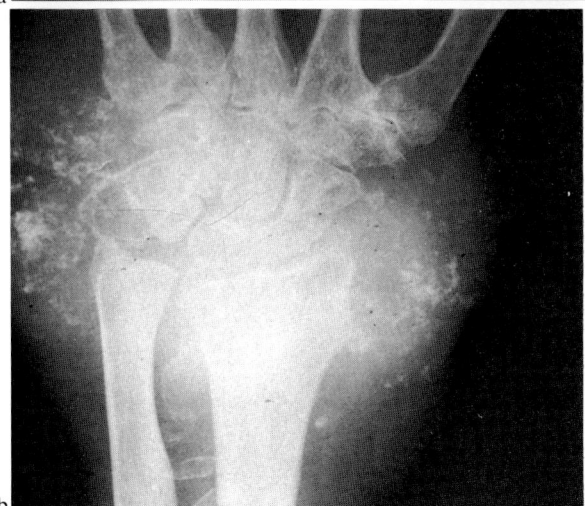

Fig. 2.1. *Malignant synovioma (synovial sarcoma) of major joints.* **a** *Ankle.* Massive soft tissue swelling around the joint in this young adult is accompanied by large and poorly defined erosions of the synovial attachments on the tibia, fibula and talus. Even on presentation a 'cannon-ball' pulmonary metastasis was present. **b** *Wrist.* Soft tissue swelling around this joint of several months' duration caused chronic pain in this elderly man. Extensive calcification is present within the mass and numerous para-articular erosions have poorly defined margins.

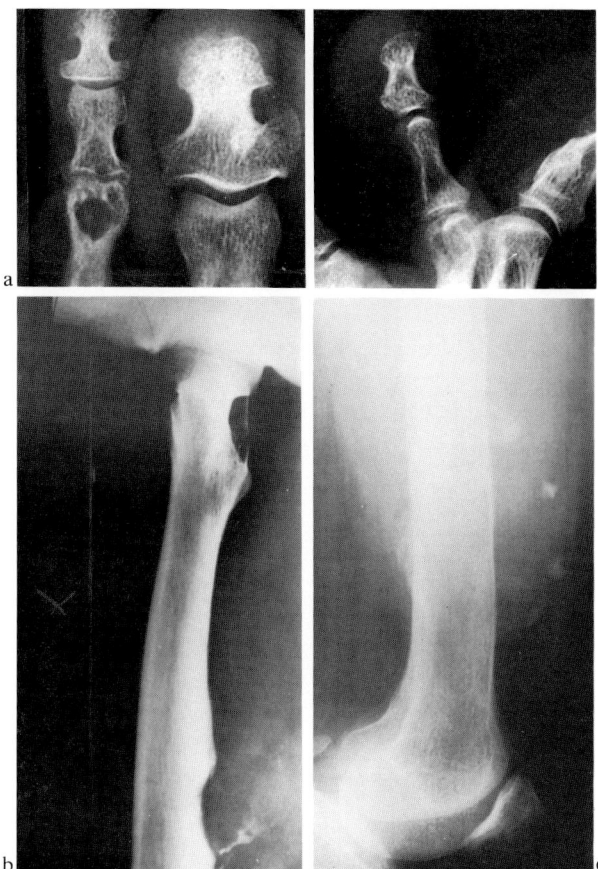

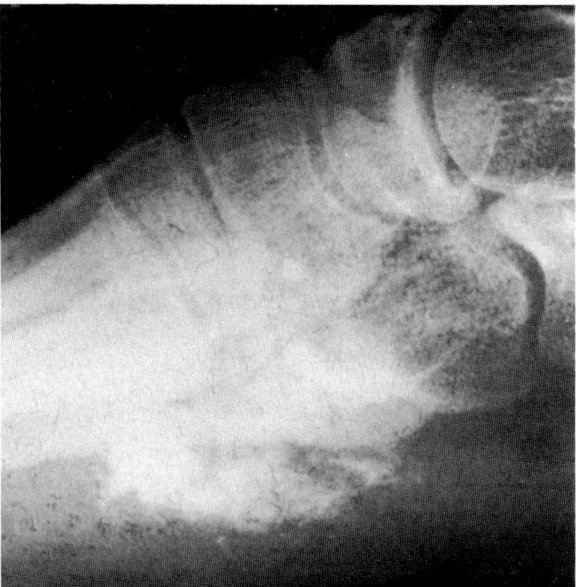

Fig. 2.3. *Malignant synovioma (synovial sarcoma)— tendon sheath.* This 19-year-old girl had complained of an intermittently painful swelling on the sole of the foot for 4 years. The irregular mass of calcification involved synovium of a tendon sheath. The synovium of bursae also may be affected.

Fig. 2.2. *Malignant synovioma (synovial sarcoma)—less common manifestations.* **a** Proximal interphalangeal joint of 2nd toe. This 49-year-old woman had a tender, painful swelling of several months' duration. In addition to the swelling, a large erosion is present on the plantar aspect of the neck of the proximal phalanx. **b** In this middle-aged female with a tender swelling in the thigh a large excavation was demonstrated on the femoral shaft. Some irregular calcification was present within the soft tissue mass. **c** Another example of an ectopic lesion causing a large soft tissue swelling containing punctate foci of calcification. A periosteal reaction is evident. In each of these cases the histological diagnosis was surprising.

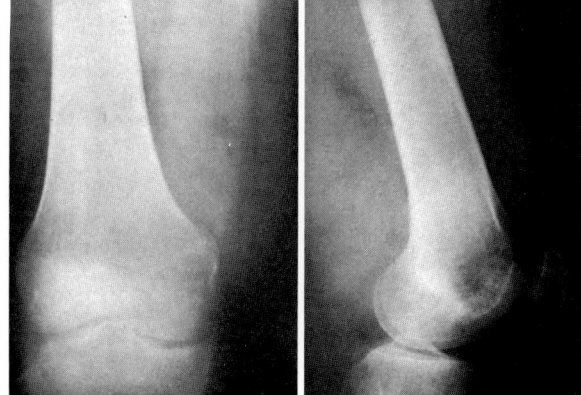

Fig. 2.4 *Malignant synovioma (synovial sarcoma) without bone involvement.* This 21-year-old man had complained of pain on the postero-medial side of the right thigh, just above the knee, for a year. During the previous 8 months a firm, slightly tender swelling had developed, with significant limitation of flexion. Differential diagnosis from other malignant soft tissue neoplasms, particularly fibrosarcoma, is impossible on radiological grounds. Radiologically the mass is well defined and dense but the bones appear normal. The lesion showed increased uptake on a radionuclide scan. Mid-thigh amputation was performed.

Q1. This 68-year-old woman complained of mild pain and swelling around the left shoulder, attributed to an injury incurred in a fall 6 months before.

Clinical examination demonstrated the presence of a large swelling approximately 10 cm in diameter, apparently related to the scapula, but tender only slightly on its lateral side. Movements of the shoulder were normal. No other significant clinical abnormality was detected.

The radiographs showed the swelling to be due to a large, expanding osteolytic lesion arising from the upper border of the scapula. The cortex had become thinned and partially destroyed. No sclerotic reaction was evident around the endosteal margin.

A biopsy was performed.

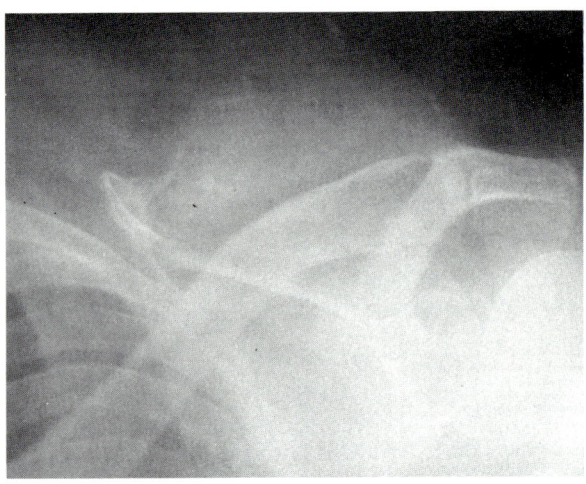

Q1a.

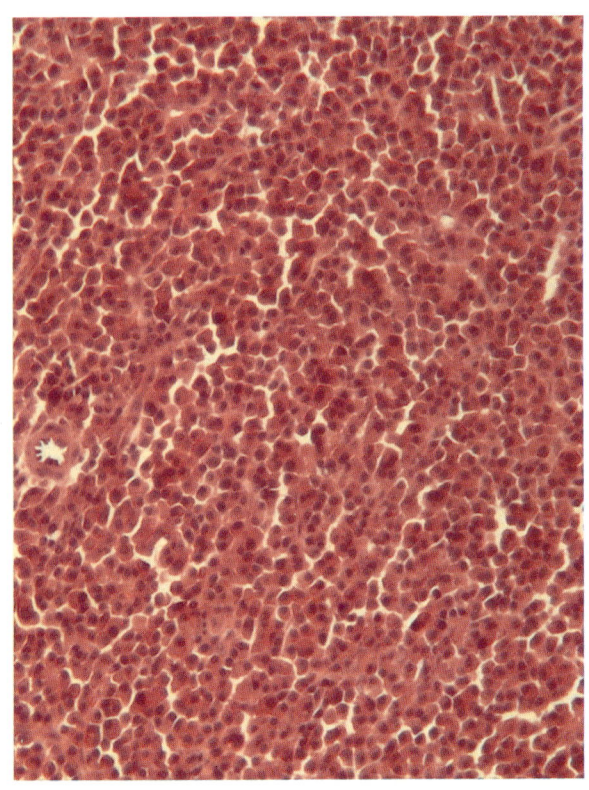

Q1b. (×210)

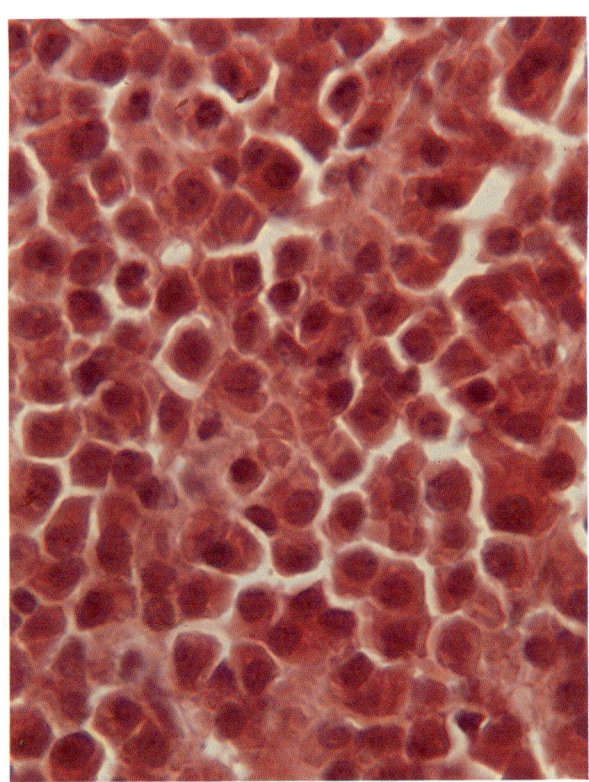

Q1c. (×775)

Q2. This patient, a man aged 60 years, presented with a history of pain in the back, of recent origin.

No clinical abnormality was found, except for localised tenderness over T8.

Radiological examination showed diffuse demineralisation of bone, collapse of the body of T7 and, to a lesser degree, of the body of T8.

Biopsy of an iliac crest was performed.

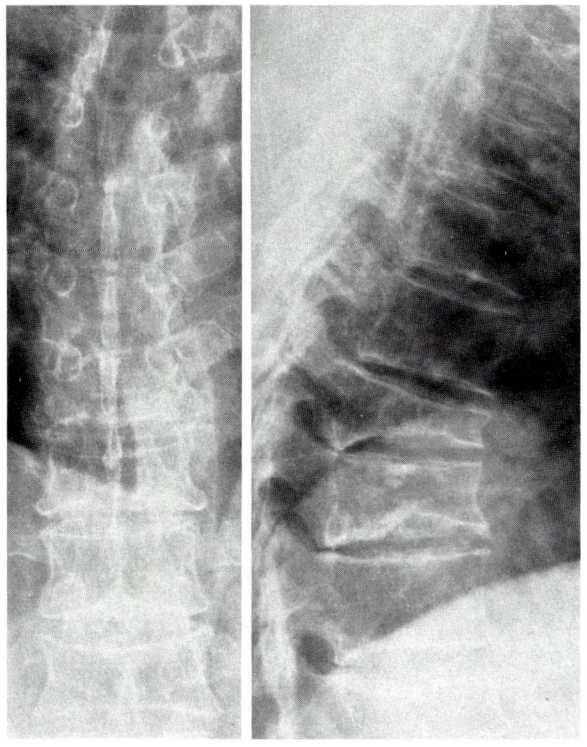

Q2a.

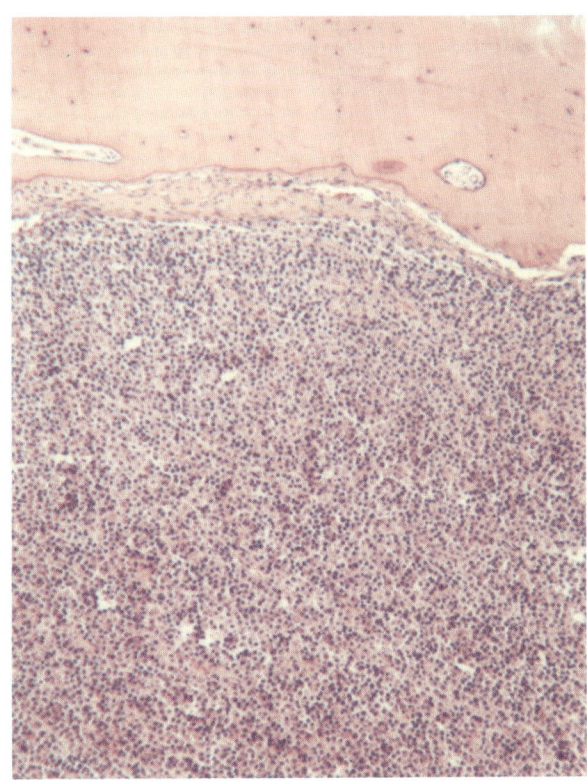

Q2b. (×41)

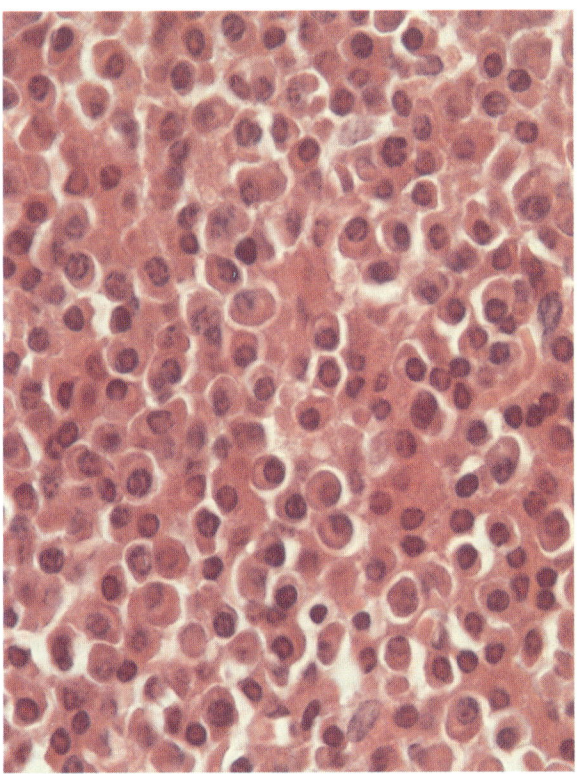

Q2c. (×610)

A1. Plasmacytoma (solitary myeloma)

The presence of such an expanding osteolytic lesion in a patient of this age suggested either a metastasis, probably from renal cancer or possibly from the thyroid (see Exercise 2), or a plasmacytoma. The latter was supported by the subsequent findings of serum electrophoresis, which showed a heavy band of γ-globulin. Skeletal survey revealed no other radiological abnormalities to suggest generalised myelomatosis.

At operation, the lesion proved to be highly vascular, but the biopsy specimen contained solid pinkish tissue in addition to blood clot and necrotic material. Histologically (Q1b and c) the tissue consisted almost entirely of 'myeloma' cells, confirming the clinical and radiological diagnosis. These neoplastic plasma cells can be recognised by their darkly staining nucleus and clear cytoplasmic outlines, and by the frequent presence of a pale juxtanuclear region. Some of the cells are binucleate and numerous mitoses could be identified in the sections. The cytology of the abnormal tissue in generalised myelomatosis is identical with that in solitary myeloma. In the present case, however, no abnormal cells were found on sternal marrow biopsy. This finding, together with the absence of radiological evidence of other lesions, was of value in excluding generalised myelomatosis.

The lesion responded excellently to a course of radiotherapy. No evidence of local recurrence or dissemination was detected 3 years later.

A2. Myelomatosis (multiple myeloma)

The radiological differential diagnosis included generalised osteoporosis (see Exercise 3) and myelomatosis, although metastatic disease could not be excluded. The presence of myelomatosis appeared to be confirmed when a skeletal survey revealed numerous areas of osteolysis in other parts of the skeleton, including the skull and the proximal ends of each femur and humerus.

The diagnosis of myelomatosis was established by the iliac crest biopsy and by the finding of an abnormal γ-globulin on serum electrophoresis. In the biopsy (Q2b and c) the normal marrow had been replaced completely by myeloma cells, the appearance resembling closely that observed in Q1.

Plasmacytoma (Solitary Myeloma) and Myelomatosis (Multiple Myeloma)

This is a malignant neoplasm of plasma cells, originating in haemopoietic bone marrow. Changes in bone tissue itself are frequently, but not invariably, present. The tumour cells frequently synthesise distinctive proteins which can be identified in the tumour tissue or in the blood or urine. Males are more commonly affected than females and it is unusual for the condition to be recognised in patients under the age of 40 years.

Clinical Features

The solitary lesion (plasmacytoma) may be found incidentally during a routine radiological examination, but its presence—as in Q1—may be indicated by mild pain and localised swelling or even by the development of a pathological fracture. Although initially the course may be benign, at least for months and in some cases prolonged for many years, ultimate dissemination to the multiple form (myelomatosis) is virtually inevitable.

In the generalised form of the disease, symptoms and signs usually become manifest and include weakness, loss of weight and unexplained anaemia. Owing to frequent involvement of the spine, back pain is a very common presenting symptom. The incidence of pathological fractures increases with severity of the disease. No indication of an antecedent solitary lesion may be found.

Certain biochemical abnormalities, particularly the reversal of the normal albumin/globulin ratio and the presence of a monoclonal γ-globulin on serum electrophoresis, are of value in diagnosis. Bence-Jones proteinuria occurs in about half the cases with disseminated disease. Hypercalcaemia is sometimes present and reflects active bone destruction, sometimes in association with impaired renal function. The serum alkaline phosphatase may be elevated, particularly when pathological fractures are healing. The diagnosis of myelomatosis is supported particularly strongly when sternal marrow puncture reveals an increased number of plasma cells.

Myelomatosis is often associated with anaemia, renal failure or amyloidosis, and with an increased susceptibility to infection.

Radiological Features

1. Site. Solitary lesions have their inception in areas of persistent haemopoiesis in adults—essentially the axial skeleton—so a plasmacytoma is encountered most commonly in the spine, ribs and pelvis.

With myelomatous dissemination the same areas are affected by myriads of lesions. While the femora and humeri occasionally may be involved, the bones distal to the knee and elbow tend to be spared.

2. Appearance. The individual foci are essentially osteolytic and expansile, thinning the cortex and being subject to pathological fractures, with a marked lack of reactive marginal sclerosis. Extensions into the adjacent soft tissues often are prominent. These features simulate very closely the pattern of an osteolytic metastasis, especially from renal or, less often, thyroid cancer.

In established myelomatosis the appearance may show considerable variation. It is possible for the disease to be present with no detectable radiological abnormality and, less rarely, generalised and severe osteoporosis may be the only positive finding (see Exercise 3). Much more usually, and generally at the first presentation, numerous discrete osteolytic lesions are widespread throughout the axial skeleton, including the calvarium, where they have been likened to 'raindrops'. Affected vertebral bodies may already have suffered some degree of collapse, representing sites of pathological fractures.

These fractures are very common, but exhibit considerable ability to repair spontaneously. Exceptionally sclerotic forms occur, characterised clinically by a peripheral neuropathy, and confused easily with osteoblastic metastases. In the absence of overt lesions, isotope scanning *may* indicate such skeletal deposits, but in general this technique is significantly less sensitive than orthodox radiography.

Pathological Features

The histological features of myeloma, whether solitary or generalised, are characteristic. The tumour cells are small and rounded; their cytoplasm is clearly outlined and their nuclei, often eccentric in position, usually show clumping of chromatin towards the periphery, as in normal plasma cells. Adjacent to the nucleus is a pale area of cytoplasm which contrasts with the prominent basophilia of the rest of the cell. Supporting stromal tissue is sparse. The cells are, on the whole, uniform in appearance, although a minority may be large and irregular, or have more than one nucleus. The distinctive cytological features of the cells, while usually evident in sections, are more clearly apparent in imprint preparations (Fig. 1.1a).

It is unusual to observe any reactive bone formation in or around myelomatous lesions.

Extraskeletal lesions are sometimes encountered, and take the form of accumulations of myeloma cells in the spleen, liver or lymph nodes. Extensive marrow involvement is usually accompanied by severe anaemia.

Myeloma is often associated with abnormalities of plasma proteins. The abnormal proteins are homogeneous (monoclonal) γ-globulins, with or without polypeptide sub-units, and are synthesised by the myeloma cells. The complete proteins are immunoglobulins (IgG, IgA and IgD): the polypeptide sub-units are referred to as light chain or heavy chain fragments. The accumulation of the abnormal proteins in the blood is indicated by an increase in the total globulin content, by reversal of the normal albumin/globulin ratio, and by the presence of a monoclonal band on serum electrophoresis. The appearance of an abnormal γ-globulin is often the first indication of the dissemination of an initially solitary plasmacytoma or myeloma. The light chain fragments, which have a relatively low molecular weight, are excreted in the urine where they are recognised as 'Bence-Jones protein'. Their presence can lead to the obstruction of renal tubules by protein casts (Fig. 1.1b) and renal failure can ensue.

Amyloidosis is a recognised complication of myelomatosis, and is present in about 10% of cases studied at autopsy. In addition it may develop in the later stages of chronic inflammatory processes, such as tuberculosis and rheumatoid arthritis. The amyloid, a protein-polysaccharide complex, is chemically related to the light chain fragments. It accumulates in a variety of tissues, including the liver, spleen, kidney, muscle and skin. Involvement of bone may occur, but is unusual. In the kidney (Fig. 1.1c) it characteristically appears as a diffuse extracellular pink-staining material in the walls of the glomerular capillaries and other small blood vessels. It can be more specifically identified by its staining reactions with Congo Red and Thioflavine S, and by its characteristic fibrillary structure on electron microscopy.

The histological diagnosis of myelomatosis is made by the examination of sternal or iliac marrow, or, less frequently, by the biopsy of a recognised bone lesion. Identification of an abnormal plasma protein by electrophoresis can be important when bone lesions are inconspicuous or when they are confused with some other condition, often metastatic carcinoma.

Treatment

Solitary lesions usually respond dramatically to radiotherapy. Multiple lesions are treated more satisfactorily with cytotoxic drugs, particularly melphalan (L-phenylalanine mustard) and cyclophosphamide. These agents produce objective and subjective remissions in approximately 80% of cases, sometimes for many years. Isolated lesions of the spine with associated paraparesis respond well to decompression through an antero-lateral or anterior approach. When stabilised by grafting, the fate of the graft appears to be unaffected by subsequent radiotherapy.

When the disease is widespread, an otherwise bedridden patient can be kept ambulant by the judicious use of internal fixation and joint replacement, even when the ultimate prognosis is poor.

References

Brown TS, Peterson CR (1973) Osteosclerosis in myeloma. J Bone Jt Surg 55B: 621–623
Christopherson WM, Miller AJ (1950) Re-evaluation of solitary plasma-cell myeloma of bone. Cancer 3: 240–252
Glenner GG, Terry WD, Isersky C (1973) Amyloidosis: its nature and pathogenesis. Semin Hematol 10: 65–86
Ludwig H, Kumpan W, Sinziger H (1982) Radiography and bone scintigraphy in multiple myeloma: a comparative analysis. Br J Radiol 55: 173–181
Snapper I, Kahn A (1971) Myelomatosis. Fundamentals and clinical features. University Park Press, Baltimore
Wright CJE (1961) Long survival in solitary plasmacytoma of bone. J Bone Jt Surg 43B: 767–771

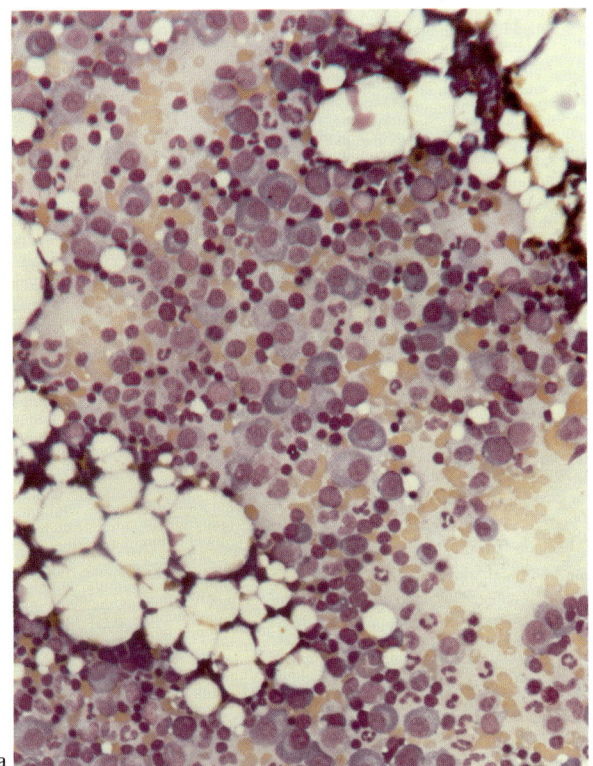
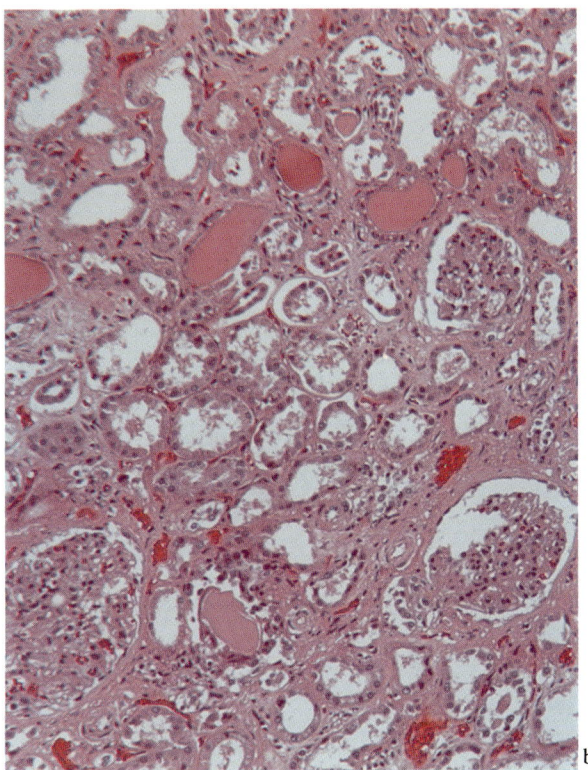
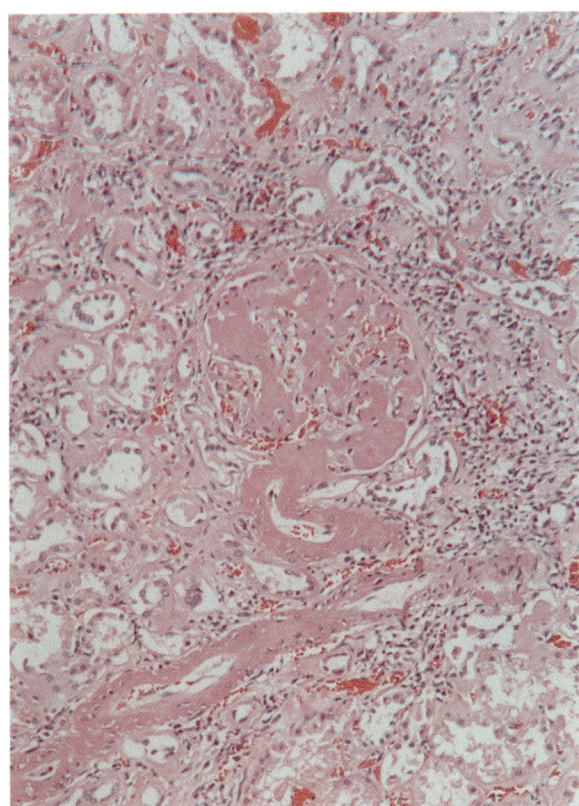

Fig. 1.1a. Giemsa-stained imprint preparation from iliac crest biopsy in Q1, showing the distinctive morphology of plasma cells with their pale juxtanuclear area. (×300). **b** Section of kidney in a case of myelomatosis, with eosinophilic casts in renal tubules ('myeloma kidney'). (×120). **c** Section of kidney in another case of myelomatosis. Pink-staining amyloid material is deposited in the walls of the capillaries of a glomerulus and its afferent arteriole. (×102)

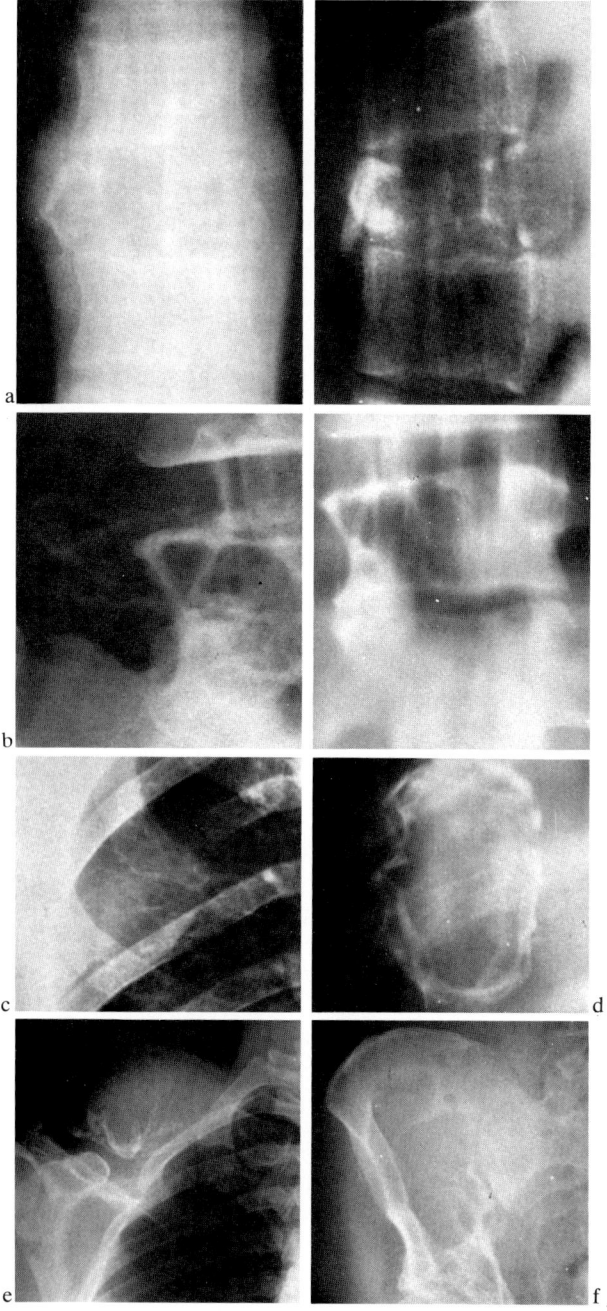

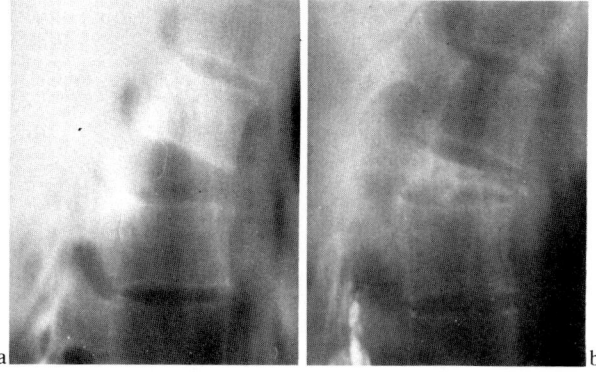

Fig. 1.3. *Plasmacytoma—severe vertebral lesions.* **a** *Body of T5* showing total destruction in a 45-year-old man. He had attributed backache for 18 months to stress while driving a bus. Apart from a localised kyphos all investigations were normal. As the patient was an immigrant to Britain from the Middle East, tuberculosis was suspected. The diagnosis was established by needle biopsy and an excellent response to radiotherapy was obtained. **b** *Body of T6.* A similar 44-year-old male immigrant developed sudden pain while lifting, with weakness of the legs. A partial block at this level was shown by myelography. Operation was refused and complete paraplegia ensued within 5 months.

Fig. 1.2. *Plasmacytoma—typical lesions in axial skeleton*, all in middle-aged patients and essentially osteolytic and expansile. **a** *Body of T8* in a 39-year-old man with increasing back pain accentuated by vertebral collapse. **b** *Body and neural arch of L5* in a 47-year-old woman also with localised pain. This patient died 3 years later of myelomatosis. **c** *Right 6th rib* in a 45-year-old man with mild pain in the chest. Radiotherapy induced excellent repair and the patient was alive and well 14 years later. **d** *Sternum* in another middle-aged patient. **e** *Clavicle* with gross expansion in a middle-aged Chinaman. Rather unusually, Bence-Jones proteinuria was present. **f** *Ilium.* This lesion was discovered incidentally and was regarded initially as fibrous dysplasia.

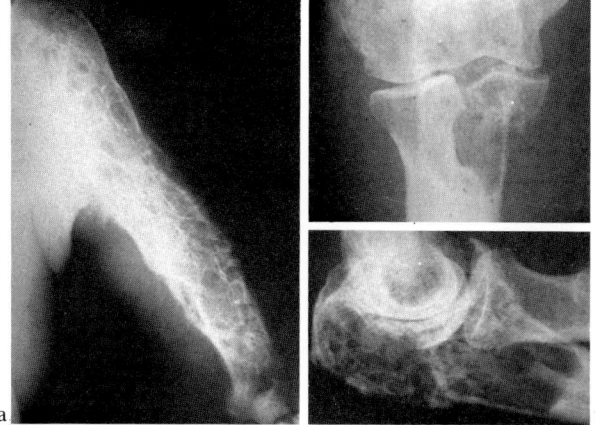

Fig. 1.4. *Plasmacytoma—unusual lesions in appendicular skeleton.* **a** *Humerus* in an elderly woman with chronic pain in the arm. This destructive lesion has a multilocular and partially sclerotic appearance. **b** *Olecranon process*, with a pathological fracture, in a 75-year-old woman with acute pain. Since she had previously an established carcinoma of an ethmoid sinus, this lesion was regarded at first as a metastasis—a common source of diagnostic confusion.

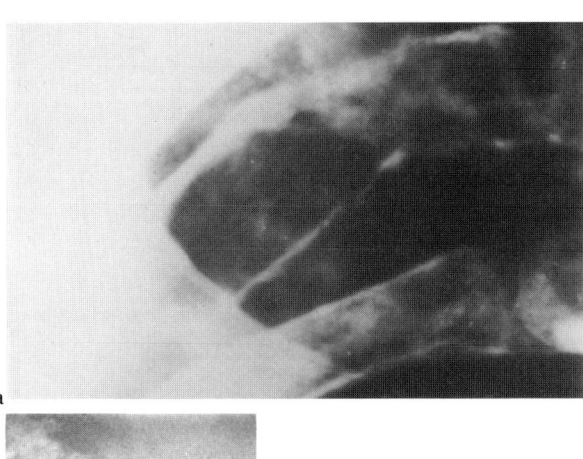

Fig. 2.1. *Plasmacytoma of rib, progressing to myelomatosis.* **a** This lytic, expanding lesion in the right 5th rib was discovered in a routine examination of the chest in a 38-year-old man. At this relatively early age the primary diagnosis was fibrous dysplasia, but biopsy disclosed its true nature (cf. Fig. 1.2c in this Exercise and Fig. 1.2c in Exercise 1.) Within 2 years widespread myelomatous dissemination had developed with classical clinical and radiological manifestations. **b** Lytic vertebral lesions with collapse. **c** Typical 'raindrop' areas of bone destruction in the calvarium. **d** Similar lesions in long bones and **e** pelvis.

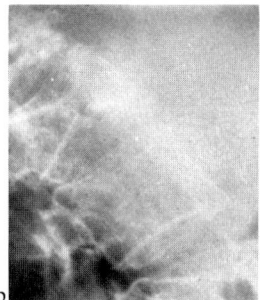

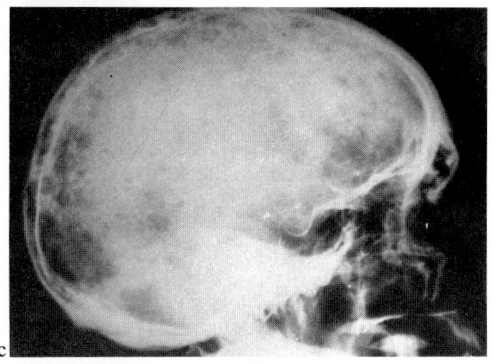

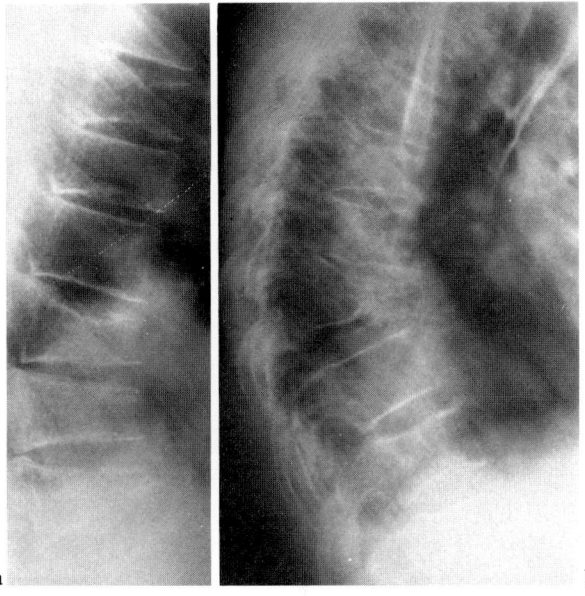

Fig. 2.2. *Myelomatosis—spine.* **a** Diffuse demineralisation with vertebral collapse is evident in this 59-year-old man with persistent backache. Areas of myelomatous replacement of marrow may be so small that the appearance simulates osteoporosis. **b** More advanced disease in an elderly woman. Numerous lytic areas are present with vertebral collapse and almost complete destruction of the body of T10. The main differential diagnosis in such a case is metastatic disease.

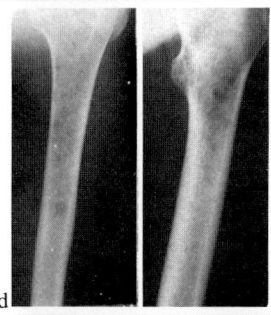

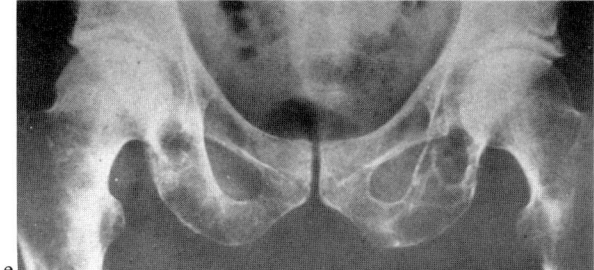

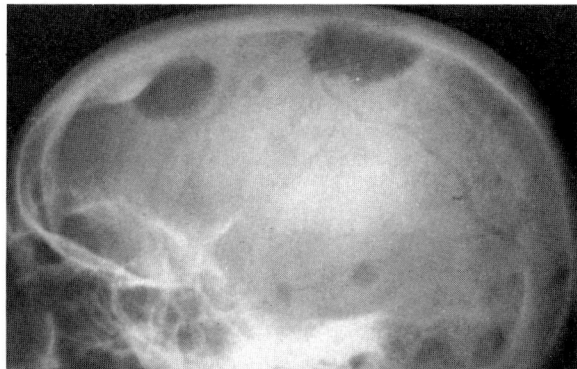

Fig. 2.3 *Myelomatosis—calvarium.* Numerous lytic lesions are present without sclerotic reaction. These are unusually large with prominent feeding vessels.

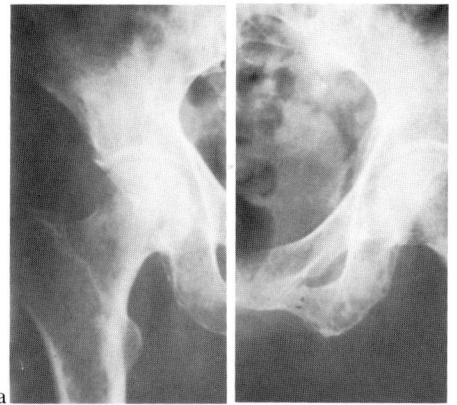
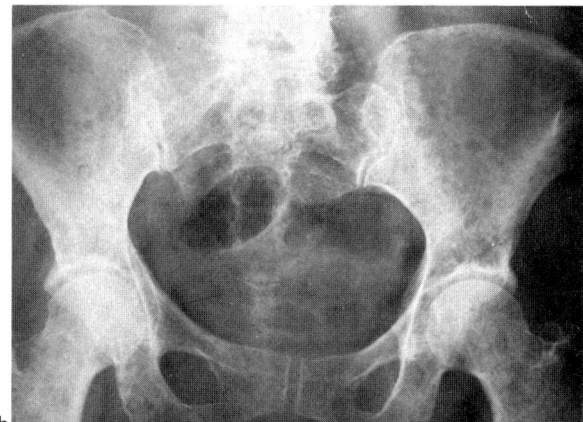
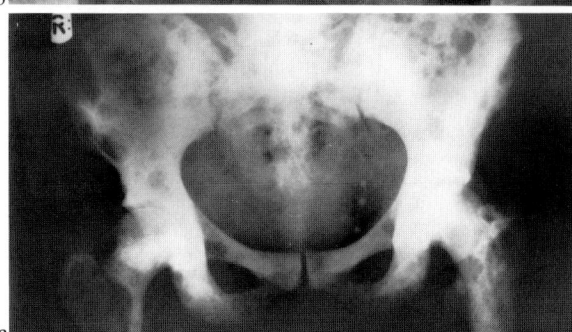

Fig. 2.4. *Myelomatosis—pelvis.* **a** This 84-year-old woman was examined to exclude a fracture. She had no symptoms of the disease, but the diagnosis was suggested by the round and oval lucencies in the proximal ends of the femora and in the pelvis with some endosteal, cortical erosions. Pathological confirmation was obtained. This case illustrates the not unknown possibility of the disease being recognised by chance. **b** A more classical example of widespread lytic lesions in a middle-aged woman. **c** These areas of destruction in the pelvis and femora were found in a 65-year-old woman investigated for respiratory symptoms. The chest film had shown patchy areas of bone density in the thorax. Most unusually these lesions are accompanied by dense sclerosis—a particularly rare type of myelomatosis which usually is associated with a peripheral neuropathy. Even more exceptionally a plasmacytoma may be sclerotic.

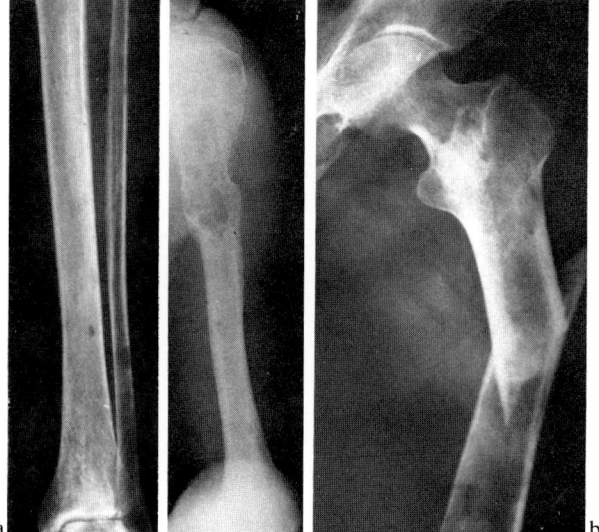

Fig. 2.5. *Myelomatosis—long bones.* **a** Typical lesions in the tibia and fibula in a patient with disseminated disease. **b** These small lytic areas in the humerus represented spread from the plasmacytoma in the proximal end of the bone in a 57-year-old man who had complained, for only 2 weeks of pain associated with a pathological fracture. **c** An oblique pathological fracture of the femur in an old woman of 85 with widespread disease.

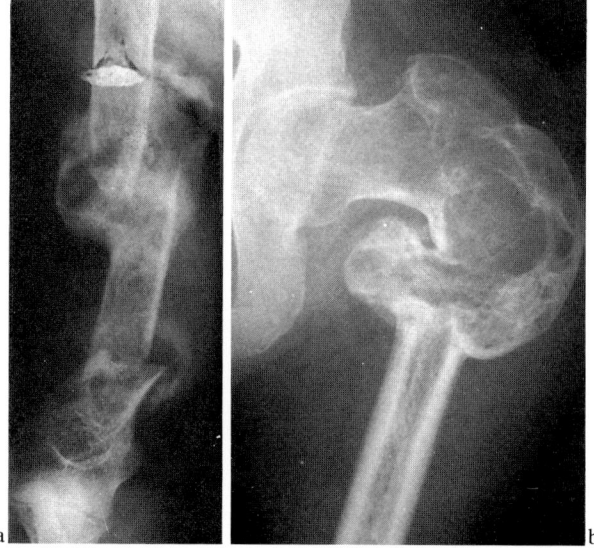

Fig. 2.6. *Myelomatosis—pathological fractures* often repair spontaneously with massive callus formation or may respond to radiotherapy. **a** Healing fractures of humerus (same patient as Fig. 2.5c). **b** This pathological fracture of the femur repaired well, but with deformity, after a course of radiotherapy. Pain was relieved. Nevertheless, lucencies in the medullary cavity were part of diffuse disease in this patient.

Exercise 38

Q1. This 12-year-old boy was brought to hospital because of a painful swelling above and behind the left knee. The swelling had been observed first 4 months previously.

Clinical examination showed a bony, hard swelling attached to the posterior surface of the lower part of the femur, but movement of the knee was full and painless.

The lateral radiograph showed a bony mass arising from the posterior cortex of the femur.

A biopsy was carried out.

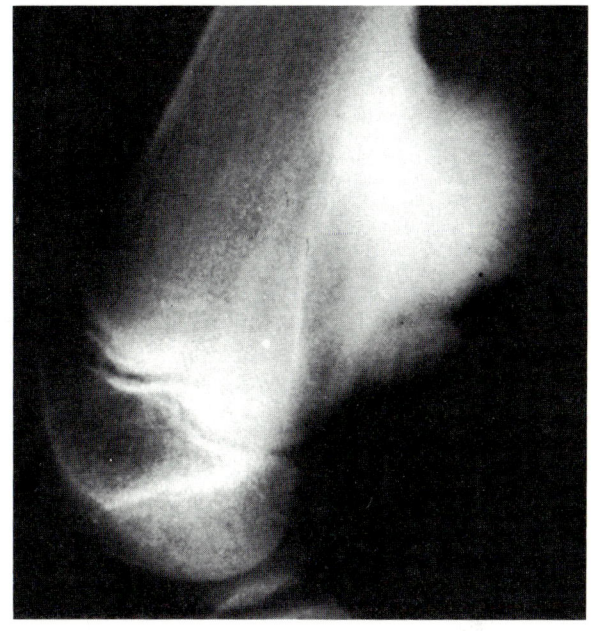

Q1a.

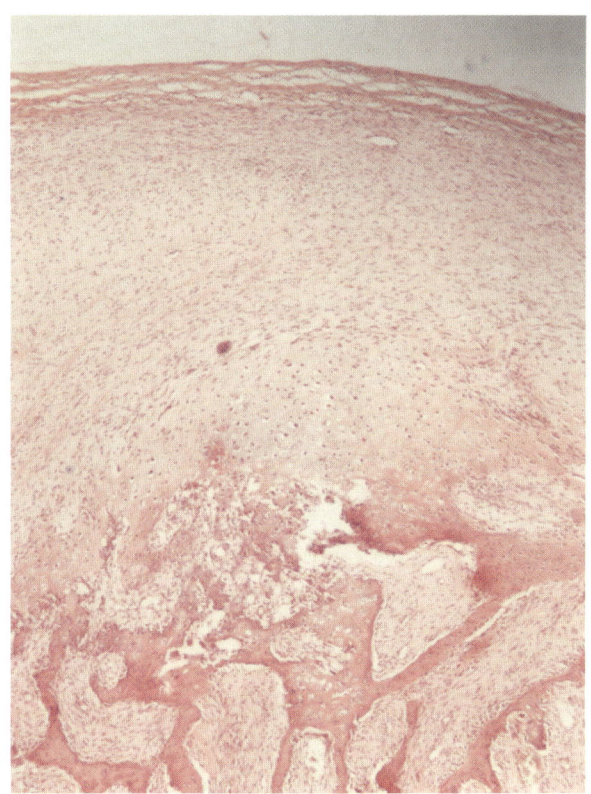

Q1b. (×40)

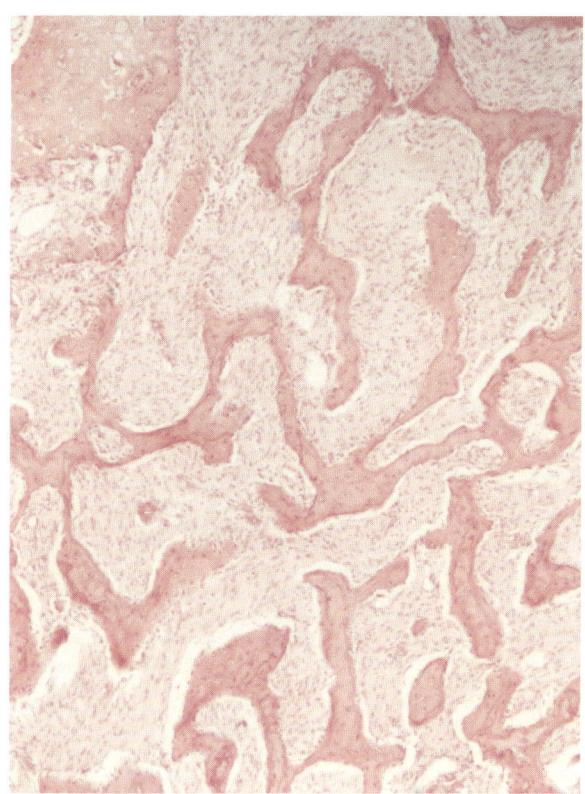

Q1c. (×55)

This exercise is continued on the following two pages ▶

Q2. A painful swelling on the medial side of the left thigh caused this young man, aged 18, to seek medical advice. The swelling had been present for 3 months and he believed it had enlarged, although it had become less painful. The patient was a keen player of field hockey, but could recall no injury to the affected area.

Apart from slight tenderness on pressure over the affected area, no abnormality was found on physical examination.

The radiograph showed a localised periosteal thickening with an irregular opacity in the adjacent soft tissues.

A block resection of the lesion was carried out.

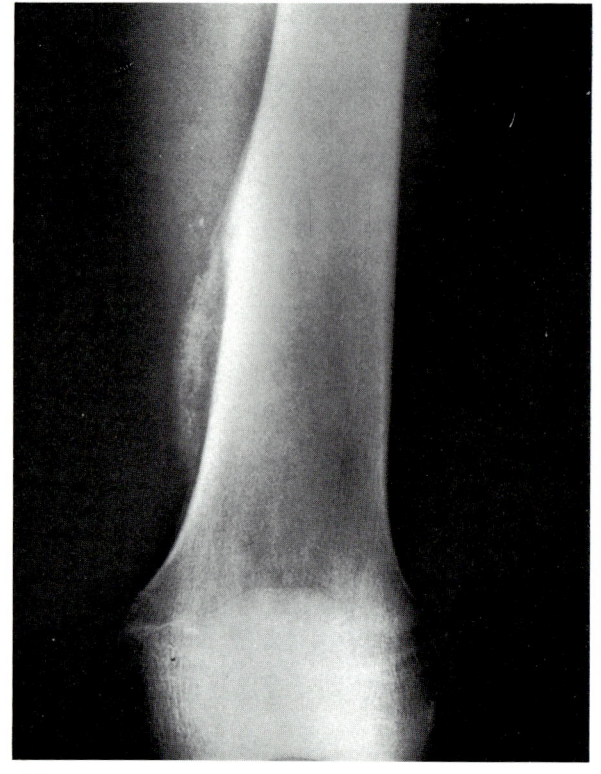

Q2a.

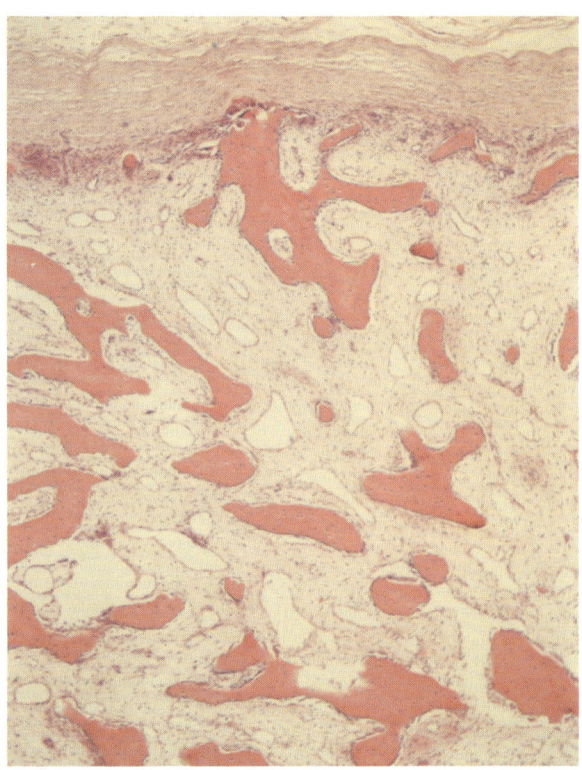

Q2b. (×35) Superficial portion

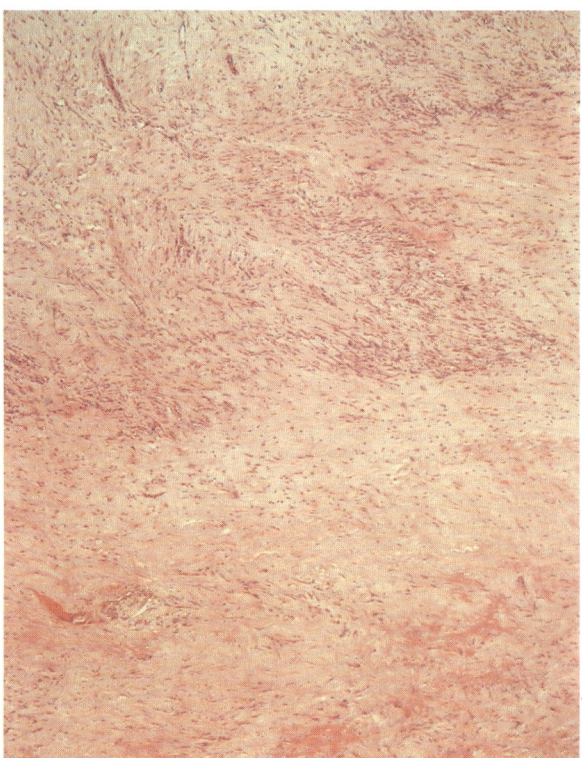

Q2c. (×35) Deep portion

Q3. This 15-year-old boy presented with a painful swelling on the antero-medial aspect of the tibia. He had noticed the swelling 2 months previously. No history of trauma was elicited.

Clinically, the swelling was barely palpable and was not significantly tender. No associated lymphadenopathy was detected. Routine laboratory investigations were normal.

Radiological examination showed segmental thickening of the soft tissue and cortex in the affected area, with the appearance of an organised periosteal reaction. In addition some increase of bone density was observed on the inner side of the cortex.

The lesion was explored.

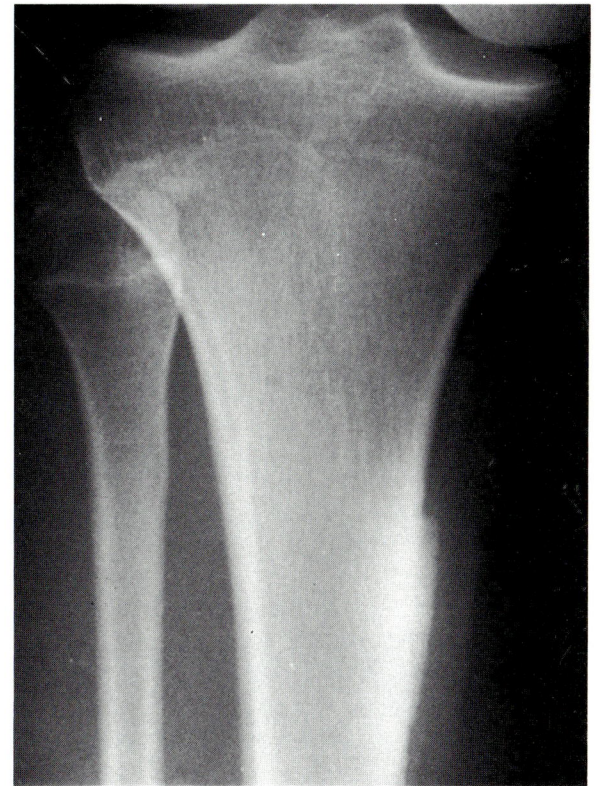

Q3a.

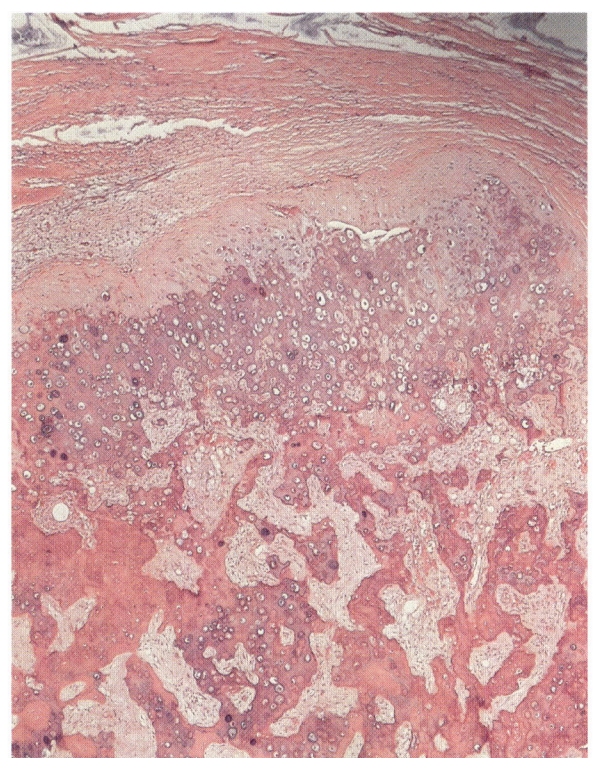

Q3b. (×35)

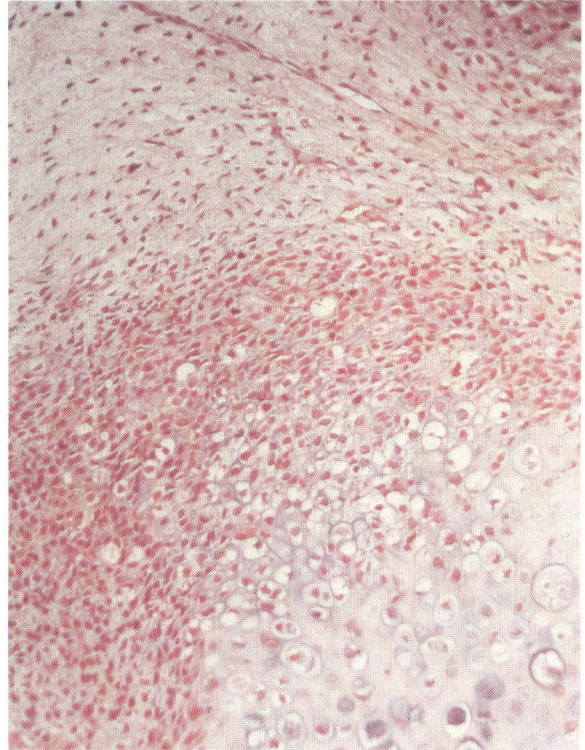

Q3c. (×140)

A1. Parosteal (juxtacortical) osteosarcoma

Although the clinical and radiological findings favoured this diagnosis, despite such an early age of the patient, hopeful consideration was given pre-operatively to the possibility of this lesion being a cartilage-capped exostosis.

The biopsy, however, established firmly the diagnosis of parosteal osteosarcoma. The tissue consists of relatively mature bone, cartilage and fibrous tissue (Q1b). On the basis of this diagnosis it was decided to treat the lesion by mid-thigh amputation. Figure 1.1a shows the gross appearance of the tumour, which appears to be restricted to the external surface of the bone. Sections from different parts of the lesion showed the same combination of mature bone and fibrous tissue illustrated in Q1c. At the base of the lesion, however, the spindle-celled tissue had invaded the cortex and was beginning to extend to the marrow spaces of the adjacent cancellous bone (Fig. 1.1b).

Ten years after amputation, the patient was alive and well with no evidence of recurrence or metastasis.

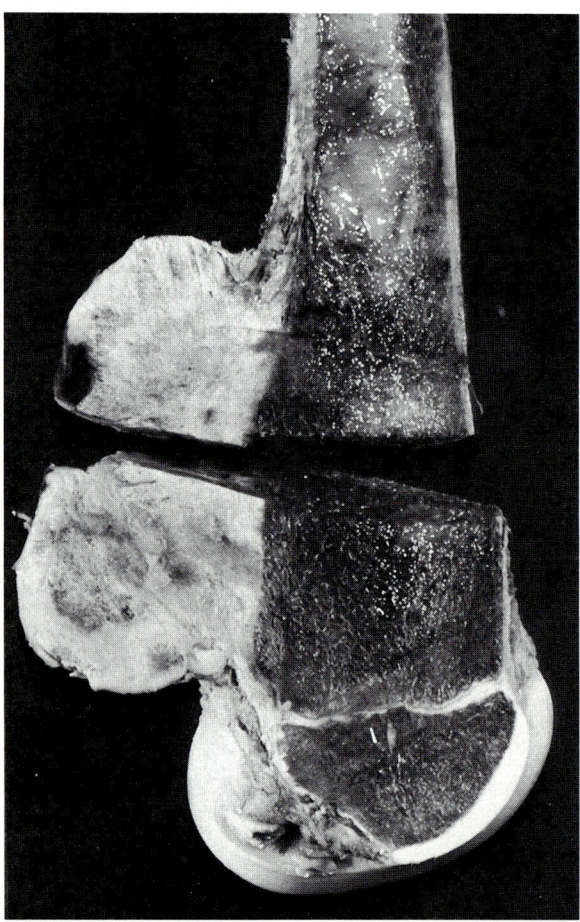

Fig. 1.1a. Appearance of tumour, restricted to the external surface of the bone, in the amputation specimen. The dark area towards the surface of the tumour indicates the site of the biopsy.

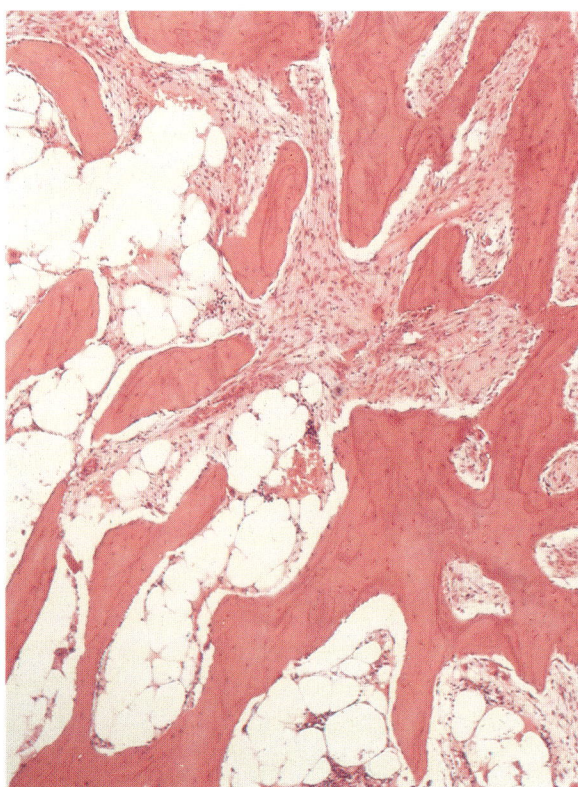

Fig. 1.1b. Extension of spindle-celled tumour tissue to the cancellous bone deep to the invaded cortex. (×110)

Parosteal Osteosarcoma

These lesions are slowly growing tumours of low-grade malignancy, which develop on the external surface of a bone. They should be distinguished from the classical 'central' osteosarcoma, because of their much better prognosis following surgical removal. The ultimate diagnosis depends on the radiologist and, in particular, the pathologist. In contrast to ordinary osteosarcoma, most of these parosteal tumours occur in individuals in their third to fifth decades. The patient illustrated in Q1 was affected at an unusually early age. Some published series show a slight female preponderance.

Clinical Features

These tumours are more indolent in their manifestations than the ordinary osteosarcoma and they are less likely to evoke pain. The patient usually is aware first of a hard swelling at the affected site. Pain, however, may be caused by impingement of the lesion on an adjacent peripheral nerve.

Radiological Features

1. Site. These cortical lesions are located, almost invariably, on a long bone, with a particular predilection for the distal end of the femur and the proximal ends of the tibia and humerus. Axial skeletal involvement is rare.

2. Appearance. A dense, bony mass grows outward from the cortex and may appear to be separated partially from the parent bone by a narrow zone of lucency. The peripheral border is usually smooth and undulating, but as growth proceeds it may become less regular and satellite areas of ossification may develop in adjacent soft tissues. The medulla initially escapes invasion, often for many years, in contrast to the periosteal sarcoma, which otherwise presents a similar radiological pattern. Diagnostic difficulty may arise in differentiation from a *sessile osteochondroma* (see Exercise 4), *hypertrophic callus* from a stress fracture (see Exercise 28) and post-traumatic ossification in soft tissues (see Q2 of this Exercise).

Pathological Features

Demonstration of the anatomical location of the tumour is critical in making a diagnosis of parosteal osteosarcoma and is more likely to be achieved by radiological examination than by the appearances in a limited biopsy. Most of these tumours, like the present example (Q1), consist of relatively mature tissue. Because of this, histological differentiation from some type of benign lesion may be difficult. The tissue can be so mature and well differentiated (see Q1b and c) that some type of benign lesion is considered. Indeed, these tumours were, for a long while, known as parosteal osteomas, until their malignant potential was realised. They differ from osteochondromas by the absence of a recognisable cap of cartilage, with regular endochondral ossification. The histological pattern of soft tissue myositis ossificans is rather different, these lesions showing a shell of condensed mature bony tissue which is lacking in a parosteal osteosarcoma.

Some osteosarcomas, undoubtedly parosteal in anatomical situation and origin, show the poorly differentiated sarcomatous tissue characteristic of the usual central osteosarcoma. These tumours have a worse prognosis than the typical well-differentiated parosteal tumours.

The cases reported by Unni et al. as *periosteal osteosarcoma* (see Q3 of this Exercise) have rather similar radiological features and even pathological distinction between the two lesions can be difficult.

Treatment

Excision of the lesion is imperative, since then survival for 5 years or longer may be expected in 75% as against 25% for the ordinary osteosarcoma. The surgical procedure undertaken may be influenced by the degree of malignancy as assessed by the pathologist. Some parosteal sarcomas have responded satisfactorily to local excision, but massive prosthetic replacement, when practicable, is favoured increasingly. Amputation, however, may be necessary. The role of cytotoxic therapy in these cases remains to be determined.

References

Ahuja SC, Villacin AG, Smith J, Bullough PG, Huvos AG, Marcove RC (1977) Juxtacortical (parosteal) osteogenic sarcoma: histological grading and prognosis. J Bone Jt Surg 59A: 632–647

Unni KK, Dahlin DC, Beabout JW, Ivins JC (1976) Parosteal osteogenic sarcoma. Cancer 37: 2466–2475

Van der Heul RO, Van Ronnen JR (1967) Juxtacortical osteosarcoma. Diagnosis, differential diagnosis, treatment and an analysis of eighty cases. J Bone Jt Surg 49A: 415–439

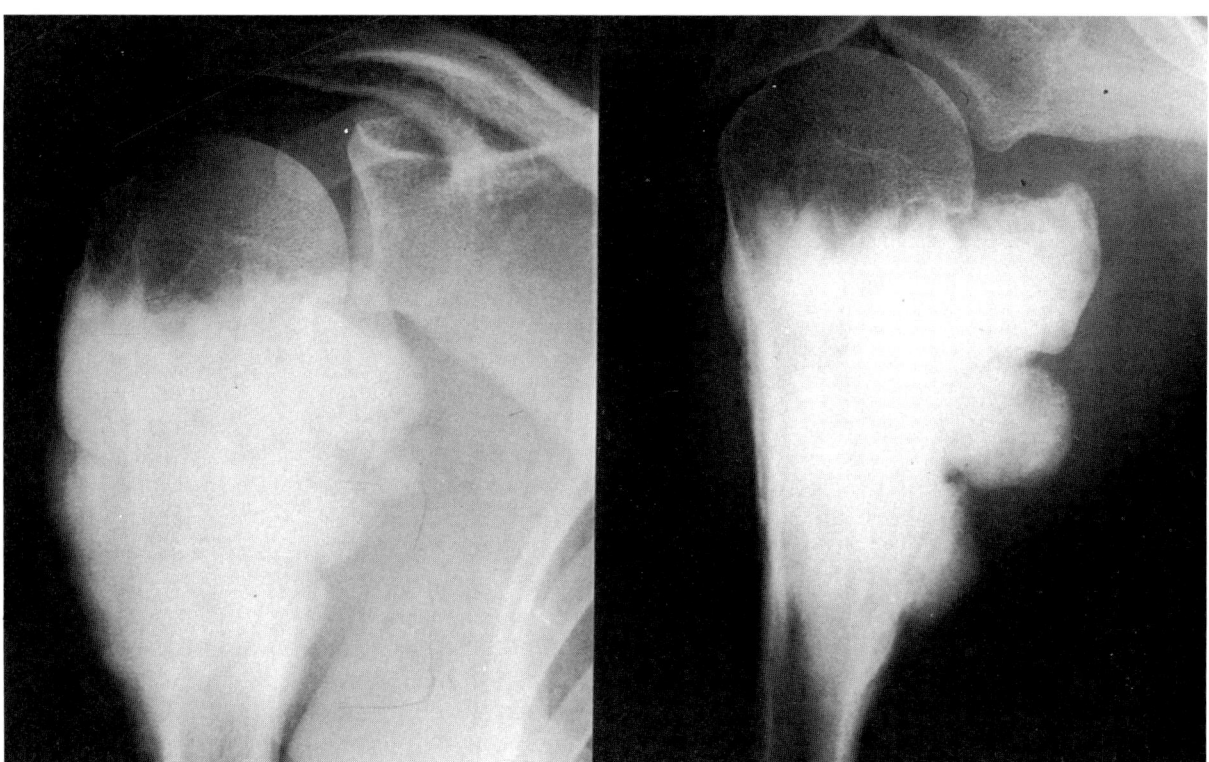

Fig. 1.2. *Parosteal sarcoma of neck of humerus.* This painless swelling originally was regarded as osteochondroma in an 18-year-old girl. The patient was alive and well 10 years later following a prosthetic replacement.

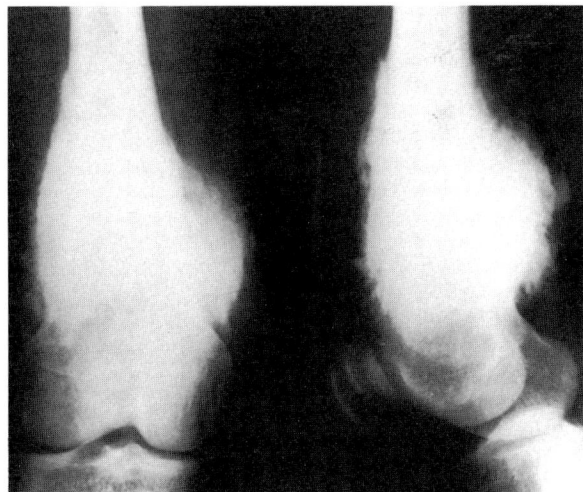

Fig. 1.3. *Parosteal sarcoma of femur.* This 18-year-old athletic man had developed a painful swelling above the left knee. A biopsy 6 months previously had been diagnosed as a stress fracture—a diagnostic error usually taking place in a reverse direction. Renewed histological studies confirmed the diagnosis.

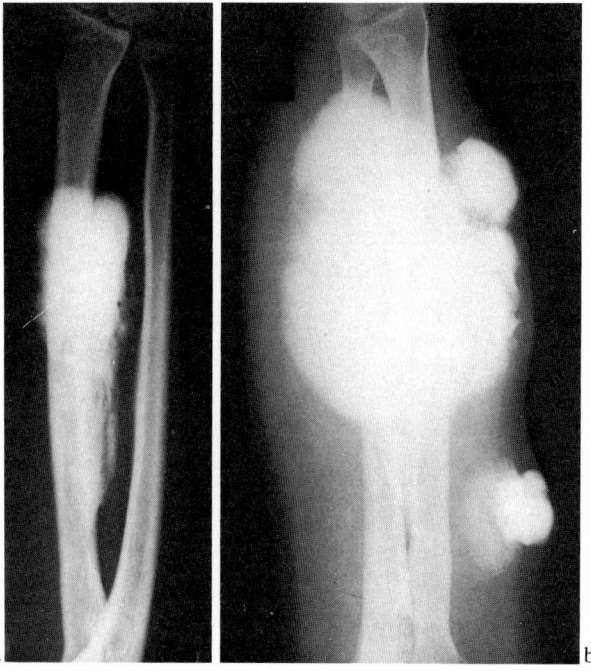

Fig. 1.5. *Aggressive parosteal sarcoma of radius.* **a** This lesion, in a young female nurse, grew rapidly and **b** satellite lesions developed in the soft tissues within 15 months. The patient died from pulmonary metastases.

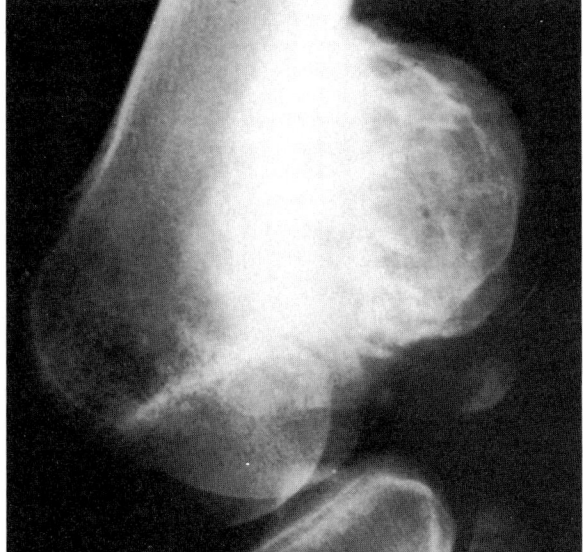

Fig. 1.4. *Parosteal sarcoma of femur.* The osseous excrescence on the posterior aspect of the distal end of the femur was found in a 26-year-old woman who complained of a painless swelling restricting flexion. An erroneous radiological diagnosis of an osteochondroma delayed definitive treatment by prosthetic replacement for 6 months. The diagnostic clue of a satellite lesion in the soft tissues was neglected.

A2. Calcified periosteal haematoma

The radiological findings of calcification in the soft tissues and a localised periosteal reaction suggested the possibility of a calcified haematoma, despite the absence of a specific history of trauma. Such an episode may be forgotten by the patient, especially if it has occurred in violent contact sports, or with suppression of pain sense by alcoholic stupor.

In this case, the surgeon considered the possibility of an early parosteal osteosarcoma and carried out a block resection of the lesion. At operation, a mass of 'pale, fleshy tissue', was encountered on the periosteal surface of the bone. Histologically, the superficial part of the specimen (Q2b) consists of bony tissue, while the deep part of the specimen (Q2c) consists of fibrous tissue, some of which is rather cellular. On closer examination, however, these cellular areas (Fig. 2.1) consist of fibrous tissue with numerous capillary blood vessels. The tissue is, in fact, an organising haematoma and not a neoplasm. The bone in Q2b is reactive, having been formed by the periosteum. Note that its pattern is different from that of the parosteal osteosarcoma (Q1b and c) and that the tissue separating the bony structures is also different.

Subperiosteal Haematoma

These lesions, which are presumed to be the result of trauma and are often related to a definite injury, sometimes are described as 'myositis ossificans'. The same term has been applied to a rather different type of lesion, occurring in muscle, which may be mistaken for a soft tissue osteosarcoma. For this the description 'pseudomalignant osseous tumour of soft tissues' is preferred, being a reminder of the need to distinguish them from malignant tumours and so avoid iatrogenic disasters. As mentioned above, a frank history of injury may not be obtained.

Clinical Features

A mildly tender swelling may be palpated, particularly in relation to a subcutaneous bone, such as the tibia, but also within the quadriceps and gluteal muscles and the flexor muscles of the arm.

Radiological Features

1. Site. Most of these lesions develop in soft tissues related to the humerus and femur.

2. Appearance. Irregular calcification develops in a few weeks, as organisation of the haematoma progresses, often followed by frank ossification. Such lesions may resolve spontaneously or persist as masses of heterotopic bone.

Pathological Features

The tissue from a subperiosteal haematoma consists, in the early stage, of organising blood clot. Later, this tissue becomes replaced by a larger or smaller mass of reactive periosteal new bone. In the case of the intramuscular pseudomalignant osseous tumour a characteristic 'zoned' structure permits its identification and differentiation from a soft tissue osteosarcoma. A lesion of this type is illustrated in Fig. 2.4. The periphery consists of relatively mature bone (Fig. 2.4a and b), while less organised spindle-celled tissue is present in the central portion (Fig. 2.4c). These lesions do not undergo malignant change; indeed, they appear to resolve with time, the peripheral bony shell being regarded as part of the process of maturation and resolution.

Treatment

Conservative measures, such as reassurance and rest, possibly with adjuvant analgesics, are usually adequate. When doubt exists it is wise to rely on serial radiographs confirming resolution and to avoid immediate surgical exploration.

References

Ackerman LV (1958) Extra-osseous localised non-neoplastic bone and cartilage formation (so-called myositis ossificans). J Bone Jt Surg 40A: 279–298

Angervall L, Stener I, Stener B, Ahren C (1969) Pseudomalignant osseous tumour of soft tissue. A clinical, radiological and pathological study of five cases. J Bone Jt Surg 51B: 654–663

Jaffe HL (1958) Pseudomalignant osseous tumor of soft tissues. In: Tumors and tumorous conditions of the bones and joints. Lea & Febiger, Philadelphia, p 526

Lewis D (1923) Myositis ossificans. JAMA 80: 1281–1287

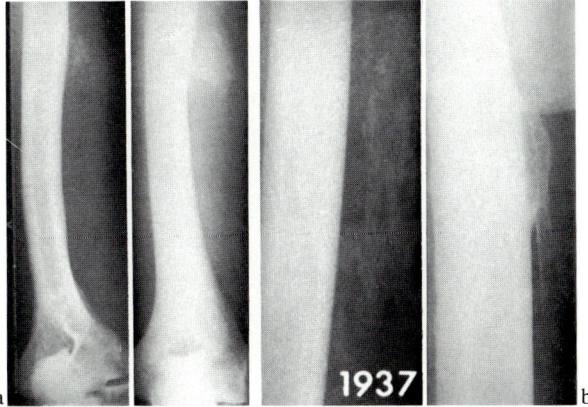

Fig. 2.2. *Organising subperiosteal haematoma.* **a** This calcifying mass presented as a painful swelling in the arm of a 23-year-old man who had forgotten sustaining an injury several weeks before; it became osseous within another 2 months. **b** At the age of 25 this man suffered a severe blow on the thigh at football. Irregular calcification in the soft tissues developed within a few days and then organised. Forty-five years later a painless bony mass persisted.

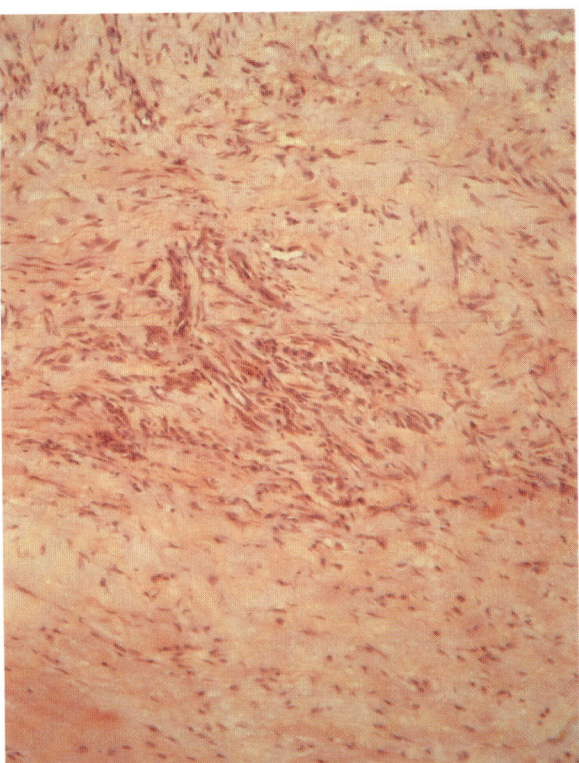

Fig. 2.1. More magnified view of tissue in Q2c, showing that the apparent cellularity is due to capillary blood vessels, formed as part of the organisation of the blood clot. (×90)

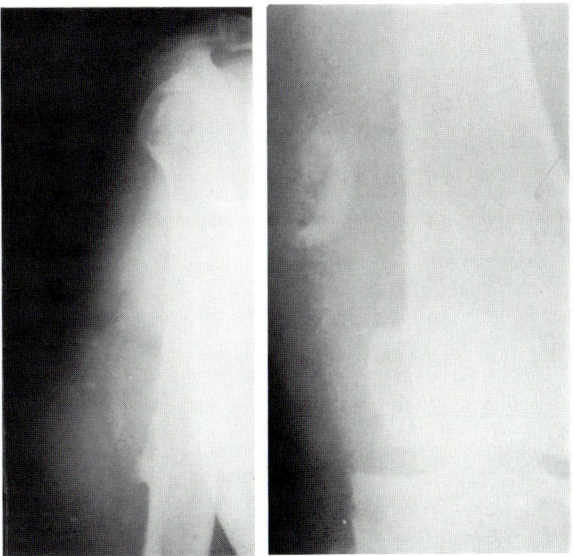

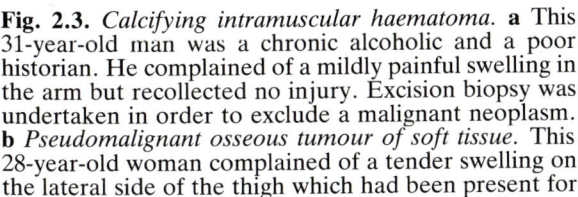

Fig. 2.3. *Calcifying intramuscular haematoma.* **a** This 31-year-old man was a chronic alcoholic and a poor historian. He complained of a mildly painful swelling in the arm but recollected no injury. Excision biopsy was undertaken in order to exclude a malignant neoplasm. **b** *Pseudomalignant osseous tumour of soft tissue.* This 28-year-old woman complained of a tender swelling on the lateral side of the thigh which had been present for several weeks. Again, no history of trauma was elicited. Although the mass is of bony texture it is more dense in its periphery. These lesions can cause radiological and histological difficulty in differentiation from the rare soft tissue osteosarcoma. They contain a core of benign fibrous tissue and have been known to follow intramuscular injections.

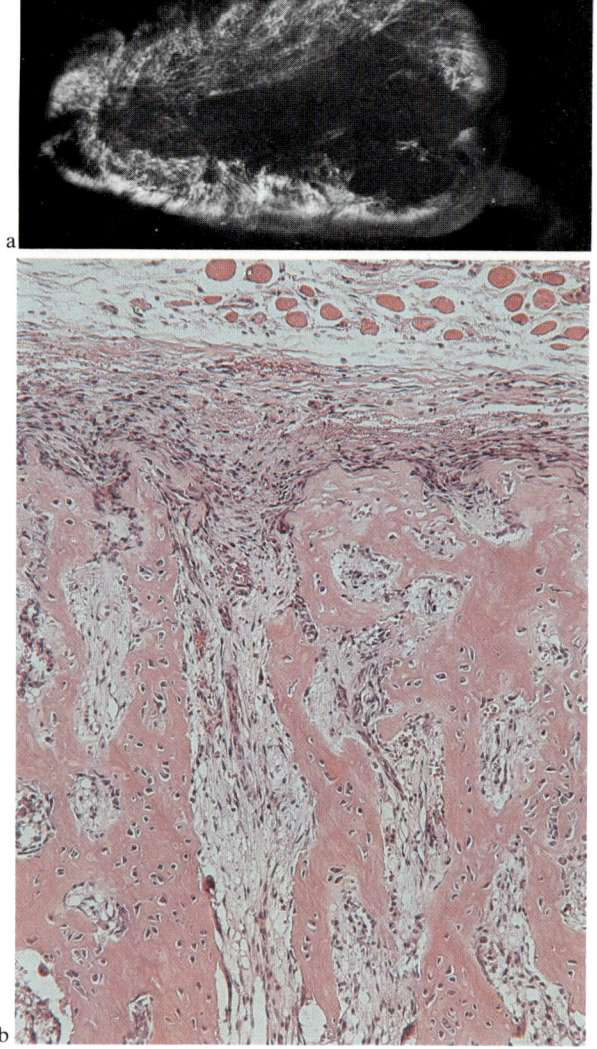
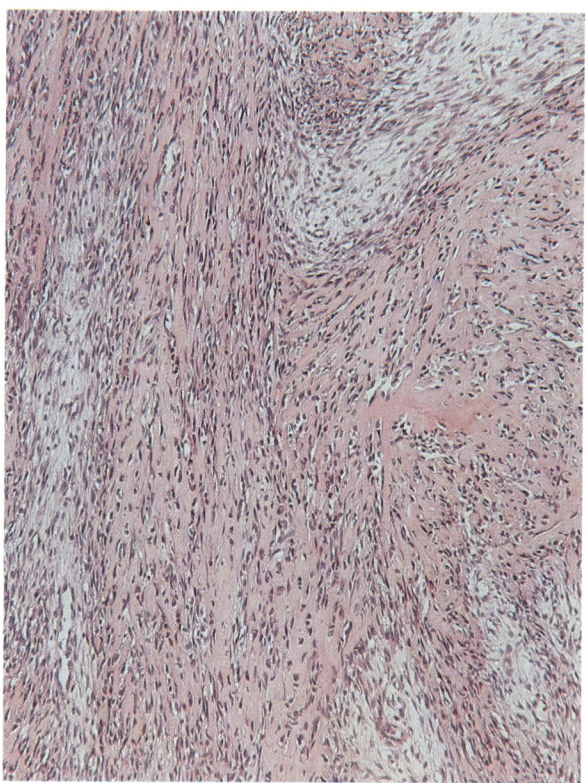

Fig. 2.4. a Slab radiograph from a surgical specimen of a pseudomalignant osseous tumour of the deltoid muscle. The patient was a woman aged 25 years, who developed a swelling of the arm 6 weeks after an anti-rubella injection. Observe the peripheral ossification. **b** The peripheral part of the lesion consists of trabeculae of relatively mature bone. (×84) **c** The deeper part of the same lesion shows benign spindle-celled tissue. (×84)

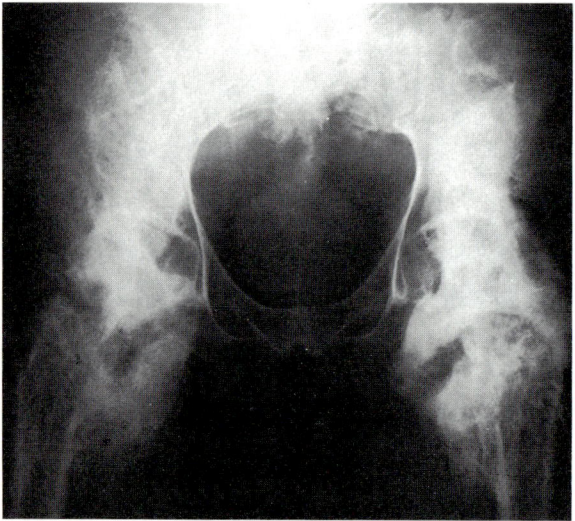

Fig. 2.5. *Paraplegic myositis ossificans.* Massive bone formation around the hips was demonstrated in a 39-year-old man 3 years after traumatic transection of the spinal cord at the T7 level. The cause is unknown.

A3. Periosteal osteosarcoma

Radiologically, the changes are equivocal. As in Q2, they might be merely reactive, but again the suspicion of malignancy led to surgical intervention.

At operation, the periosteal tissues were diffusely replaced by firm whitish fibrous tissue. The gross appearance confirmed the suspicion of malignancy, and a block excision of the lesion was performed.

The sections show bone, fibrous tissue and cartilage (Q3b), and some of the cartilage is decidedly cellular (Q3c). Superficially, the appearances resemble those encountered in parosteal osteosarcoma (Q1b and c), but the tumour has, in fact, certain characteristics which more closely resemble the cases described by Unni et al. as *periosteal osteosarcoma*. Although some bone is present, much of the tissue is cartilaginous (Figs. 3.1a and 3.1b) and the lesion has the 'mushroom' outline which is regarded as characteristic of these tumours. In the deeper part of the specimen the tumour tissue was invading the cancellous bone adjacent to the cortex (Fig. 3.1c). Not all authorities are agreed that the distinction between 'parosteal' and 'periosteal' osteosarcomas is valid.

Reference

Unni KK, Dahlin DC, Beabout JW (1976) Periosteal osteogenic sarcoma. Cancer 37: 2476–2485

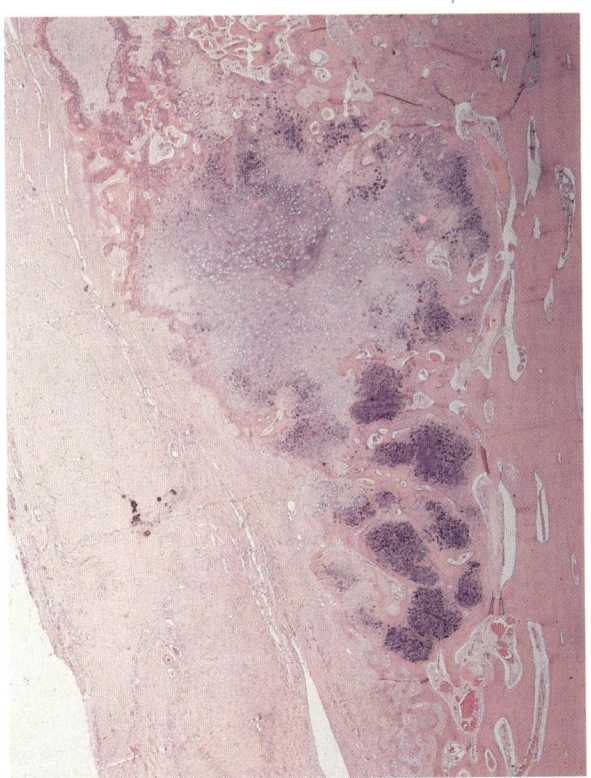

Fig. 3.1a. Low-power view of part of the block excision specimen. Much of the tumour tissue consists of cartilage. (×7)

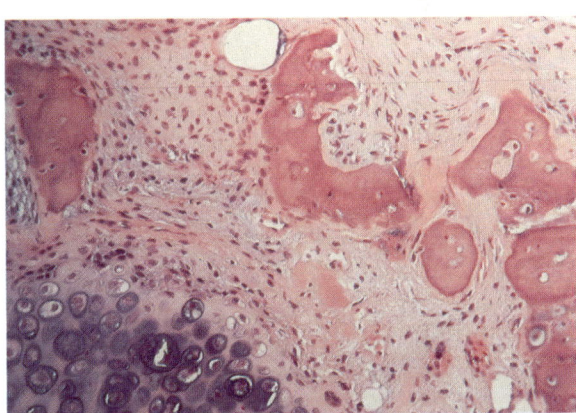

Fig. 3.1b A more magnified view, showing the appearance of the bone, cartilage and fibrous tissue making up the tumour. (×94)

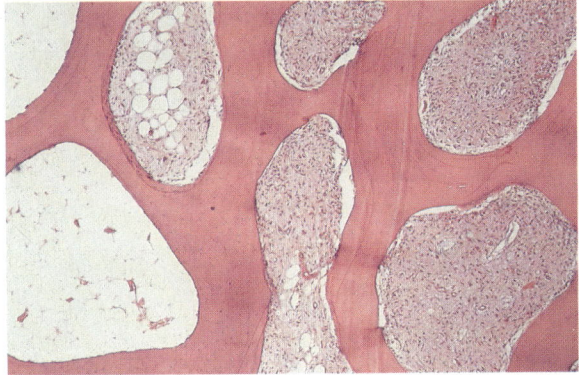

Fig. 3.1c. Invasion of the marrow spaces of the cancellous bone by spindle-celled tumour tissue. (×35)

Q1. **This 35-year-old woman had been aware of a painless swelling on the medial side of her left thigh for 15 years. It had enlarged slowly and had caused mild discomfort during the previous year.**

Clinically, on palpation the mass was found to be firm, slightly tender and immobile. No other physical abnormality was detected.

The radiographs showed the mass to be clearly delineated with peripheral and central strands of density enclosing areas of increased lucency. The mass merged into the medial cortex of the femur.

Local excision was performed.

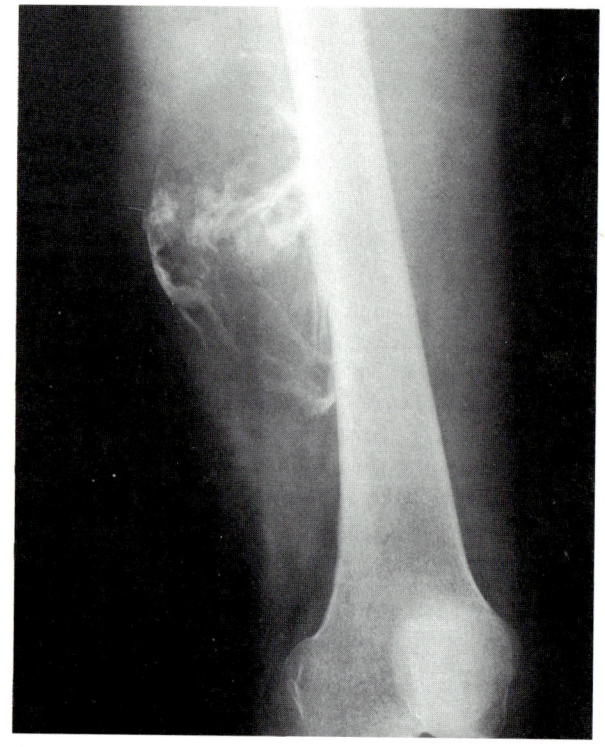

Q1a.

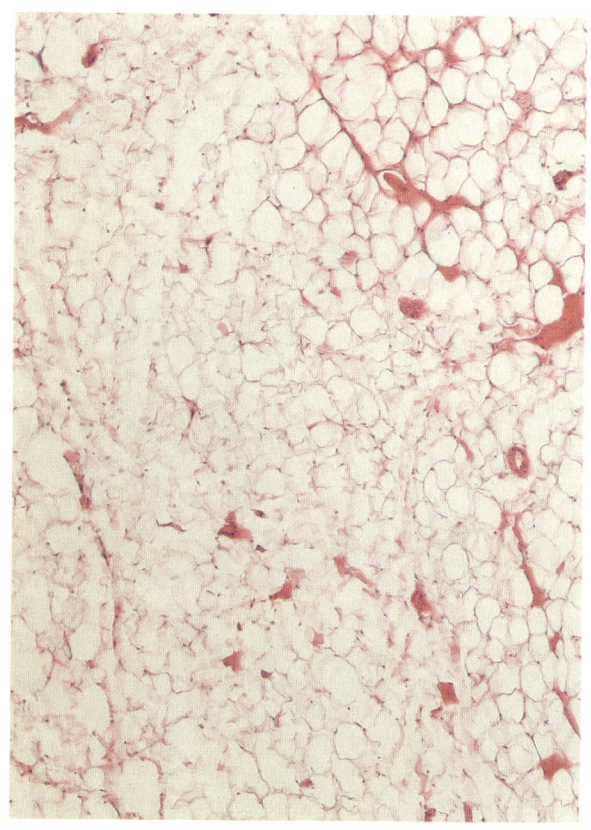

Q1b. (×45)

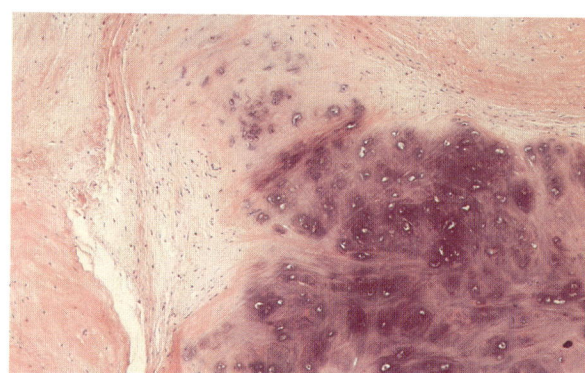

Q1c. (×52)

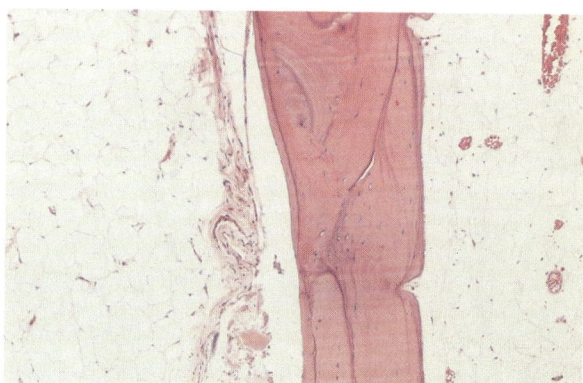

Q1d. (×52)

Q2. This 47-year-old woman was deaf and dumb. She was brought to hospital by a friend who had observed a large swelling of the right thigh to increase in size during the previous 3 months.

Clinical examination of the swelling showed it to be firm, immobile and slightly tender. The skin over it was stretched, but no other abnormality was detected.

The radiographs revealed the mass to be dense with peripheral and central strands of calcification. The adjacent femoral cortex appeared to have been attenuated by pressure erosion.

A biopsy was performed.

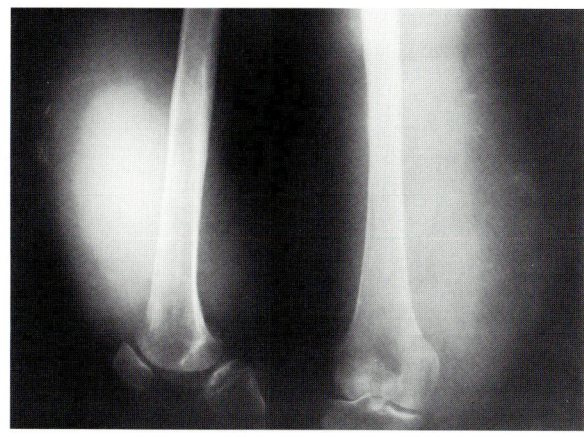

Q2a.

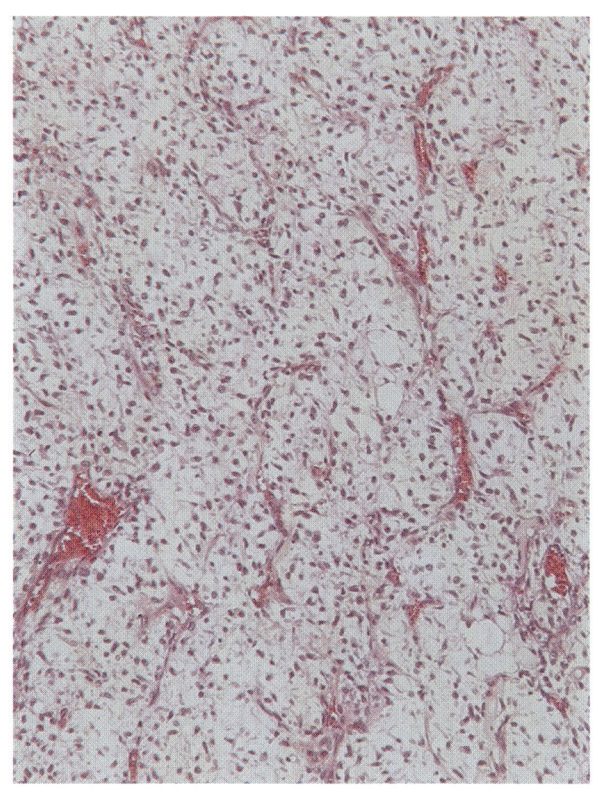

Q2b. (×106)

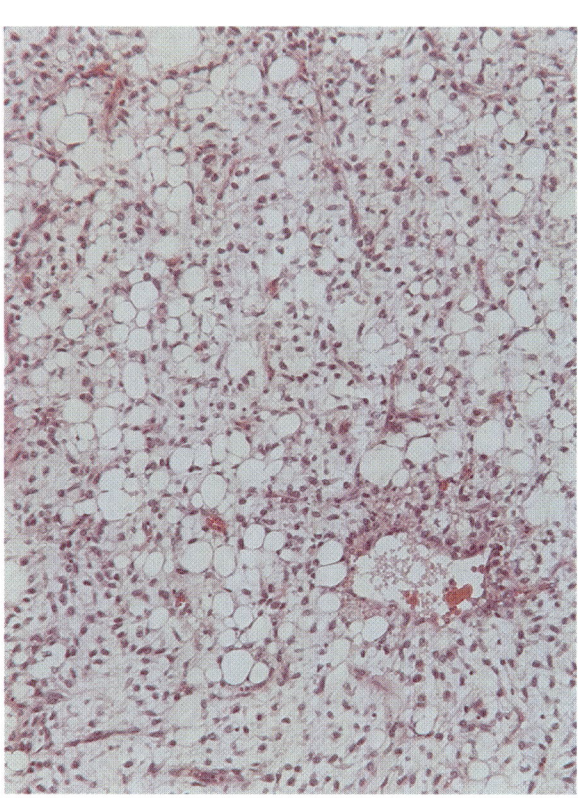

Q2c. (×106)

A1. Parosteal lipoma of femur

The clinical history and the radiological appearance both suggested a benign lesion. The lucent areas were of fatty density and represented lipomatous lobules. These lobules were surrounded characteristically by intervening capsules which were partially calcified or ossified. This radiological pattern was so characteristic that the diagnosis of a fatty tumour alone was offered. Despite the clinical history of recent enlargement, malignant change was considered to be very unlikely in view of the fatty lucencies.

The specimen removed at operation did consist of a lobulated mass of fatty tissue. Q1b confirms the lesion to be a lipoma. Much of it represents mature adipose tissue, being made up of rounded fat cells. The contents of these cells have been removed during histological processing and they consequently appear as empty spaces in the illustration. Strands of fibrous tissue are present and contain a ramifying network of mature cartilage (Q1c) and bone (Q1d). These structures account for the linear densities in the radiographs.

Excision of the tumour was curative, no recurrence developing within the subsequent 5 years.

A2. Liposarcoma of thigh

The clinical history of relatively rapid enlargement of the mass together with its radiological density made consideration of a malignant soft tissue tumour imperative. The strands of calcification caused a pre-operative radiological diagnosis of a liposarcoma to be offered, but such calcifications may be observed also in other malignant tumours of soft tissue, such as malignant synovioma or fibrosarcoma.

The biopsy specimen had the naked-eye appearance of fleshy tissue, and was not obviously fatty. Histological sections show an appearance which is characteristic of the type of liposarcoma known as myxoid liposarcoma. Much of the tumour tissue (Q2b) consists of myxoid tissue made up of spindle-shaped cells and showing a prominent network of capillary blood vessels. Relatively few lipoblasts—the fat-forming cells which are diagnostic for liposarcoma—are present in these areas, although these cells can be found in other parts of the biopsy specimen (Q2c). Slight nuclear pleomorphism is present, but there is little or no evidence of mitotic activity.

Lipomatous Tumours

Orthopaedic surgeons may encounter patients with symptoms and signs attributable to a variety of neoplasms, either benign or malignant, arising in soft tissues. Pre-operative assessment of such lesions by orthodox radiological procedures has been limited in the past to recognition of the spectrum of lipomatous tumours and the phleboliths which are so characteristic of a vascular tumour (see Exercise 34). To a large extent these methods have been reinforced by the use of the other techniques of diagnostic imaging, including ultrasound, radionuclide studies and CT scanning.

Clinical Features

Benign fatty tumours are common, but often are so small that they cause neither discomfort nor significant cosmetic deformity, so that their presence frequently is neglected. A predilection for females exists and the majority are recognised in middle life. Larger lesions may alarm affected individuals and occasionally provoke mild localised pain, possibly due to pressure on nerves. When such tumours enlarge, even over many years, malignant change must be considered, in which case diagnostic imaging is of great value.

Radiological Features

1. Site. Lipomas may occur anywhere in soft tissues. Those arising within the neural canal are of special interest. A small number have been reported to arise within bone.

2. Appearance. The typical, simple lipoma is shown as a clearly defined lucency, possibly having a racemose pattern, resembling a bunch of grapes. Adjacent bones may develop slight pressure erosions or periosteal reactions. As the tumour matures, calcification and ossification often occur around the lobules, as illustrated in the relatively unusual example of the parosteal type in Q1. Loss of the classical lucency of the fatty element of these neoplasms reflects an increase of the fibrous tissue content and should cause malignant change to be considered.

Pathological Features

Histologically, a typical lipoma consists of an encapsulated lobulated mass of mature fat, sometimes containing strands of fibrous or fibrovascular tissue. Some types of fatty tumour, previously included in the group of well-differentiated liposarcomas, are now regarded as benign and referred to by terms such as 'atypical lipoma', 'pleomorphic lipoma' or 'spindle-cell lipoma'.

The diagnosis of liposarcoma depends on the identification, in a malignant soft tissue tumour, of fat-forming lipoblasts. A number of histological types of liposarcoma—well-differentiated, myxoid, pleomorphic and mixed—are recognised. The well-differentiated and myxoid varieties have a better prognosis than the pleomorphic and mixed types. Well-differentiated liposarcomas, at least in some areas, can show a close resemblance to the normal adipose tissue of a lipoma, but more cellular areas are present to indicate the sarcomatous nature of the tumour. Myxoid liposarcomas, the commonest type, have a characteristic histological structure which is illustrated in Q2b and c. In addition to lipoblasts containing recognisable fat droplets, they contain myxoid tissue made up of spindle-shaped cells and show a characteristic pattern of capillary blood vessels. The histological appearance of more malignant pleomorphic liposarcomas, with bizarre multinucleated tumour giant cells as well as fat-containing lipoblasts, is illustrated in Figs. 2.3 and 2.4.

Treatment

For most lipomas in the soft tissues simple excision is curative and recurrences are rare. Those arising in the lumbosacral portion of the neural canal, however, are so interspersed with nerve roots that complete excision is technically difficult.

Liposarcomas, like other malignant soft tissue tumours, should be treated by widespread resection including a generous margin of normal tissue. For the more malignant types of liposarcoma, surgical resection or amputation is commonly combined with chemotherapy.

Radiotherapy is of little value.

References

Allen PW (1981) Tumors and proliferations of adipose tissue. Monographs in Diagnostic Radiology, vol I. Masson, New York
Bassett RC (1950) Neurologic deficit associated with lipomas of cauda equina. Ann Surg 131: 109–116
Enzinger FM, Winslow DJ (1962) Liposarcoma: a study of 103 cases. Virchows Arch. 335: 367–388
Jacobs P (1972) Parosteal lipoma with hyperostoses. Clin Radiol 23: 196–198
Reszel PA, Soule EH, Coventry MB (1966) Liposarcoma of the extremities and limb girdles. J Bone Jt Surg 48B: 229–244

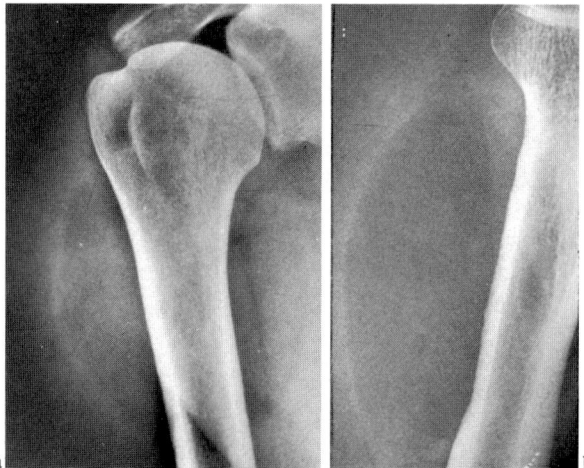

Fig. 1.1. *Lipoma of soft tissues.* **a** This 49-year-old man complained of discomfort in the right shoulder during his occupation as a truck driver. A rather solid painless swelling was palpated. It shows the typical well-defined lucency of a lipoma. Histologically it consisted entirely of mature fat. **b** This lipoma of the forearm was tender and caused mild pain in this young man. Observe pressure erosion of the superficial cortex of the adjacent radius.

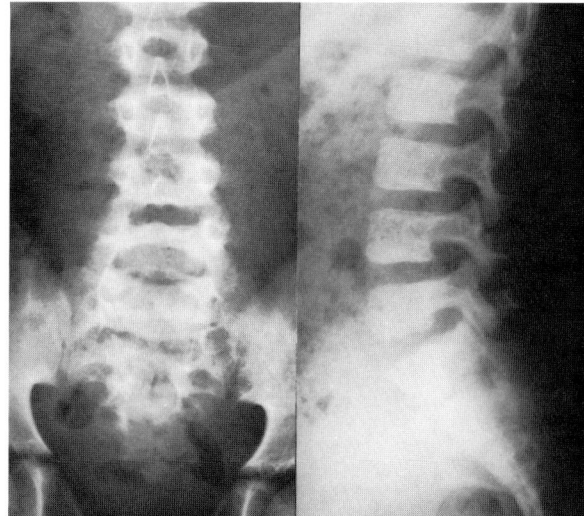

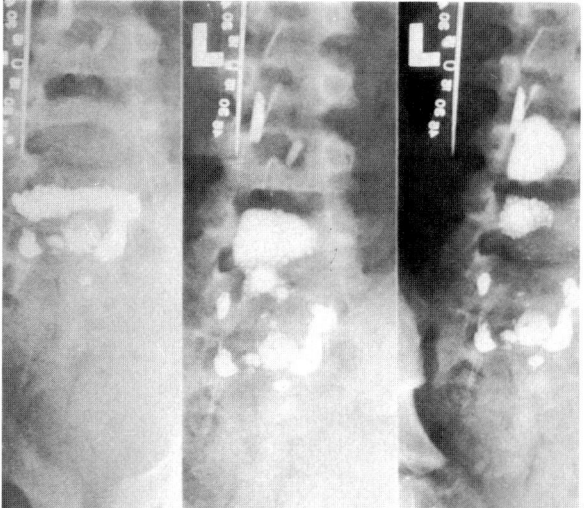

Fig. 1.3. *Lipoma of neural canal.* **a** This 7-year-old boy with bilateral pes cavus and enuresis was examined to exclude spina bifida. The extreme widening of the neural canal in the lumbosacral region, with erosion of the posterior aspects of the body of L5 and the upper sacral segments, indicated a space-occupying lesion. **b** Myelography showed the lobulated pattern of the lipoma, of which the nature was confirmed histologically. The predilection of this site has long been known to neurosurgeons.

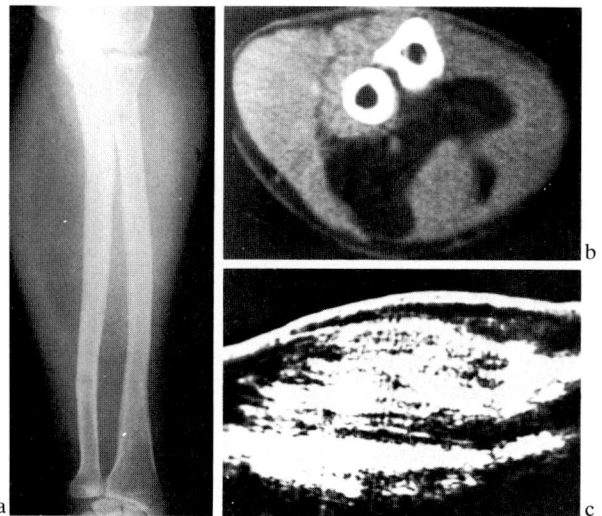

Fig. 1.2. *Lipoma of soft tissues.* **a** This painless swelling in the forearm of a young man is shown clearly in the radiograph and also **b** in the CT scan, illustrating low density of the tumour, and **c** in this longitudinal ultrasound section of the forearm, demonstrating displacement of the normal muscle planes by an echogenic lobulated mass.

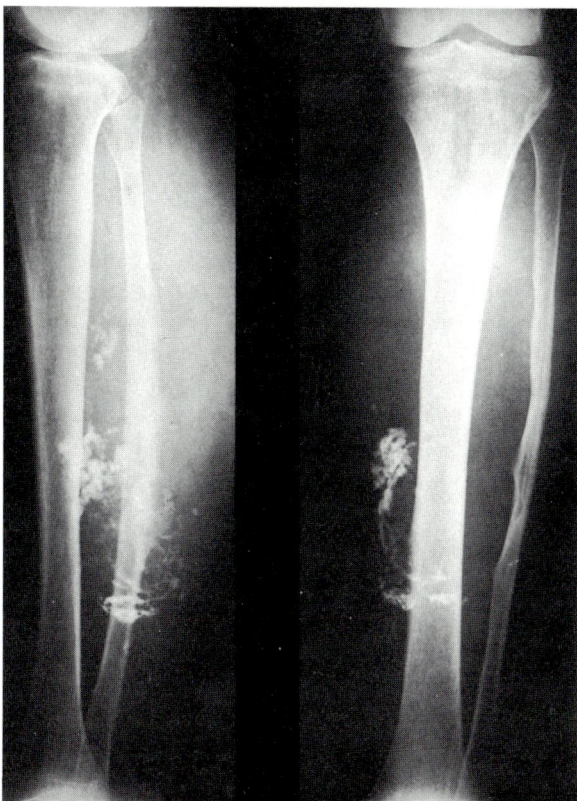

Fig. 2.1. *Liposarcoma*. This huge soft tissue mass was found in the leg of a 66-year-old woman, who had observed it to grow slowly during the previous 6 years. Irregular strands of calcification, comparable to those illustrated in Q1a, are present and extensive pressure erosions have affected the fibula. The lucency of benign fatty tissue, however, is absent, a radiological feature suggesting malignancy.

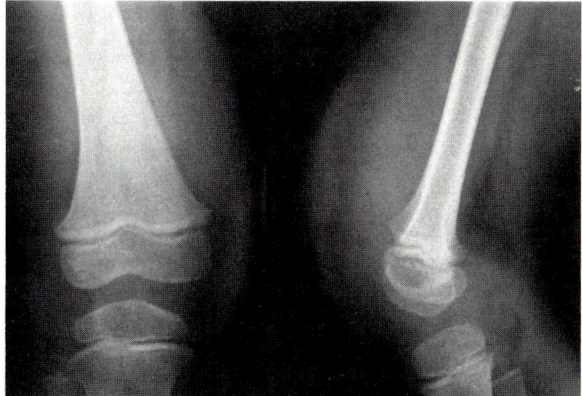

Fig. 2.2. *Liposarcoma*. An aggressive and painful soft tissue swelling developed above the right knee within a few months in this 4-year-old boy. The dense soft tissue mass suggested a malignant tumour, but the exact diagnosis was established only by biopsy. Despite amputation survival was limited to 14 months.

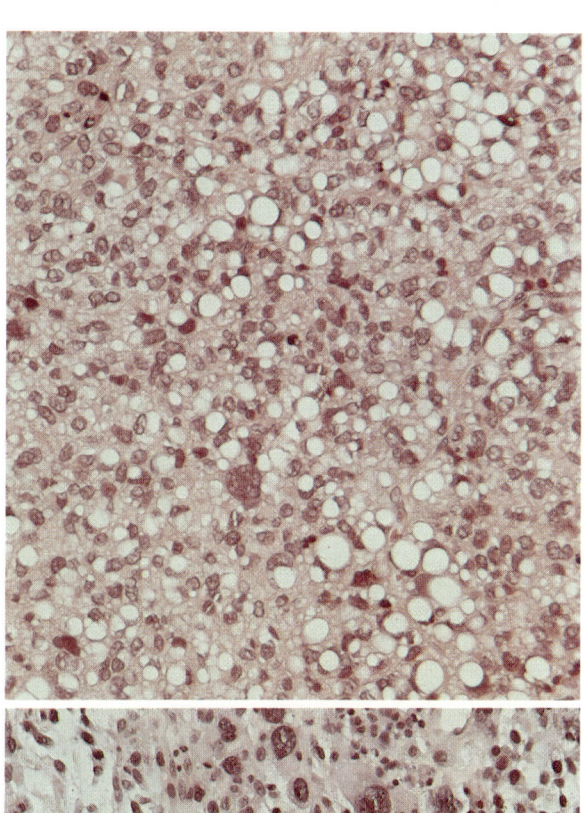
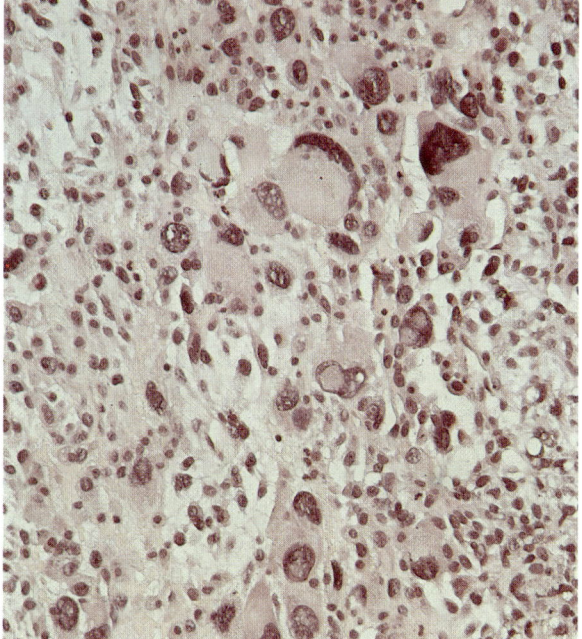

Fig. 2.3a. *Pleomorphic liposarcoma*. A field from a case of this more aggressive form of this malignant tumour shows many lipoblasts, with empty fat droplets. A considerable degree of nuclear pleomorphism is present. (×200). **b** Another field from the same tumour, showing bizarre multinucleated giant cells. (×150)

Exercise 40

Q1. This 32-year-old woman presented with a large, painless swelling of the tip of the left middle finger.

This swelling had developed during the previous year and had impaired function. Clinical examination revealed no other abnormality. Q1a is a photograph of the affected finger.

The radiograph shows the distal phalanx to be expanded with a coarse trabecular pattern in the medullary cavity. The overlying soft tissues were swollen. No other bony abnormality was detected.

Because of the functional disability, the terminal phalanx was amputated.

Q2. This 64-year-old man sought advice on account of a persistent swelling on the tip of his right thumb.

On clinical examination a small firm mass lay under the nail. No other abnormality was detected.

The radiographs showed a small lytic area in the tuft of the terminal phalanx. Its margin was sharply defined with a narrow zone of transition.

This area was curetted.

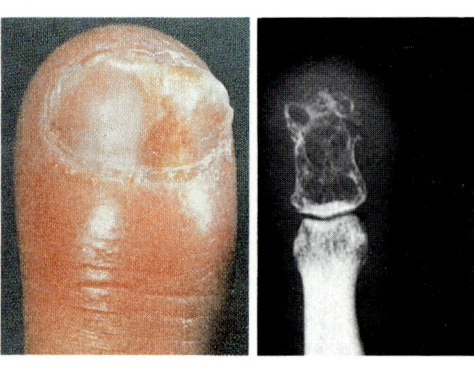

Q1a. **Q1b.**

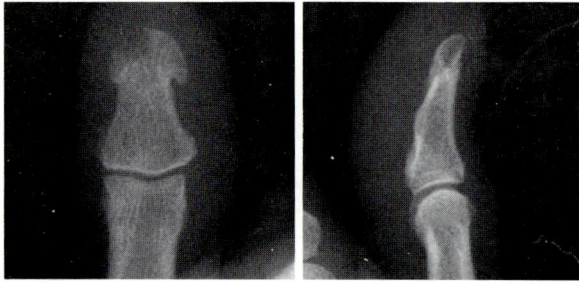

Q2a.

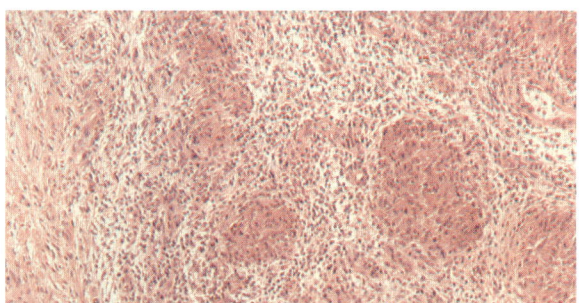

Q1c. (×90)

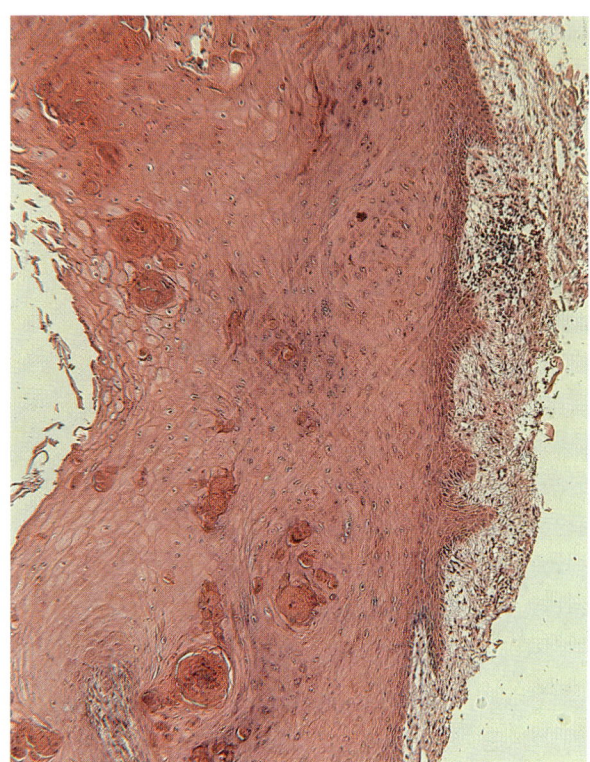

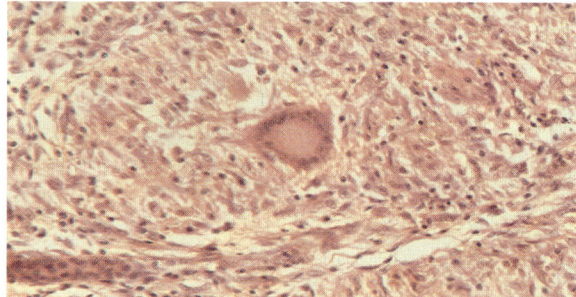

Q1d. (×130)

Q2b. (×58)

Q3. This patient, a 49-year-old woman, complained of intermittent pain at the tip of the middle finger for many years.

On clinical examination the tip of the finger was swollen, and the tissue under the nail was red and exquisitely tender.

Radiological examination showed a clearly defined lytic area involving the radial aspect of the tuft of the terminal phalanx.

The lesion was explored.

Q4. This 66-year-old man complained of a swelling of the tip of the little finger.

This swelling had become increasingly painful during the previous 4 months and was interfering with function. The swelling was palpable and tender on clinical examination and radiological examination was requested.

The radiograph revealed almost complete destruction of the 5th terminal phalanx.

The histological appearance is illustrated below.

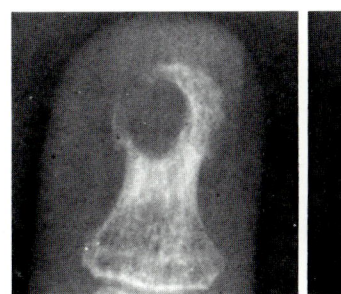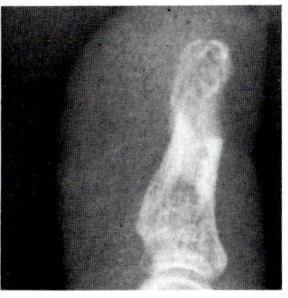

Q3a.

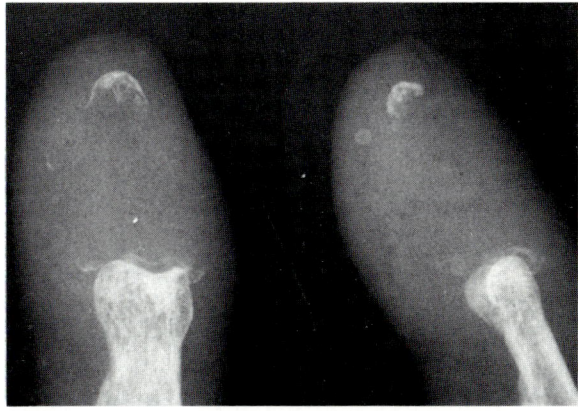

Q4a.

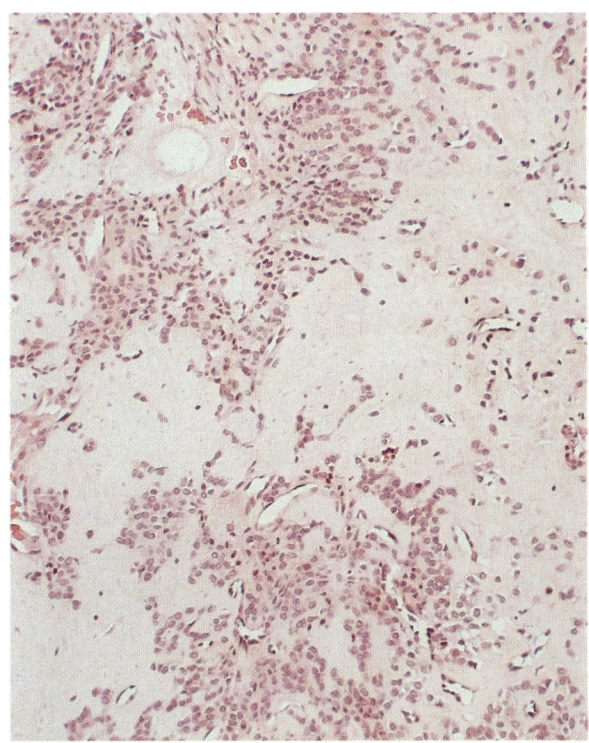

Q3b. (×140)

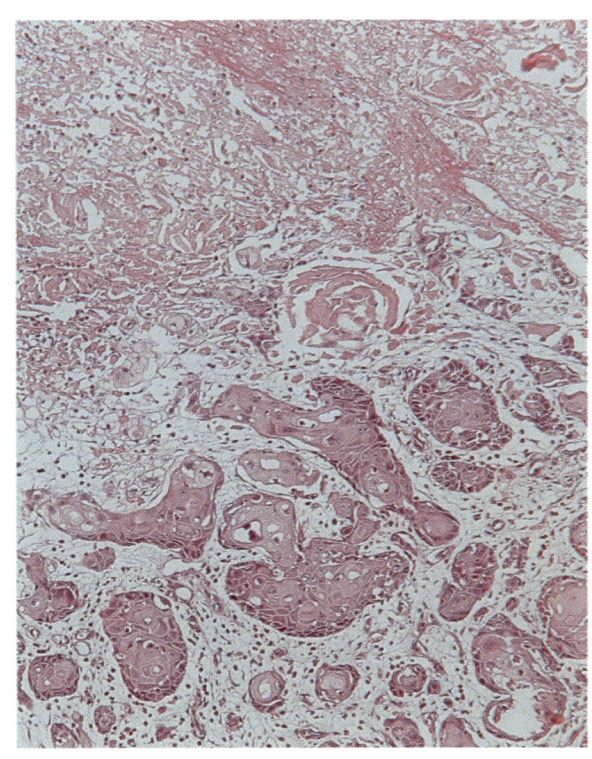

Q4b. (×88)

A1. Sarcoidosis of terminal phalanx

A number of lesions affecting this particular segment of the skeleton are illustrated in this Exercise. The clinical photograph of this patient shows the erythematous swelling which suggested chronic inflammation. The reticular pattern of bone destruction in this terminal phalanx is accompanied by enlargement of the entire bone and marked thinning of the cortex, representing one of the several types of bone involvement which can occur in this disease.

Pathological examination of the specimen showed expansion and replacement of the bone by a mass of firm greyish material. Q1c shows granulomatous tissue containing tubercle-like clusters of epithelioid cells, but without any of the caseous necrosis that would be expected in tuberculosis (see Exercise 13). Some of the cell clusters (Q1d) contain large multinucleated giant cells with peripherally arranged nuclei, known as Langhans' (or foreign body) giant cells. Although these findings are not specific, they are typical of sarcoidosis. A diagnosis of tuberculosis was excluded, not only because of the lack of caseation, but by the absence of acid-fast bacilli and by the patient's negative tuberculin reaction. The diagnosis of sarcoidosis was supported by a previous history of indurated plaques on the skin of the face. These plaques actually had regressed before the development of the bone lesion.

Sarcoidosis

Sarcoidosis is a generalised granulomatous disease of undetermined aetiology. It occurs mainly in adults during the first half of life and exhibits a remarkable predilection for the black races. The disease commonly begins in, and remains confined to, the lungs, but many other tissue systems, including the lymph nodes, liver, spleen and skin are often affected. Involvement of the skeleton, considered here, is confined to fewer than 10% of all cases.

Clinical Features

The disease may be mild and frequently attention to its presence is drawn by a symmetrical hilar adenopathy in a routine chest film, possibly with pulmonary densities, all of which tend to resolve spontaneously. In more severe cases it provokes constitutional symptoms and signs such as mild pyrexia and chronic cough, possibly accompanied by hepatomegaly and splenomegaly. Skin lesions are often present. When bones are involved, arthralgia, swelling and localised bone pain usually develop. Affected digits may become significantly deformed. A positive Kveim test, consisting of a non-caseating granulomatous response to an intracutaneous injection of an extract of sarcoid tissue, can be obtained in many cases.

Radiological Features

1. Site. The vast majority of osseous lesions, usually multiple, due to sarcoidosis occur in the small bones of the hands and feet. Less commonly other bones may be affected, including the carpus and tarsus and, exceptionally, the major long bones, the axial skeleton and even the skull.

2. Appearance. The lesions are largely osteolytic and are usually associated with soft tissue swelling. They may present a variety of radiological patterns in the phalanges of the hands and feet, including the lacework or reticular type illustrated in Q1b, multiple rounded foci of destruction in the phalangeal necks, due to granulomatous disease at sites of nutrient foramina, expansile lucent areas simulating enchondromas, resorption of phalangeal tufts and cortical erosions. Medullary sclerosis and neuropathic-like joints may be observed. Rare involvement of other portions of the skeleton usually offers considerable diagnostic difficulty. Although largely osteolytic, as in the spine, where they may resemble a tuberculous infection, widespread sclerosis is observed exceptionally.

Pathological Features

The clusters of epithelioid cells detected within granulomatous tissue, together with the large multinucleated giant cells, which have their nuclei distributed around their margins, indicate a low-grade inflammatory process. This characteristic histological finding of epithelioid tubercles without necrosis, however, is not specific, and tuberculosis, fungal infection and other causes must be excluded. In the past, indeed, sarcoidosis was regarded as having a relation to tuberculosis, but this hypothesis has never been substantiated.

Treatment

In that the cause of sarcoidosis is unknown, treatment is essentially non-specific. Symptoms of early inflammatory manifestations are controlled by anti-inflammatory agents such as aspirin, phenylbutazone and indomethacin. The active granulomatous phase is suppressed by the use of steroids. In the majority of patients only minimal therapy is required as the natural course of the disease is toward resolution with minimal disability.

Specifically, intrathoracic sarcoidosis requires treatment when respiratory function is affected. Further, uveitis and hypercalcaemia require control as a matter of urgency. Hypercalcaemia and hypercalcuria may respond to vitamin D and control of calcium intake.

References

Holt JF, Owens WI (1949) Osseous lesions of sarcoidosis. Radiology 53: 11–19

Longcope WT, Foreman DG (1952) A study of sarcoidosis based on a combined investigation of 160 cases, including 30 autopsies from the Johns Hopkins Hospital and the Massachusetts General Hospital. Medicine 31: 1-132

Mitchell DN, Scadding JG, Heard BE, Hinson KFW (1977) Sarcoidosis: histopathological definition and clinical diagnosis. J Clin Pathol 30: 395–398

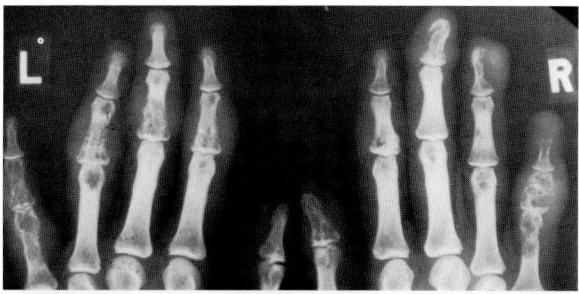
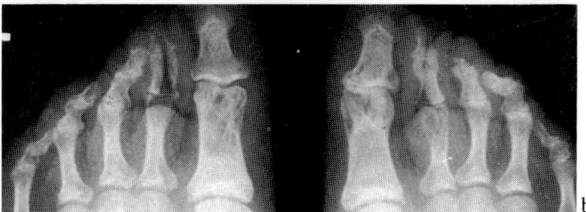
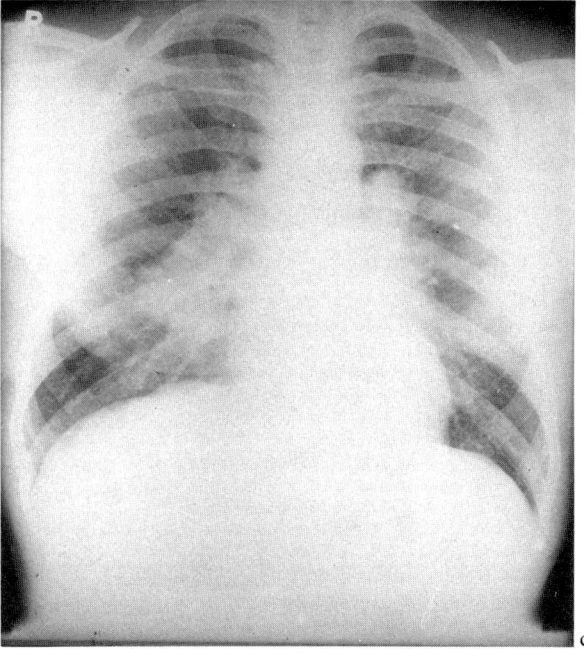

Fig. 1.1. *Sarcoidosis* in a 38-year-old man with painful swellings and deformities of the fingers developing during the previous 2 years. **a** *Hands*—the typical reticular destructive form of the disease has involved many phalanges. Circular lytic lesions in the phalangeal necks reflect granulomatous deposits in nutrient foramina. Some are large enough to resemble enchondromas. Resorption of some phalangeal tufts, areas of medullary sclerosis and soft tissue swellings are present. **b** *Feet*. Although asymptomatic, similar reticular lesions were demonstrated in the heads of both 1st proximal phalanges. **c** *Chest* examination revealed the classical hilar adenopathy of the disease.

A2. Epidermal (implantation dermoid) cyst of terminal phalanx

This lesion radiologically appeared to be benign. The diagnosis of an epidermal cyst certainly deserved consideration, but, as is usually the case, no history of a previous penetrating injury was obtained.

Material curetted from the bone consisted of fragments of squamous epithelium with foci of keratinisation (Q2b). This tissue is quite foreign to bone, and its presence establishes a diagnosis of epidermal cyst.

Epidermal Cyst of Phalanx

The aetiology of these cysts is not completely understood. They occur, as rare lesions, in the terminal phalanges of the fingers or thumbs. This anatomical location, together with an occasional confirmatory history of a former penetrating injury to the affected digit, has suggested that they are due to trauma. Epithelium from the overlying skin or nail bed is assumed to have become separated and implanted in the bone, giving rise to the descriptive term 'implantation dermoid'. When this tissue remains viable and continues to grow, slow erosion of the bone appears to follow.

Clinical Features

These rare lesions may be detected incidentally by radiological examination, although they may be recognised by the occurrence of a pathological fracture. Only occasionally, as in the present case, do they cause enough swelling and pain for medical advice to be required.

Radiological Features

Lytic lesions in terminal phalanges, as illustrated in this Exercise, may be caused by a variety of conditions. The solitary epidermal cyst of a terminal phalanx may be difficult to differentiate from an enchondroma, but usually the appearance is benign.

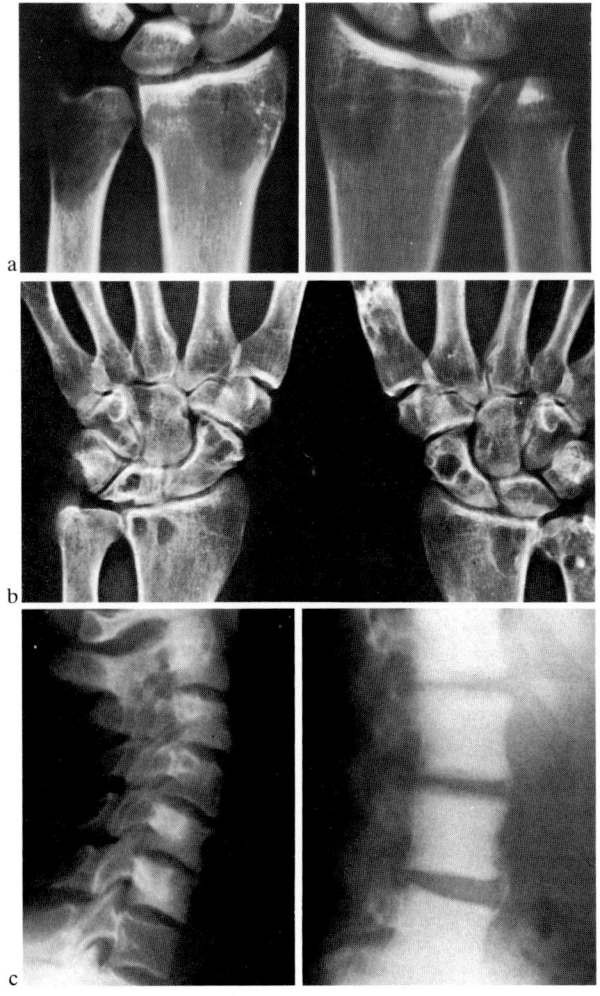

Fig. 1.2. *Sarcoidosis—unusual sites and manifestations.* **a** *Forearms.* This 24-year-old man sustained a pathological fracture through a well-defined lytic lesion in the distal end of the left radius. He was otherwise in excellent health. A similar lytic lesion was evident in the distal end of the left ulna. Skeletal survey revealed a symmetrical appearance in the right ulna, but no other bony abnormality was detected. A wide differential diagnosis was offered prior to biopsy, but without mention of sarcoidosis. Histologically non-caseating granulomatous tissue was found, comparable to that illustrated in Q1c and d. Following healing of the fracture, the patient was without symptoms of the disease 3 years later. **b** *Wrists.* Multiple lytic lesions in the carpal bones and several metacarpals in a 34-year-old black woman with pain and limitation of movement. Marginal sclerosis in some bones suggests healing. In this patient the diagnosis had been established on other grounds and bone biopsy was not performed. **c** *Spine.* These exceptional sclerosing lesions in many vertebrae were found in a 43-year-old man who presented with dyspnoea and back pain. Such an appearance is very unusual. Biopsy confirmation was obtained.

Treatment

If symptomatic, firm curettage of the affected bone is curative, almost always without recurrence.

Reference

Byers P, Mantle J, Salm R. (1966) Epidermal cyst of phalanges. J Bone Jt Surg 48B: 577–581

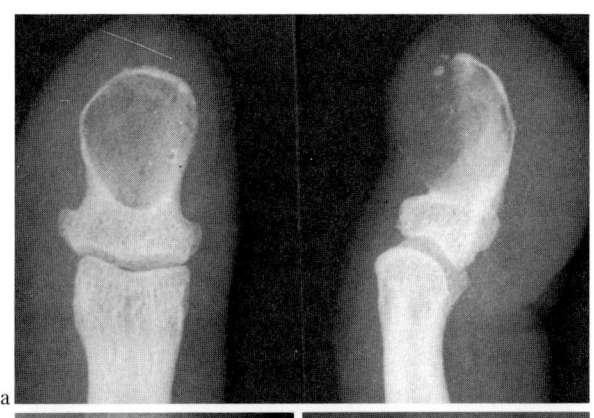
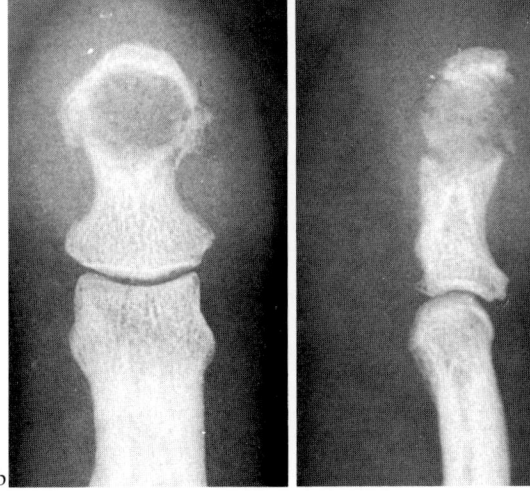

Fig. 2.1. *Epidermal cysts.* Further examples with a history of trauma. **a** This elderly woman gave a history of injury to the left thumb many years before. The osteolytic erosion of the dorsal side of the distal phalanx is sharply demonstrated. **b** This cyst was encountered because of a pathological fracture. The patient was an elderly seamstress who recalled having pricked this finger with a needle several years previously.

A3. Glomus tumour of terminal phalanx

The clinical history in this entity is particularly important, the diagnosis being supported strongly by the well-demarcated lytic lesion in the bone, with significant swelling of the soft tissues.

The involved part of the terminal phalanx was excised. The section shows (Q3b) a lesion consisting of rounded cells with abundant intercellular material. The cells are clustered around small blood vessels. These appearances are characteristic of a glomus tumour.

Glomus Tumour of Bone

A glomus tumour is a specific type of benign vascular neoplasm with a histological structure which resembles that of a normal 'glomus' or arteriovenous anastomosis.

Clinical Features

Adults, usually females, are especially affected, often with a long history. These uncommon lesions usually involve the skin and subcutaneous tissue, particularly that of the fingers and toes. They are small and often are associated with intermittent and severe localised pain, which occurs either spontaneously or as a result of pressure. Rarely, they are encountered in the skeleton, most of the reported cases involving the terminal phalanx of a finger.

Radiological Features

1. Site. These lesions are classically confined to terminal phalanges.

2. Appearance. The abnormality consists of a non-specific and rounded area of bone destruction with a sharply defined margin. As mentioned above, differentiation from other lytic lesions, of which some are described in this Exercise, may be suggested clinically, but ultimately the diagnosis depends on histological assessment.

Pathological Features

These tumours consist of small vascular channels surrounded by characteristic glomus cells, which are believed to be derived from the walls of blood vessels. They are generally accepted as variants of haemangiopericytoma (see Exercise 34.)

Treatment

Excision of a bony lesion usually is completely effective, but recurrences are not unknown.

References

Lattes R, Bull DC (1948) A case of glomus tumor with primary involvement of bone. Ann Surg 127: 187–191

Lehman W, Kraissl C (1949) Glomus tumor within bone. Surgery 25: 116–121

Mackenzie DH (1962) Intraosseous glomus tumours. Report of two cases. J Bone Jt Surg 44B: 648–651

Siegel MW (1967) Intraosseous glomus tumor. A case report. Am J Orthop 9: 68–69

A4. Osteolytic metastasis from bronchogenic carcinoma

Metastatic lesions distal to the elbow and knee are, in contradistinction to earlier reports, not exceptionally rare (see Exercise 2). In a patient of this age the appearance primarily demanded further investigation to confirm or exclude this diagnosis. Examination of the chest revealed an opaque mass and on skeletal survey another osteolytic bone lesion was found in the left tibia.

The histological illustration (Q4b) is from the tumour of the 5th distal phalanx, the specimen being obtained at autopsy. It shows a well-differentiated squamous carcinoma, recognised by the presence of rounded epithelial formations, each of which contains large pale keratinising cells. These epithelial formations are separated by a delicate stromal connective tissue containing capillary blood vessels and a few 'inflammatory' cells. In the field shown, some of the tissue has undergone necrosis and appears as a network of pink-staining material which is relatively devoid of cells. The microscopic appearance of the lesion is utterly different from that of a primary bone tumour.

Possible sites for a primary tumour with this squamous structure include skin, oesophagus and lung. In the present case, the tumour originated in the lung. This diagnosis was suggested by the appearances in the chest film and was confirmed by the findings at autopsy.

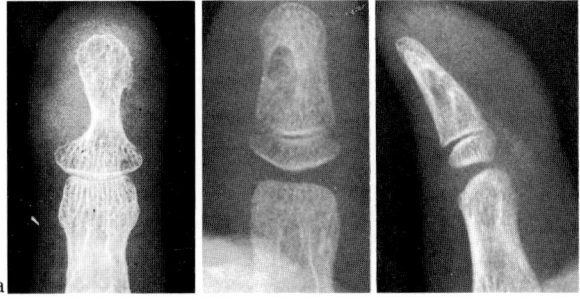

Fig. 3.1. *Glomus tumour—further examples.* **a** This 57-year-old female secretary had not used the left ring finger when typing for 30 years, because of a slowly enlarging swelling. This swelling was intermittently and acutely painful. A soft tissue mass, clearly delineated, had eroded the ulnar side of the distal phalanx. Relief was obtained by curettage, but 2 years later the tumour recurred. The histological appearance was typical. **b** This lesion, which was confirmed histologically, occurred in an 8-year-old boy, an exceptionally early age, with a typically tender swelling of the tip of the thumb. The lytic defect has a sharp endosteal margin and is associated with swelling of the soft tissues.

Some Other Lesions of Digits

In order to emphasise the difficulty in differentiating the variety of abnormalities detected radiologically, the following examples are illustrated.

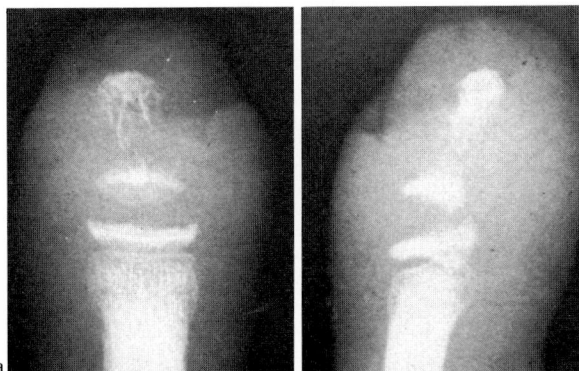

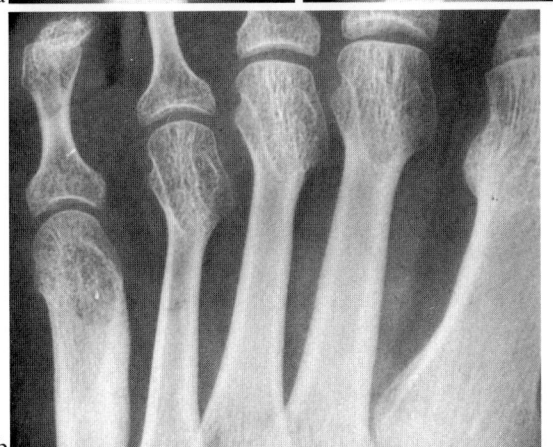

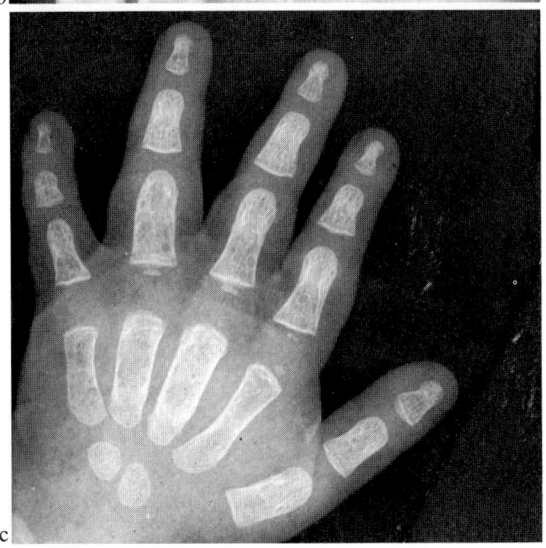

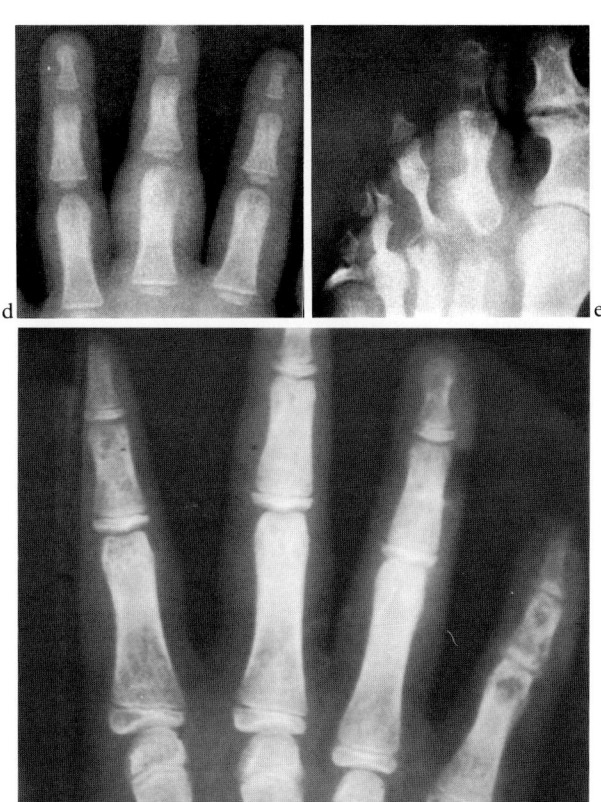

Fig. 4.1. *Infections.* **a** *Acute osteomyelitis* complicating a whitlow in a 15-year-old boy. Despite separation of the growth plate the joint has escaped involvement. Marked soft tissue swelling is present, with destruction of the shaft of the terminal phalanx (cf. Fig. 1.5 in Exercise 10). **b** *Chronic osteomyelitis* with a typical Brodie's abscess in the neck of the 5th metatarsal. An organised periosteal reaction is present. Culture showed the infecting organism to be *typhoid*. Radiological differentiation is impossible. **c** *Tuberculous dactylitis*, now very rare. Multiple expanding lytic lesions are demonstrated in varying stages of aggression and repair (see Exercise 13). **d** *Torulosis of 3rd proximal phalanx.* This destructive lesion developed in a few weeks, causing a painful and tender swelling in a 2-year-old child in Australia, where this fungus infection is well recognised. It simulates closely a tuberculous infection. **e** *Leprosy—neuropathic form* with typical destruction of the metatarso-phalangeal joints and the 1st interphalangeal joint. Secondary infection through trophic ulcers is a common complication. **f** *Leprosy—lepromatous form*, causing painful swellings of the fingers in a Chinese child. The nutrient foramina of the phalanges of the little finger are enlarged by granulation tissue, the appearance resembling sarcoidosis.

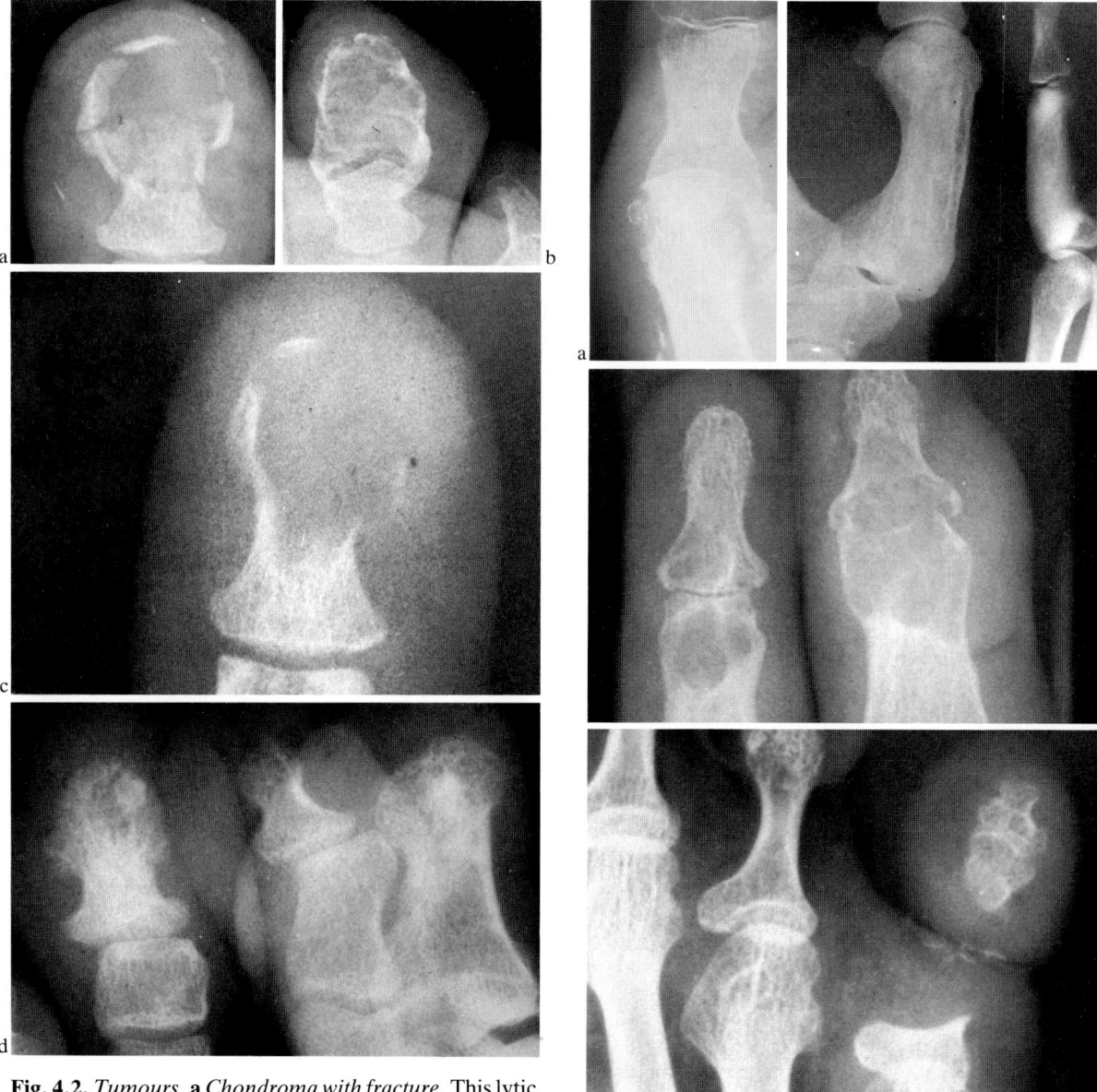

Fig. 4.2. *Tumours.* **a** *Chondroma with fracture.* This lytic expanding lesion was detected only after a mild injury in a young adult man. **b** *Chondroma* with gross expansion of the distal phalanx. **c** *Aneurysmal bone cyst* in the terminal phalanx of the index finger in a 26-year-old woman with localised pain. Histological studies established the diagnosis. (cf. Fig. 1.8a in Exercise 22) **d** *Osteoid osteoma of 3rd terminal phalanx of toe.* This 24-year-old man complained of chronic pain, attributed at first to implantation of a fragment of coral. The whole bone is enlarged and dense with a lytic area containing a classically dense nidus (cf. Fig. 1.8b in Exercise 21).

References

Cole GJ (1965) Ainhum. J Bone Joint Surg [Br] 47: 43–51

Reinhardt K (1981) Healed diabetic arthropathies. Skeletal Radiol 7: 167–172

Fig. 4.3. *Other causes.* **a** *Diabetes.* This disintegration of the 1st metatarso-phalangeal joint was found incidentally in a 55-year-old man with a painless trophic ulcer. Diabetes is the commonest cause of such neuropathies and the diagnosis is supported by premature and extensive vascular calcification. **b** *Paget's disease.* Examples, discovered incidentally, of the mixed form in a 1st metacarpal and the amorphous form in a proximal phalanx (see Exercise 8). **c** *Gout.* Two digits with characteristic tophi caused by urate deposits in an elderly man with long-established disease. Isolated lesions may cause diagnostic difficulty (cf. Fig. 1.4d in Exercise 33). **d** *Ainhum.* An example of this extraordinary entity of unknown aetiology which affects middle-aged blacks living in hot climates. Observe the soft tissue contracture, which is likely to culminate in auto-amputation of the little toe.

Q1. This 38-year-old man had complained of increasing pain in the left shoulder for a year.

On clinical examination a tender swelling was palpated on the lateral side of the proximal end of the humerus. All movements of the shoulder joint were restricted and some wasting of the muscles of the upper arm was evident.

Radiographs revealed a large osteolytic area in the head and neck of the humerus with a wide zone of transition. A periosteal reaction was evident on the lateral aspect of the neck of the humerus. Situated centrally within this osteolytic lesion a number of irregular opacities were detected. The articular surfaces of the glenohumeral joint appeared normal and this joint space was of normal width. A further zone of subchondral osteolysis, slightly loculated in appearance and having a sharply defined endosteal margin, was present in the subglenoid portion of the scapula.

A biopsy of the lesion in the humerus was performed.

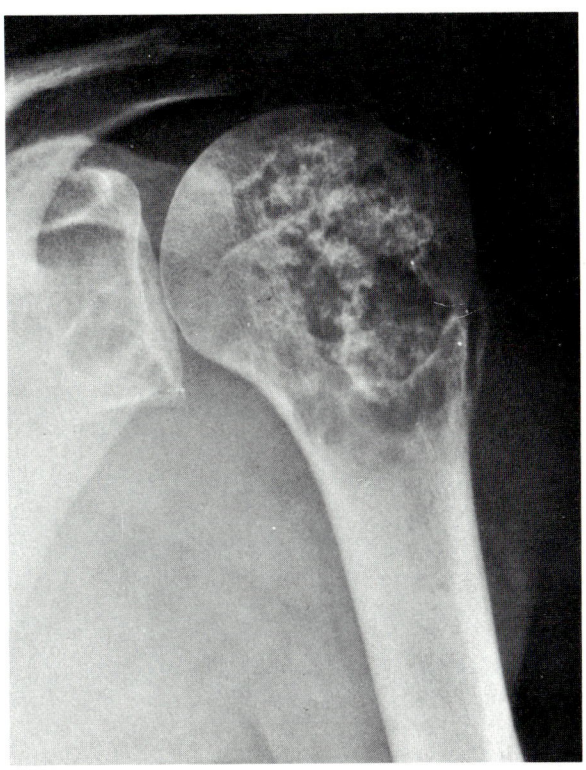

Q1a.

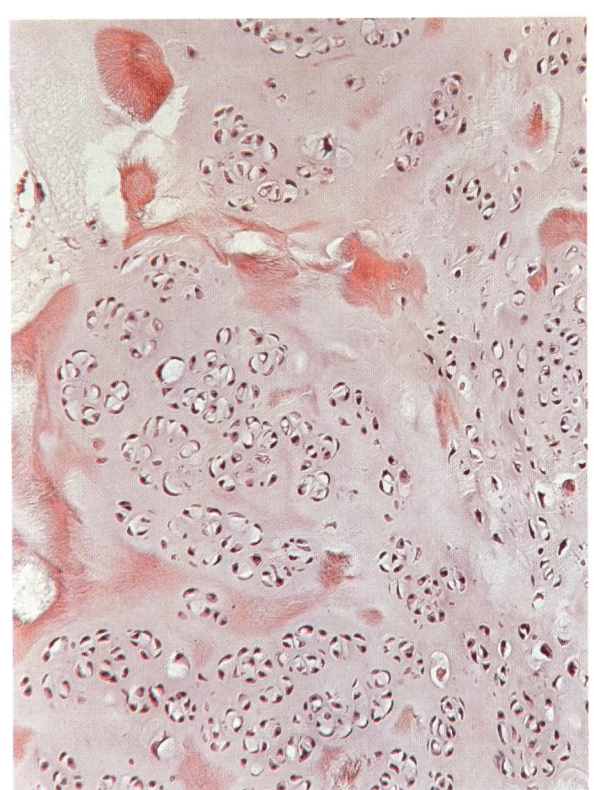

Q1b. From the central portion of the lesion. (×90)

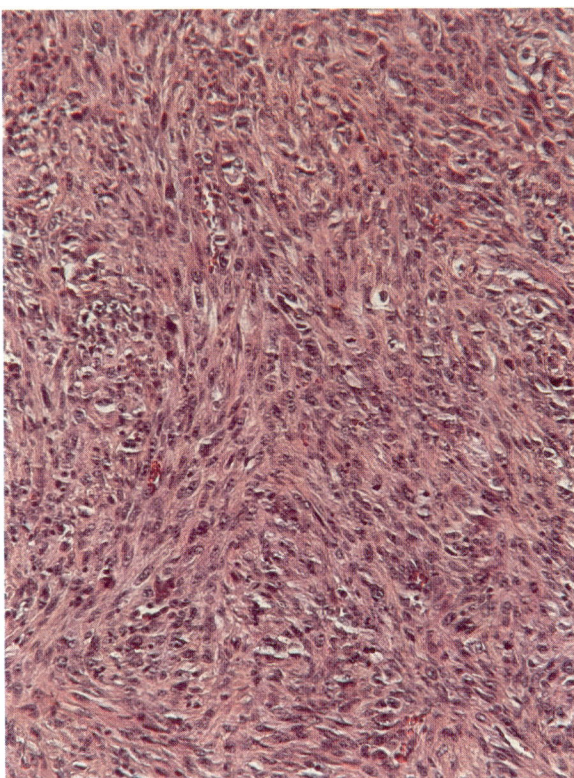

Q1c. From the peripheral portion of the lesion. (×125)

A1. Dedifferentiated chondrosarcoma of humerus

The clinical evidence of a tender swelling, coupled with radiological evidence of scattered calcification in an osteolytic lesion, strongly suggested a cartilaginous tumour. Its poorly outlined margin and the periosteal reaction on its lateral aspect indicated it to be malignant.

The lesion in the adjacent portion of the scapula raised a number of possibilities, including a similar cartilaginous focus (enchondromatosis), pigmented villonodular synovitis, a ganglion of bone or even a direct extension of the primary tumour.

The histological appearances of the lesion in the humerus confirmed this diagnosis. They established further the specific diagnosis of a dedifferentiated chondrosarcoma.

Q1b, from the central portion of the lesion, shows moderately cellular cartilaginous tissue interspersed with pink-staining areas of amorphous calcification, corresponding to the opacities evident in the radiograph. The bluish intercellular matrix and the rounded cell spaces are the features which indicate cartilage. This pattern is consistent with a low-grade chondrosarcoma. Obvious cytological evidence of malignancy is not present (cf. Q1b and c in Exercise 16).

Q1c, on the other hand, was derived from the peripheral portion of the lesion and shows an entirely different appearance. This field consists of highly cellular spindle-celled tissue, without any indication of cartilage, but with numerous pleomorphic and mitotic cells. This combination of histological features is characteristic of a 'dedifferentiated' chondrosarcoma, namely a slowly growing cartilaginous tumour which has become transformed into a rapidly growing and highly malignant neoplasm. Histologically, the aggressively malignant component of a dedifferentiated chondrosarcoma (see Exercise 16) can have the structure of a fibrosarcoma, an osteosarcoma or a malignant fibrous histiocytoma. The mildly storiform pattern of the tumour tissue in Q1c suggests the last of these possibilities.

Following biopsy, the patient was treated by a radical resection of the proximal end of the humerus and scapula (the Tikhoff-Linberg procedure). The gross appearance of the tumour is illustrated in Figures 1.1 and 1.2. Most of the tumour tissue consists of cartilage, as indicated by its nodular appearance and by the presence of scattered calcification. The dedifferentiated part of the tumour, which has extended through the cortex to form a periosteal mass, presents a totally different appearance. It demonstrates instead many of the characteristics of a malignant fibrous histiocytoma (see Exercise 29).

The incidental lesion of the scapula is a smooth-walled cyst, a so-called intra-osseous ganglion (synovial cyst: subchondral cyst) (cf. Q2c in Exercise 5).

Dedifferentiated Chondrosarcoma

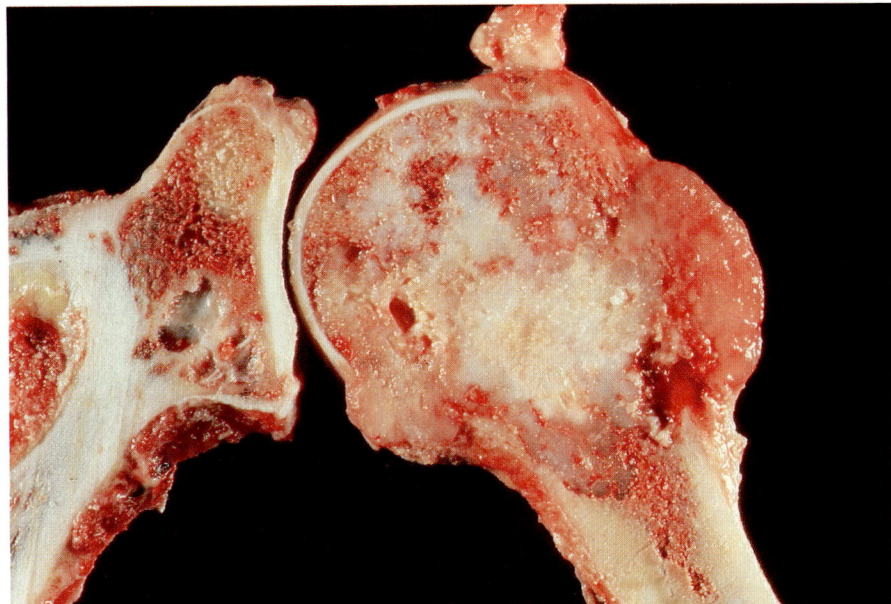

Fig. 1.1. The cut surface of the resection specimen shows that the tumour has replaced the cancellous bone of the humerus and has extended into the soft tissues medially and laterally. The medial extension was not apparent in the pre-operative radiograph. The lesion in the scapula is a cyst ('intra-osseous ganglion').

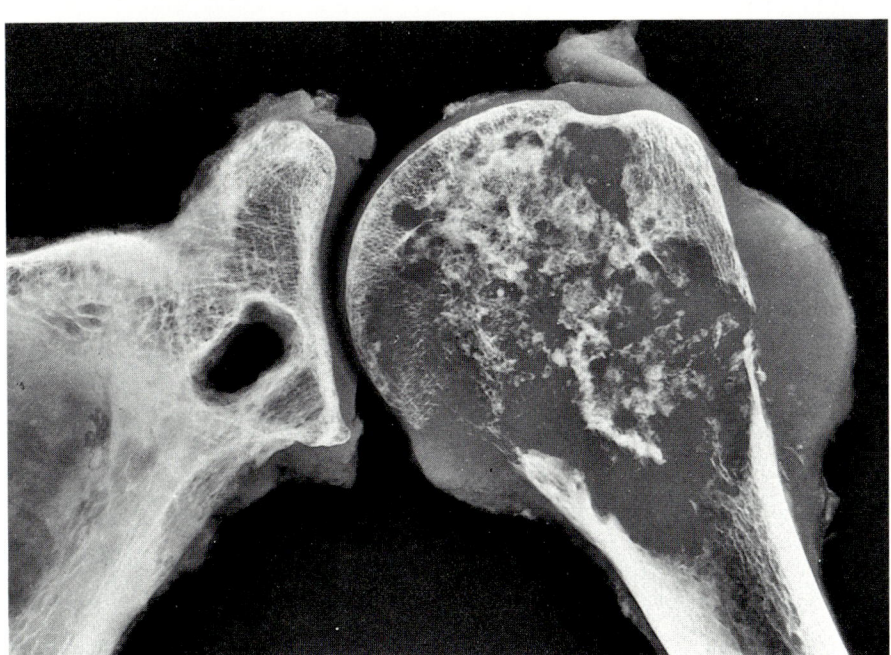

Fig. 1.2. A radiograph of a slab of tissue from the same specimen. The central portion shows the scattered areas of calcification characteristic of cartilaginous tumours.

Dedifferentiated Chondrosarcoma

Tumours of cartilage sometimes undergo conversion to a more malignant and more rapidly growing type of neoplasm. These 'dedifferentiated chondrosarcomas', which amount to about 10% of all chondrosarcomas, occur in rather older patients than ordinary chondrosarcomas and have a decidedly worse prognosis. In reported series, some of the cases have the histological structure of osteosarcomas, while others are fibrosarcomas or malignant fibrous histiocytomas. Most of these tumours occur in individuals over 50 years of age. Like other chondrosarcomas, they usually involve the proximal bones of the limbs, the pelvis, the scapula and the axial skeleton. Irrespective of treatment, most patients die from early metastatic spread to the lungs.

References

Bauer TW, Dorfman HD (1982) Intraosseous ganglion. A clinicopathologic study of 11 cases. Am J Surg Pathol 6: 207–213

Dahlin DC, Beabout JW (1971) Dedifferentiation of low-grade chondrosarcomas. Cancer 28: 461–466

Linberg BE (1928) Interscapulo-thoracic resection for malignant tumour of the shoulder joint region. J Bone Joint Surg 10: 344–349

McCarthy EF, Dorfman HD (1982) Chondrosarcoma of bone with dedifferentiation. A study of 18 cases. Human Pathol 13: 36–40

Exercise 42

Q1. This 39-year-old woman complained of a painful swelling on the lateral side of the right thigh, just above the knee.

This swelling had been present for 4 months and was found clinically to be firm, slightly tender and warm. The patient had a history of hypertension and diabetes for 7 years.

Radiological examination disclosed the presence of symmetrical and abnormal densities with serpiginous margins in the medullary cavities in the distal end of each femur. Similar densities were detected in the proximal end of each tibia. In addition, however, the lateral cortex of the right femur, at the site of the swelling, had been breached by a poorly defined area of destruction which extended to the edge of the medullary lesion and which had provoked a periosteal reaction.

A biopsy was performed.

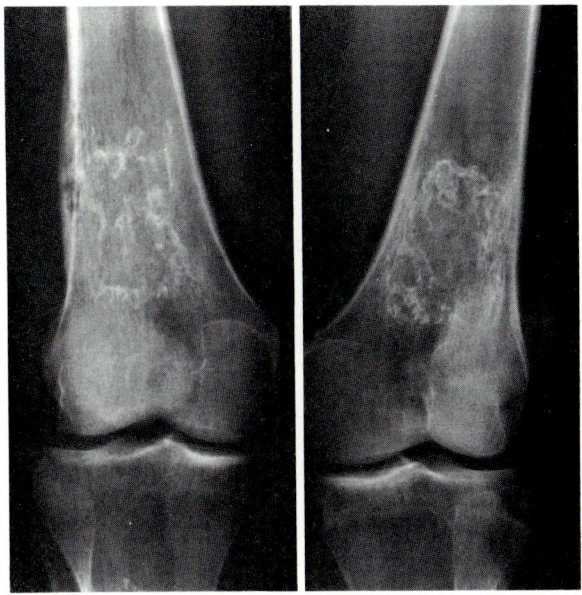

Q1a.

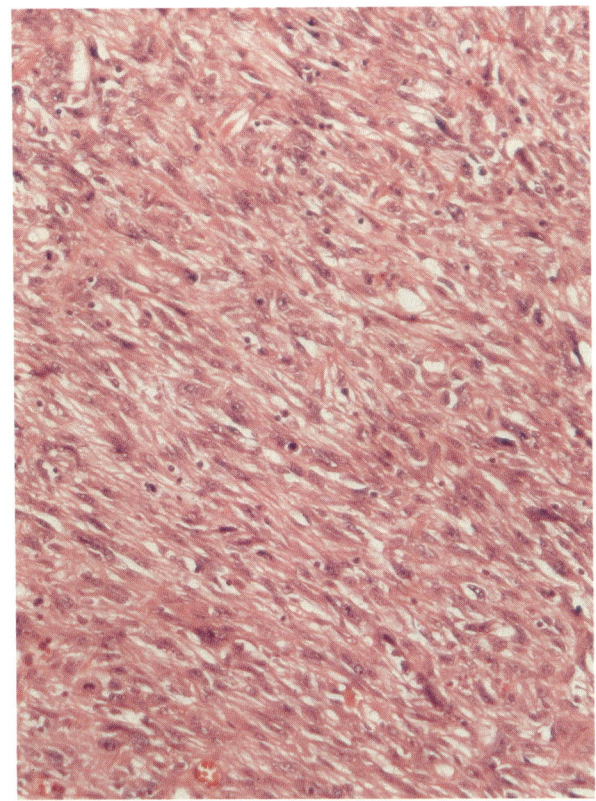

Q1b. (×145)

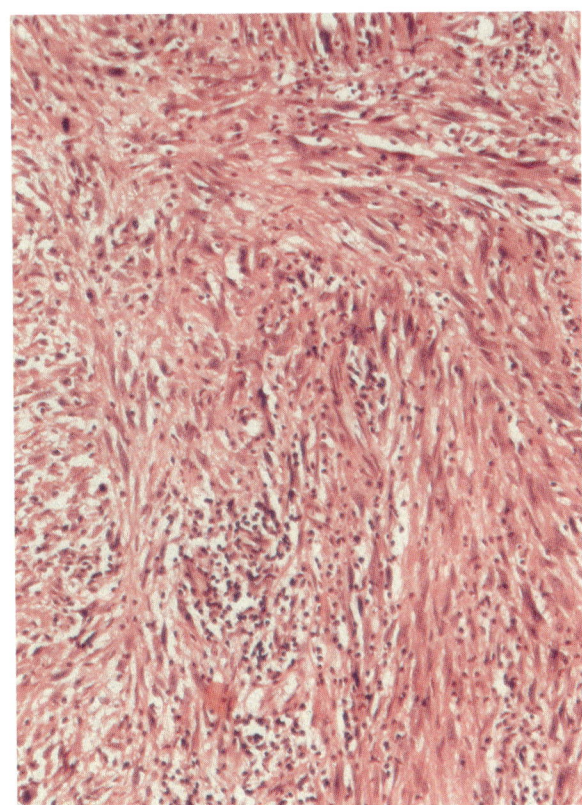

Q1c. (×145)

A1. Malignant fibrous histiocytoma arising in relation to a bone infarct

Interpretation of the original films of the right knee alone had suggested a malignant tumour complicating an enchondroma, but the subsequent demonstration of the other symmetrical abnormalities clearly indicated these lesions to be infarcts (see Exercise 7). The pattern of peripheral calcifications around areas of necrotic bone is typical. An enchondroma usually shows more irregular and central calcification. Such lesions, moreover, even when multiple, are rarely symmetrical (see Exercise 12). The development of a malignant tumour in relation to a bone infarct, although rare, is a well-recognised complication and this diagnosis was proposed.

The biopsy (Q1b and c) confirmed the diagnosis of a malignant tumour. It consists of pleomorphic spindle-celled tissue with some intercellular collagen. In some areas (Q1c) the tumour tissue is arranged in a storiform pattern of interweaving bundles and shows infiltration by lymphocytes. The tumour has, in fact, the histological features of a malignant fibrous histiocytoma. In addition to fibroblastic cells, it contains rounded histiocytic cells. In other areas the histiocytic nature of these cells was shown by their phagocytosis of haemosiderin pigment (see Exercise 29).

No tissue from the underlying bone infarct was included in the biopsy, but this part of the lesion, and its anatomical relation to the malignant tumour, can be seen in the photograph (Fig. 1.1) and the slab radiograph (Fig. 1.2) from the amputation specimen. The infarct appears as a white opaque area in the cancellous bone of the femoral metaphysis. Adjacent to it, and extending through the overlying cortex to produce a large soft tissue mass, is the malignant tumour. The dark area of haemorrhage towards the upper part of the specimen indicates the site of the biopsy.

Figures 1.3 and 1.4 illustrate the histological features of the infarct. Figure 1.3 shows necrotic bone trabeculae surrounded by poorly cellular fibrous tissue which is undergoing calcification. This calcification is evident in the slab radiograph (Fig. 1.2) and is responsible for the distinctive radiological appearance of the lesion in Q1a. Figure 1.4 shows the appearance of the necrotic bone, with empty osteocyte lacunae, and also includes an area of calcification beginning in the adjacent fibrous tissue.

As already indicated, the tumour was treated by amputation. The patient died 2 months later, with evidence of widespread metastases. In this case, the cause of the multiple bone infarcts, presumably present for a long time without symptoms, is not known. None of the usual factors which are known to predispose to bone infarcts (alcoholism, steroid therapy, hyperbaric exposure, sickle cell trait) were present.

Bone Tumours Associated with Infarcts

Quite a number of cases are now on record where a malignant bone tumour has originated in the neighbourhood of a bone infarct. This does not appear to be the result of chance, and it is generally accepted that the tumours have had their origin in the reparative tissue which develops in and around the area of infarction. A further point of interest is that most of the tumours have been diagnosed as malignant fibrous histiocytomas, although some have been described as fibrosarcomas or osteosarcomas.

References

Galli SJ, Weintraub HP, Proppe KH (1978) Malignant fibrous histiocytoma and pleomorphic sarcoma in association with medullary bone infarcts. Cancer 41: 607–619

Mirra JM, Bullough PG, Marcove RC, Jacobs B, Huvos AG (1974) Malignant fibrous histiocytoma and osteosarcoma in association with bone infarcts. J Bone Jt Surg 56A: 932–940

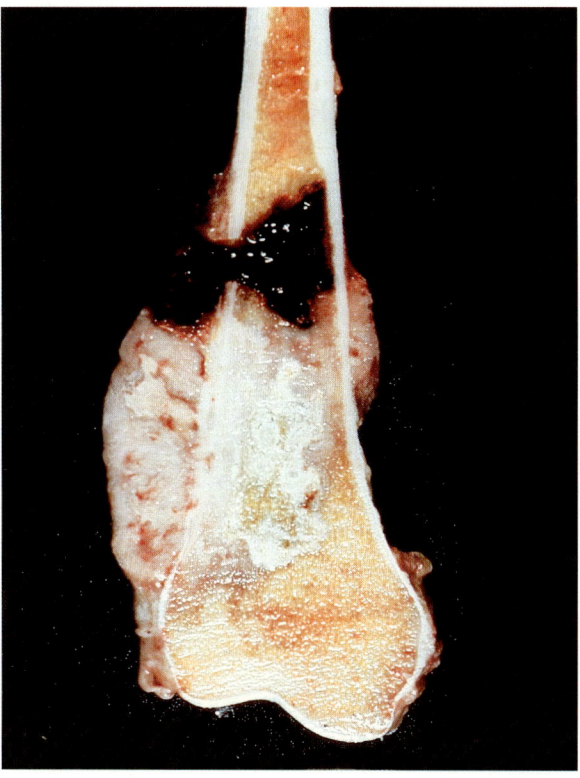

Fig. 1.1. Photograph of longitudinally divided specimen, showing central area of bone infarction, with adjacent tumour.

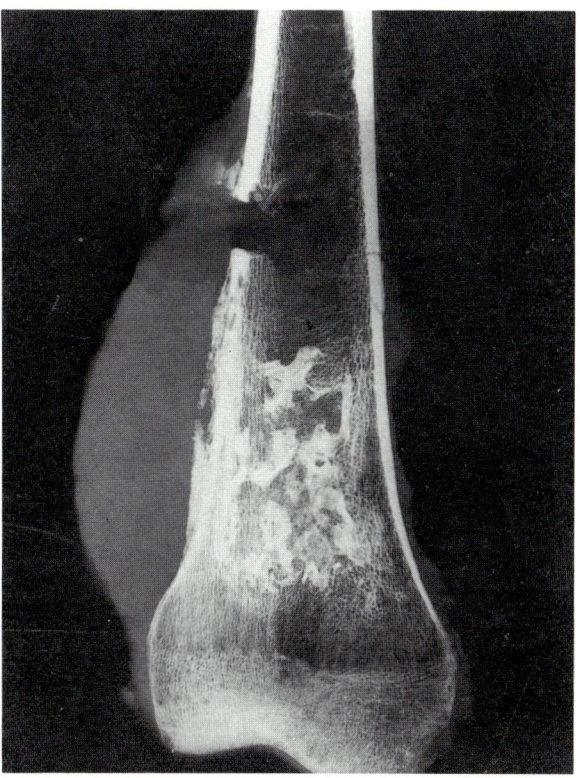

Fig. 1.2. Radiograph of a slice of tissue from the surface of the specimen shown in Fig. 1.1. Note the patchy calcification in the area of infarction, the periosteal reaction and the subperiosteal tumour mass.

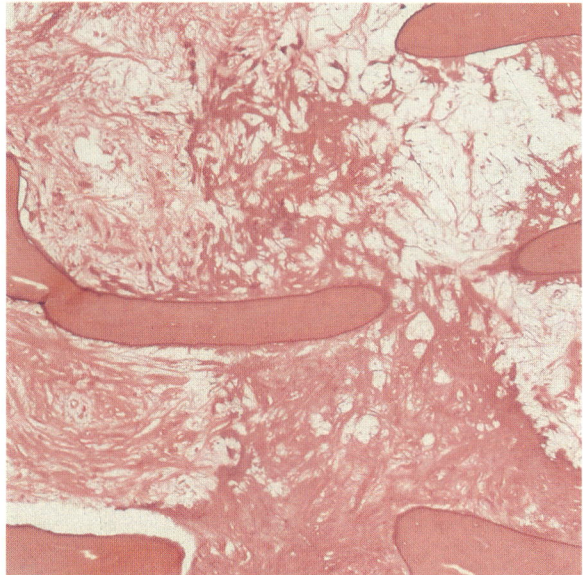

Fig. 1.3. The appearance of the area of infarction. The bone trabeculae are necrotic: the marrow spaces are occupied by poorly cellular fibrous tissue, some of which is heavily calcified, as indicated by its darker staining. (×58)

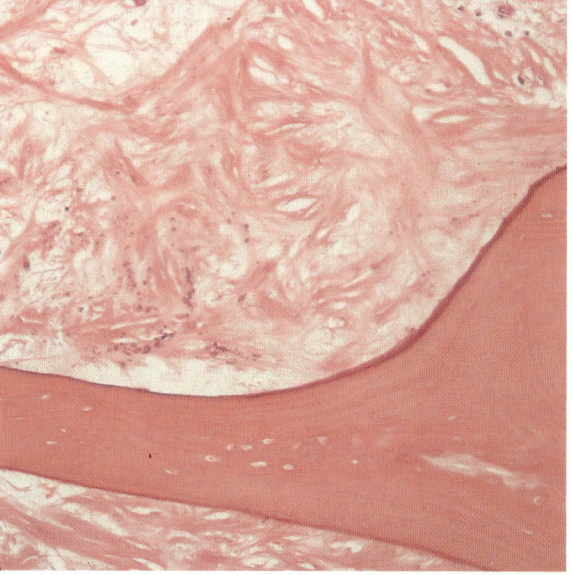

Fig. 1.4. At a higher degree of magnification, the empty osteocyte lacunae of the necrotic bone trabeculae can be identified. Granular basophilic material indicates early calcification of the fibrous tissue. (×117)

Q1. This 11-year-old boy presented with a painless and hard swelling of the left shin, which had been observed only recently.

Clinical examination revealed no other abnormality.

Radiological examination showed an expanded area of sclerosis within the anterior cortex which contained numerous lucencies. This lesion had a well-defined endosteal margin and had encroached on and narrowed the medullary cavity. The posterior cortex in this portion of the tibia was unusually thick.

Partial excision was performed.

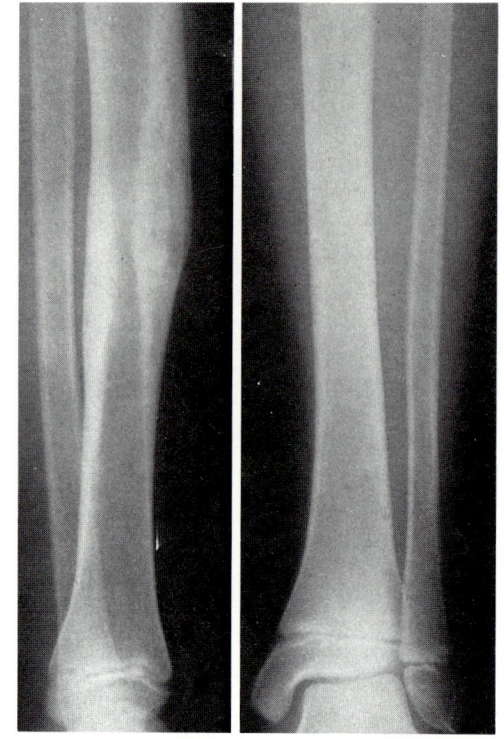

Q1a.

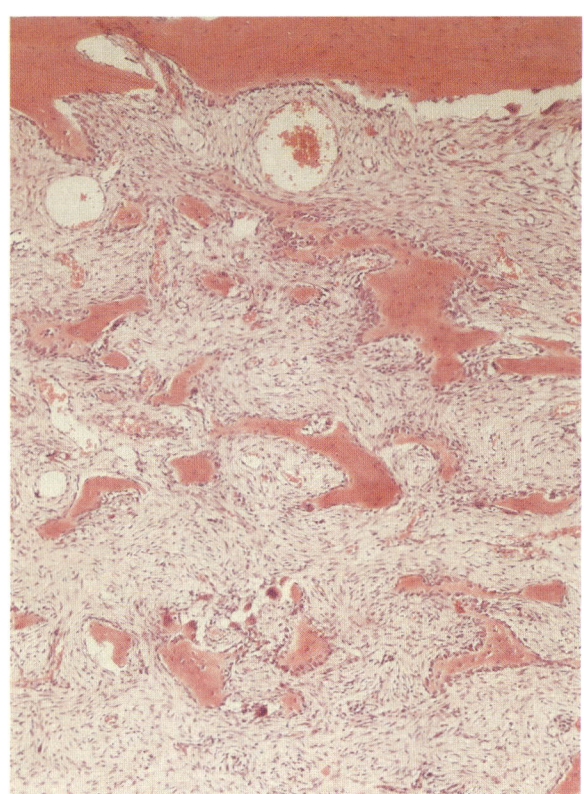

Q1b. (×53)

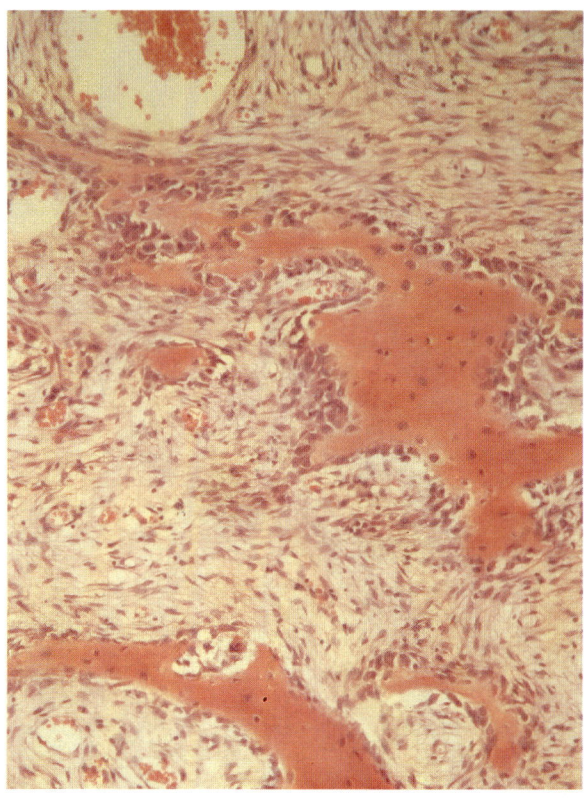

Q1c. (×53)

Q2. This 7-year-old boy presented because of pain in the right wrist following a fall.

On clinical examination the right forearm was shortened and bowed medially. Acute tenderness was elicited on pressure over the distal end of the ulna.

On radiological examination the clinical deformity was shown to be associated with a sharply defined osteolytic lesion in the distal end of the ulna. Punctate densities were evident within this area. The overlying cortex had been thinned and expanded. An oblique undisplaced fracture was present.

The distal end of the ulna was excised.

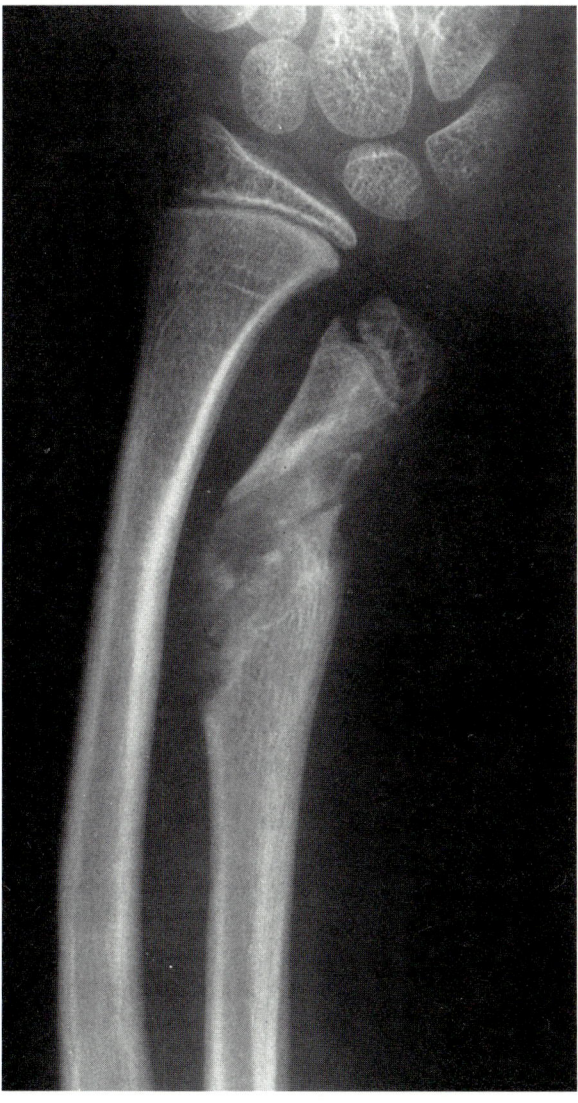

Q2a.

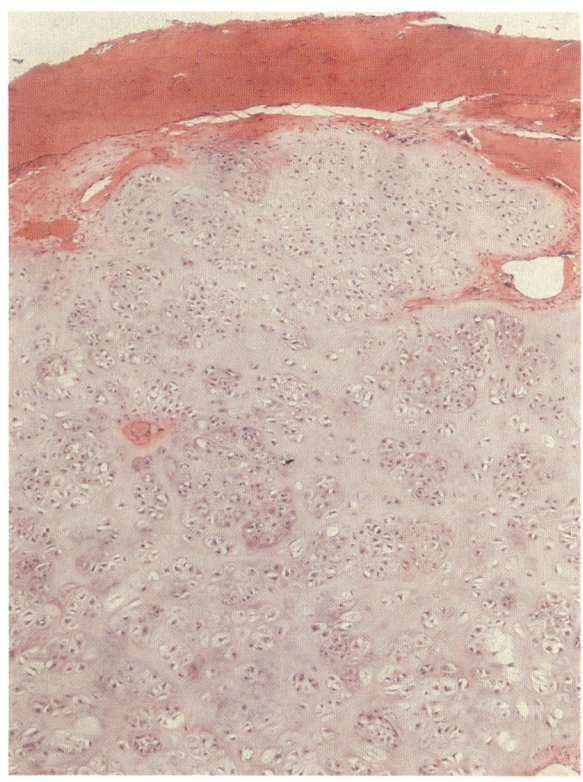

Q2b. (×45)

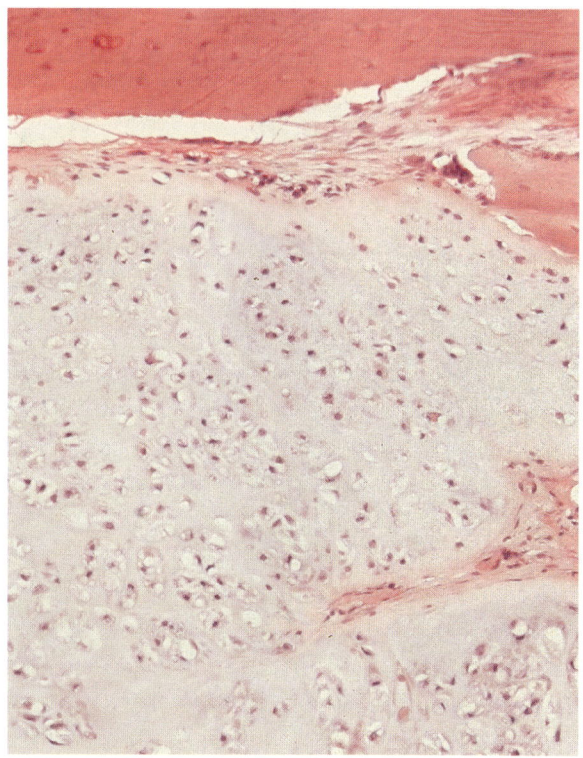

Q2c. (×120)

A1. Osteofibrous dysplasia of tibia

The pre-operative diagnosis, based primarily on the radiological appearance, was fibrous dysplasia (cf. Fig. 1.3a, Exercise 1). Nevertheless, the operation was undertaken to exclude the possibility of an adamantinoma (see Exercise 27), a diagnosis unlikely at this age.

Gross examination of the resected specimen showed that the thickened cortical bone indeed contained confluent pockets of fibrous tissue. Histologically, the fibrous tissue contains trabeculae of woven bone (Q1b and c), but in contrast to typical fibrous dysplasia these structures are covered by layers of prominent osteoblasts.

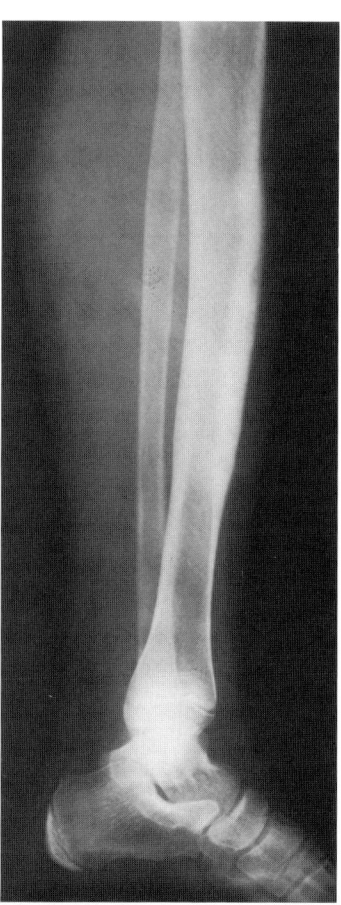

Fig. 1.1. *Osteofibrous dysplasia.* Two years later the lesion had regressed, leaving only some residual sclerosis—a finding characteristic of this entity and entirely unlike fibrous dysplasia.

Osteofibrous Dysplasia

This term has been suggested recently for a group of lesions, all very similar to the present case, which were regarded previously as fibrous dysplasia (see Exercise 1). The same type of abnormality has been reported also as 'ossifying fibroma'. The term osteofibrous dysplasia, however, is preferred because of the general similarity of the lesions to fibrous dysplasia.

The lesions in question almost invariably involve the tibia, particulary the middle third, although in a few cases the fibula has been affected. The condition is detected usually at birth or in early childhood. A slight male preponderance has been observed .

Clinical Features

A hard swelling, usually painless, is palpated easily. The bone may be bowed slightly, particularly in an antero-lateral direction. In about a third of cases attention to the abnormality is drawn by the pain of a pathological fracture, either complete or incomplete. These fractures almost invariably repair rapidly, unlike those in neurofibromatosis (cf. Fig. 1.12 in Exercise 28).

Pseudarthrosis of the tibia is most exceptional. Unlike classical fibrous dysplasia, in which the lesions are usually recognised later in childhood, spontaneous regression may be expected in the course of a few years.

Radiological Features

1. Site. Tibia and, rarely, fibula; occasionally both bones.

2. Appearance. Mixed areas of sclerosis and lucency are evident, primarily involving the anterior cortex and extending into and narrowing the medullary cavity. (Contrast the medullary location of classical fibrous dysplasia.) Normal bone architecture is restored in serial studies, but bowing deformities may persist.

Pathological Features

The lesions consist of fibrous tissue containing trabeculae of woven bone which are covered by osteoblasts. The fibrous tissue is relatively mature and may have a whorled storiform pattern reminiscent of fibrous histiocytoma (see Exercise 29). Multinucleate giant cells may be present, probably related to haemorrhage and resorption of bone.

Treatment

If the diagnosis on radiological grounds can be made with reasonable confidence, surgical intervention should be avoided if possible. Pathological fractures usually respond well to immobilisation in plaster. On the other hand, very large lesions, even in early childhood, may require curettage or resection, with or without grafting, but such procedures have a tendency to be followed by recurrence. Osteotomy to correct a residual curvature may be indicated after growth is complete.

References

Campanacci M, Laus M (1981) Osteofibrous dysplasia of the tibia and fibula. J Bone Jt Surg 63A: 367–375

Campbell CJ, Hawk T (1982) A variant of fibrous dysplasia (osteofibrous dysplasia). J Bone Jt Surg 64A: 231–236

Kempson RL (1966) Ossifying fibroma of the long bones. Arch Pathol. 82: 213–233

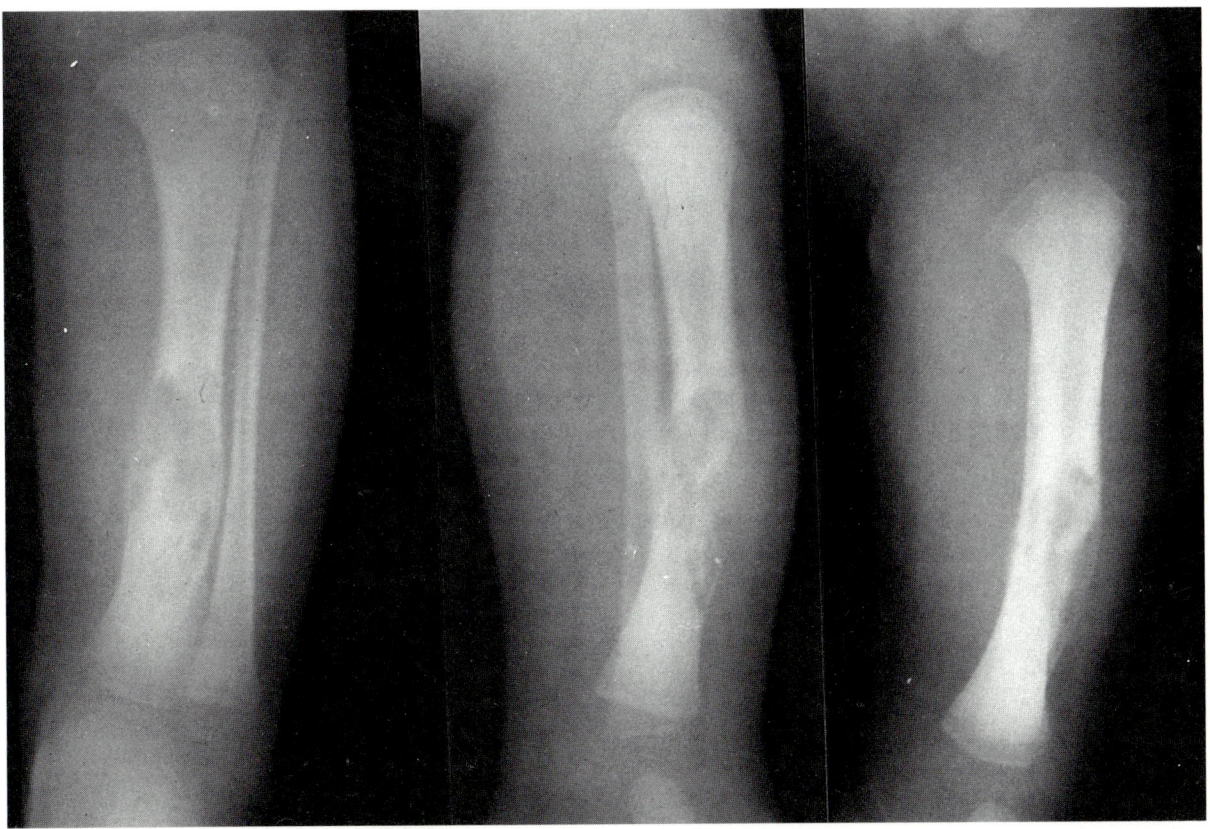

Fig. 1.2. *Osteofibrous dysplasia*. In this 9-day-old female infant a prominent swelling of the left leg was observed. It was obviously tender. The expanding lytic lesion in the tibia was regarded radiologically and, initially histologically, as fibrous dysplasia. Subsequent review of the sections altered the diagnosis. The lesion was curetted, but a recurrence a year later required repetition of the procedure. Thereafter a normal texture developed with only slight residual anterior bowing of the tibia. No further recurrence had taken place at the age of 9 years.

A2. Multiple enchondromas (dyschondroplasia; Ollier's disease)

The deformity of the forearm had caused clinical suspicion of a developmental abnormality. On demonstration of the lytic lesion, which had all the radiological characteristics of an enchondroma, a skeletal survey was carried out and other typical chondromas were found in the right humerus, left ulna, ribs, pelvis and the phalanges of the toes. The diagnosis of multiple enchondromata was thus established. Of interest was the presence of a soft tissue swelling in the right axilla. This was biopsied and found to be a haemangioma, but radiological examination had not shown any associated phleboliths. The combination of multiple enchondromata and soft tissue haemangioma constitutes Maffucci's syndrome (see Exercise 12).

Histologically, the excision specimen (Q2b and c) showed expansion of the cortex by a mass of cartilaginous tissue. The moderate cellularity of this tissue is consistent with a diagnosis of enchondromatosis (see Exercise 12). The cellular pleomorphism and mitotic activity that would be expected in a chondrosarcoma (see Exercise 16) are lacking.

Q1. This 29-year-old man had complained of mild pain in the left groin for 4 years. During recent months the pain had been accentuated by exercise.

Clinical examination failed to reveal any significant abnormality. Movement of the left hip was full and unrestricted.

Radiological examination disclosed extensive and confluent areas of osteolysis involving the left superior and inferior pubic rami. The medial portion of the superior pubic ramus had undergone significant attenuation. Minimal sclerotic reaction was evident in relation to the osteolytic areas.

A biopsy was performed.

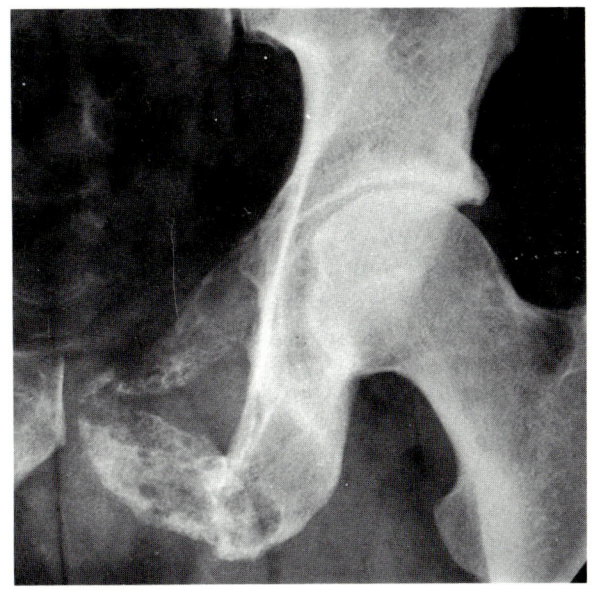

Q1a.

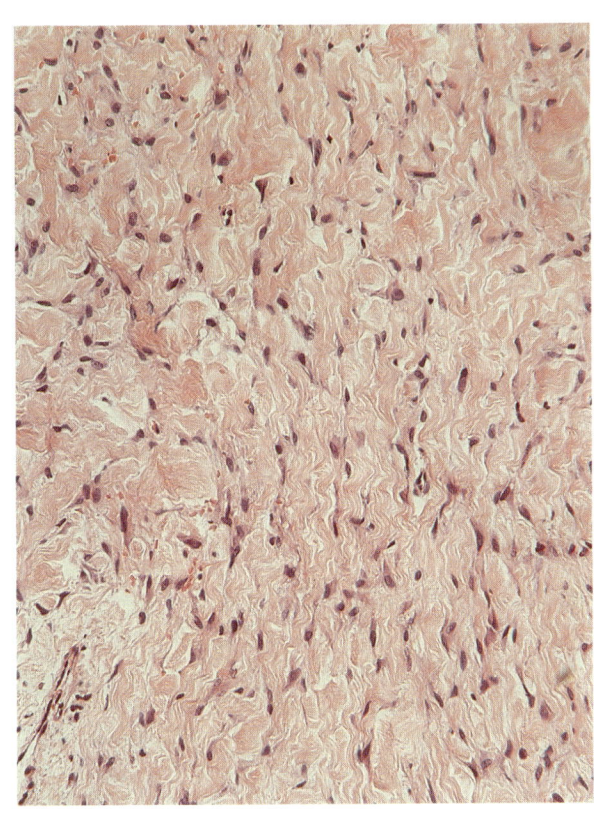

Q1b. (×150)

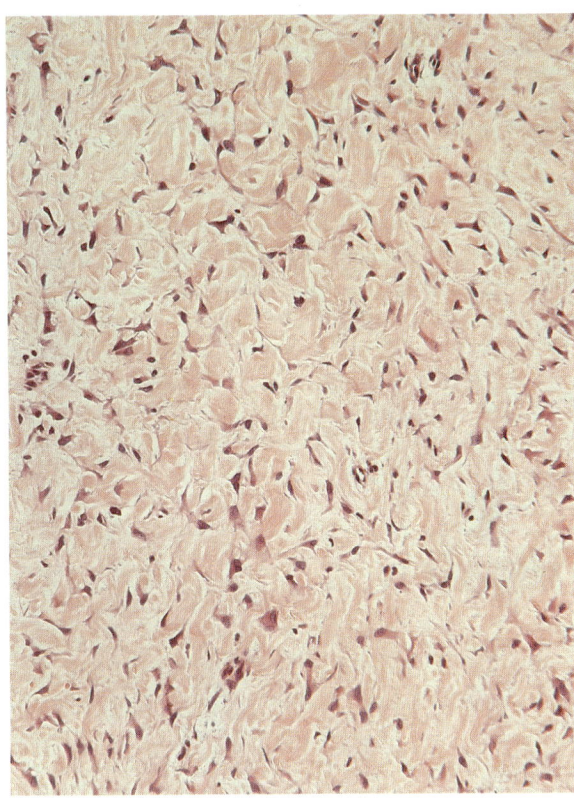

Q1c. (×150)

A1. Desmoplastic fibroma of pubis and ischium

Although the clinical findings had not given rise to anxiety, the radiological appearance of the lesion caused considerable concern. The aggressive appearances of the large destructive lesion raised a number of different diagnostic possibilities. Pre-operatively, a malignant tumour, possibly fibrosarcoma (see Exercise 29) or malignant round cell tumour (see Exercise 31), was favoured strongly. Less sinister suggestions had included fibrous dysplasia (see Exercise 1) and haemangiomatosis (see Exercise 40).

Histologically, material from the biopsy (Q1b and c) shows poorly cellular fibrous tissue characterised by regular bundles of collagen fibres and mature spindle-shaped cells. These are the features of the benign bone tumour known as desmoplastic fibroma.

Following biopsy, the lesion was treated by local resection. The patient was alive and well, without evidence of recurrence or metastasis, 6 years later.

Desmoplastic Fibroma of Bone

Desmoplastic fibroma of bone is an extremely rare type of skeletal neoplasm, encountered very occasionally in children and young adults. Malignant transformation has not been reported. The importance of recognising this entity lies in its differentiation, almost entirely on histological grounds, from other fibrous lesions of bone, both benign and malignant.

Clinical Features

Mild pain and localised tenderness, often of several months' or years' duration, are the usual presenting complaints. No specific abnormalities are detected clinically, but a pathological fracture through an area of weakened bone may draw attention to this lesion.

Radiological Features

1. Site. The small number of cases which have been reported in the literature indicate a number of flat bones to have been affected, including particularly the pelvis, scapula and clavicle, but a predilection has been recognised for the ends of long bones.

2. Appearance. The lesions are eventually destructive and expansile, the lucent areas frequently being interspersed with bony strands resembling exceptionally coarse trabeculae. The resulting appearance may simulate a particularly aggressive focus of fibrous dysplasia or, more commonly, as indicated in A1, a malignant neoplasm.

Pathological Features

The histological appearance of this unusual tumour bears a distinct resemblance to certain neoplastic processes in skin and soft tissue—desmoid tumours and certain varieties of fibromatosis—which are outside the scope of this work. Poorly cellular fibrous tissue consisting of bundles of collagen fibres and mature spindle-shaped cells is typical. This pattern, particularly in a biopsy sample which is limited, may make differentiation from other fibrous lesions, especially a low-grade fibrosarcoma, difficult. It has been suggested, indeed, that misinterpretations of this type may have been responsible for unusually long-term survivals in patients in whom fibrosarcoma has been diagnosed. Unlike malignant fibrous histiocytoma, which has been described in Exercise 29, sections of desmoplastic fibroma do not show the storiform appearance encountered in that entity and in non-ossifying fibroma of bone (see Exercise 6).

Treatment

Thorough curettage and packing with bone chips is the minimum required, since recurrences are common when removal is incomplete. Total excision, when practicable, is desirable.

References

Jaffe HL (1958) Tumors and tumorous conditions of the bones and joints. Lea and Febiger, Philadelphia
Rabhan WN, Rosai J (1968) Desmoplastic fibroma. J Bone Jt Surg 50A:487–502
Whitesides TE, Ackerman LV (1960) Desmoplastic fibroma. A report of 3 cases. J Bone Jt Surg 42A: 1143–1150

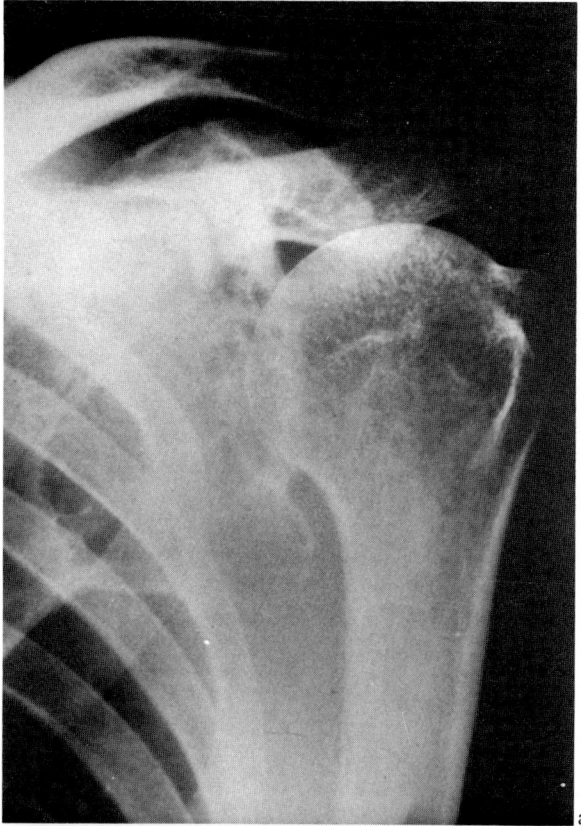

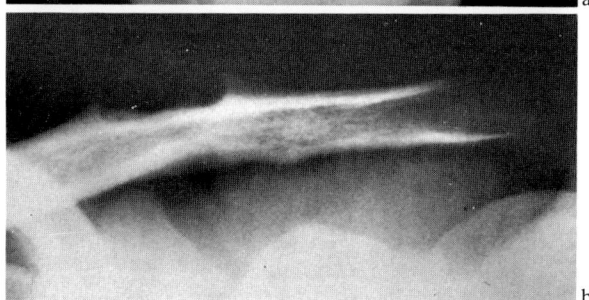

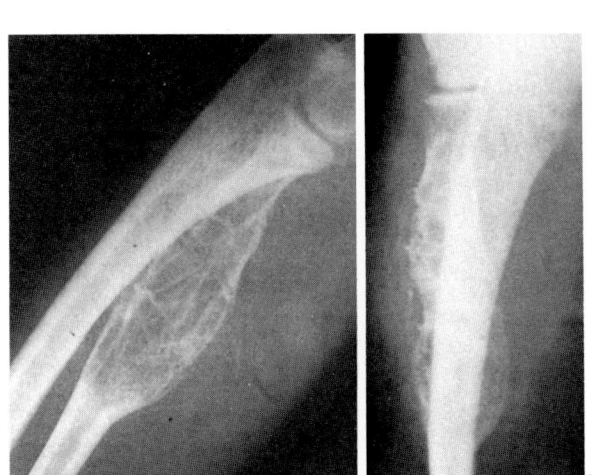

Fig. 1.1. *Desmoplastic fibroma of bone. Radius.* This lesion in the proximal end of this long bone had caused localised pain for only 3 months in this 19-year-old man. The coarse trabeculation within the expanded segment of the radius simulated an unusual fibrous lesion or even a haemangioma (see Exercise 34).

Fig. 1.2. *Desmoplastic fibroma of bone—flat bones.* **a** *Scapula.* This expansile lytic lesion in the subglenoid portion of the scapula was found in a 31-year-old man who had developed pain in the left shoulder for several months. The pain was accentuated by his occupation as a jazz drummer. Observe the resemblance to fibrous dysplasia and to an aneurysmal bone cyst (compare Fig. 1.5a in Exercise 22). **b** *Clavicle.* This 16-year-old boy had observed a painless swelling to develop over the left clavicle. An irregular texture of the mid-shaft of the bone was associated with an area of expansion which again appeared to be cystic. Solid tissue only was encountered on biopsy.

The remaining Exercises illustrate diagnostic
problems of particular interest.
Reference to each of the problems concerned
has been made already in the preceding
pages of this book.

Exercise 45

Q1. This 32-year-old man complained of chronic pain in the back which had become increasingly severe during the previous 4 years.

On clinical examination a mild kyphos was observed in the upper lumbar area. Minor neurological deficits were elicited, including impaired dorsiflexion of the feet.

The radiographs showed marked density and deformity of the body of L1, with some flattening and anterior protrusion. Myelography was normal.

Laminectomy was performed.

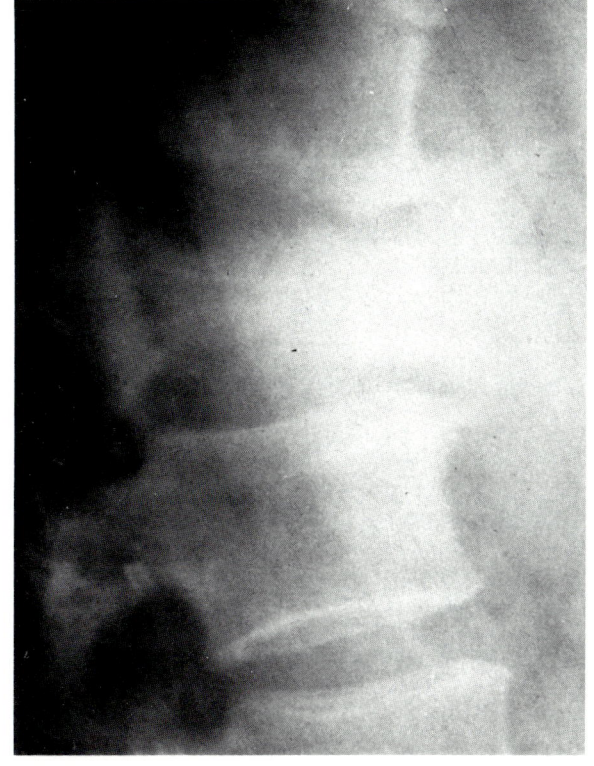

Q1a.

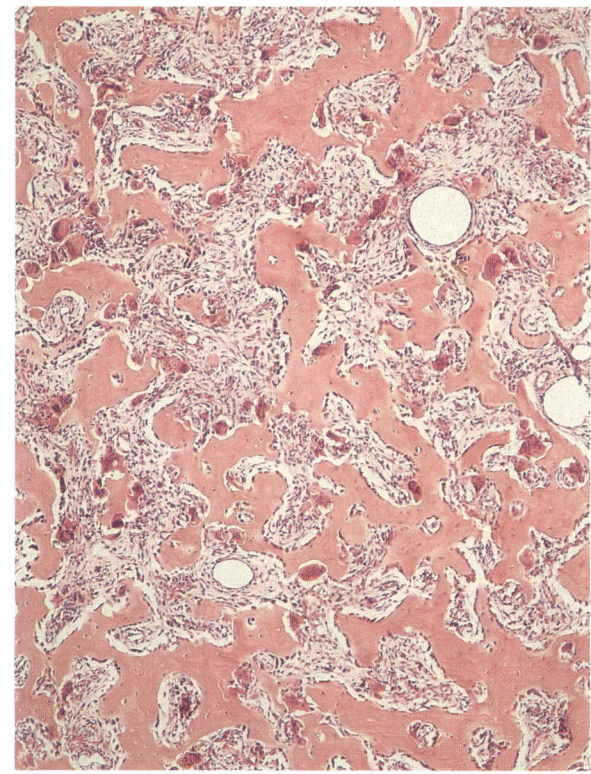

Q1b. (×50)

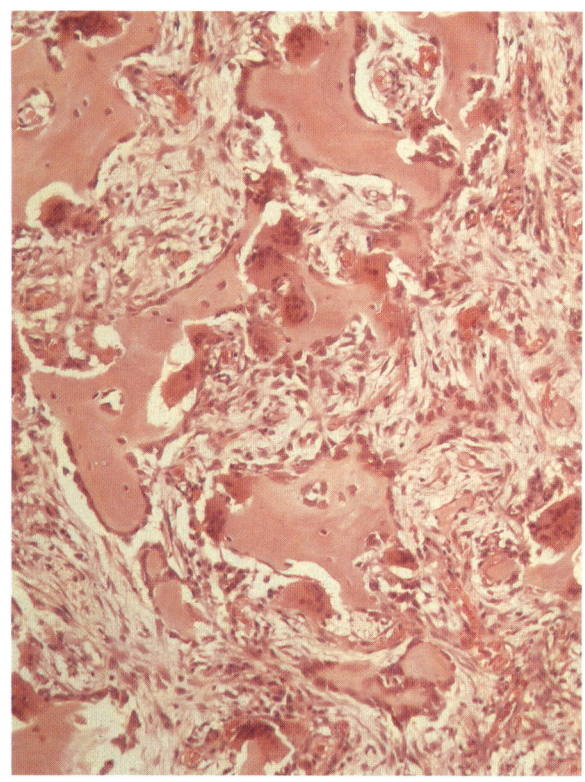

Q1c. (×120)

A1. Paget's disease of L1

This extremely unusual case is presented to emphasise some rare aspects of this common disease. The recognition of the disorder under the age of 40 years is itself so unusual that this diagnosis would be unlikely even to be considered radiologically. The biochemical investigations were helpful, in that the serum calcium (10.0 mg%; 2.5 mmol/litre) and the serum phosphate (3.1 mg%; 1.0 mmol/litre) were normal, whereas the alkaline phosphatase was significantly elevated (58 KA units; 420 IU/litre).

At operation, part of the affected vertebral body was resected. The histological sections show evidence of intensely active bone remodelling (Q1b and c). The normal cancellous bone is replaced by a close network of bone trabeculae, the surfaces of which are covered by active osteoclasts and osteoblasts. Vascular fibrous tissue occupies the marrow spaces.

These changes are not specific for Paget's disease and could, for example, be encountered in hyperparathyroidism (see Exercise 23). In conjunction with the clinical and radiological findings, however, they point strongly to Paget's disease. The more specific histological feature of this condition, the 'mosaic' pattern of cement lines (see Exercise 8), can be found elsewhere in the specimen (Fig. 1.1). The trabeculae in Q1b and c are newly formed structures which have not yet undergone sufficient remodelling to show the typical histological pattern of the disease.

The subsequent history of this patient, who was affected by Paget's disease at such an exceptionally early age, is of interest. The neurological symptoms resolved after the laminectomy and pain was relieved by calcitonin therapy. Six years later the patient suffered a compression fracture of L1 with neurological complications following a fall. Calcitonin therapy then was ineffective but diphosphonate treatment produced a good response. Ten years later more widespread disease was shown radiologically.

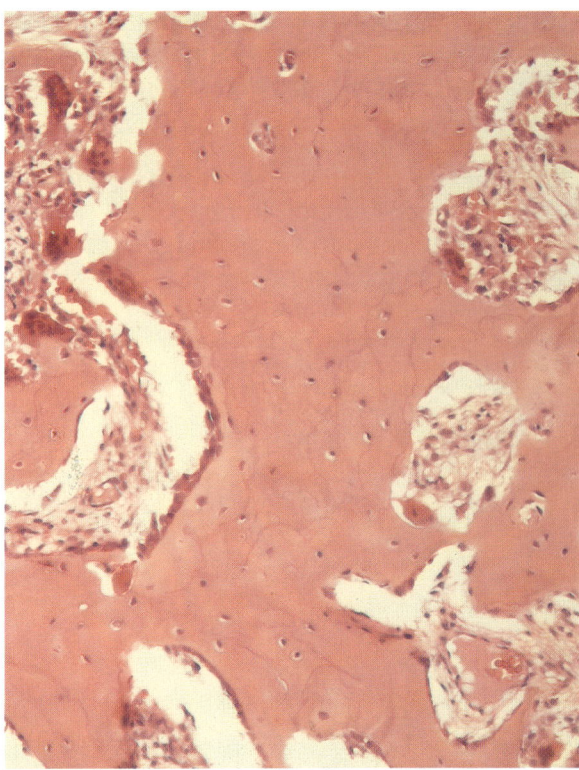

Fig. 1.1. A thicker bone trabecula, from the same specimen, shows the 'mosaic' pattern of cement lines, which indicates earlier osteoclastic and osteoblastic remodelling and which establishes conclusively the diagnosis of Paget's disease. (×144)

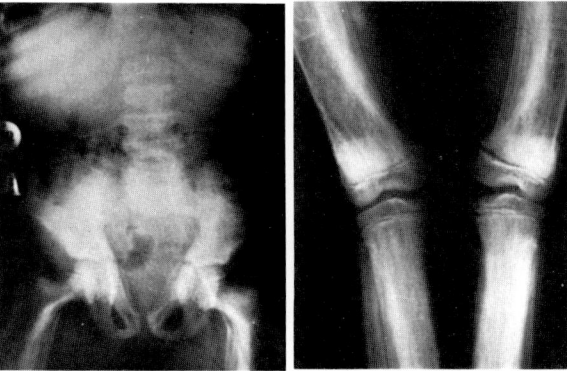

Fig. 1.2. *Hyperphosphatasia.* This rare and unique familial disorder deserves mention at this point since the radiological findings may cause confusion with Paget's disease. Clinically, bowing deformities and enlargement of long bones occur early in life and are accompanied by pain and muscular weakness. Alkaline phosphatase values are very greatly increased. Pathologically, primitive fibrous bone fails to mature into compact bone. A classical 'mosaic' pattern of cement lines is not present. Radiologically the bones are thickened with a coarse pattern simulating the spongy texture of active Paget's disease. Nevertheless, importantly, the epiphyses are not affected. This case illustrates severe changes of this type in a young child. All the bones, with the exception of the epiphyses, are affected. The long bones are widened in diameter. Lateral bowing of the femora and a trifoliate pelvis reflect the generalised bone softening. The alkaline phosphatase level was extremely elevated—920 KA units.

References

Caffey J (1972) Familial hyperphosphatasemia with ateliosis and hypermetabolism of growing membranous bone: Review of the clinical, radiographic and chemical features. Bull Hosp Joint Dis 33: 81–110

Lancu TC, Almagor G, Friedman E, Hardoff R, Front S (1978) Chronic familial hyperphosphatasemia. Radiology 129: 669–676

Murray RO, Jacobson HG (1977) In: Radiology of skeletal disorders, 2nd edn. Churchill Livingstone, Edinburgh, p 1056

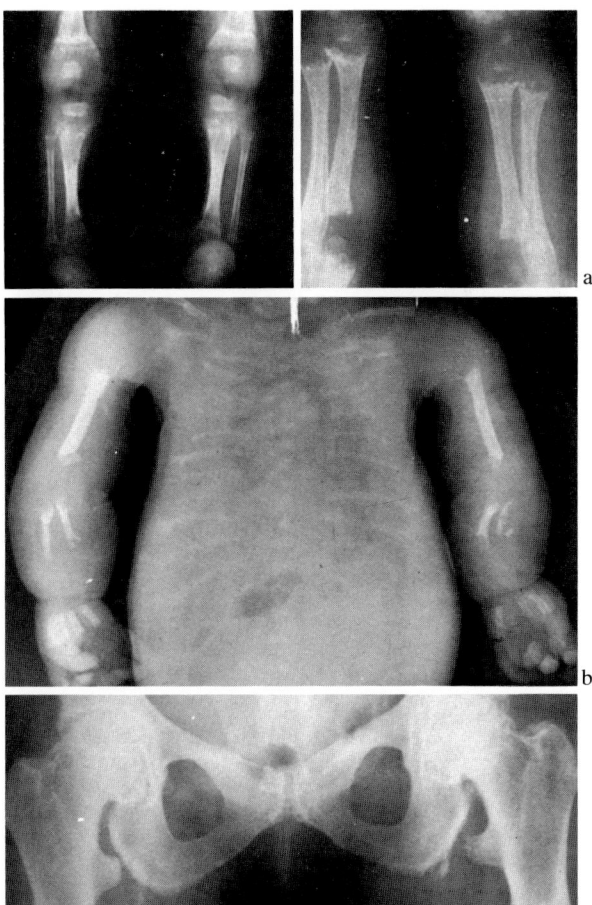

Fig. 1.3. *Hypophosphatasia.* This contrasting hereditary disorder is considered here briefly. It appears that deficiency of alkaline phosphatase inhibits the deposition of calcium phosphate in osteoid, essentially causing rickets and osteomalacia (see Exercise 3). The gravity of the disorder varies greatly, from causing foetal death to the recognition of minor osteomalacic stigmata in siblings of individuals more frankly affected. These examples illustrate **a** gross failure of metaphyseal ossification, comparable to exceptionally severe rickets, in an 8-month-old baby girl; **b** enormously reduced skeletal mineralisation in a stillborn infant, both of whose parents had a congenitally low alkaline phosphatase, and **c** Looser's zones in each femur of an elderly woman with osteomalacia due to hypophosphatasia. Bone biopsies in such patients show the same increase in osteoid tissue seen in other types of osteomalacia and illustrated in Q2 of Exercise 3.

Q1. This 63-year-old woman, known to have suffered from ankylosing spondylitis for many years, presented again, complaining of constant pain above the right thigh.

Clinical examination revealed no gross abnormality apart from limited spinal motion due to her former ankylosing spondylitis.

Radiological examination showed a large osteolytic lesion, with a loculated pattern, in the right ilium. This extended into the sacrum across the remnant of one of the ankylosed sacro-iliac joints.

A biopsy of the lytic area was performed.

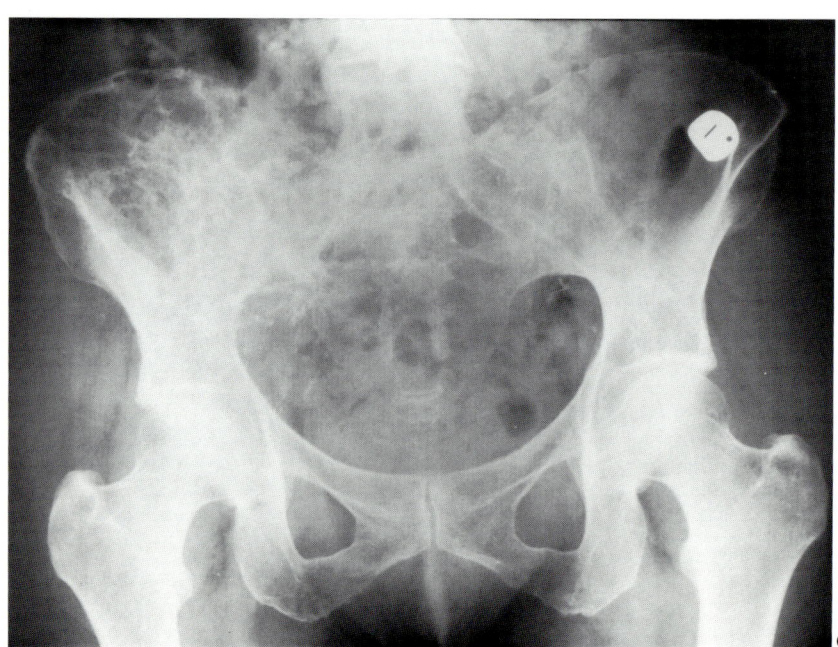

Q1a.

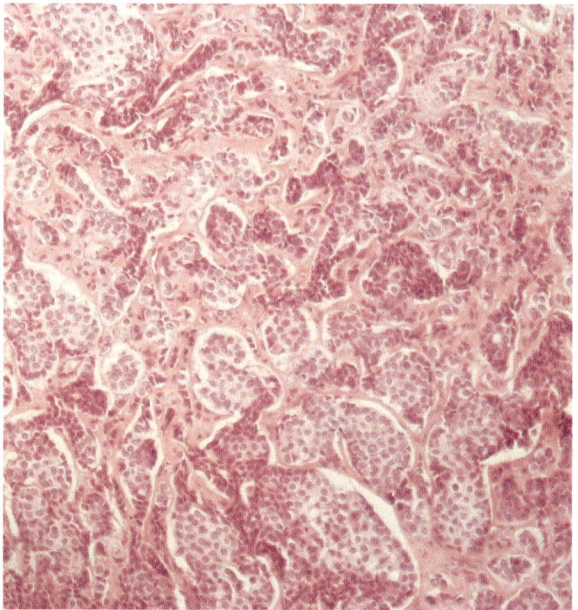

Q1b. (×140)

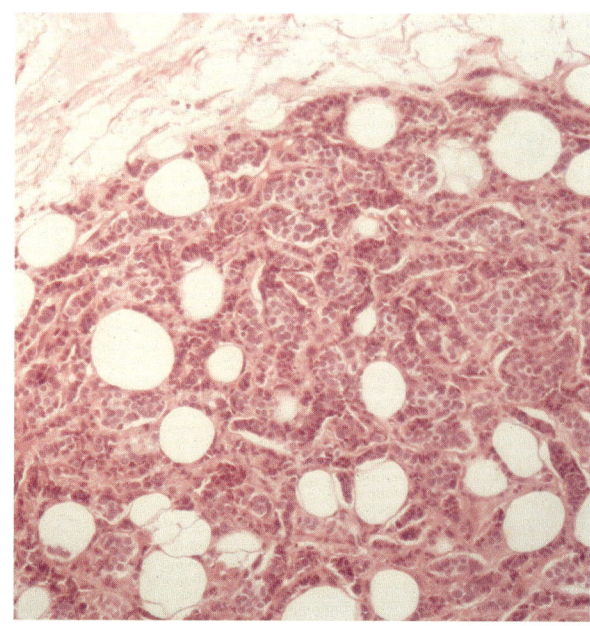

Q1c. (×140)

Q2. This 61-year-old man complained of pain in the left hip. Symptoms had begun 4 months before and pain had increased progressively.

Clinical examination revealed localised tenderness and pain which limited movement of the left hip.

Radiological examination showed the presence of a large osteolytic lesion, having a poorly defined endosteal margin, with minimal sclerotic reaction, in the lateral part of the left ilium. Destruction of the cortex was associated with a swelling extending into the soft tissues and containing hazy densities.

A biopsy was performed.

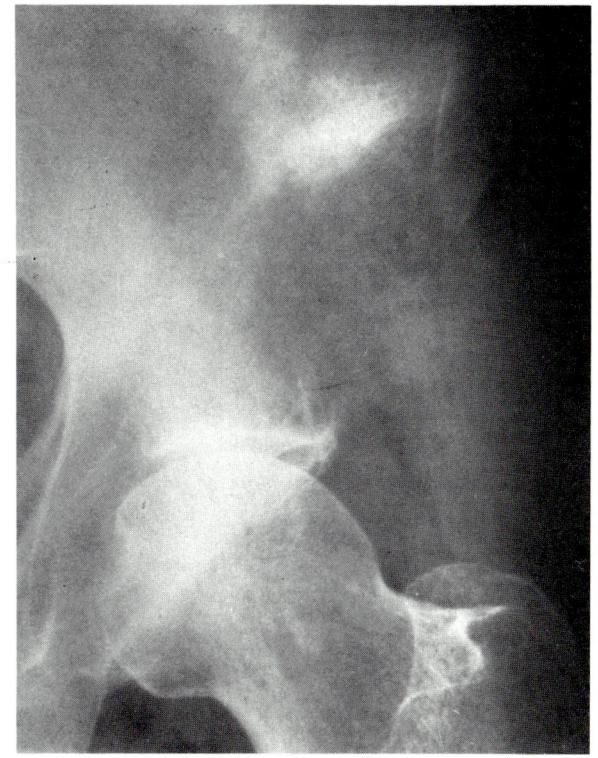

Q2a.

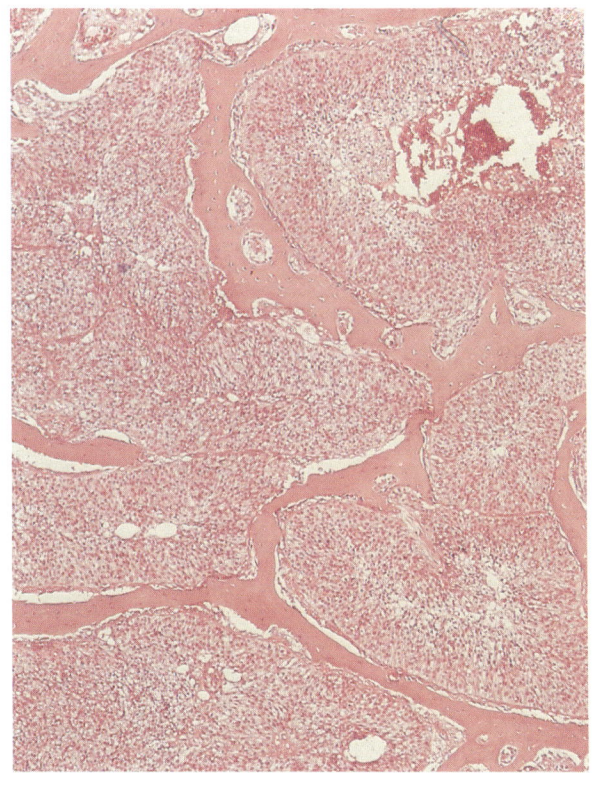

Q2b. (×50)

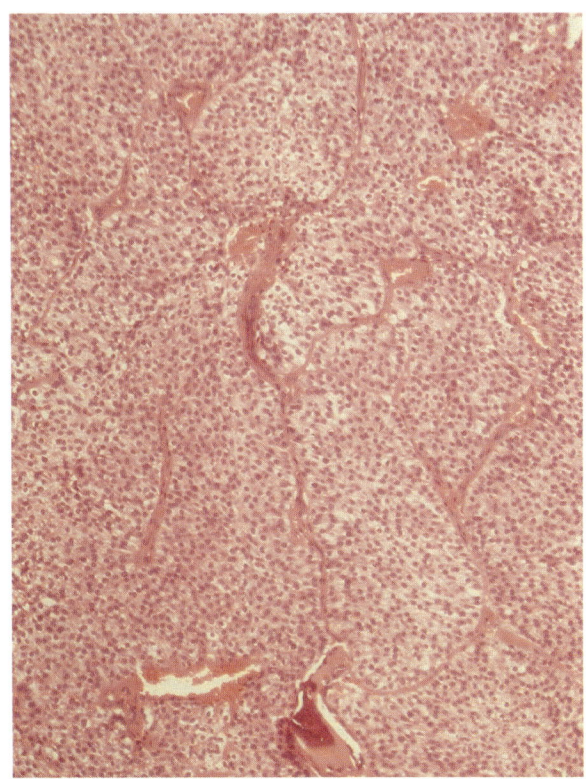

Q2c. (×110)

A1. Metastasis from carcinoma of breast

Any bizarre skeletal lesion in the elderly, especially if lytic in type, must arouse suspicion of a metastasis. In the present case this suspicion was strengthened by the knowledge that 7 years earlier a mastectomy had been performed for carcinoma of the breast. Such a history, however, is not always available, and in its absence enquiries and investigations must be directed to a range of possible primary tumours (see Exercise 2).

Q1b and Q1c show the histological appearance in the biopsy from the lesion of the ilium. This is clearly a malignant tumour, and the presence of solid strands and clusters of cells establish that it is epithelial. This pattern is completely consistent with the diagnosis of carcinoma of the breast. In Q1c the tumour cells are invading adipose tissue at the margin of the lesion. In keeping with its osteolytic character, most of the tumour tissue is devoid of bone, but Fig. 1.1 includes a few bony structures which persist towards the margin of the lesion.

A section from the primary tumour of the breast was available (Fig. 1.2) and shows exactly the same histological appearance as the bone metastasis.

The tumour of the ilium was treated with radiotherapy, with marked symptomatic relief.

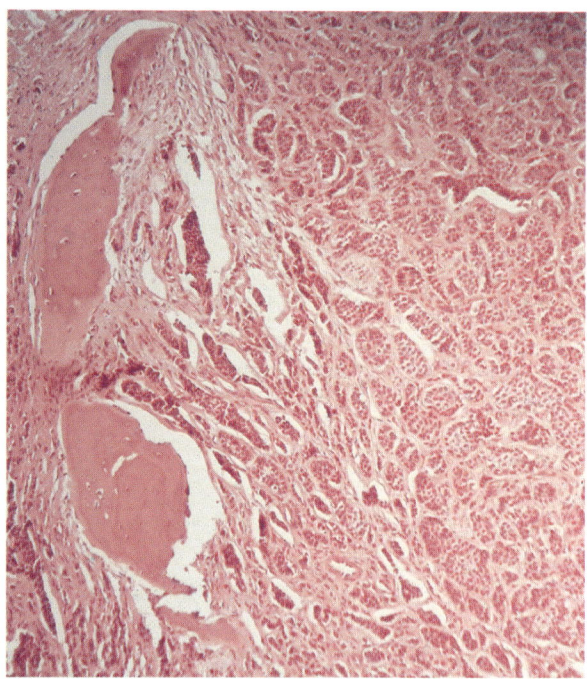

Fig. 1.1. Another field from the biopsy of the lesion of the ilium in Q1. Two bony structures, not yet completely resorbed, are present in the tumour tissue. (×90)

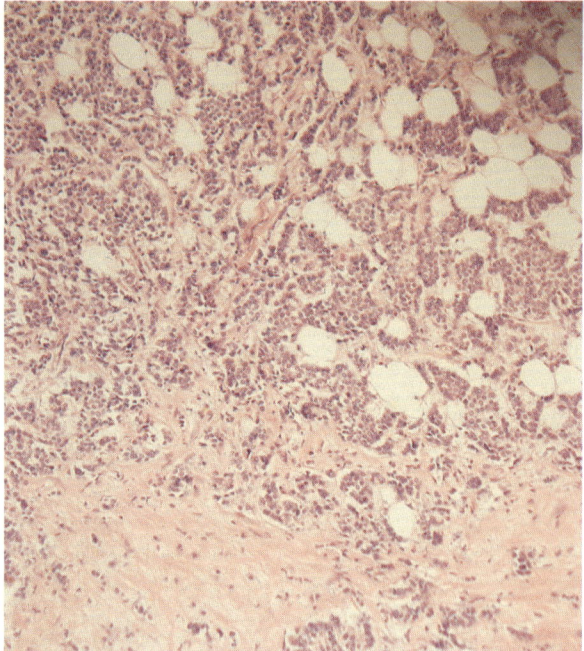

Fig. 1.2. The histological structure of the primary tumour of the breast in the case illustrated in Q1. The appearance is identical to that of the bone metastasis. (×90)

A2. Metastasis from papillary carcinoma of bladder

Pre-operatively, the clinical and radiological findings strongly suggested that the lesion was a metastasis. The expansile nature of the lesion raised the possibility of a renal carcinoma for the primary tumour, but the much rarer carcinoma of the thyroid also was considered. The alternative diagnosis of plasmacytoma (see Exercise 37) was thought less likely in view of the wide zone of transition that was present.

As in Q1, the appearance in the biopsy indicated the lesion to be a malignant epithelial tumour. Q2b is from part of the tumour where bone trabeculae are still present, although the lesion is predominantly osteolytic. The tumour has a papillary structure (Q2c), which suggested the possibility of an origin from urinary epithelium. The epithelial structure of the tumour is apparent even more clearly in Figure 2.1, where the masses of neoplastic cells are shown to be separated by strands of reticulin fibres. Appropriate investigations established the presence of a primary carcinoma of the bladder (cf. Q2 in Exercise 2).

The reticulin staining technique demonstrates the arrangement of reticulin and fine collagen fibres in the tissue being studied. As in the present case, it is sometimes of help when a diagnosis of metastasic carcinoma is suspected and where the pattern of stromal collagen confirms this by demonstrating the glandular pattern of the tumour tissue. It may also aid the diagnosis of certain primary bone tumours, such as osteosarcoma and reticulosarcoma, by showing the morphological pattern of the reticulin and collagen fibres produced by the tumour cells themselves (see Exercise 31).

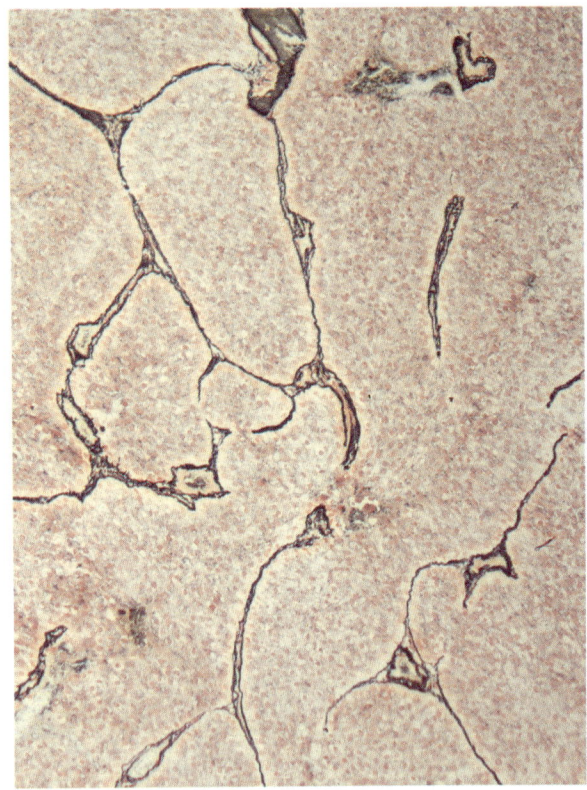

Fig. 2.1. *Reticulin stain.* Another section from the lesion in Q2. Masses of neoplastic cells are separated by strands of reticulin fibres. (×110)

Q1. This 15-year-old girl gave a history of intermittent episodes of pain in the left clavicle, with the slow development of swelling of this bone during the preceding 2 years.

Asymmetrical enlargement of the left clavicle was obvious on clinical examination, causing a mild cosmetic deformity. Significant tenderness was elicited on palpation and movements of the shoulder were limited by pain. The skin appeared normal and no local increase in warmth was detected.

The radiograph revealed fusiform expansion of almost the entire shaft of the clavicle and generalised increase of density. Organised periosteal reactions were present.

The clavicle was resected.

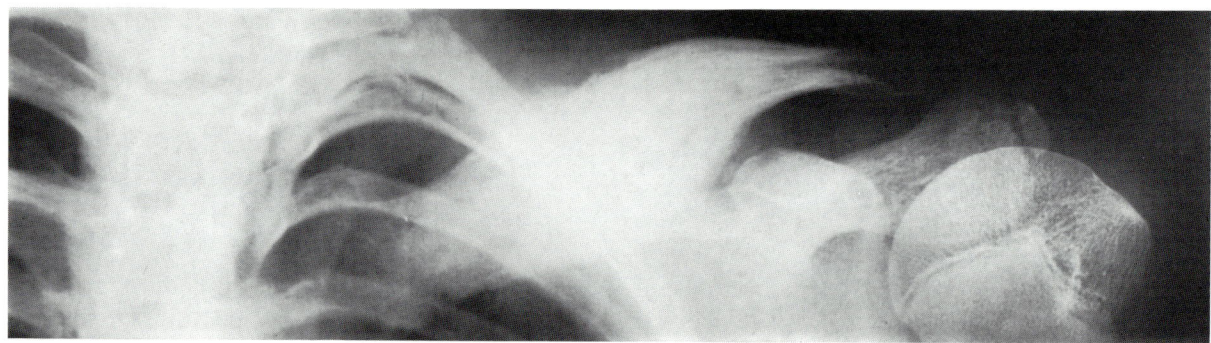

Q1a.

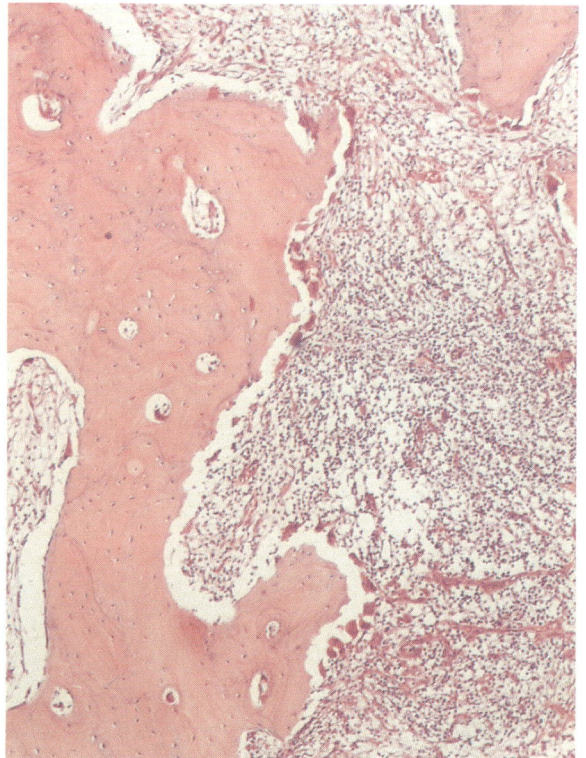

Q1b. (×63)

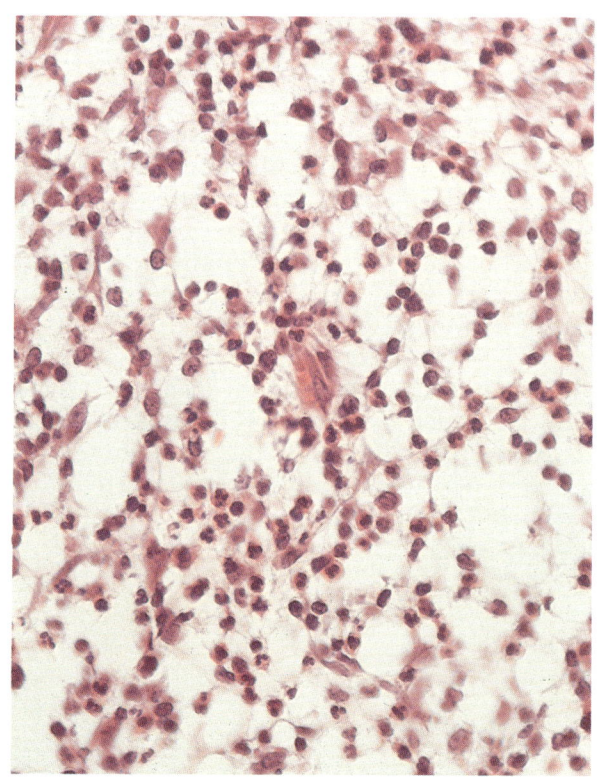

Q1c. (×380)

Q2. This 35-year-old woman had complained of pain and swelling over the middle of the right clavicle for several months.

No history of injury was obtained and clinical examination revealed no abnormality apart from mild tenderness on palpation of the painful area. No localised swelling was detected.

The radiograph disclosed an oval area of osteolysis in the mid-shaft of the clavicle. This portion of the bone was slightly expanded, with erosion and thinning of the cortex on both sides of the lesion. The zone of transition was narrow. No other bony abnormality was detected in the remainder of the skeleton.

The lesion was explored.

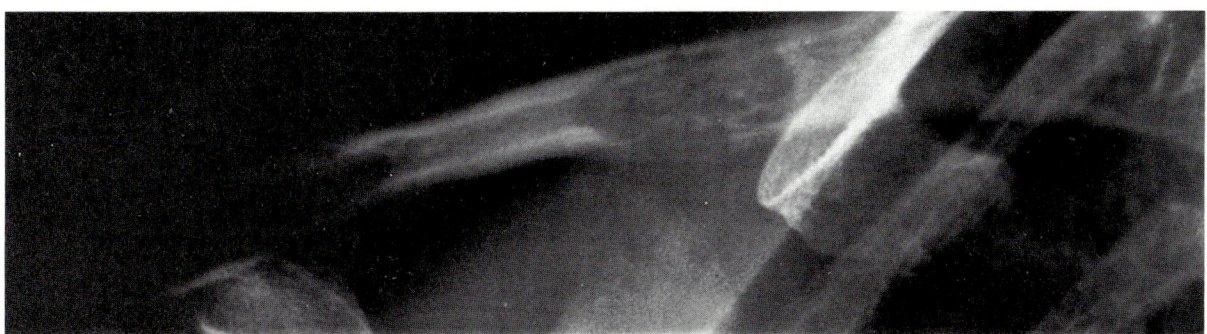

Q2a.

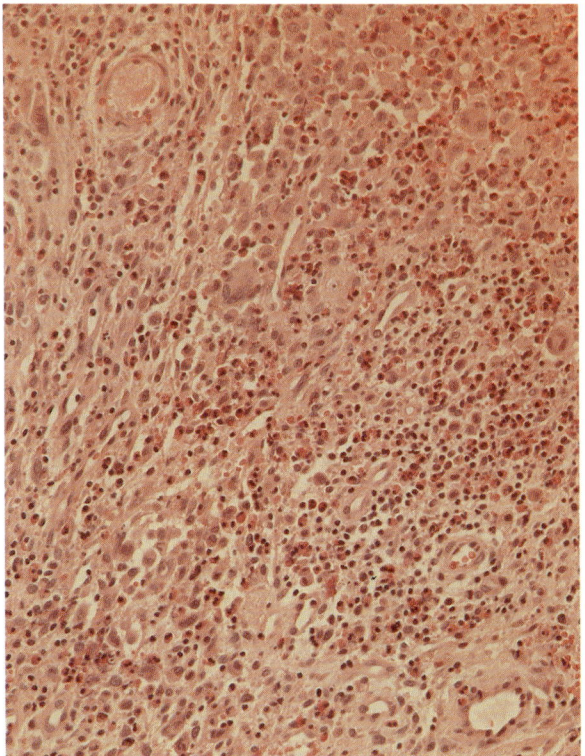

Q2b. (×160)

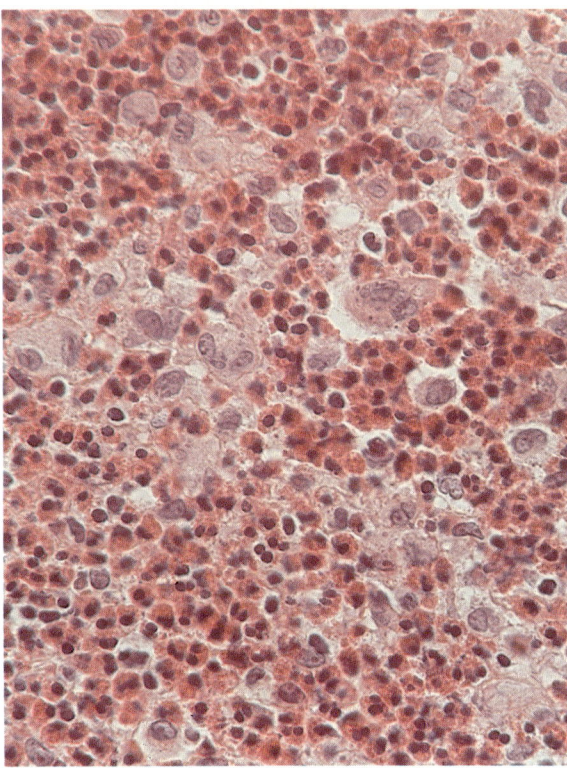

Q2c. (×480)

A1. Chronic sclerosing osteomyelitis of clavicle

Both the clinical and radiological findings in this case suggested a low-grade and chronic inflammatory process. In addition to the possibility of infection, an eosinophil granuloma was considered. A malignant tumour, particularly in view of the length of history, was considered to be very unlikely.

The resected clavicle was grossly thickened. Its cut surface showed coarsely trabeculated bone with scattered focal areas of bone destruction.

Q1b and c are from one of these foci of bone destruction. Thickened trabeculae, with an irregular outline, are undergoing active osteoclastic resorption on their surfaces. Between these trabeculae Q1c illustrates, at higher magnification, granulation tissue containing occasional capillary blood vessels and numerous inflammatory cells. Most of these cells can be identified, from their multilobed nuclei, as polymorphonuclear leucocytes, but small and large mononuclear cells (lymphocytes, histiocytes and fibroblasts) also are present. The focal areas of bone destruction are, in fact, micro-abscesses, and the lesion is an example of chronic sclerosing osteomyelitis.

In other parts of the lesion (Fig. 1.1), reactive bone formation is evident. Here, new trabeculae, covered with active osteoblasts, are forming in fibrous tissue. The maturation and remodelling of these trabeculae has led to the radiographic appearance of increased bone density. Because of the coarsely trabecular bony architecture, this type of lesion is sometimes referred to as 'pagetoid osteomyelitis'. Histologically, however, although the thickened trabeculae do show a few cement lines (Q1b), the typical 'mosaic' pattern which these structures exhibit in true Paget's disease is not present. This hypertrophic response to infection is common in the clavicle.

Despite this histological evidence of an active chronic inflammatory process, all methods of culture were negative. This type of chronic recurrent osteomyelitis, without obvious bacteriological cause, may be responsible for multiple bone lesions. In addition to the clavicle, the metaphyses of long bones can be affected. These cases may have a very prolonged course, but the ultimate prognosis is good. The aetiology is obscure. Attention to these relatively rare manifestations of osteomyelitis has been drawn already in Exercise 10.

Reference

Björksten B, Boquist L (1980) Histopathological aspects of chronic recurrent multifocal osteomyelitis. J Bone Jt Surg 62B: 376–380

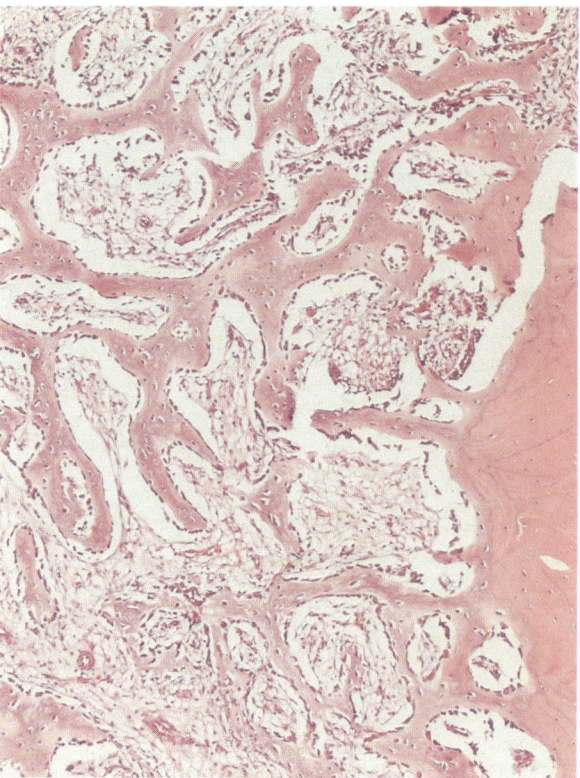

Fig. 1.1. Trabeculae of reactive bone at the margin of an inflammatory focus. (×63)

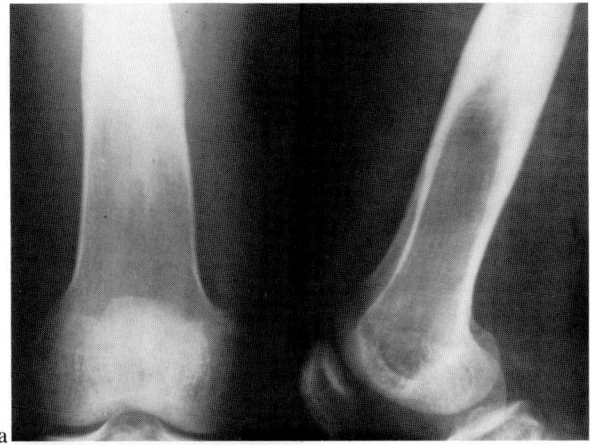
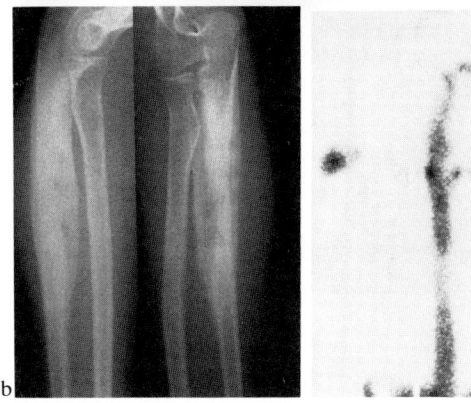
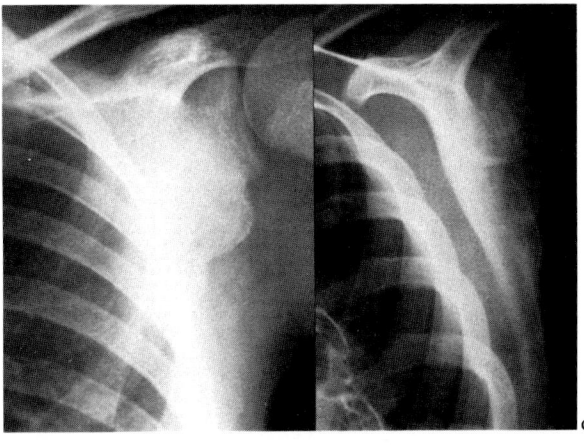

Fig. 1.2. *Chronic osteomyelitis of femur—reactivation.* **a** This 34-year-old man had complained of an ache above the left knee for 2 months. The sclerotic lesion in the femoral shaft was surrounded by fusiform cortical thickening due to an organised periosteal reaction and had narrowed the medullary cavity. The diagnosis was simplified by recognition of a 'ghost' shadow in the former distal femoral epiphysis, corresponding to the size of this structure at the time of the original infection at the age of 8 years. **b** A similar example in the right ulna of a 14-year-old girl with chronic pain for 1 year. In the same patient a radionuclide scan **c** demonstrated activity not only at this site, but also in the right scapula, where a further, but asymptomatic lesion **d** was present. The diagnosis of the ulnar lesion was confirmed histologically after biopsy.

A2. Eosinophil granuloma of clavicle

A wide differential diagnosis existed radiologically for this type of lesion, a problem arising frequently in such bones as the clavicle and ribs. No definite pre-operative diagnosis was offered.

A 'brown tumour' of hyperparathyroidism was excluded by normal blood investigations and the absence of other radiological abnormalities (see Exercise 23). The age of the patient made a metastasis or a plasmacytoma unlikely. The clinical history did not suggest an inflammatory process.

The histological illustrations are from material curetted from the lesion of the clavicle, which at operation appeared as a solid mass of rather vascular tissue. Q2b shows 'granulomatous' tissue with numerous capillary blood vessels; many 'inflammatory' cells are present, including small round cells with dark nuclei, larger spindle-shaped cells and occasional giant cells with multiple nuclei. In Q2c many of the smaller cells can be identified as polymorphonuclear leucocytes because of their lobed (apparently multiple) nuclei and granular cytoplasm. The larger mononuclear cells with pale cytoplasm are histiocytes. The intense eosinophil staining of the cytoplasmic granules of the polymorphs identifies these cells as eosinophil polymorphs. The lesion is, in fact, an eosinophil granuloma. This entity, and its associated manifestations of histocytosis, has been described in Exercise 20.

Q1. This 13-year-old girl had been aware of mild and intermittent pain in the left arm during the previous 6 weeks. This pain suddenly had become acute and severe during vigorous dancing on the previous day.

On clinical examination a diffuse tender swelling was detected around the proximal end of the humerus. All movements of the arm were restricted by pain.

Radiological examination revealed a large expanding lytic lesion in this area with marked attenuation of the cortex, which showed an infraction on the lateral side. The endosteal margin was clearly defined with a narrow zone of transition.

A biopsy was performed.

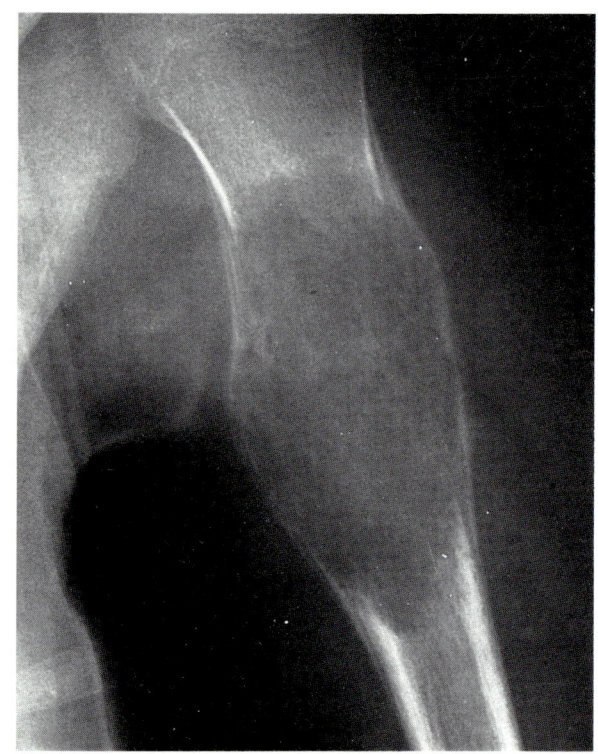

Q1a.

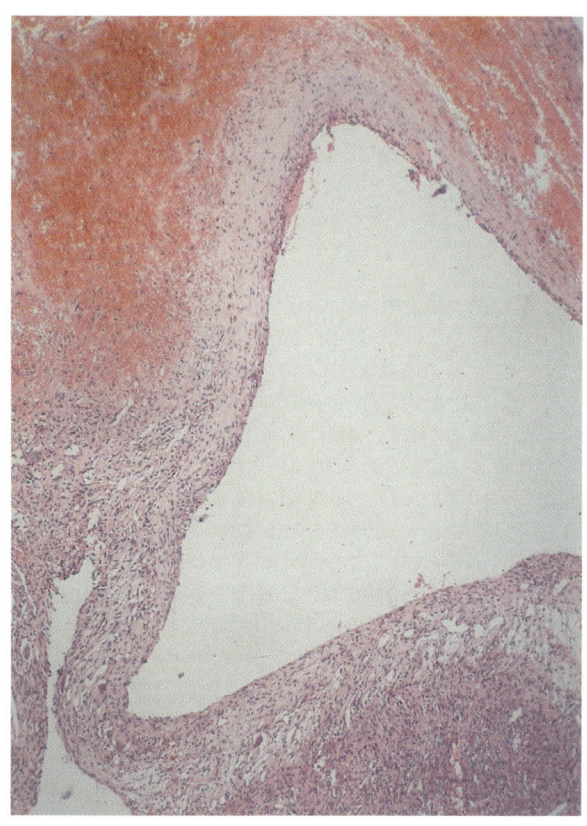

Q1b (×56)

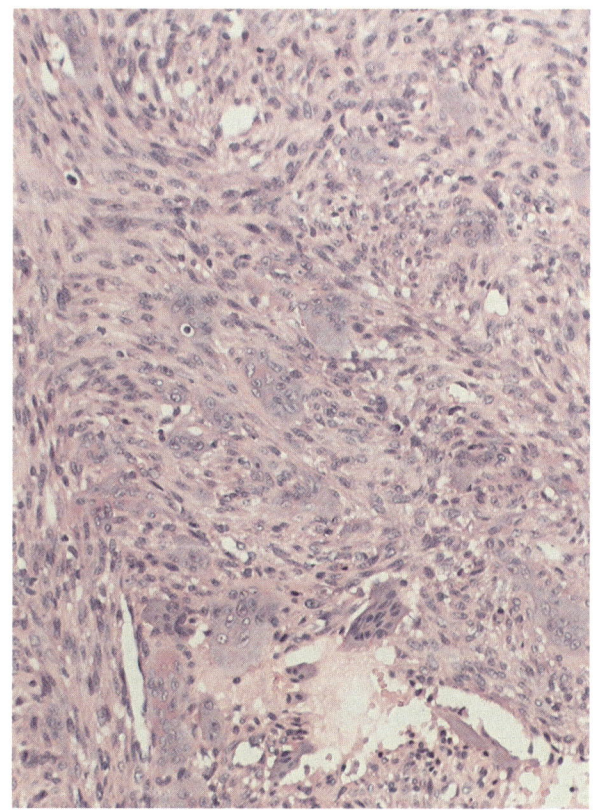

Q1c. (×170)

Q2. This 12-year-old boy was examined as an emergency, having developed acute pain in the arm after a fall.

Clinically, all movements of the arm were limited by pain. A fracture of the humerus was suspected and radiological examination was requested.

The radiograph at the time of presentation showed the proximal portion of an expanding lytic lesion in the shaft of the humerus. Its extent can be appreciated more accurately in the subsequent examination undertaken after application of a light plaster cast.

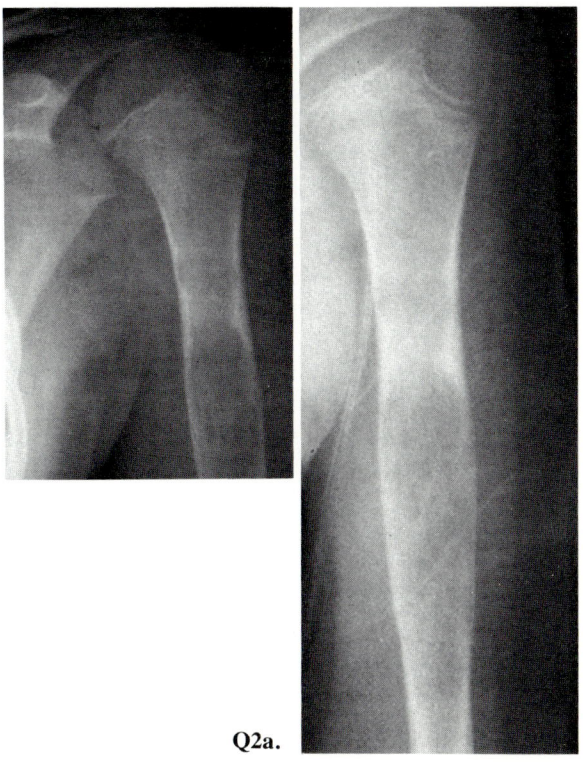

Q2a.

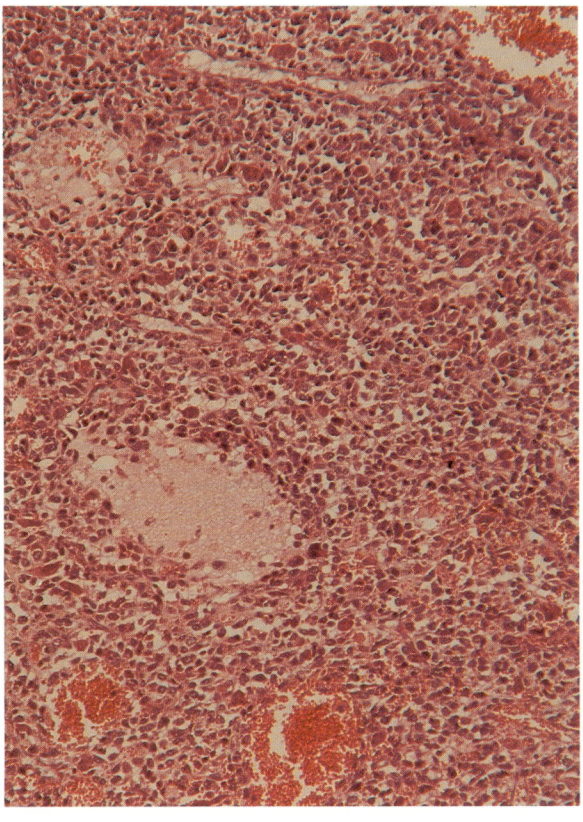

Q2b. (×94)

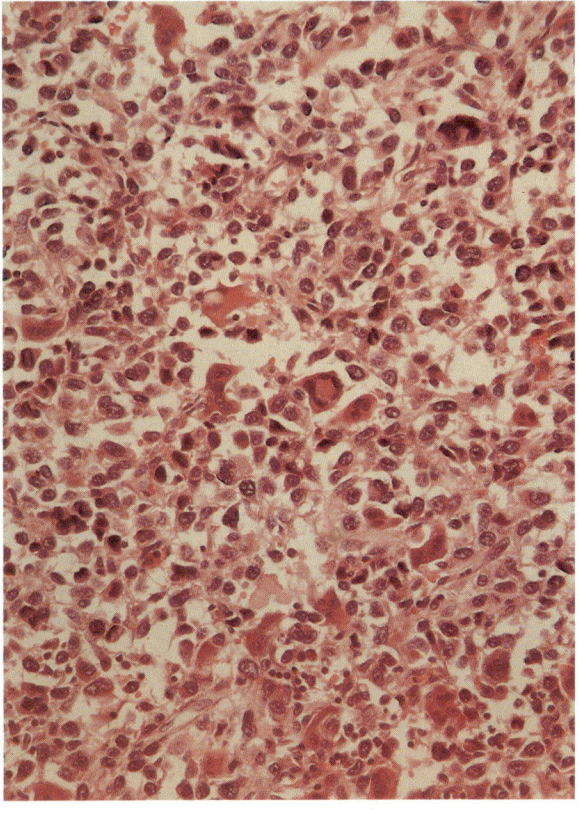

Q2c. (×170)

A1. Aneurysmal bone cyst of humerus

This diagnosis was suggested pre-operatively although in long bones these tumours more commonly develop in metaphyseal areas than in diaphyses (see Exercise 22). At operation much vascular tissue was encountered which bled profusely. Q1b shows characteristic cystic spaces separated by septae of solid tissue, within which areas of recent haemorrhage are present. At a higher magnification (Q1c) it is evident that the solid tissue contains many giant cells and areas of reactive bone formation. The combination of these features typifies an aneurysmal bone cyst. Despite curettage the lesion continued to enlarge during the following 4 months (Fig. 1.1a). Radiotherapy—3000 rads—then was administered with an excellent response, the tumour contracting and becoming sclerotic (Fig. 1.1b). The patient then was asymptomatic.

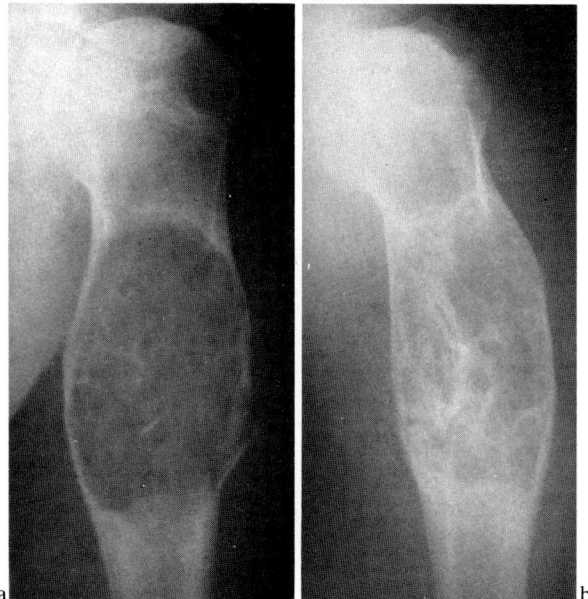

Fig. 1.1. **a** Four months after curettage the tumour had enlarged. **b** One year later, following radiotherapy, the lesion had contracted and developed considerable sclerosis.

A2. Osteosarcoma of humerus

The abnormality was considered to represent a unicameral bone cyst, an entity which has a particular affinity for this anatomical site (see Exercise 19). Curettage and bone grafting of the lesion were planned. At operation no trace of a cyst was found. Only solid haemorrhagic tissue was encountered. Despite this finding, the surgeon adhered to his planned procedure. Pain persisted during the post-operative period and further radiographs obtained after intervals of 2 and 4 months respectively (Figs. 1.1a and b) indicated the lesion to enlarge progressively and to develop central strands of bony density. The patient was referred at this stage for a second opinion.

The histological appearance of the material obtained by the original curettage is illustrated in Q2b and c. The lesion consisted of highly cellular tumour tissue. The cells showed a marked degree of nuclear pleomorphism, with numerous mitoses. Many giant cells are present. Some of these cells, with centrally placed uniform nuclei, have the appearance of osteoclasts. Others, with more irregular darker nuclei, are tumour giant cells. No particular pattern of differentiation is evident to justify a specific diagnosis. These findings indicate an 'undifferentiated malignant tumour arising in bone'.

As a result of these findings forequarter amputation was performed, permitting further histological study. Residual tumour tissue was present. Some had the same undifferentiated appearance as in the earlier specimen, but in other areas (Fig. 2.2) abundant tumour bone was evident, establishing conclusively the diagnosis of osteosarcoma (see Exercise 14). The patient succumbed from pulmonary metastases within a year, despite continuous chemotherapy.

This case illustrates a most unusual presentation of an osteosarcoma simulating a unicameral or simple bone cyst. It emphasises also that the correct histological diagnosis of a malignant bone tumour must depend on the provision of a representative sample of tissue from it.

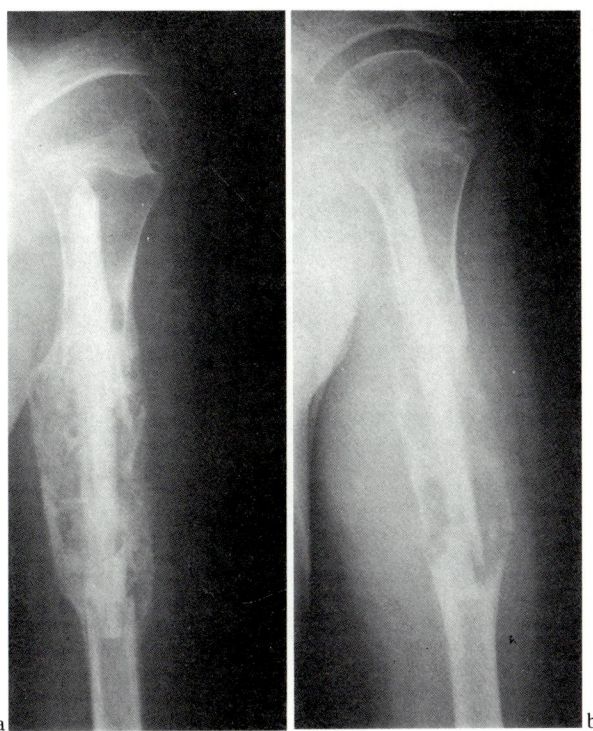

Fig. 2.1. Radiographs obtained **a** 2 months after the operation show the graft in situ and expansion of the cortex due to growth of the tumour, with evidence of new bone formation. **b** After 4 months both this new bone and the graft had been eroded, and a large and clearly defined extension of the tumour into the adjacent soft tissues had developed.

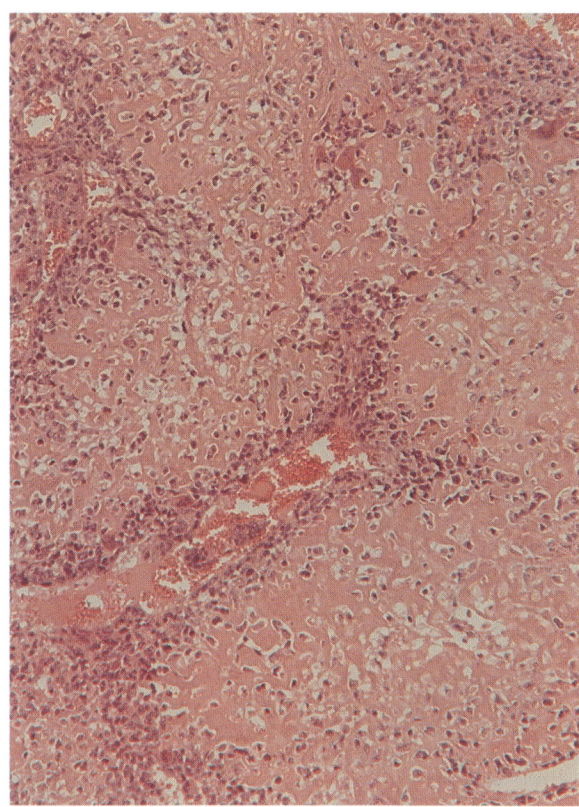

Fig. 2.2. Characteristic tumour bone from the amputation specimen with many mitoses and numerous giant cells. (×94)

Q1. **This 16-year-old boy had complained for 4 months of intermittent pain in the left thigh. The pain was aggravated by exercise and was worse at night.**

On clinical examination a tender mass was palpated on the antero-lateral aspect of the proximal end of the femoral shaft. The mass appeared to be fixed to the bone. No other abnormality was detected. Movements of the left hip were full and painless. No lymphadenopathy was found.

The radiographs showed a diffuse area of destruction in the medulla of the femur with no clear marginal definition. Overlying this area laminated periosteal reactions had developed. No enlargement of the adjacent soft tissues was detected.

Surgical exploration was undertaken.

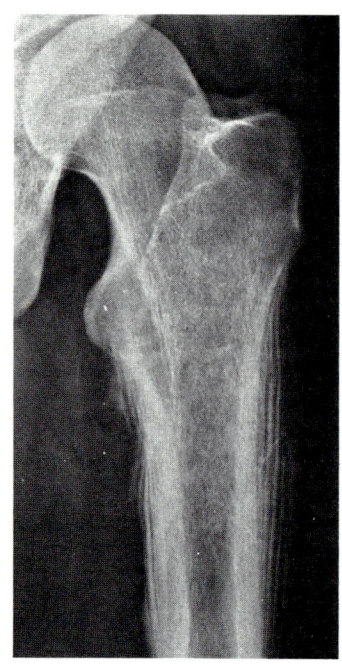

Q1a.

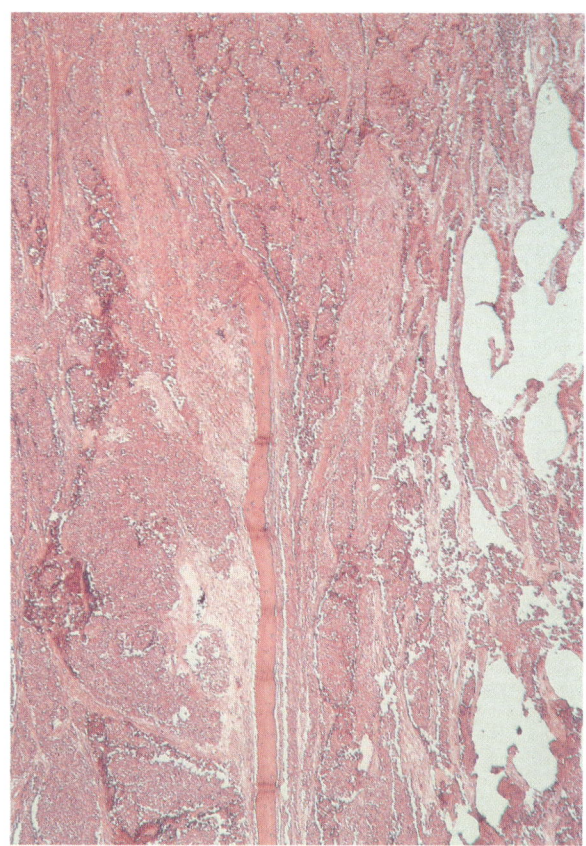

Q1b. (×35)

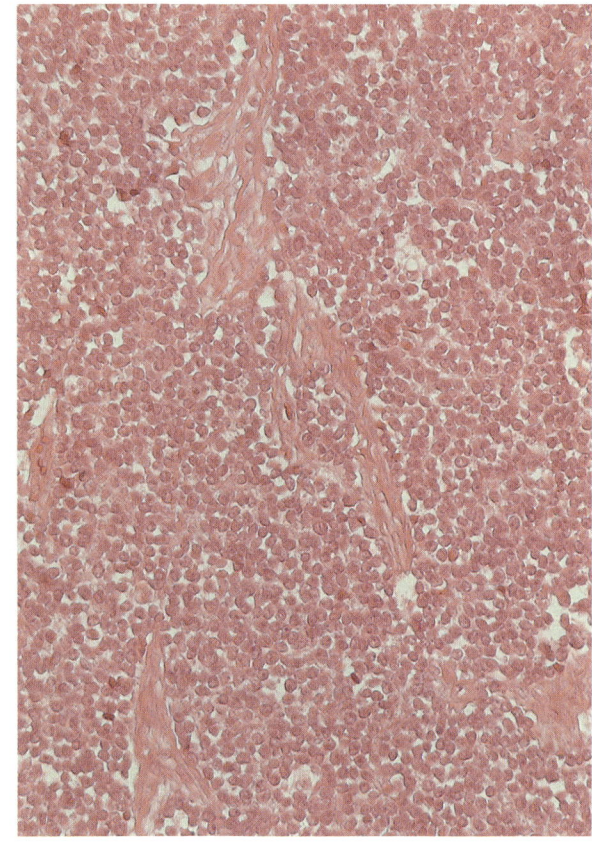

Q1c. (×220)

Q2. This 19-year-old man complained of a chronic ache in the right thigh, which had been present for approximately 2 months.

Slight swelling of the thigh, with deep tenderness on palpation, was observed clinically. The patient was apyrexial, but some enlargement of the right inguinal lymph nodes was detected. Biochemical and blood investigations were normal, except for an elevated ESR.

Radiological examination revealed rather irregularly defined lucencies in the long axis of the medullary cavity of the femur. A segment of the medial cortex showed diminished density and around this area a periosteal reaction was evident.

A biopsy was performed.

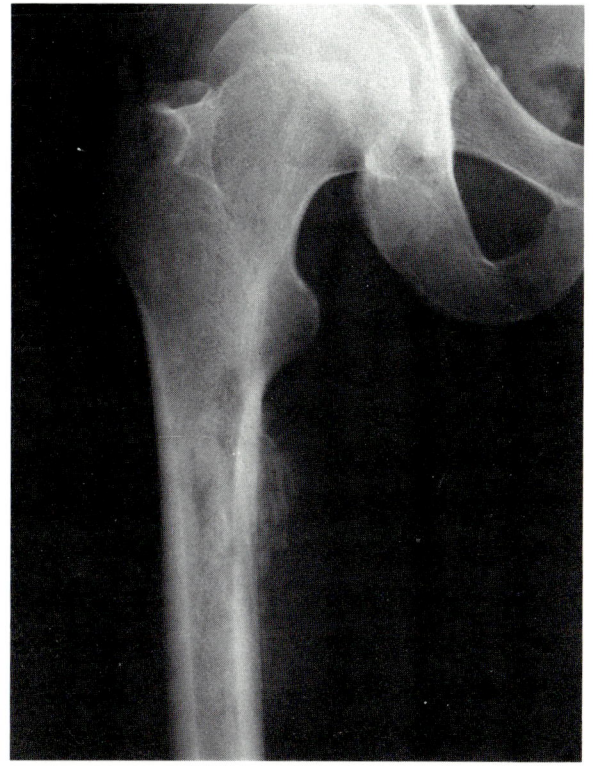

Q2a.

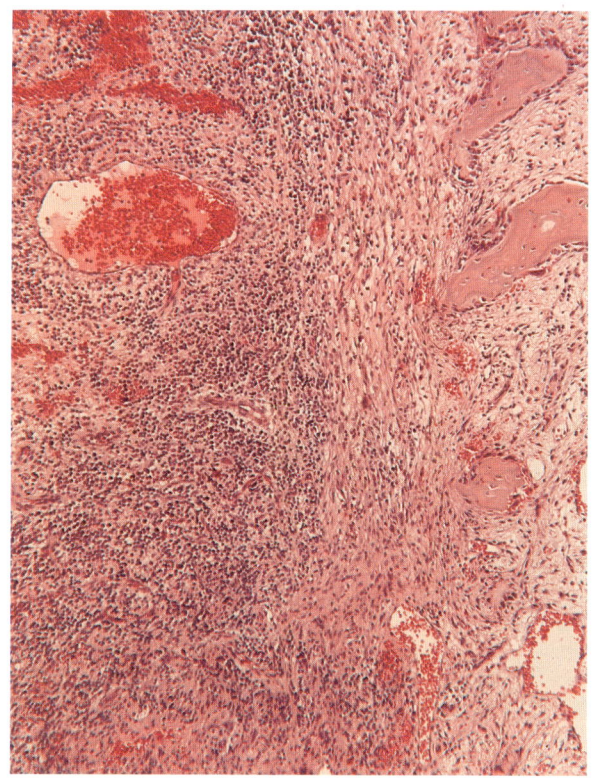

Q2b. (×40)

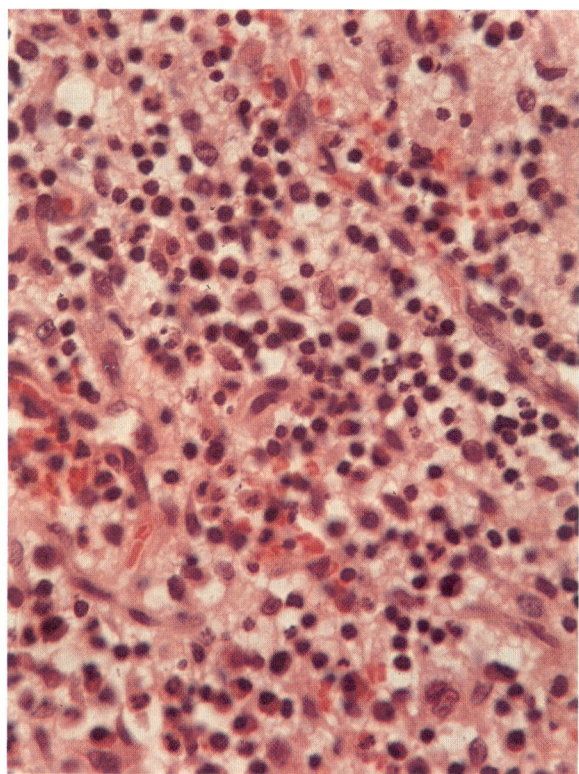

Q2c. (×320)

A1. Ewing's sarcoma of femur

Clinically the possibilities of a malignant round-cell tumour and of a focus of pyogenic infection were considered. Radiologically, however, the pattern conforms to the classical findings in a Ewing's sarcoma, consisting of ill-defined medullary destruction in the diaphysis of a major long bone, with an overlying or 'onion-peel' periosteal reaction.

At operation, the soft tissue mass was found actually to surround the shaft of the femur. The sections showed the histological features of a malignant round-cell tumour (Q1b and c). The nuclei of the tumour cells show little pleomorphism, and numerous mitoses could be identified when the sections were examined. Appropriate staining procedures for glycogen and reticulin (see Exercise 31) confirmed the diagnosis of Ewing's sarcoma.

A disarticulation through the hip joint was carried out, and preparations from the amputation specimen show very beautifully the histological basis of the conspicuous periosteal lamination that was apparent in the radiograph. Figures 1.1a and b show the bony structures as they appear in radiographs of longitudinal and transverse slabs of tissue from the specimen. Figures 1.2a and b show the microscopic structure of the periosteal bone. Vertical bone spicules have been produced as the periosteum has been displaced by the growth of the tumour, and, in the deeper part of the mass, the bony structures adjacent to the cortex have been remodelled to form a series of thick horizontal layers of bone. This appearance, although regarded as characteristic of Ewing's sarcoma, is not specific, and can be found in other conditions. The reason for the arrangement of the deep bone into separate horizontal layers is not known, but the intermittent nature of the growth and remodelling processes may be concerned.

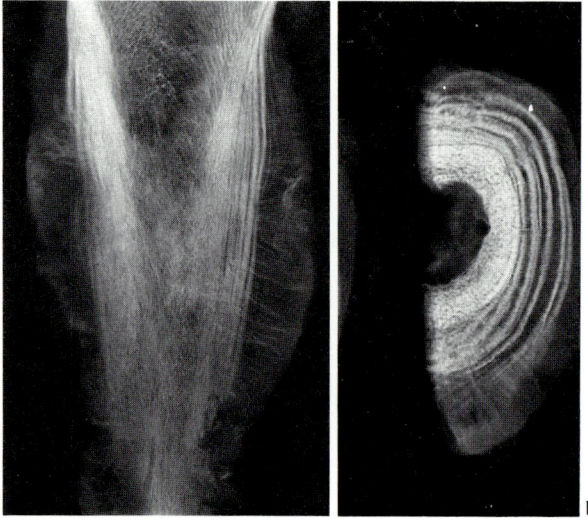

Fig. 1.1. Radiographs of **a** longitudinal and **b** transverse slabs of tissue from the specimen showing the vertical bony spicules and the laminated periosteal reactions.

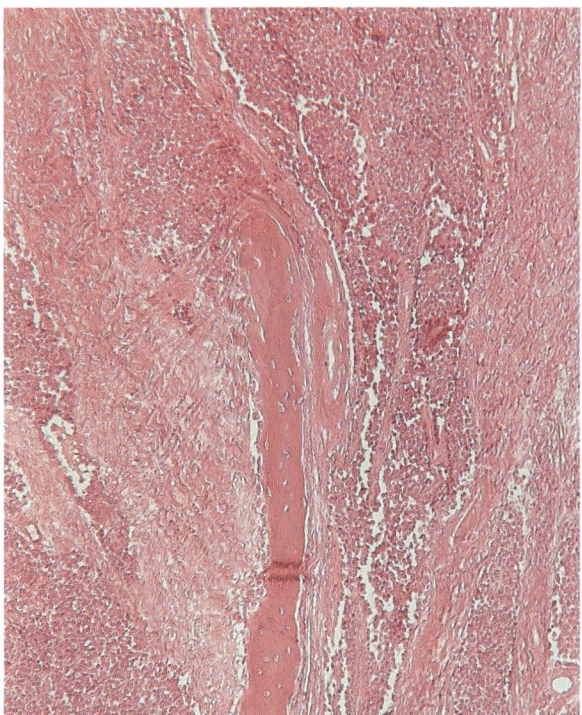

Fig. 1.2a. One of the vertical spicules of bone produced by the displacement of the periosteum. Note the osteoblasts on the surface of the bony structure. (×85)

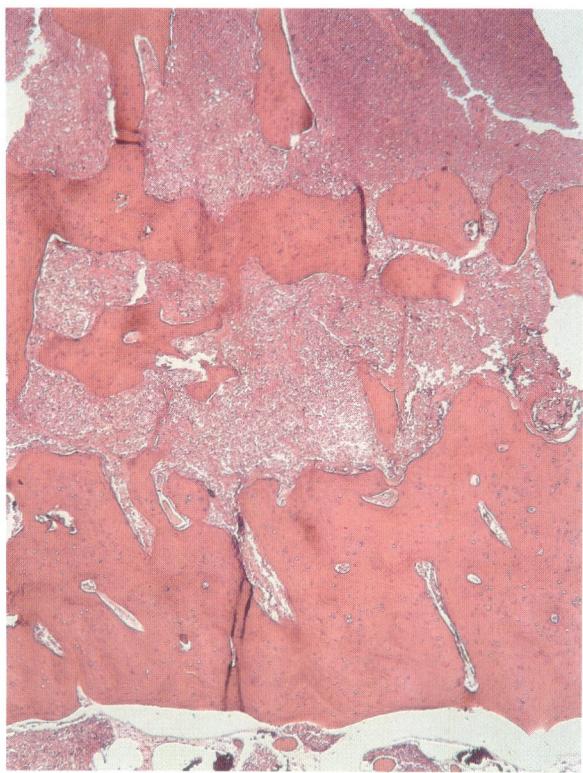

Fig. 1.2b. A section through two of the horizontal layers of bone nearer the surface of the cortex. (×37)

A2. Subacute pyogenic osteomyelitis of femur

In this case also the differential diagnosis lay primarily between an infection and a malignant neoplasm. In such cases both the clinical and the radiological findings may cause difficulty in making a correct decision. Once the acute phase of a pyogenic infection has subsided, routine haematological investigations are rarely helpful. A significant radiological feature, however, was relatively clear definition of the linear lucency on the medial side of the medullary cavity, giving the appearance of 'tunnelling', which has been described in Exercise 10.

At operation, the periosteum was found to be displaced by material which, although not recognised as pus, gave a positive culture for *Staphylococcus aureus*. The histological sections showed chronic inflammatory tissue with reactive bone. In Q2b this inflammatory tissue can be recognised, together with some newly formed bony trabeculae which represent a portion of the periosteal reaction which was apparent in the radiograph. At a higher magnification (Q2c), these inflammatory cells which are scattered throughout the tissue can be identified as lymphocytes (small round cells with dark nuclei), plasma cells (larger cells with dark nuclei, sometimes showing a pale juxtanuclear area in the cytoplasm) and polymorphonuclear leucocytes (smaller cells with multilobular nuclei). In addition to these cells the field contains some mononuclear cells with large pale nuclei (fibroblasts or histiocytes) and the endothelial lining cells of capillary blood vessels.

The histological findings indicate an inflammatory process which has commenced acutely (polymorphs), but which is now becoming chronic (lymphocytes and plasma cells) (cf. Fig. 1.1, Exercise 10) This is in keeping with the staphylococcal aetiology. The patient was treated with penicillin, to which the cultured organism was sensitive. The wound healed well with no subsequent complications.

In such cases antibiotic therapy must be maintained for a minimum of 3 months after the erythrocyte sedimentation rate has returned to normal.

Exercise 50

Q1. This 62-year-old woman complained of increasing pain in the right hip. The pain had developed and had become progressively severe during the preceding year. Even with the use of a cane walking was restricted to short distances.

On clinical examination the patient was observed to be obese and movement of the right hip was limited in all directions. No other abnormality was detected. All routine investigations were normal.

Radiographs of the right hip revealed obvious degenerative change in this joint, to which her symptoms and signs were attributed (see Exercise 5). In addition, however, a large lucent area was evident in the intertrochanteric portion of the femur, extending proximally into the neck and distally into the shaft of the bone. The margins of this lesion were defined sharply by a narrow zone of increased density.

Histological sections from this lesion are illustrated below.

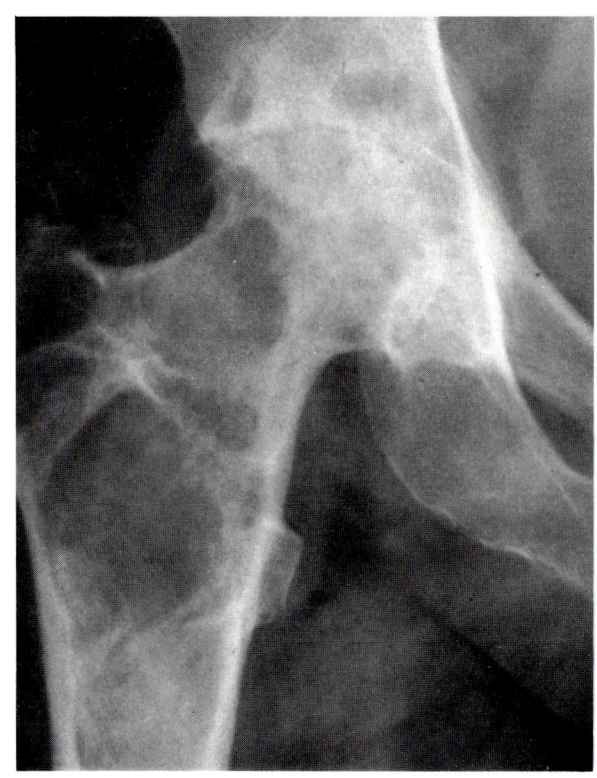

Q1a.

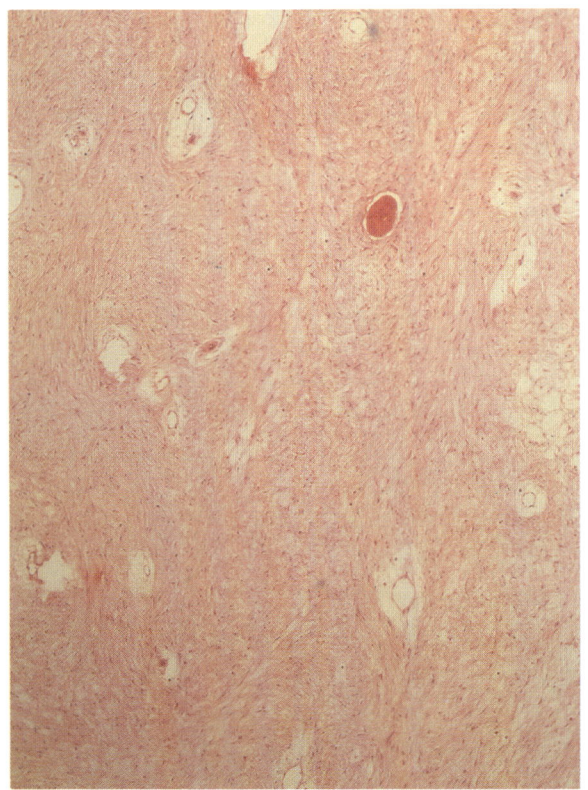

Q1b. (×44)

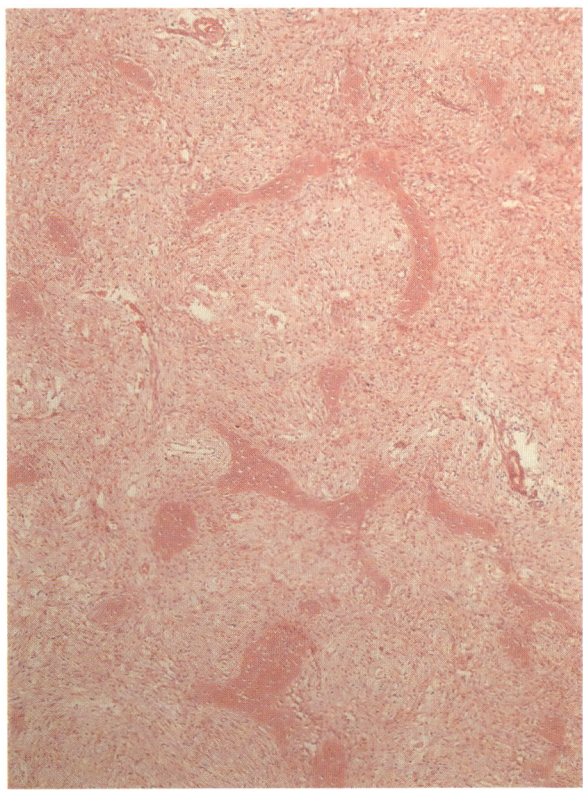

Q1c. (×44)

Exercise 50

Q2. This 54-year-old man sought medical advice because he had been aware of mild discomfort in the upper part of the left thigh for 2 years.

No abnormal physical signs were detected clinically and the symptoms were suspected to be due to prolapse of an intervertebral disc.

Radiological examination demonstrated the presence of a lytic lesion of the femoral neck and intertrochanteric area, interspersed with hazy densities. The endosteal margin was minimally irregular and the lateral cortex had been eroded on its internal surface. Organised periosteal reactions could be discerned on each side of the femur at the level of the lesser trochanter.

This lesion was explored.

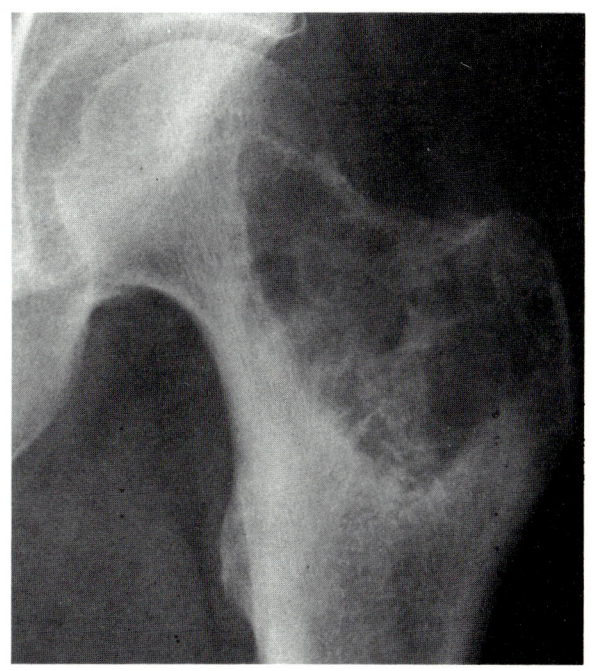

Q2a.

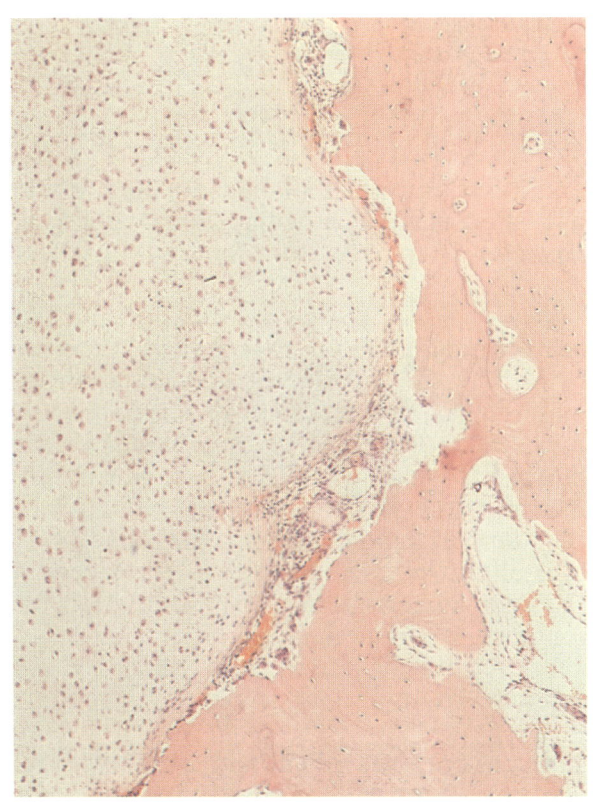

Q2b. (×62)

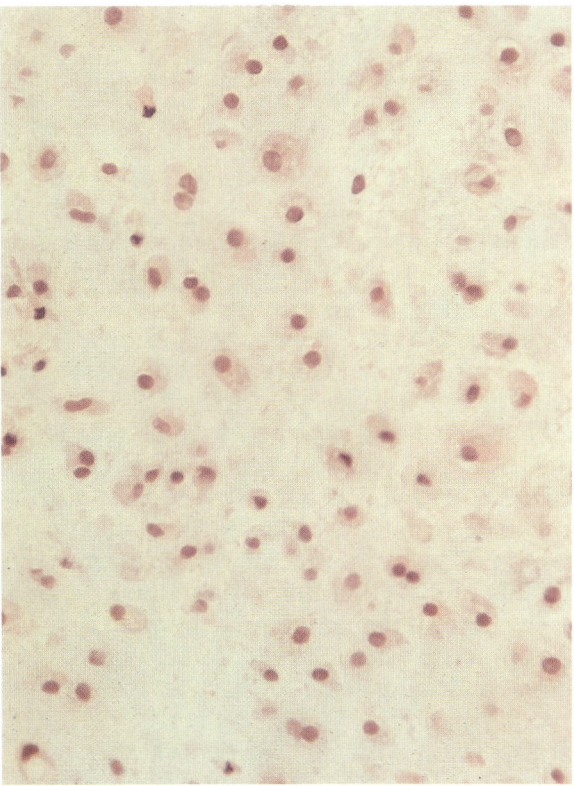

Q2c. (×335)

A1. Fibrous dysplasia of femur

In view of the clinical opinion that the symptoms and signs in this patient were due to degenerative changes in the hip, total prosthetic replacement of this joint was undertaken. The lytic area, demonstrated radiographically, in the femur was regarded confidently as an unimportant focus of fibrous dysplasia. Because of the potential weakening of this portion of the femur a custom-built prosthesis was employed, so that the entire lesion could be resected. Q1b and c are histological sections from this specimen and confirm the diagnosis of fibrous dysplasia. Part of the abnormal tissue (Q1b) consists of nondescript fibrous tissue, interspersed with small vascular channels. Elsewhere in the specimen (Q1c) a characteristic combination of rather cellular fibrous tissue and trabeculae of woven (non-lamellar) bone presents a diagnostic appearance. These trabeculae are arranged in an open network. At a higher magnification (Fig. 1.1) the non-lamellar structure of the bone is more evident and the trabeculae lack a covering layer of osteoblasts (see Exercise 1).

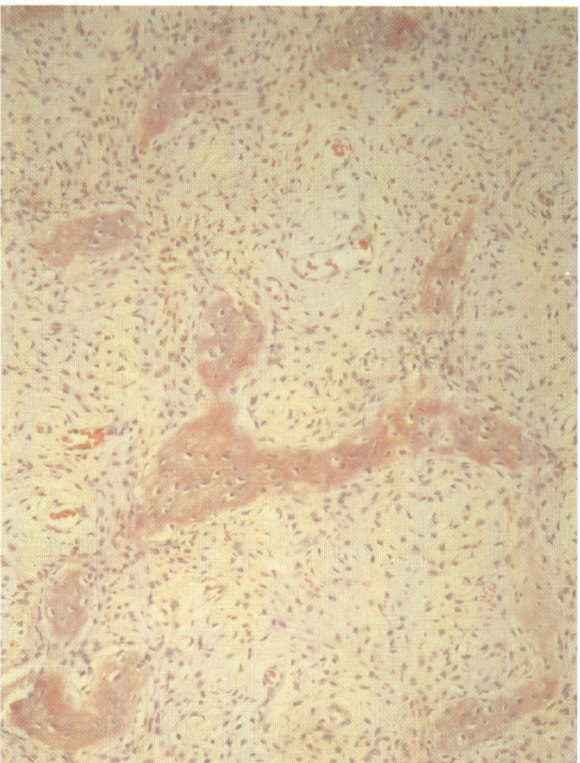

Fig. 1.1. A more magnified view of the abnormal tissue, showing more clearly the trabecular network of woven (non-lamellar) bone. (×100)

A2. Low-grade chondrosarcoma of femur

The mild symptoms engendered by this lesion and the relatively long history, coupled with the radiological appearance, caused this diagnosis to be considered. Biopsy was mandatory and Q2b and c illustrate its histological appearance. Q2b shows it to consist of cartilaginous tissue which is eroding the overlying cortical bone. This tissue is moderately cellular, but lacks the pleomorphism that might be expected in a malignant tumour. The diagnosis of a well-differentiated or low-grade chondrosarcoma, however, is indicated with higher magnification in Q2c by the presence of a considerable number of large and binucleate cells. This degree of cellularity in the tumour tissue in a cartilaginous lesion of this type, together with evidence of growth—in the form of invasion of cortical bone at its margin—represent additional indications of malignancy and would not be expected in a benign chondroma (see Exercise 12).

The tumour was treated by local resection and replacement of the proximal end of the femur by a metallic prosthesis. Examination of material from the resection specimen showed the same histological features noted in the biopsy. No highly malignant chondrosarcomatous tissue was encountered, but much of the tumour margin showed the same bony erosion and local extension that was evident in the biopsy specimen. The features of this relatively common, low-grade type of chondrosarcoma have been discussed in Exercise 16.

The patient was alive and well, without evidence of recurrence or metastasis, 5 years after operation.

Exercise 51

Q1. This 11-year-old girl complained of pain in the right foot of several weeks' duration following determined gymnastic exercises.

Clinically a tender swelling was felt over the third metatarsal head. The initial radiograph suggested a stress fracture and no special treatment was given. Some weeks later the lesion had increased in size and uncertainty was expressed about its nature, on which account a biopsy was performed.

The first radiograph (Q1a) revealed considerable new bone formation in relation to the head and neck of the third metatarsal. The later study, (Q1b), obtained after 5 weeks, showed the new bone to have become much more prominent.

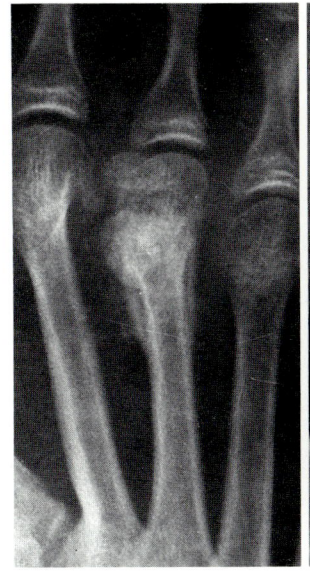 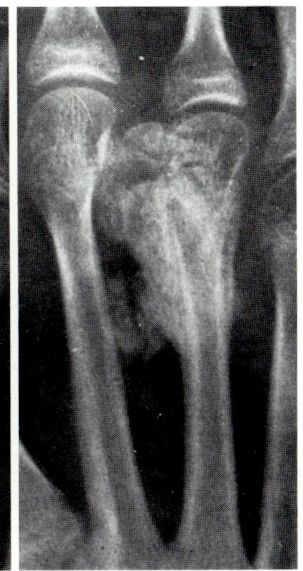

Q1a. Q1b.

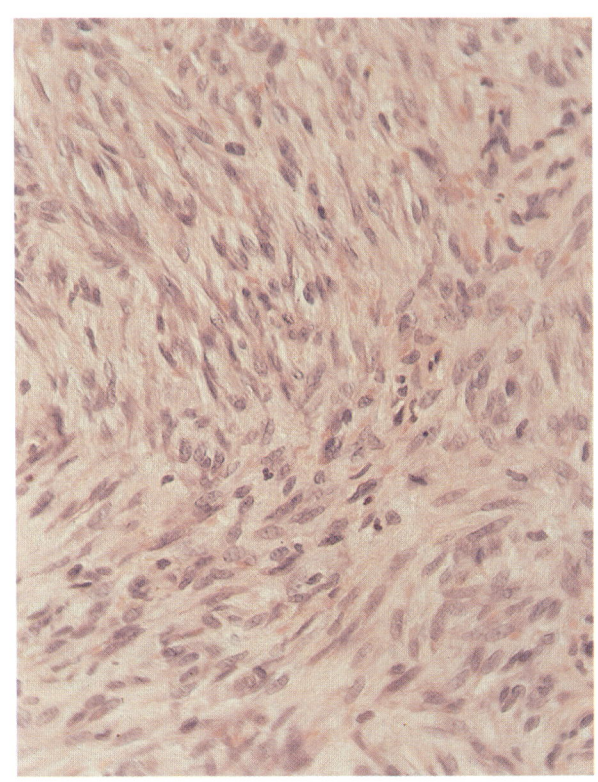

Q1c. (×240)

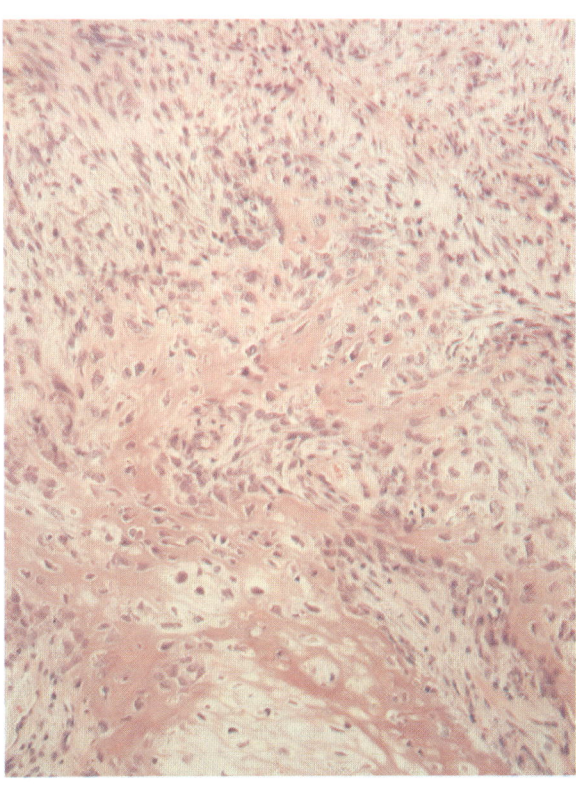

Q1d. (×110)

A1. Stress fracture of neck of third metatarsal

In this case it is not only the radiological appearances but also the biopsy findings which are liable to misinterpretation. On radiological grounds alone the hyperplastic callus formation around the neck of the third metatarsal was accompanied by a mild, but definite, valgus displacement of the metatarsal head so that the diagnosis of a stress fracture was justified entirely, particularly as another hairline fracture of the neck of the fourth metatarsal was evident, but without significant reactive bone formation. The development of still more opaque callus in the later examination (Q1b) should not have altered the diagnosis and an expectant line of treatment should have been adopted, as illustrated in Fig. 1.1.

Histologically, the presence of actively mitotic spindle-celled tissue with areas of bone and cartilage (Q1c and d) was, in fact, wrongly interpreted by an inexperienced pathologist as indicating an osteosarcoma. On consultation, however, careful examination of the sections showed areas of maturing cartilage with endochondral ossification (Fig. 1.2). Such an appearance is *not* a feature of osteosarcoma (see Exercise 14), but indicates that the tissue *is* reparative callus (see Exercise 28).

It is important to realise how closely the histological appearance of callus tissue can resemble that of a malignant tumour. Such errors have, in the past, been responsible for the iatrogenic tragedy of unnecessary amputation.

References

Daffner RH (1978) Stress fractures: Current concepts. Skeletal Radiol 2: 221–229

Levin DC, Blazina ME, Levine E (1967) Fatigue fractures of the shaft of the femur: simulation of malignant tumour. Radiology 89: 883–885

Murray IPC (1980) Bone scanning in the child and young adult. Part II. Skeletal Radiol 5: 65–76

Sevitt S (1981) Bone repair and fracture healing in man. Churchill Livingstone, Edinburgh

Wilson ES, Katz FN (1969) Stress fracture. An analysis of 250 consecutive cases. Radiology 92: 481–486

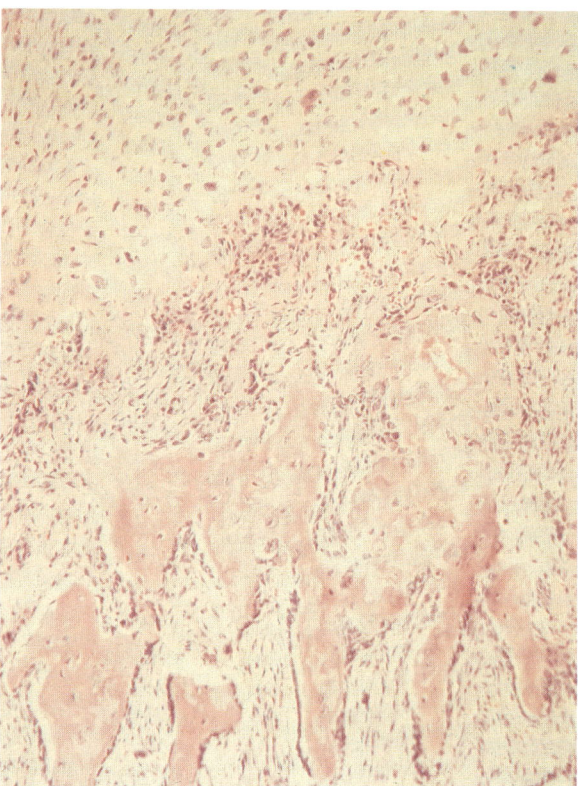

Fig. 1.1. Six months later the stress fracture had consolidated. Despite further increase in size the reparative callus had organised, but its bulk had caused pressure erosion on the shaft of the adjacent second metatarsal. The fracture of the neck of the fourth metatarsal had fused soundly without displacement.

Fig. 1.2. Areas of maturing cartilage with endochondral ossification. (×85)

Exercise 52

Q1. This 27-year-old woman had complained of mild, but persistent, pain in the left hip for more than a year.

On clinical examination movement of this hip was found to be restricted in all directions by pain. No other abnormality was detected.

The radiographs revealed destructive, but clearly defined, lesions on the medial side of the acetabulum and on the neck of the femur. The articular surfaces appeared normal, but the joint space was minimally narrowed. No significant osteoporosis was evident. Arthrography was performed and showed marked expansion of the joint cavity with numerous diverticular extensions.

At operation, material was removed for histological study.

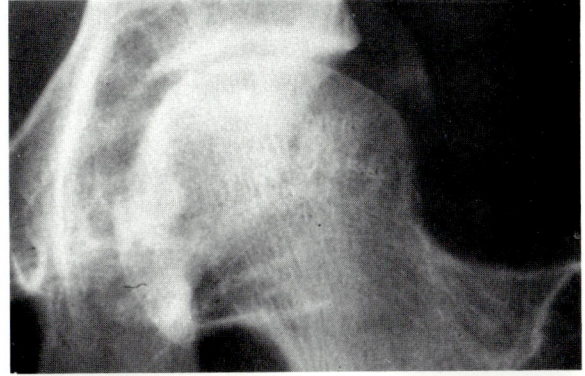
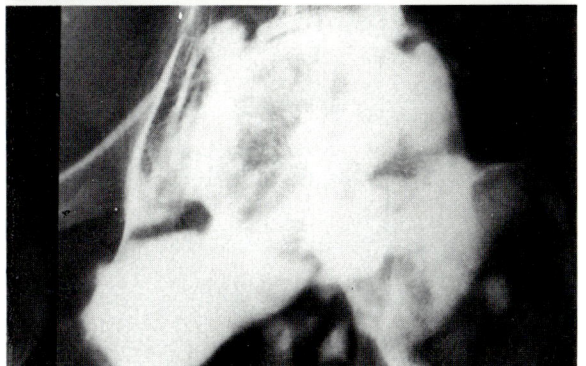

Q1a.

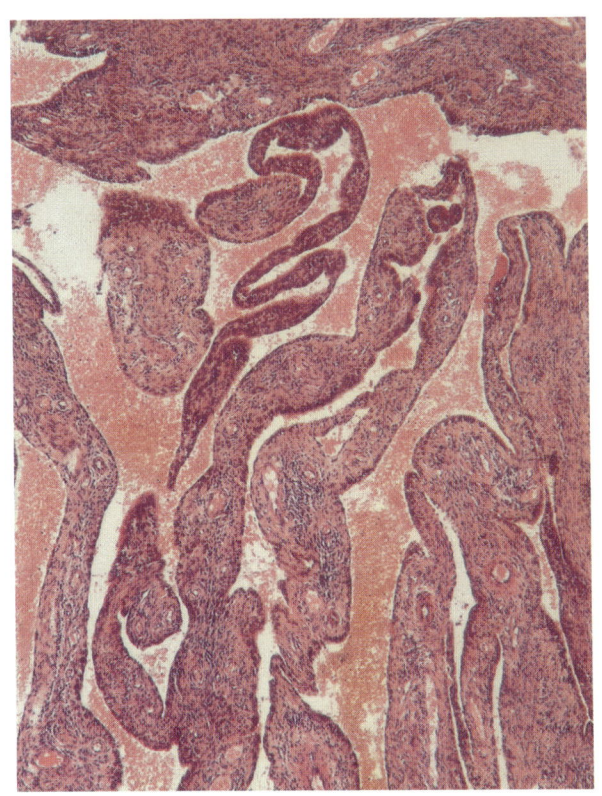

Q1b. (×52)

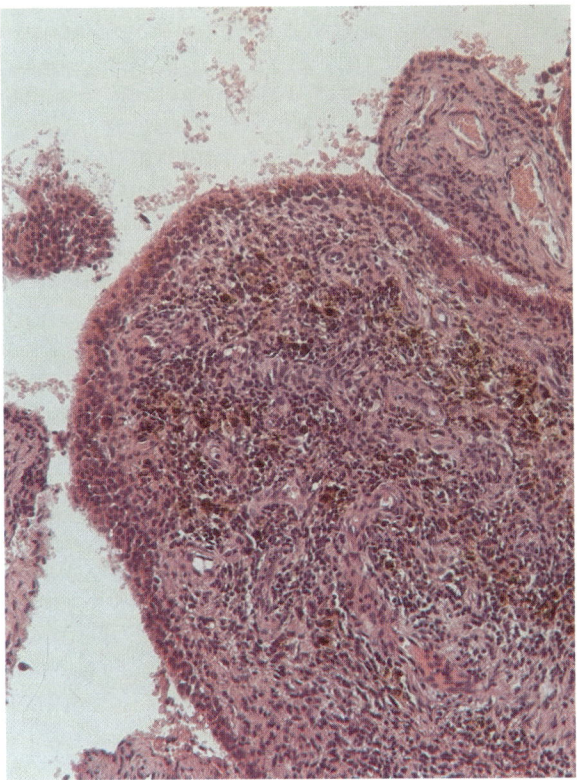

Q1c. (×125)

A1. Pigmented villonodular synovitis of hip

Clinical examination had failed to establish a diagnosis, but the radiological appearance was characteristic of a synovial disorder. The erosions on both sides of the joint indicated involvement of this tissue. Their clearly defined margins made a malignant process, such as a synovioma, unlikely. Preservation of the articular surfaces excluded an infective process and the subarticular osteoporosis of rheumatoid arthritis was lacking. Pigmented villonodular synovitis was favoured preoperatively. Since similar para-articular erosions, however, may occur in the early stages of synovial chondromatosis (see Exercise 9), arthrography was undertaken. The expanded joint cavity with diverticular extensions corresponding to the sites of bony erosion provided a conclusive diagnostic appearance.

Synovectomy was performed. During this operation, once the capsule of the hip joint had been opened, massive nodular proliferation of the synovium became evident. These nodules displayed the classical pigmentation of the disease, attributable to their haemosiderin content, varying from bright yellow to dark brown (Fig. 1.1). An unusual feature was attenuation of the articular cartilage of the femoral head, accounting for the narrowing of the joint space noted in the original radiograph.

Further confirmation of the diagnosis was provided by study of the excised synovium (Q1b and c). The combination of villous and nodular synovial projections, with numerous small round cells and abundant haemosiderin pigment, is characteristic of pigmented villonodular synovitis.

Synovectomy around the hip is rarely complete, so that recurrences are not infrequent. Nevertheless, this procedure can delay progression of the disease (see Exercise 36). In this instance the patient's symptoms were relieved completely. No recurrence had developed during the subsequent 2 years.

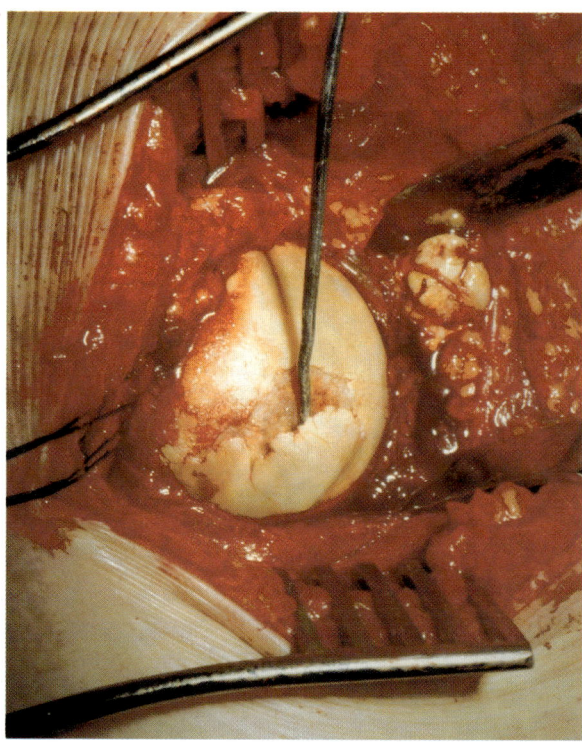

Fig. 1.1. The characteristic pigmented nodules are demonstrated clearly, especially on the right side of the femoral head, in this operative photograph. The rather unusual attrition and partial separation of the articular cartilage is evident.

Exercise 53

Q1. This 50-year old woman had been aware of a hard swelling in the right lumbar area for many years. During recent months this swelling had enlarged and, for the first time, had become painful.

Clinical examination confirmed the presence of a large solid mass which appeared to be attached to the right iliac crest. It extended proximally almost to the lower costal margin. Further swellings of firm consistency were detected elsewhere, including the posterior side of the right hemithorax and the inferior portion of each scapula. In addition the right forearm was deformed, being short and bowed.

Radiographs of the lumbar lesion showed the mass to contain numerous opacities. Displacement of the intestinal gas shadows indicated its retroperitoneal location. Bony excrescences were demonstrated at the sites of the swellings palpated clinically.

A biopsy of the lumbar mass was performed.

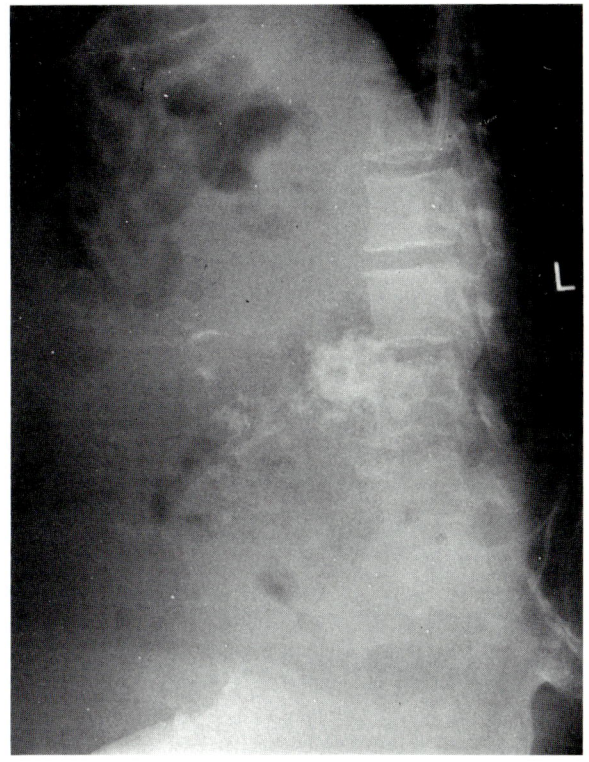

Q1a.

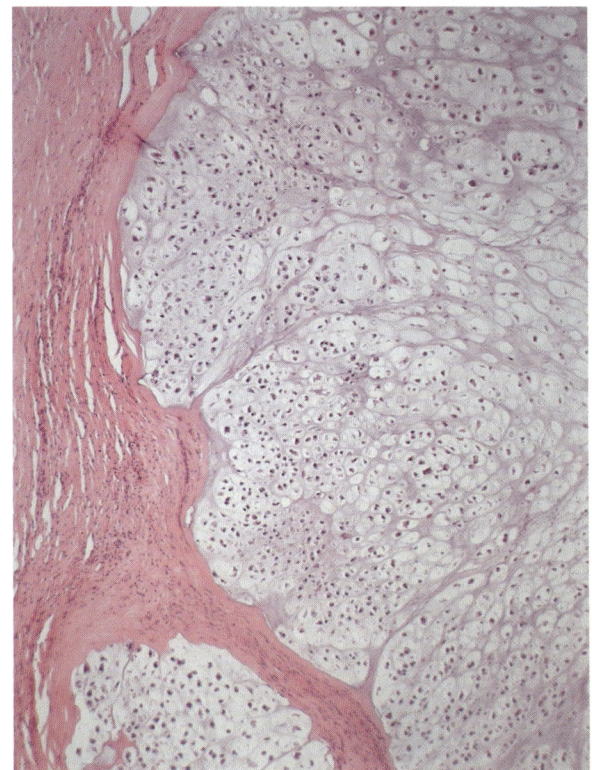

Q1b. (×56)

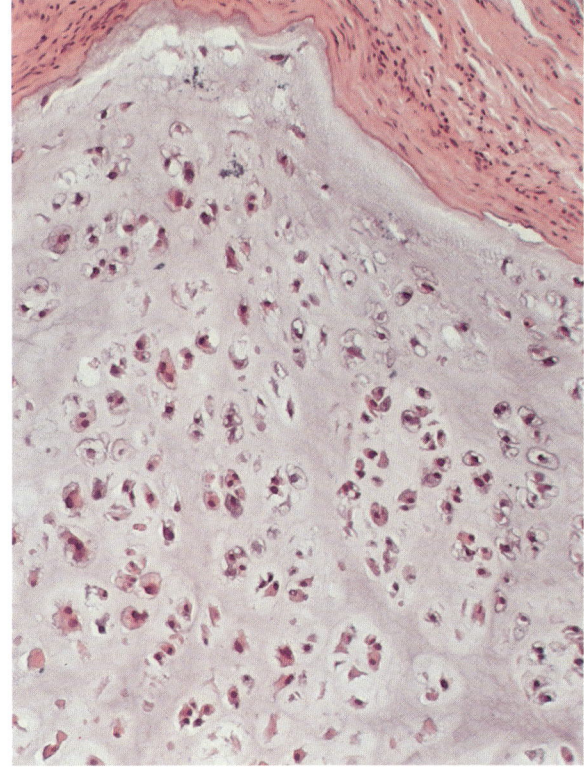

Q1c. (×160)

A1. Chondrosarcoma complicating diaphyseal aclasia (multiple exostoses)

The clinical diagnosis of the generalised and hereditary skeletal disorder of diaphyseal aclasis (see Exercise 4) was confirmed by the radiological examination. Figure 1.1 illustrates the osteochondromas which were present on each scapula and on the right 5th and 6th ribs, and in Fig. 1.2 modelling deformities of the radius and ulna were evident, being accompanied by another exostosis on the radius.

The history of slow but progressive enlargement of the lumbar lesion strongly suggested chondrosarcomatous change in the cartilage cap of another exostosis arising from the right iliac crest. This suspicion was augmented by the radiological appearance of diffusely scattered calcifications within the mass. As has been mentioned in Exercise 4, this complication occurs in approximately 10% of individuals affected by diaphyseal aclasis.

The diagnosis was established finally by the histological appearance of the material obtained by the biopsy of the bulky lesion arising from the right ilium. Q1b and c showed the tumour to consist essentially of cartilage, recognised from the rounded cells and cell spaces and also from the bluish staining of the intercellular matrix in the haematoxylin and eosin stained sections. Unlike the cartilaginous components of the benign neoplasms described in Exercises 4 and 12, however, the increased cellularity of the tissue, containing large bizarre cells with binucleate and mitotic features, left no doubt that the lesion was malignant.

Resection of the neoplasm was attempted at operation, but was inevitably incomplete. The huge retroperitoneal mass was confirmed to have originated in the ilium, but extended proximally to compress the right kidney and was related closely to the abdominal aorta. Palliative radiotherapy proved to be of little value and death from pulmonary metastases followed 7 months later.

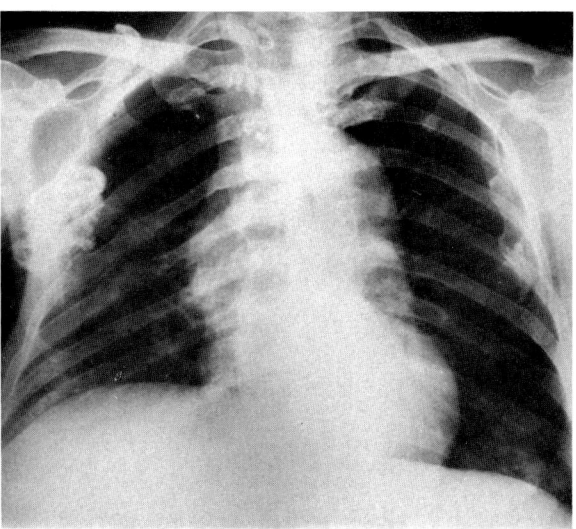

Fig. 1.1. Multiple exostoses on the ribs and scapula of the same patient.

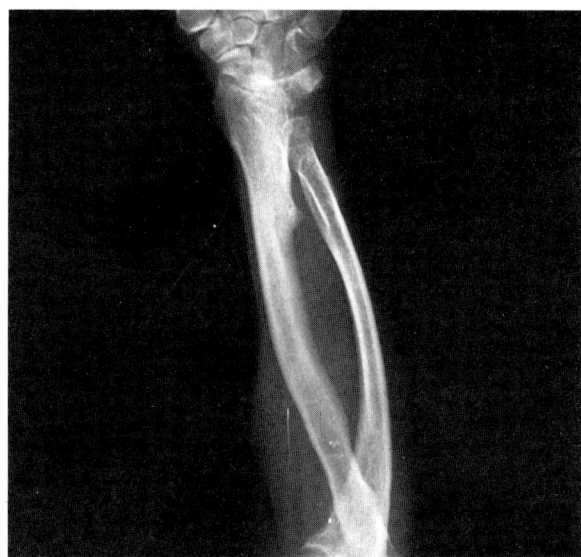

Fig. 1.2. Modelling deformities of the right radius and ulna. The latter bone is short and bowed and another exostosis is present on the radius.

Q1. This 52-year-old woman presented with a history of pain in the back for 8 months, with loss of weight of 16 kg and recent difficulty in walking.

On clinical examination tenderness was elicited over T6, with evidence of sensory and motor deficits in the lower limbs.

Radiological examination revealed extensive destruction of the body of T6 and of the adjacent portions of the bodies of T5 and T7. Bilateral paraspinal soft tissue masses were present. No other bony abnormality was detected in the remainder of the skeleton.

Laboratory investigations: Hb 11 g, ESR 45 mm/h, Mantoux positive at 1:5000, serum proteins and electrophoresis normal.

The lesion was explored.

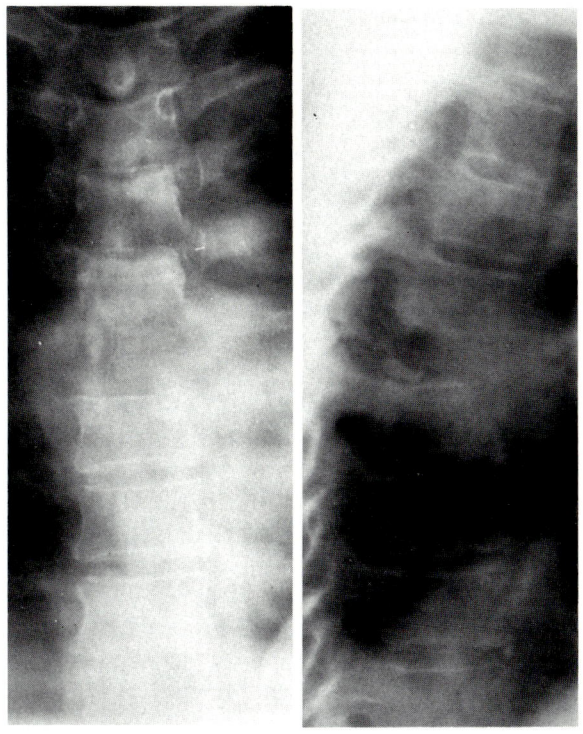

Q1a.

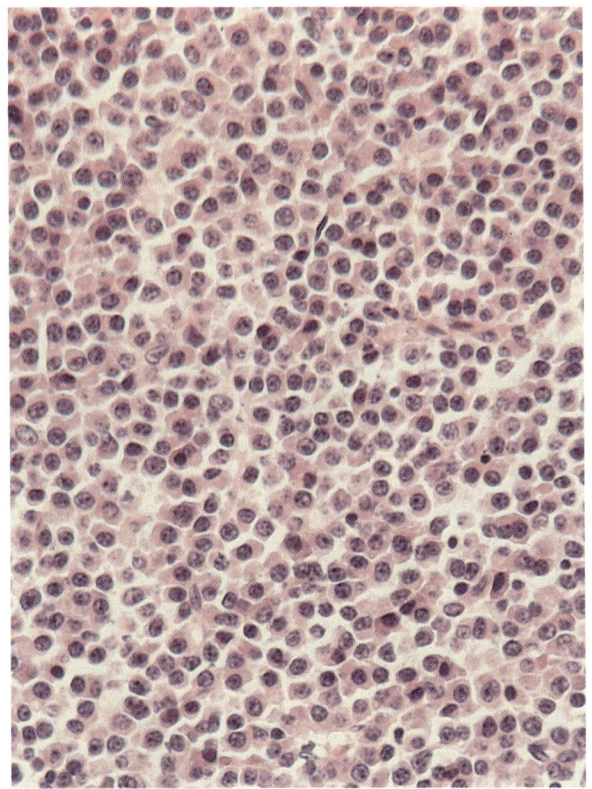

Q1b. (×350)

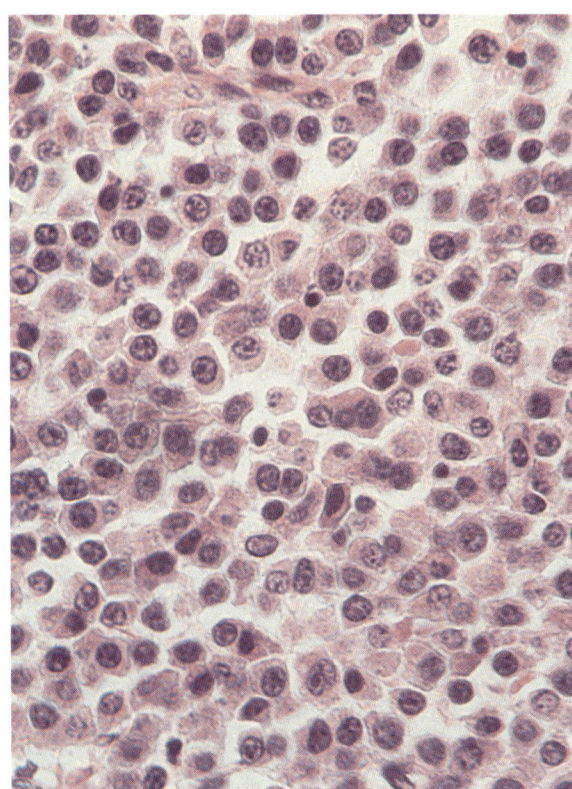

Q1c. (×610)

A1. Myelomatosis

A confident pre-operative diagnosis of tuberculosis (Pott's disease) was made, because of the radiological evidence of the involvement of three vertebral bodies, together with the strongly positive tuberculin test (Mantoux reaction) and the normal serum proteins. The paravertebral opacities were regarded as tuberculous abscesses.

Costo-transversectomy was undertaken to decompress the spinal cord and to obtain material for diagnosis. Instead of pus or granulation tissue, the surgeon was surprised to encounter a solid fleshy mass. This mass was biopsied. The sections (Q1b and c) show the unmistakable appearances of myeloma (plasmacytoma). The entire tissue consists of plasma cells. The presence of binucleate and mitotic cells indicates clearly the neoplastic nature of the lesion (see Exercise 37). No tuberculous or other inflammatory tissue was present.

A section from part of the 6th rib, removed during the course of the operation (Fig. 1.1), shows a lesser degree of involvement of the bone marrow by myeloma cells, which are apparent as small dark structures lying between the larger rounded outlines of fat cells. This pattern constitutes definite evidence of generalised marrow involvement. At this stage, no radiological or biochemical evidence of myelomatosis was present, but 1 year later the patient returned to hospital with disseminated bony lesions of myelomatosis.

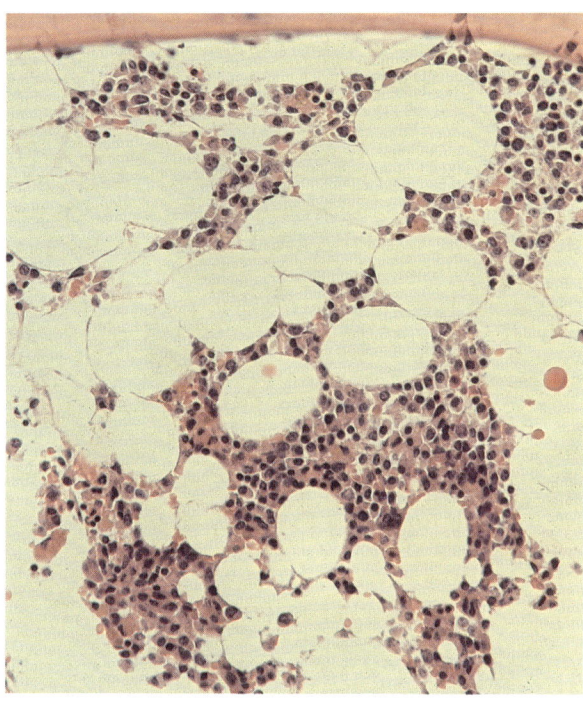

Fig. 1.1. Diffuse infiltration of bone marrow of rib by myeloma cells. (×210)

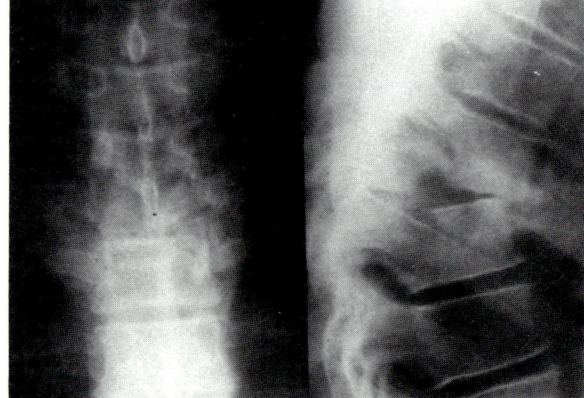

Fig. 1.2. *Myeloma of thoracic spine.* This 43-year-old farm labourer had complained of mid-thoracic pain for 1 year. The body of T8 had undergone complete attrition with extensive destruction of the adjacent portions of the bodies of T7 and 9. Not surprisingly, Pott's disease was suspected in view of a positive Mantoux test and an ESR of 40, despite partial preservation of the vertebral end-plates and anterior new bone formation. Other laboratory investigations, including serum electrophoresis, were negative. At operation the lobulated paravertebral masses were found to consist of solid tumour tissue identical to that in Q1. Excellent recovery followed radiotherapy, the patient being alive and well 6 years later.

Exercise 55

Q1. This 51-year-old woman presented with a history of recent back pain.

On clinical examination marked tenderness was elicited over L2. No other significant abnormality was detected.

The radiographs showed confluent lytic areas involving the body and neural arch of L2.

A biopsy was performed.

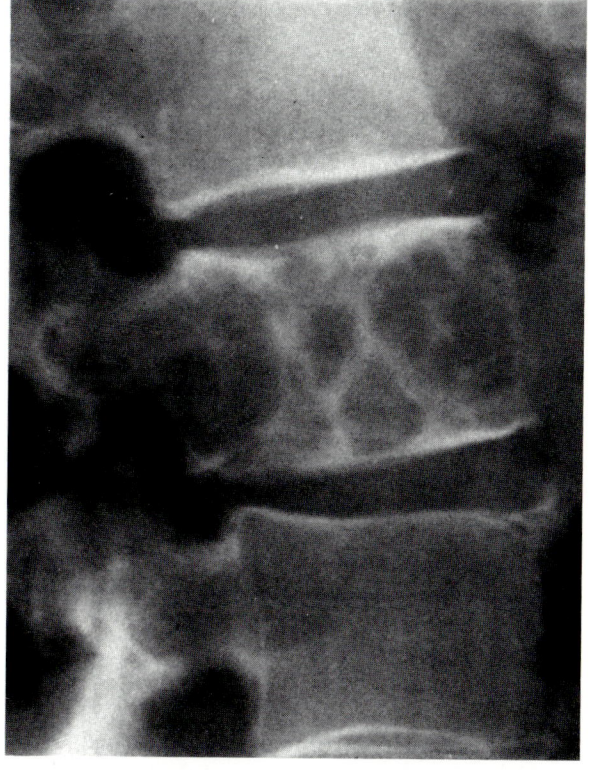

Q1a.

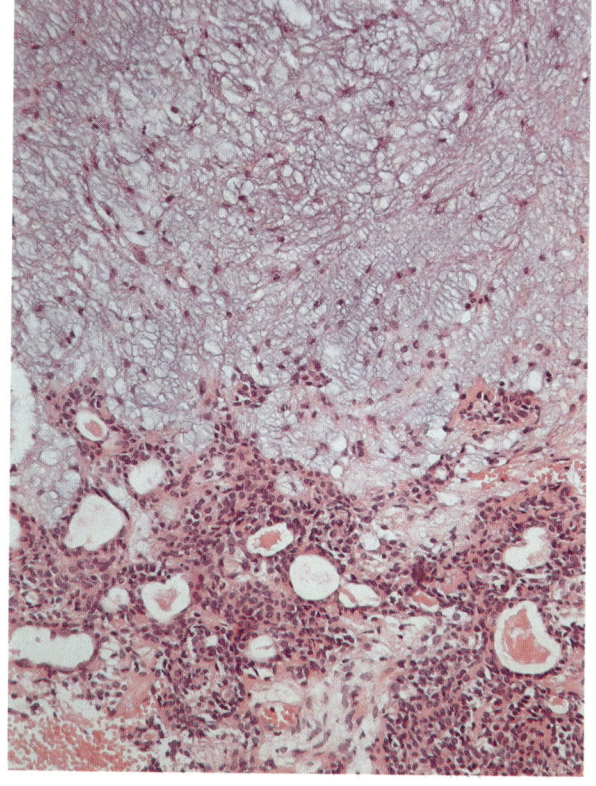

Q1b. (×110)

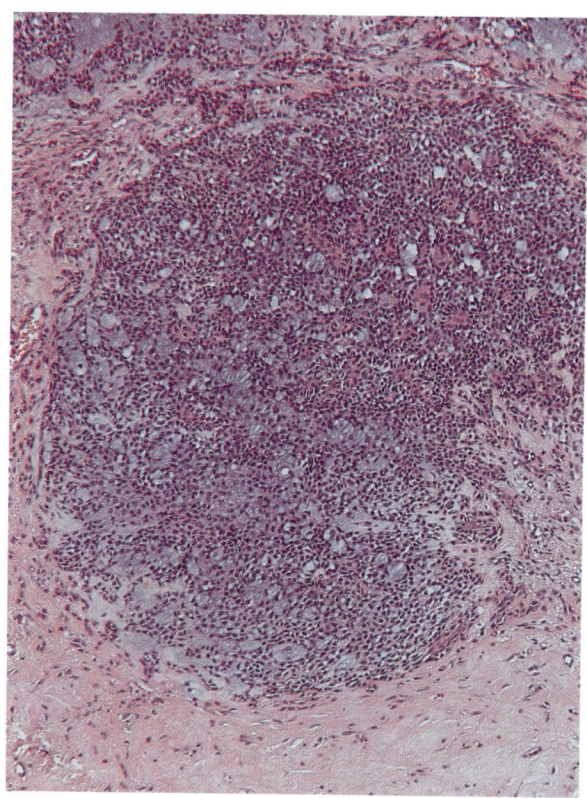

Q1c. (×85)

A1. Metastasis from 'mixed tumour' of parotid

The correct diagnosis was not suggested pre-operatively. A haemangioma of cavernous type was favoured (see Exercise 34) and the possibility of fibrous dysplasia was considered. Despite the apparently benign radiological appearance a metastasis could not be excluded at this age.

The biopsy shows a decidedly unusual histological appearance. In Q1b the upper part of the field consists of poorly cellular tissue with abundant bluish-staining myxoid or chondroid intercellular material. In the lower part of the field tongues of more cellular tissue contain rounded spaces. Q1c demonstrates a rounded mass of cellular tissue which contains the same bluish intercellular material as that evident in Q1b. It might be thought that the lesion was a primary bone tumour with an unusual type of cartilage matrix. It is, however, a metastasis from a 'mixed tumour' of the parotid. The primary tumour had been excised 20 years before. Examination of the original sections of the parotid tumour (Figs. 1.1a and b) shows the same histological features as the bone lesion. The histological appearance is, in fact, quite characteristic of this type of salivary tumour, sometimes described as a 'pleomorphic adenoma'. The epithelial nature of the lesion is readily apparent in Fig. 1.1a and the chondroid material is seen to develop from the stromal connective tissue. In Fig. 1.1b, the chondroid material, with its diffuse basophilic staining and its round cell spaces, exhibits a close resemblance to normal cartilage. Histological evidence of malignancy is not present, either in the primary tumour or in the spinal lesion.

This type of salivary tumour, usually involving the parotid, is a slowly growing and usually benign lesion. Local recurrence, following incomplete excision, is not uncommon. Exceedingly rarely, as in the present case, a tumour of this type has been reported to metastasise without any histological evidence of malignant change. Salivary tumours usually metastasise to the lungs, although other tissues, including bone, can be involved.

Treatment posed a problem in this unusual case. Since histological study had excluded the usual types of malignant metastatic tumours, and further operative intervention at this level was considered to be hazardous, the patient was treated empirically by low dose radiation therapy.

References

Gerughty RM, Scofield HH, Brown FM, Hennigar GR (1969) Malignant mixed tumours of salivary gland origin. Cancer 24: 471–486

Thackray AC, Lucas RB (1974) Tumors of the major salivary glands. Atlas of Tumor Pathology (2nd Series, Fascicle 10). AFIP Washington

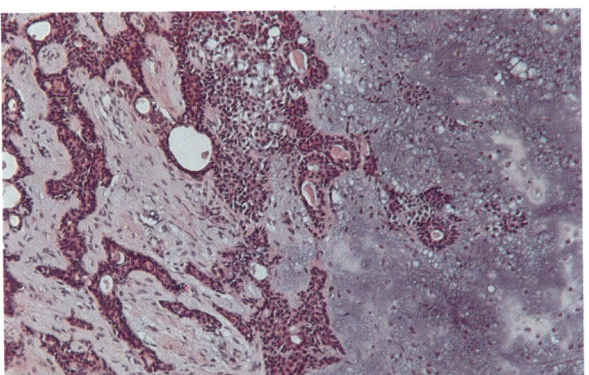

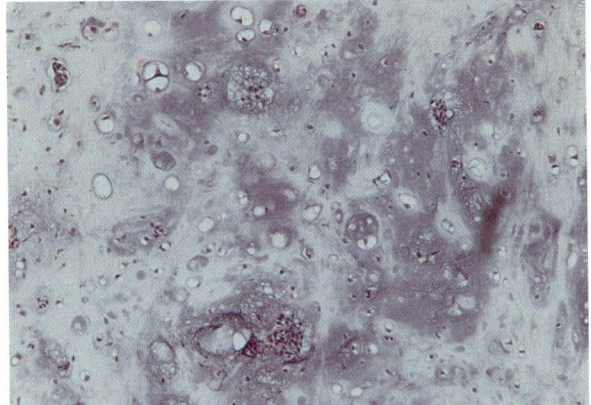

Fig. 1.1a The histological appearance of the primary tumour of the parotid in this case. The epithelial nature of the cellular tissue is apparent. (×80). b Another field from the primary tumour. The chondroid intercellular material closely resembles normal cartilage. (×80)

Exercise 56

Q1. This 54-year-old woman attended hospital because of a chronic ache in the left hip. This discomfort had been present for some months.

On clinical examination some restriction of movement of the left hip was detected. No other abnormality was found.

Radiological examination showed a large osteolytic lesion in the head and neck of the femur. Its margin was clearly defined. It contained interspersed densities.

A biopsy was performed.

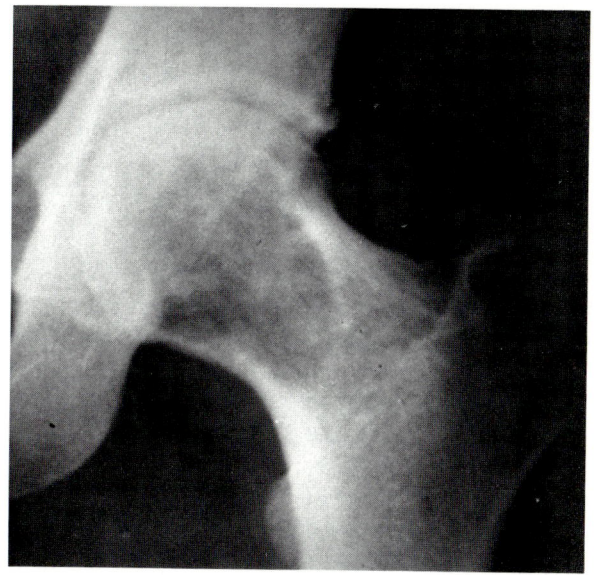

Q1a.

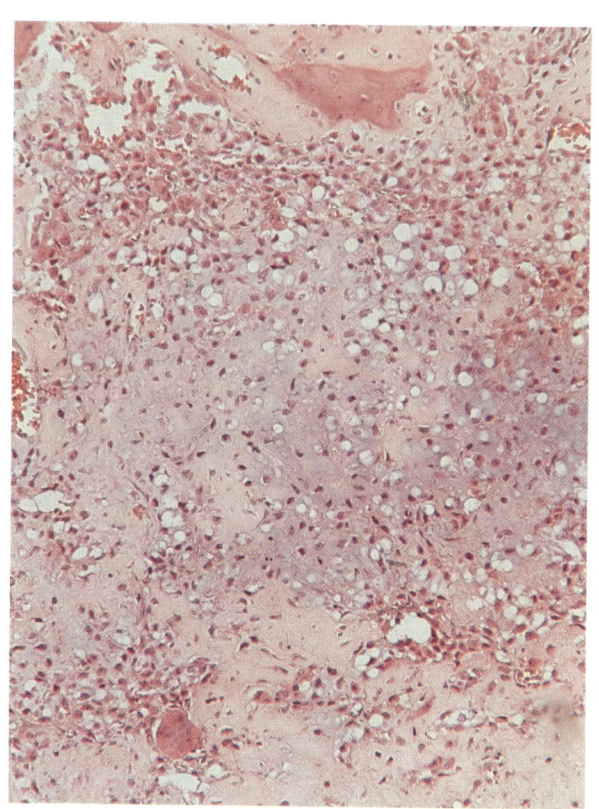

Q1b. (×105)

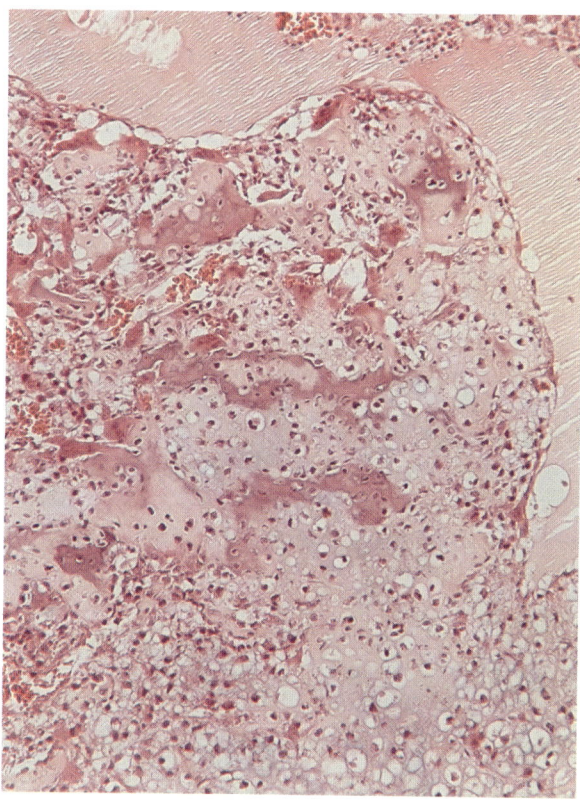

Q1c (×105)

A1. Clear-cell chondrosarcoma of femur

The relatively minor clinical abnormalities were associated with a radiological pattern which suggested a benign lesion, and a pre-operative diagnosis of fibrous dysplasia was offered.

Histologically, the biopsy material (Q1b and c) shows a lesion consisting of rounded cells, the nuclei of which are surrounded by a conspicuous clear, or vacuolated, space. The intervening matrix has a cartilaginous or chondroid appearance. Scattered osteoclast giant cells and occasional bone trabeculae are present. The appearances are, in fact, those of the rare form of malignant cartilaginous neoplasm known as the 'clear-cell chondrosarcoma'. The matrix and the rounded cells are thought to be the essential part of the lesion, while the osteoclasts and bony structures are regarded as part of the reaction to it by the host tissues. The term 'clear-cell chondrosarcoma', although a good description of the appearance of the tumour in conventional histological preparations, may be something of a misnomer. In imprint preparations (Fig. 1.1) and in electron micrographs, the tumour cells are not vacuolated, the clear spaces involving the intercellular matrix surrounding the cells.

The lesion was treated first by curettage, but this procedure was followed by local recurrence, treated in turn by local resection and prosthetic replacement of the proximal end of the femur. Six years later an osteolytic lesion developed in the right ilium. This, too, was resected and showed exactly the same histological structure as the original lesion of the left femur. Later, further tumours developed in the left humerus and the skull, and the patient died with evidence of pulmonary metastases 8 years after presentation of the original tumour.

Clear-cell chondrosarcoma is a rare variety of chondrosarcoma (See Exercise 16). As in the present case, it is often regarded, clinically and radiologically, as a benign lesion. It typically involves the ends of the long bones in adult patients. Growth is slow, but metastases may occur. Treatment is similar to that of other types of chondrosarcoma and depends essentially on the size and site of the lesion.

Reference

Unni KK, Dahlin DC, Beabout JW, Sim FH (1976) Chondrosarcoma: clear cell variant. A report of sixteen cases. J Bone Jt Surg 58A:676–683

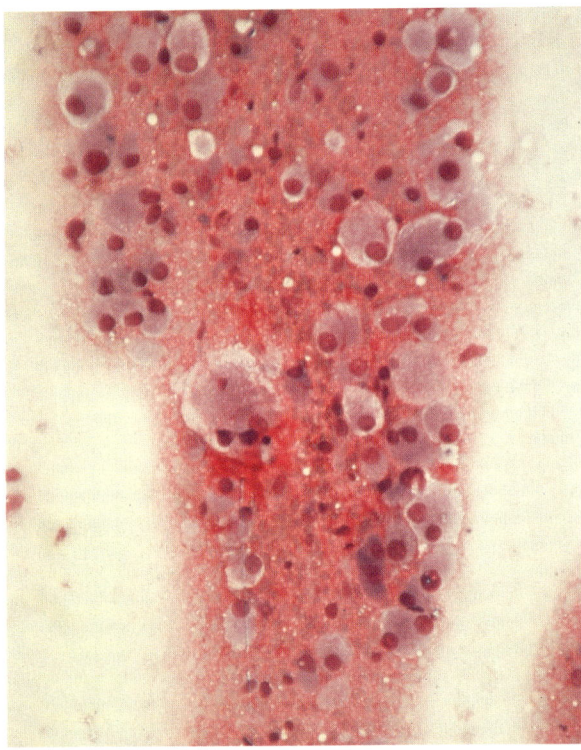

Fig. 1.1. An imprint preparation from the tumour in Q1. In contrast to the appearance in sections, the rounded tumour cells are clearly outlined and their cytoplasm is not vacuolated (×350)

Exercise 57

Q1. This 26-year-old woman had been aware of mild and intermittent pain in the right knee for 3 years. These symptoms had increased in severity during the previous 6 months.

On clinical examination a firm and slightly tender swelling of the proximal end of the tibia was present. The overlying skin was normal and no other clinical abnormality was found. The results of routine laboratory investigations were normal.

Radiological examination revealed a grossly expansile lytic lesion involving the proximal end of the tibia. Coarse linear densities were present within the osteolytic area. The expanded cortex was reduced to the thickness of an eggshell. The endosteal margin was clearly defined, with a narrow zone of transition. Partial collapse of the tibial plateau had occurred.

A biopsy was performed.

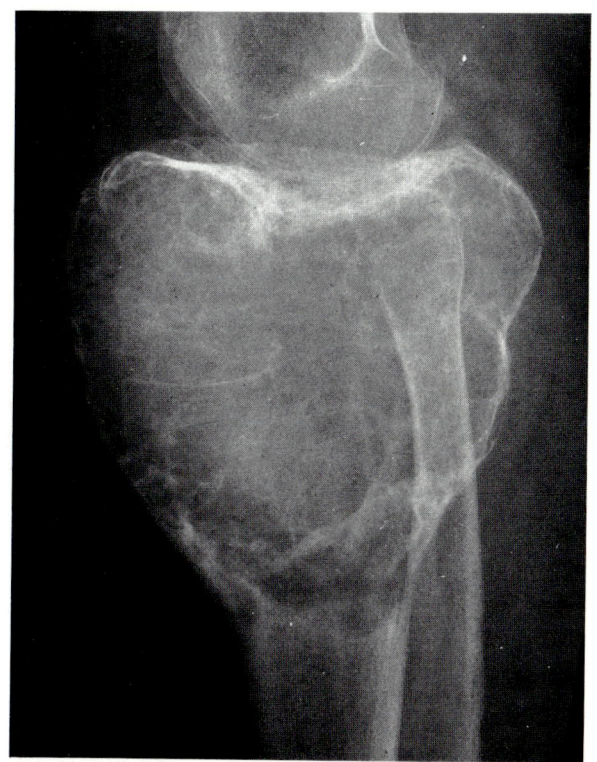

Q1a.

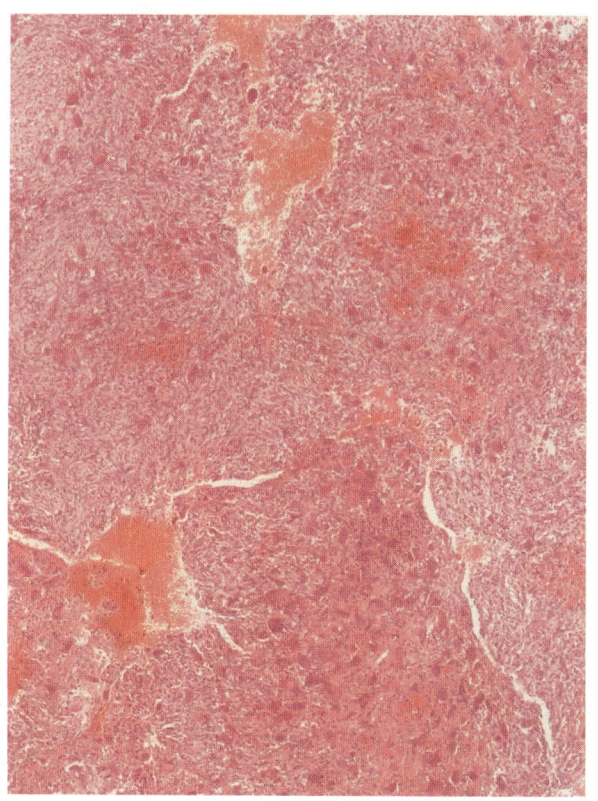

Q1b. (×46)

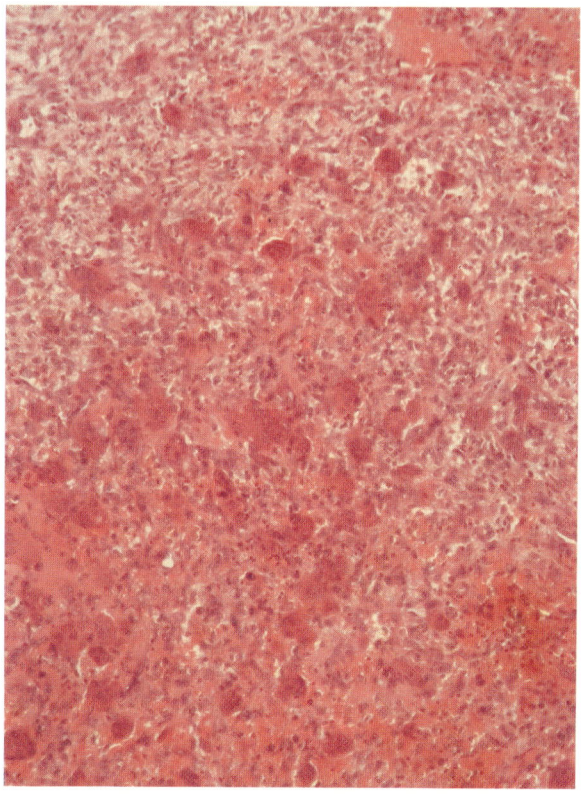

Q1c. (×120)

A1. Secondary aneurysmal bone cyst (developing in giant-cell tumour of tibia)

The clinical and radiological features in this patient caused both aneurysmal bone cyst and giant-cell tumour to be considered as preoperative diagnoses. The radiological difficulty of distinguishing between these two conditions has been emphasised in Exercises 15 and 22. In the present case the lesion is situated in a common location for a giant-cell tumour and the age of the patient is appropriate. On the other hand the gross enlargement of the affected portion of the bone, the collapse of the tibial plateau and the sharply defined and narrow zone of transition are more characteristic of an aneurysmal bone cyst.

A limited biopsy from the lesion produced solid tissue, the histological appearance of which is shown in Q1b and c. The presence of a large number of evenly distributed osteoclast giant cells, separated by spindle-celled stromal tissue, established a diagnosis of giant-cell tumour and appeared to resolve the diagnostic problem.

It was decided to treat the lesion by local resection. The appearance of the longitudinally divided surgical specimen is shown in Fig. 1.1. In contrast to the biopsy findings, the lesion was predominantly cystic. It contained only a small amount of solid tissue, most of it appearing as narrow partitions between the cystic spaces. Many of these spaces (see Fig. 1.2a and b) contained blood and were lined by flattened endothelial cells. They have all the features of the spaces observed in aneurysmal bone cyst (see Exercise 22). Some of the few solid areas have, like the biopsy, the characteristic histological features of giant-cell tumour (Fig. 1.2c), while others show the collections of lipid-filled histiocytes not infrequently encountered in giant-cell tumour and in aneurysmal bone cyst (Fig. 1.2d).

This combination of the histological features of giant-cell tumour and aneurysmal bone cyst is not unusual, and is explained by the concept of a secondary cystic change occurring in the original giant-cell tumour. (See Exercise 22 for other examples of secondary aneurysmal bone cyst).

Reference

Bonakdarpour A, Levy WM, Aegerter E (1978) Primary and secondary aneurysmal bone cyst. A radiological study of 75 cases. Radiology 126: 75–83

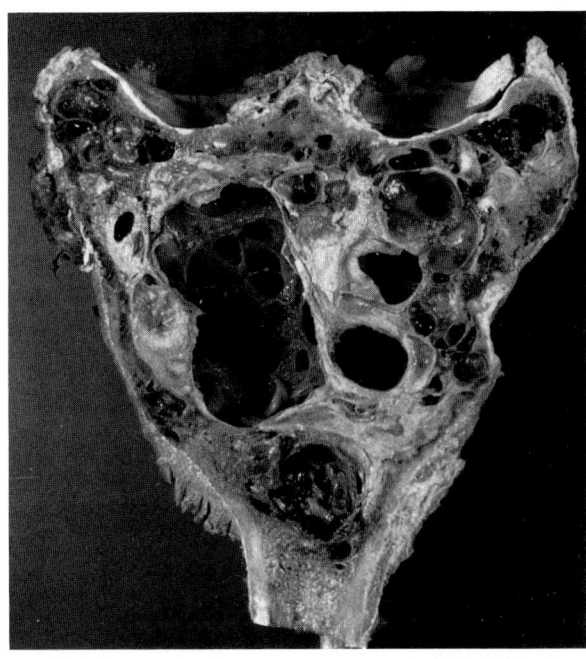

Fig. 1.1. Longitudinally divided resection specimen from the case in Q1. The lesion is predominantly cystic.

Opposite page ⎯⎯⎯⎯⎯⎯⎯⎯→

Fig. 1.2. Histological preparations from different parts of the resection specimen shown in Fig. 1.1. **a** From a cystic part of the lesion, showing prominent spaces separated by relatively small amounts of solid tissue, some of it staining darkly because of its cellularity (×6). **b** Further cystic spaces containing blood and lined by flattened endothelial cells. The thinned and expanded cortex can be seen above and to the right (×43). **c** An area of solid tissue, with numerous giant cells (×120). **d** Another area of solid tissue, with numerous pale rounded lipid-containing histiocytes (×120).

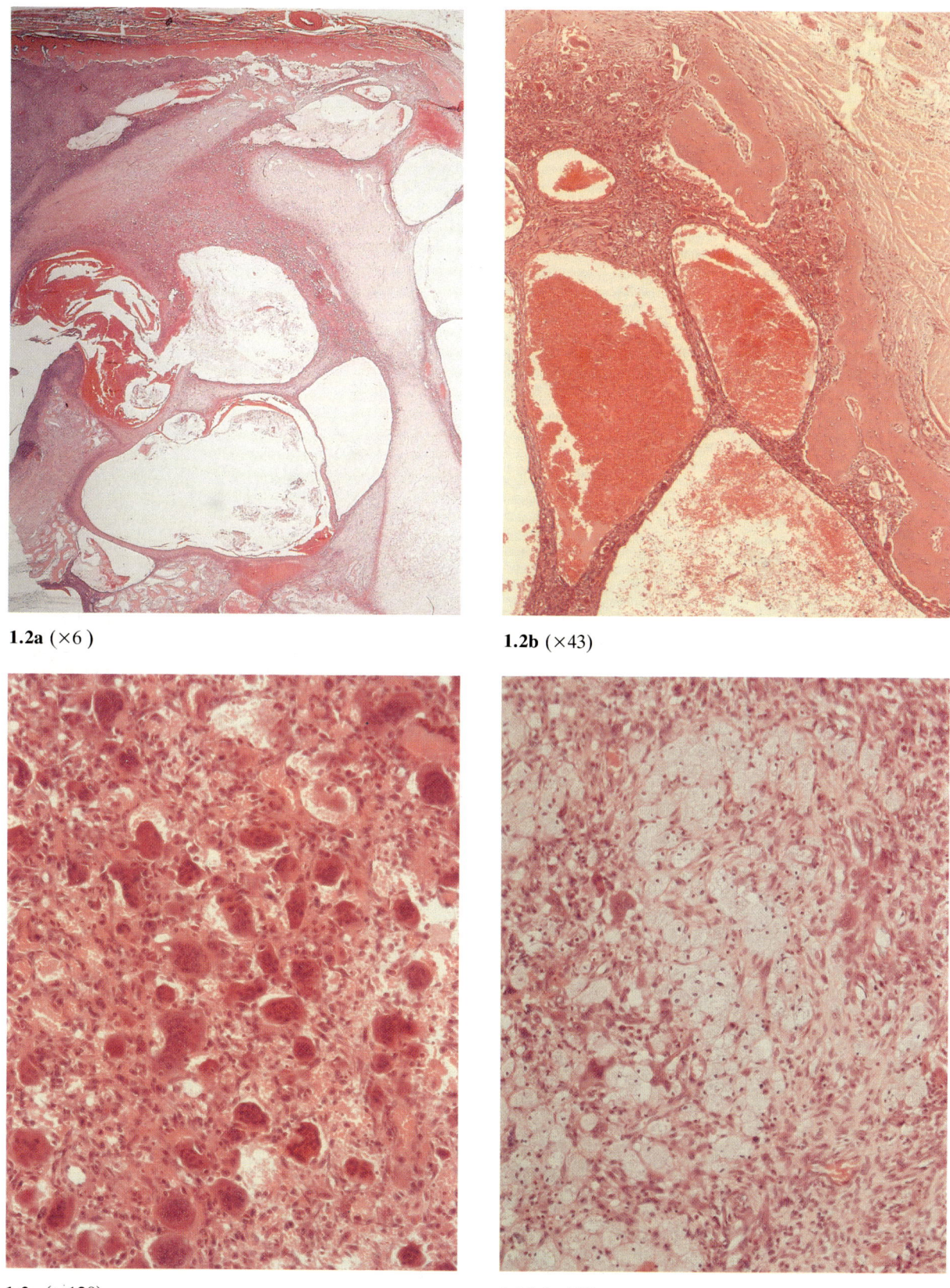

1.2a (×6)

1.2b (×43)

1.2c (×120)

1.2d (×120)

Index

Page references in bold type indicate main descriptions
Page references in roman type indicate answers to questions and supplementary mentions
Page references in italic type indicate clinical, radiological and pathological illustrations
Generalities, such as infections and neoplasms, are listed individually.

Abscess, Brodie's 87, *90–91*
Acetabular dysplasia 44
   secondary osteoarthritis in *47*
Adamantinoma of long bones 229, **230–231**, *231*
Ainhum 344
Albright's syndrome 2
Alcoholism, chronic 64
   infarcts in *67*
Alkaptonuria (ochronosis) 277, *277*
Ameloblastoma 231
Amyloidosis
   in rheumatoid arthritis 156
   in myelomatosis 314, *315*
Anaemia
   due to iron deficiency 295
   in Gaucher's disease 296
   in myelomatosis 313
   in sickle cell disease 292
   thalassaemia (Cooley's, Mediterranean) 295
Andersson lesion 163, *166*
Aneurysm, arterio-venous 289, *289*
Aneurysmal bone cyst *194–196*, **197–198**, *198–201, 344, 372, 374, 374*
   secondary to chondroblastoma 195, 196
   secondary to giant-cell tumour 395, 396, *396–397*
Angiomatosis, cystic **287**, *287*
Ankylosing spondylitis **163–164**, *164–166*, 364
   Andersson lesion in 163, *166*
   HLA antigen in 163
   Romanus lesion in 163, *166*
   syndesmophytes in 163, *164*
Anorexia nervosa 19, *23*
Anticonvulsant therapy in epilepsy 25, 29
Antigens, HLA in seronegative spondyloarthropathies 154, 162
Arterio-venous aneurysm 289, *289*

Arthritis
   degenerative—*see under* osteoarthritis
   erosive (inflammatory) osteoarthritis **169**, *169*
   infantile septic 86, *91*
   psoriatic **167**, *167*
   rheumatoid 152, **154–156**, *157–161*
      juvenile (Still's disease) 154, *161–162*
   tuberculous *94–97, 96–97*, **98–99**, *99–101*
Arthropathy
   iatrogenic 20, 23, 45, *51*
Atrophy
   disuse 20, *24*
   Sudeck's 19, *24*

Baker's cyst, synovial chondromatosis in *77, 78*
Behçet's syndrome **169**
Benign chondroblastoma 213, **214–215**, *215*
Benign osteoblastoma 185, **190–191**, *191–193, 365, 367, 367*
Bladder, metastasis from *7, 8, 12*
Blastomycosis 92
Bone cyst
   aneurysmal *194–196*, **197–198**, *198–201, 344, 372, 374, 374*
   secondary to chondroblastoma 195, 196
   secondary to giant-cell tumour 395, 396, *396–397*
   simple (unicameral) 171, **172–173**, *173–174*
   subchondral, post-inflammatory 44, *47, 49*
   post-traumatic *41–43*, 155, *159, 161*
Bone tumours, *see specific types*
   complicating infarcts *349*, **350**
Bouchard nodes 46

Breast, metastasis from *8, 12, 13, 364, 366, 367*
Brodie's abscess 87, *90–91*, 343
Bronchus, metastasis from *8–9, 13–14, 337, 342*
'Brown' tumours in hyperparathyroidism 202–203, 204–208, *209–211*
Burns 67

Caisson disease (dysbaric necrosis) 59, 61, 64, *67*
Calcium pyrophosphate deposition disease (CPDD) 269, **275–276**, *276*
   pyrophosphate crystals in 269, 275
Cartilage-capped exostosis (osteochondroma) 30–33, **34–35**, *35–37*
   secondary chondrosarcoma in 137, *144*
Cherubism 2, **5**
Chondroblastoma, benign 213, **214–215**, *215*
Chondrocalcinosis, polyarticular 269, **275–276**, *276*
   hyperparathyroidism in 208, *211*
   pyrophosphate crystals in 269, 275
Chondroma 102, 103, **104–105**, *106–107, 344*
   multiple (enchondromatosis, Ollier's disease) 104, *107, 353, 356*
   Maffucci's syndrome in **105**
   secondary chondrosarcoma in 144
   parosteal 106
Chondromatosis, synovial 77, **78–79**, *80–83*
   Baker's cyst in *77, 78*
   chondrosarcoma in 78–79, *83*
Chondromyxoid fibroma 247, **248–249**, *250–251*
Chondrosarcoma 135, 136, *136*, **137–139**, *140–143, 381, 382*

Chondrosarcoma—*continued*
    clear cell   138, *393*, **394**, *394*
        imprint preparation in   *394*
    dedifferentiated   138, *345*, 346, **347**, *348*
    mesenchymal   138
    secondary to
        benign enchondroma   137
        cartilage-capped exostosis   137, *144*
        diaphyseal aclasis   *387*, 388
        Maffucci's syndrome   137, *144*
        synovial chondromatosis   78–79, 83
        soft tissue, in   *144*
Chordoma   265, **266–267**, *267*
Chronic granulomatous disease   87, **182**, 183
Clear cell chondrosarcoma   138, *393*, **394**, *394*
    imprint preparation in   *394*
Coccidioidomycosis   92
Codman triangle in Ewing's sarcoma   255, *258–259*
    in osteosarcoma   124, *126*
Colon, metastasis from   8, *14*
Cooley's anaemia (thalassaemia)   295
Coxa valga magna luxans   99
Cushing's syndrome (hypercorticism)   19, *23*, 45
    iatrogenic   20, *23*
    stress fractures in   234, *239*
Cyst
    aneurysmal bone   *194–196*, **197–198**, *198–201*, *344*, 372, 374, *374*
    secondary to
        chondroblastoma   *195*, 196
    secondary to giant-cell tumour   *395*, 396, *396–397*
    epidermal (implantation dermoid)   *336*, **340**, *341*
    simple (unicameral)   *171*, **172–173**, *173–174*
    semimembranosus (Baker's), synovial chondromatosis in   77, 78
    subchondral post-inflammatory   44, *47*, 49
    subchrondral post-traumatic   *41–43*, 155, *159*, *161*
Cystic angiomatosis   **287**, *287*
Cystinosis   25

Dactylitis, tuberculous   112, *115*, *343*
Diabetic neuropathy   344
Dedifferentiated chondrosarcoma   138, *345*, 346, **347**, *348*
Degenerative joint disease (osteoarthritis)   *40–41*, *42–43*, **44–45**, *46–50*, 153, 162, *380*
    post-inflammatory   *41*, *42–44*, *43*, *159*, *161*
    post-traumatic   40, *42*, *46–49*
    secondary to
        acetabular dysplasia   44, *47*
        athletic stress   44, *46–47*
        Perthes' disease   44, *49*
        slipped upper femoral epiphysis   44, *48*
    spinal   44, *50*

Desmoplastic fibroma   357, **358–359**, *359*
Diaphyseal aclasis (multiple hereditary exostoses)   34, **38–39**, *387*, *388*, *388*
    chondrosarcoma in   *387*, *388*, *388*
Diffuse idiopathic skeletal hyperostosis (DISH, Forestier's disease)   **170**, *170*
Disc, intervertebral, degeneration of   44, *50*
Discitis, infective   *109*, **116–117**, *116*, *118–119*
Disuse osteoporosis   20, *24*
Dysbaric necrosis (caisson disease)   59, 61, 64, 67
Dyschondroplasia (enchondromatosis, Ollier's disease) 104, *107*, *353*, 356
    with haemangiomas (Maffucci's syndrome)   105, *107*, 356
    secondary chondrosarcoma in   137, *144*
Dysplasia
    acetabular   44, 47
    epiphysealis hemimelica (Trevor's disease)   34, *39*
    fibrous   1, **2–3**, *4–5*, *380*, 382, *382*
        monostotic   *1*, 2, *3–5*, *380*, 382, *382*
        polyostotic   2, *4–5*
        sarcoma in 2, 5
    osteofibrous   2, *4*, *352*, **354–355**, *354–355*
Dystrophy, reflex sympathetic   19

Enchondroma *102–103*, **104–105**, *106–107*, *344*
Enchondromatosis (multiple enchondroma, Ollier's disease)   104, *107*, *353*, 356
    secondary chondrosarcoma in   137, *144*
Eosinophil granuloma   *175*, 176, **177**, *179–181*, *369*, 371
Epidermal cyst   *336*, **340**, *341*
Epilepsy, anticonvulsant therapy in   25, *29*
Erosive (inflammatory) osteoarthritis   **169**, *169*
Ewing's sarcoma   252, **254–256**, *256–259*, 376, 378, *378–379*
    Codman triangle in   255, *258–259*
    intracellular glycogen in   254–255, *256*
    saucerisation defect in   259
Exostosis, cartilage-capped (osteochondroma)   *30–31*, 32, 33, *32–33*, **34–35**, *35–39*
    secondary chondrosarcoma in   137, *144*

Fanconi syndrome   25, *29*
Fibroma
    chondromyxoid   247, **248–249**, *249–251*
    desmoplastic   357, **358–359**, *359*
    non-ossifying   *52–54*, 54, **55**, *56–57*

Fibrosarcoma   240, **242–243**, *243–244*
    associated with infarcts   350
    in fibrous dysplasia   5
    of soft tissues   242, *244*
Fibrous cortical defects (non-ossifying fibroma)   *52–54*, 54, **55**, *56–57*
Fibrous dysplasia   1, **2–3**, *4–5*, *380*, 382, *382*
    monostotic   *1*, 2, *3–5*, *380*, 382, *382*
    polyostotic   2, *4–5*
    sarcoma in   2, 5
Forestier's disease (diffuse idiopathic skeletal hyperostosis, DISH)   **170**, *170*
Frostbite   67
Fungus infection   88, *92*
    blastomycosis   92
    coccidioidomycosis   92
    mycetoma   92
    torulosis   343

Gaucher's disease   291, **296–297**, *297–299*
    anaemia in   296
    infarcts in   296, *297*
    osteomyelitis in   299
Giant-cell tumour   129, **130–131**, *132–134*
    secondary aneurysmal bone cyst in   *395*, 396, *396–397*
Glomus tumour   288, *337*, **341–342**, *342*
Glycogen, intracellular in Ewing's sarcoma   254–255, *256*
    Schiff technique for   *256*, 262
Gorham's syndrome (haemangiomatosis, massive osteolysis, vanishing bone disease)   **286**, *286*
Gout   *268*, **270–272**, *344*
    urate crystals in   271, *272*
    pseudotumours in   271, *274*
Granuloma, eosinophil   *175*, 176, **177**, *179–181*, *369*, 371

Haemangioma of bone   *278–279*, **281–282**, *283–285*
    capillary   280
    cavernous   280
    associated with dyschondroplasia (Maffucci's syndrome)   105, *107*
    secondary chondrosarcoma in   *144*
Haemangiomatosis (Gorham's syndrome, massive osteolysis, vanishing bone disease)   **286**, *286*
Haemangiopericytoma   **288**, *288*
    associated with osteomalacia   288
Haematoma
    intramuscular calcifying   *327*
    subperiosteal   *320*, **326**, *327*
Haemopoiesis, extramedullary
    in sickle cell disease   292, *295*
    in thalassaemia   295
Hand-Schüller-Christian disease   **177**, *181*
Heberden nodes   46

Hepato-lenticular degeneration (Wilson's disease) **277**, *277*
Histiocytic lymphoma 260
Histiocytoma, malignant fibrous *241*, **245–246**, *246*
　associated with bone infarct 349, **350**, *351*
　of soft tissue 246
Histiocytosis *175–176*, **177–178**, *179–181*
Hodgkin's disease *223*, **224–225**, *226–228*
Human leucocyte antigens (HLA) 154
　in seronegative spondyloarthropathies 162
Hypercalcaemia
　in hyperparathyroidism 206
　in myelomatosis 313
Hypercorticism (Cushing's syndrome) *19*, *23*, 45
　iatrogenic 20, *23*
　stress fractures in 234, *239*
Hyperparathyroidism *202–203*, *204–205*, **205**, **206–208**, *209–211*
　'brown' tumours in *202–203*, *204–208*, *209–211*
　chondrocalcinosis in 208, *211*
　primary *202*, 204, 206, 207–208, *209–211*
　secondary in osteomalacia *203*, *204–208*, *211*
　tetany, post-operative in 210
　tertiary 207
　urinary calculi in 206
Hyperphosphatasia *363*
Hypophosphatasia 25, *363*

Iatrogenic arthropathy 20, *23*, 45, 51
Implantation dermoid cyst *336*, **340**, *341*
Imprint preparation in clear cell chondrosarcoma *394*, *394*
Infantile septic arthritis *86*, *91*
Infarcts of bone *59*, *61*, **64**, *67*, *292*, *294*, *296*, *297*, *349*, *350*
　bone tumours associated with 349, 350
　caisson disease (dysbaric osteonecrosis) in *59*, *61*, *64*, *67*
　chronic alcoholism in *64*, *67*
　Gaucher's disease in *291*, *296*, *297–299*
　idiopathic 64
　malignant fibrous histiocytoma in *349*, *350*
　sickle cell disease in *290*, *292*, *294*
Infective discitis *109*, *116*, **116–117**, *118–119*
Inflammatory (erosive) osteoarthritis **169**, 169
Intervertebral disc, degeneration of 44, 50

Juvenile rheumatoid arthritis (Still's disease) 154, *161–162*
Juxtacortical (parosteal) chondroma 105, *106*

Juxtacortical (parosteal) osteosarcoma *319*, 322, **323–324**, *324–325*

Kidney, metastasis from *8*, *10*, *13*
Kienbock's disease (post-traumatic necrosis of lunate) *63*, *216*, 218

'Lazy leucocyte' syndrome **182**, *183*
Leontiasis ossea *2*, *5*
Leprosy
　lepromatous *343*
　neuropathic *343*
Letterer-Siwe disease 177, *181*
Lipomatous tumours *330–331*, **332–333**, *334–335*
　lipoma of neural canal *334*
　parosteal 330
　of soft tissues *334*
　liposarcoma *331*, *335*
　of soft tissues *335*
Looser's zones *17*, *25–26*, *27–28*
Lung, metastasis from *8*, *9*, *13–14*, *337*, *342*
Lymphoma
　histiocytic 260
　malignant 260

Maffucci's syndrome 105, *107*, *356*
　chondrosarcoma in 137, *144*
Malignant fibrous histiocytoma *241*, **245–246**, *246*, *349*, *350*, *351*
　associated with bone infarct 349, 350, *351*
　of soft tissues 246
Malignant lymphoma 260
Malignant round cell tumour 254, *264*
Malignant synovioma (synovial sarcoma) *301*, **307–308**, *308–309*
　of soft tissues *309*
Massive osteolysis (haemangiomatosis, Gorham's syndrome, vanishing bone disease) **286**, *286*
Mediterranean anaemia (thalassaemia) *295*
Metastases, skeletal *6–7*, **8–11**, *11–15*, *364–365*, *366–367*, *366–367*, *391*, *392*, *393*
　from breast *8*, *12–13*, *364*, *366*, *366*
　bronchus *8–9*, *11*, *13–14*, *337*, 342
　colon 8, *14*
　Ewing's sarcoma 255, *258*
　kidney 8, *13*
　lung *8–9*, *11*, *13–14*, *337*, 342
　neuroblastoma *14*
　osteosarcoma 123
　Paget's disease 128
　parotid gland *391*, *392*, *393*
　prostate *6*, *8–9*, *11–12*, *14–15*
　reticulum cell sarcoma *264*
　salivary gland *14*, *391*, *392*, *393*
　skin 10, *14*
　stomach *8*, *12*
　thyroid *8*, *13*

　urinary bladder *7*, *8*, *12*, *365*, *367*, *367*
Mycetoma *92*
Myeloma, solitary (plasmacytoma) *310*, **312–314**, *316*
　progressing to myelomatosis *317*
Myelomatosis (multiple myeloma) *311*, **312–314**, *317–318*, *389*, *390*, *390*
　amyloidosis in 314, *315*
　hypercalcaemia in 313
　resembling Pott's disease *389*, 390, *390*
Myositis ossificans *320*, *326*
　paraplegic *328*

Necrosis of bone
　post-traumatic *58*, *60–62*, **62**, *65–66*, *217*, **220–221**, *222*
　due to congenital dislocation of hip 66
　due to Perthes' disease 65
　subarticular (osteochondritis dissecans) *217*, **220–221**, *222*
　systemic *59*, *61*, **64**, *67*, *290–291*, *292–293*, *294*, *296–297*, *297–299*
　alcoholism in *64*, *67*
　blood disorders in *64*, *290–291*, *292–293*, *294*, *296–297*, *297–299*
　dysbaric (caisson disease) *59*, *61*, *64*, *67*
　idiopathic 64
　poisoning in *64*
　post-radiation *64*, *67*
　thermal injuries in *64*, *67*
Nephrolithiasis in hyperparathyroidism 206
Neuroblastoma
　metastases from *14*
　catecholamines in urine in *254–255*
Neurofibromatosis, pseudarthrosis of tibia in *238*, *354*
Neuropathic joint disease
　diabetic *344*
　iatrogenic 20, *23*, 45, *51*
Non-ossifying fibroma *53–54*, **55**, *56–57*

Ochronosis (alkaptonuria) **277**, *277*
Ollier's disease (enchondromatosis) 104, *107*, *353*, *356*
　secondary chondrosarcoma in 137, *144*
Osteitis fibrosa cystica 207
Osseous syphilis *88*, *92*
　Wimberger sign in *92*
Osseous tuberculosis **111**, *115*
　cystic 112, *115*
　dactylitis 112, *115*
　Pott's puffy tumour 112, *115*
　spinal (Pott's disease) *108*, **110–112**, *110*, *111*, *113*, *114*
　subligamentous of spine 112, *114*
Osteoarthritis (degenerative joint disease) *40–41*, *42–43*, **44–45**, *46–50*, *153*, *162*, *380*

Osteoarthritis—continued
  with chondrocalcinosis 275
  inflammatory (erosive) **169**, *169*
  post-inflammatory *41*, 42–44, *43*, *159*, *161*
  post-traumatic *40*, *42*, 46–49
  secondary to
    acetabular dysplasia 44, *47*
    athletic stress 44, *46–47*
    Perthes' disease 44, *49*
    slipped upper femoral epiphysis 44, *48*
  spinal 44, *50*
Osteoblastoma, benign *185*, **190–191**, *191–193*
'Osteochondritis' **218–219**
Osteochondritis dissecans *217*, **220–221**, *222*
Osteochondroma (cartilage-capped exostosis) *30–33*, **34–35**, *35–37*
  secondary chondrosarcoma in *137*, **144**
Osteofibrous dysplasia *2*, *4*, *352*, **354–355**, *356*
Osteogenesis imperfecta *19*, *145–147*, **147**, *149*
  pseudotumours in *150*
Osteoid osteoma *184*, **186–187**, *188*, *189*, *344*, *368*, *370*, *370–371*, *377*, *379*
Osteolysis, massive (Gorham's syndrome, haemangiomatosis, vanishing bone disease) **286**, *286*
Osteoma
  ivory *34*, *39*
  osteoid *184*, **186–187**, *188*, *189*, *344*, *368*, *370*, *370–371*, *377*, *379*
Osteomalacia *17*, **25–26**, *27–29*
  haemangiopericytoma, associated with 288
  rickets in *25*, *28–29*
    dietetic *28–29*
    vitamin D resistant *29*
  steatorrhoea in *27*
  stress fractures (Looser's zones) in *26*, *27*, *234*, *238*
Osteomyelitis, pyogenic *84*, **86–88**, *88–91*
  acute *343*
  chronic sclerosing type *368*, *370*, *370–371*
  complicating Gaucher's disease *299*
  subacute *377*, *379*
  'tunnelling' in *87*, *90*, *377*, *379*
Osteonecrosis, see Necrosis of bone
Osteopetrosis, stress fractures in *238*
Osteophyte *42*, *44*, *50*
Osteoporosis *16*, *18*, **19–21**, *21–24*
  Cushing's syndrome in *19*, *23*
  disuse *20*, *24*
  iatrogenic *20*, *23*
  idiopathic *19*, *23*
  localised *19*, *24*
  post-radiation *19*, *24*
  senile *19*, *23*
  transient *19*, *24*
Osteoporosis circumscripta (Paget's disease) *71*, *76*
Osteosarcoma *120*, *122*, **123–125**, *123*, *126–127*, *233*, *239*, *373*, *374*, *375*
  Paget's disease, in *121*, **128**, *128*
  parosteal (juxtacortical) *319*, *322*, **323–324**, *324–325*
  periosteal *321*, **329**, *329*
  post-radiation *127*

Paget's disease *68–69*, **70–73**, *74–76*, *234*, *238*, *344*, *361*, *362*
  cement lines in *68*, *70*, *72*
  osteoporosis circumscripta in *71*, *76*
  sarcoma in *121*, **128**, *128*
  stress fractures in *234*, *238*
  unusual *361*, *362*
Paraplegic myositis ossificans *328*
Parosteal (juxtacortical) chondroma *105*, *106*
Parosteal (juxtacortical) osteosarcoma *319*, *322*, **323–324**, *324–325*
Pellegrini-Stieda lesion *47*
Periosteal osteosarcoma *321*, **329**, *329*
Perl's reaction for iron *302*, *302*
Perthes' disease *49*, *62*
  post-traumatic necrosis in *65*
Pigmented villonodular synovitis *79*, *301*, *302*, *302*, **303–304**, *304–306*, *385*, *386*, *386*
  Perl's reaction for iron in *302*, *302*
Plasmacytoma (solitary myeloma) *310*, **312–314**, *316*
  progressing to myelomatosis *317*
Polyarticular chondrocalcinosis (pseudogout) *269*, **275–276**, *276*
  pyrophosphate crystals in *269*, *275*
Post-radiation effects
  necrosis *64*, *67*
  sarcoma *127*
  stress fracture *238*
Post-traumatic necrosis *58*, *60–62*, **62**, *65–66*, *217*, **220–221**, *222*
  due to congenital dislocation of hip *66*
  due to Perthes' disease *65*
  of individual bones *216*, **218–219**, *218–219*, *270*
    lunate (Kienbock's disease) *216*, *218*
    metatarsal (Freiberg's disease) *270*
    navicular (Kohler's disease) *219*
  subarticular (osteochondritis dissecans) *217*, **220–221**, *222*
Pott's disease (spinal tuberculosis) *108*, **110–111**, *110–111*, *113–114*
  subligamentous *112*, *114*
Pott's puffy tumour *115*
Prostate, metastasis from *6*, *8–9*, *11–12*, *14–15*
Pseudarthrosis of tibia (in neurofibromatosis) *238*, *354*
Pseudofractures (Looser's zones) in osteomalacia *17*, *25–26*, *27–28*

Pseudogout (polyarticular chondrocalcinosis) *269*, **275–276**, *276*
  pyrophosphate crystals in *269*, *275*
Pseudomalignant osseous tumour of soft tissues *326*, *327–328*
Psoriatic arthritis **167**, *167*
  syndesmophytes in *167*, *167*
Pyogenic osteomyelitis *84*, **86–88**, *88–91*, *343*, *368*, *370*, *370–371*, *377*, *379*
  acute *343*
  chronic sclerosing type *368*, *370*, *370–371*
  subacute *377*, *379*
  'tunnelling' in *87*, *90*, *377*, *379*

Reflex sympathetic dystrophy (Sudeck's atrophy) *19*, *24*
Reiter's syndrome **168**, *168*
  syndesmophytes in *168*
Renal tubular disorders *25*, *29*
Reticulin fibres *261*, *262*
  staining technique *367*, *367*
Reticulum cell sarcoma *85*, *93*, *93*, *253*, **260–261**, *262–264*
  secondary to lymph node involvement *264*, *309*
  sclerotic form *263*
Rheumatoid arthritis *152*, **154–156**, *157–161*
  juvenile (Still's disease) *154*, *161–162*
  secondary osteoarthritis in *44*
  subcutaneous nodules in *156*, *157*
Rickets *25*, *28–29*
  vitamin D resistant *29*
Romanus lesion *163*, *166*

Salivary gland, metastasis from *14*
Salmonella infection in sickle cell disease *292*, *294*
Sarcoidosis *336*, **338–339**, *339–340*
Sarcoma
  Ewing's *252*, **254–256**, *256–259*, *376*, *378*, *378–379*
    Codman triangle in *255*, *258–259*
    intracellular glycogen in *254*, *256*
    Schiff technique for *256*
    'saucerisation' defect in *255*, *258–259*
  in Paget's disease *121*, **128**, *128*
  reticulum cell *85*, *93*, *93*, *253*, **260–261**, *262–264*
    secondary to lymph node involvement *264*
  sclerotic form *263*
  synovial *301*, **307–308**, *308–309*
  of soft tissue *309*
'Saucerisation' defect in Ewing's sarcoma *255*, *258–259*
Scheuermann's disease *51*
Scurvy *19*, *22*
  Wimberger sign in *22*
Septic arthritis, infantile *86*, *91*
Seronegative spondyloarthropathies **162**

Sickle cell disease   290, **292–293**, 294–295
  anaemia in   292
  crises in   293
  extramedullary haemopoiesis in   292, 295
  infarction in   290, 292, 294
  salmonella infection in   293, 294
Simple (unicameral) bone cyst   171, **172–173**, *173–174*
Skeletal metastases   6–7, **8–11**, *11–15, 364–365, 366–367, 366–367, 391, 392, 393*
  from breast   8, *12–13, 364,* 366, *366*
  bronchus   8–9, *11, 13–14, 337,* 342
  colon   8, *14*
  Ewing's sarcoma   255, *258*
  kidney   8, *13*
  lung   8–9, *11, 13–14, 337,* 342
  neuroblastoma   *14*
  osteosarcoma   123
  Paget's disease   128
  parotid gland   *391, 392, 393*
  prostate   6, 8–9, *11–12, 14–15*
  reticulum cell sarcoma   264
  salivary gland   *14, 391,* 392, *393*
  skin   10, *14*
  stomach   8, *12*
  thyroid   8, *13*
  urinary bladder   7, 8, *12,* 365, *367, 367*
Slipped upper femoral epiphysis   44, *48,* 62
  secondary osteoarthritis in   *48*
Spinal tuberculosis (Pott's disease)   108, **110–111**, *110–111, 113–114*
  subligamentous   112, *114*
Spondylitis, ankylosing   **163–164**, *164–166,* 364
  Andersson lesion in   163, *166*
  HLA antigens in   163
  Romanus lesion in   163, *166*

syndesmophytes in   163, *164*
Starvation   19, 25, *27*
Steatorrhoea in osteomalacia   25, *27*
Steroids   20, 87, *239*
Still's disease (juvenile rheumatoid arthritis)   154, *161–162*
Stress fracture   232, **234–235**, *236–239, 383, 384, 384*
  pathological   234, *238–239*
Subperiosteal haematoma   320, **326**, *327*
Sudeck's atrophy   19, *24*
Syndesmophytes
  ankylosing spondylitis, in   163, *164*
  psoriasis, 'floating', in   167, *167*
  Reiter's syndrome, in   168
Synovial chondromatosis   77, **78–79**, *80–83*
  chondrosarcoma in   78–79, *83*
  semimembranosus (Baker's) cyst in   77, *78*
Synovial sarcoma   301, **307–308**, *308–309*
  of soft tissues   309
Synovitis, pigmented villonodular   79, *301–302,* 302, **303–304**, *304–306, 385, 386, 386*
  Perl's reaction for iron in   302, *302*
Syphilis, osseous   88, *92*
  Wimberger sign in   92
Systemic necrosis of bone   *59,* 61, **64**, *67, 290–291,* 292–293, *294, 296–297, 297–299*
  alcoholism in   64, *67*
  blood disorders in   64, *290–291, 292–293, 294, 296–297, 297–299*
  dysbaric (caisson disease)   *59,* 61, 64, *67*
  idiopathic   64
  poisoning in   64
  post-radiation   64, *67*
  thermal injuries in   64, *67*

Tetany, post-operative after parathyroidectomy   208, *210*
Thalassaemia (Mediterranean or Cooley's anaemia)   295
Thermal injuries   64, *67*
  burns   *67*
  frostbite   *67*
Thyroid, metastasis from   8, *13*
Thyrotoxicosis, osteoporosis in   19
Torulosis   343
Traction spur   50
Transient osteoporosis   20, *24,* 79
Trevor's disease (dysplasia epiphysealis hemimelica)   34, *39*
Tuberculosis, osseous   108, **110–113**, *110–115*
  cystic   112, *115*
  dactylitis   112, *115,* 343
  skull (Pott's puffy tumour)   115
  spinal (Pott's disease)   108, **110–111**, *110–111, 113–114*
  subligamentous   112, *114*
Tuberculous arthritis   94–97, *96–97,* **98–99**, *99–101*
Typhoid osteomyelitis   343

Unicameral (simple) bone cyst   171, **172–173**, *173–174*
Urinary bladder, metastasis from   7, 8, *12, 14*

Vanishing bone disease (Gorham's syndrome, haemangiomatosis, massive osteolysis)   **286**, *286*

Wilson's disease (hepato-lenticular degeneration)   **277**, *277*
Wimberger sign
  in osseous syphilis   92
  in scurvy   *22*

Springer Orthopaedics
New and Recent Titles

K. Kozlowski, P. Beighton,
Gamut Index of Skeletal Dysplasias
An Aid to Radiodiagnosis
Foreword by F. N. Silverman
1984. Approx. 150 pages. ISBN 3-540-12825-5

Gamut Index **of Skeletal Dysplasias** concerned with the radiological diagnosis of genetic disorders of the skeleton. It is presented in the form of 'gamut lists' which will enable the practising radiologist to reach a diagnosis following the observation of abnormalities is bone radiographs. The lists are constructed in two ways – in terms of specific types of bone abnormality and also on an anatomic basis. The final section of the book provides, together with key references, brief outlines of the manifestations of each genetic condition. Cross references are given for each section.

L. Jeanmart, A. L. Baert, A. Wackenheim
Computer Tomography of Neck, Chest, Spine, and Limbs
With the collaboration of M. Osteaux
1983. 545 figures. XI, 194 pages. (Atlas of Pathological Computer Tomography, Volume 3). ISBN 3-540-11439-4

Computer Tomography of Neck, Chest, Spine, and Limbs is the final volume in a highly successful radiology series. Like its predecessors, it provides clinicians with a wealth of information on the diagnostic advantages of CT. The authors illustrate the interpretation of CT findings in pathologic abnormalities in the lungs, mediastinum and pleura, in morphologic and traumatic malformations in the limbs and spine, and in the orthopedic evaluation of limb function.

J. Koebke
A Biomechanical and Morphological Analysis of Human Hand Joints
1983 50 figures. VI, 85 pages. (Advances in Anatomy, Embryology and Cell Biology, Volume 80). ISBN 3-540-12438-1

Results of studies into the relationship between the morphology and the normal and pathologic function of three important joints of the human hand are recorded in this volume. The author's investigations of the proximal wrist joint focus on the transfer of kinetic energy from the arm to the hand, leading to a new understanding of degeneration and lesions of the articular disc and of typical radius fractures. Photoelastic experiments on the articular surfaces and capsular ligaments of the saddle joint of the thumb were studied in order to identify and characterize mechanical factors leading to the frequently observed arthrotic alterations of the joint. Finally, the author details his conclusion as to the special functions of the metacarpophalangeal joints as indicated by their particular morphologic features.

P. G. J. Maquet
Biomechanics of the Knee
With the Application to the Pathogenesis and the Surgical Treatment of Osteoarthritis
2nd edition, expanded and revised. 1984. 243 figures.
XVIII, 306 pages. ISBN 3-540-12489-6

Hailed the word over for its clarity and innovative scientific approach, Maquet's classic explanation of the biomechanical forces acting upon the knee and their application to the treatment of osteoarthritis is now in its second edition. For this revised and expanded edition, the author has updated the data on biomechanical stresses and analyzes the results of recently developed surgical procedures based on them.

W. Müller
The Knee
Form, Function, and Ligament Reconstruction
Translated from the German by T. C. Telger
Foreword by J. C. Hughston
Illustrations by R. Muspach
1983. 299 figures in 462 partially coloured separate illustrations.
VIII, 314 pages. ISBN 3-540-11716-4

"This is an excellent book which is addressed to the problems of ligament injury and reconstruction. Published by Springer-Verlag, to their usual high standard, the format is of beautiful illustrative diagrams, combined with operative photographs and where appropriate, dissected specimens. ... Part I deals with anatomy, kinematics and the examination of the injured knee. Part II describes injuries of the ligaments and capsule, general operative technique, primary repair, secondary repair, rehabilitation and results...
The book concludes with an excellent review of results. The bibliography is first rate, and the index adequate. The literature review throughout was easily the best I have ever read in this vast and complicated area of orghopaedic surgery."
British Journal of Sports Medicine

Springer-Verlag
Berlin
Heidelberg
New York
Tokyo

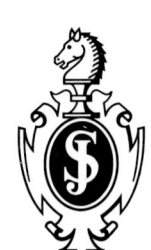

E. W. Somerville
Displacement of the Hip in Childhood
Aetiology, Management and Sequelae
1982. 262 figures. XIII, 200 pages. ISBN 3-540-10936-6

"Mr. Somerville's lucid arguments and well-selected case histories are a delight to read, his touch of evangelical zeal adding zest to our pleasure ... In all it forms a most stimulating monograph that needs no recommendation beyond the name of its author." *British Medical Journal*

B. J. Cremin, P. Beighton
Bone Dysplasias of Infancy
A Radiological Atlas
Foreword by R. O. Murray
1978. 55 figures in 124 separate illustrations, 4 tables.
XIII, 109 pages. ISBN 3-540-08816-4

"The recent explosion of publications on general skeletal dysplasias is continued in this admirable and profusely illustrated little book emanating from the Departments of Radiology and of Human Genetics in the University of Cape Town. ... a most successful venture and a useful reference book on a subject uncommonly seen outside specialists units; we look forward to further contributions from this very progressive school". *The Journal of Bone and Joint Surgery*

J. M. Connor
Soft Tissue Ossification
Foreword by V. A. McKusick
1983. 50 figures. XIII, 146 pages. ISBN 3-540-12530-2

"... The merit of this monograph is that it brings together the orthopaedic, radiographic, and pathological aspects of these uncommon disorders under one cover in greater detail than in the standard textbook of these specialties.
Soft Tissue Ossification begins logically with a chapter devoted to the distinction between soft tissue calcification and ossification... The remainder of the book deals exclusively with soft tissue ossification, with chapters devoted to trauma, tumour, myositis (fibrodysplasia) ossificans progressiva, and neurological and other causes ...
It is clearly written, well laid out, and uses tables and illustrations wisely. It will be a useful addition to many hospital and department libraries, and to the shelves of those few specialitsts with a particular interest in such disorders." *British Medical Journal*

P. Beighton, R. Grahame, H. Bird
Hypermobility of Joints
Foreword by E. Bywaters
1983. 101 figures. XIII, 178 pages. ISBN 3-540-12113-7

A wide ranging review of medically important aspects of hypermobility of joints is provided in this work. The authors bring together current knowledge in the light of their personal interest and experience and present it in a coherent form. Among the implications of hypermobility which are discussed are the basic pathogenesis, epidemiology and clinical significance, as well as the role of hypermobility in sport and the performing arts. In the final section of the book, genetic syndromes in which hypermobility is a major component are described in detail.

H. A. Keim
The Adolescent Spine
With contributions by J. R. Denton, H. M. Dick
J. G. McMurty III, D. P. Roye, Jr
2nd edition. 1982. 366 pages. XV, 254 pages. ISBN 3-540-90612-6

"... a readable account in simple terms of the spinal problems encountered in adolescents.
The first half of the book deals with spinal embryology, anatomy, congenital lesions, tumours, infections and trauma. Two new chapters 'The cervical adolescent spine' and 'Biomechanics of the adolescent spine' have been added.
The whole of the second half is devoted to spinal deformities, probably the commonest spinal problem presenting in adolescence ...
The book is well illustrated with clear line diagrams and photographs. A comprehensive list of up-to-date references appears in each chapter. This second edition is a worthy successor to the very popular first edition." *South African Medical Journal*

F. Horan, P. Beighton
Orthopaedic Problems in Inherited Skeletal Disorders
Foreword by W. J. W. Sharrard
1982. 98 figures. XVI, 142 pages. ISBN 3-540-11311-8

"Although this is a small volume it contains a wealth of well presented concisely written material. Frank Horan and Peter Beighton have chosen the clinically important members of the rare group of inherited skeletal disorders and presented them mainly for the benefit of the busy practising orthopaedic surgeon. They have achieved their goal with distinction..." *Journal of the Royal Society of Medicine*

P. Beighton, B. J. Cremin
Sclerosing Bone Dysplasias
Foreword by H. G. Jacobson
1980. 62 figures in 218 separate illustrations. IX, 191 pages
ISBN 3-540-09471-7

"Professors Beighton and Cremin have done it again! The University of Cape Town team of medical geneticist and radiologist have produced another excellent book, which is a worthy successor to their *Bone Dysplasias of Infancy* published in 1978 and widely acclaimed. No fewer than 17 sclerosing bone dysplasias are treated in separate chapters..." *South African Medical Journal*

Springer-Verlag
Berlin
Heidelberg
New York
Tokyo

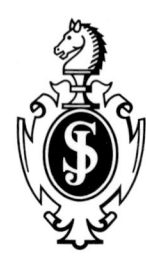